Gordis Epidemiology

Gordis Epidemiology

6th Edition

David D. Celentano, ScD, MHS
Dr. Charles Armstrong Chair and Professor
Department of Epidemiology
Johns Hopkins Bloomberg School of Public Health
Baltimore, Maryland

Moyses Szklo, MD, MPH, DrPH
University Distinguished Professor
Department of Epidemiology
Johns Hopkins Bloomberg School of Public Health
Baltimore, Maryland

ELSEVIER

ELSEVIER

1600 John F. Kennedy Blvd.
Ste 1600
Philadelphia, PA 19103-2899

Library of Congress Cataloging-in-Publication Control Number: 2018949544

Publisher: Elyse O'Grady
Senior Content Development Specialist: Deidre Simpson
Publishing Services Manager: Catherine Jackson
Book Production Specialist: Kristine Feeherty
Design Direction: Ryan Cook

Cover credit:
**An original watercolor "Remembering Baltimore" by
Haroutune K. Armenian, MD, DrPH**
Professor Emeritus
Department of Epidemiology
Johns Hopkins Bloomberg School of Public Health

Printed in Canada

Last digit is the print number: 9   8   7   6   5   4   3   2   1

In Memoriam

LEON GORDIS, MD, MPH, DrPH

1934–2015

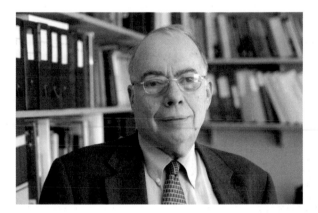

Preface

Epidemiology is one of the foundational disciplines underlying public health. Clinical research relies heavily on epidemiologic methods and contemporary medical care research, particularly in comparative effectiveness studies and statistical approaches to "big data" (as in the use of the electronic medical record for health studies). As Dr. Leon Gordis wrote in his preface to the fifth edition, "Epidemiology is the basic science of disease prevention and plays major roles in developing and evaluating public policy relating to health and to social and legal issues." There are many uses of epidemiology today. The majority of epidemiologic research focuses on establishing etiologic associations between putative risks and health outcomes. However, epidemiology is also widely used in the evaluation of primary and secondary prevention programs, comparisons of interventions, and the evaluation of policy at the population level. Epidemiologic findings commonly find their way into public media, providing the public and policy makers with data to guide personal decisions regarding their behavior. Increasingly, the scrutiny focused on epidemiology may cause researchers and practitioners some discomfort, as the interpretation of basic epidemiologic principles can be subject to considerable error. Our task is to make the thinking underlying epidemiology transparent.

This book is intended to be a basic introduction to the definitions, logic, and use of the epidemiologic method to elucidate factors influencing health and disease. We have tried to illustrate the principles with examples of how epidemiology is applied in the real world. The examples selected include both "classic examples" from the early days of the development of the discipline of epidemiology to contemporary examples. Where appropriate, we draw on examples pertaining to clinical practice.

Upon the passing of Dr. Gordis in 2015, the sixth edition of this book has been revised by two new authors, both of whom worked with and under Professor Gordis and have been actively engaged in teaching epidemiology at Johns Hopkins for over four decades. We have generally retained the structure and organization of the previous edition. In the fifth edition, learning objectives were inserted in most chapters, and we have revised these and updated the examples throughout. Additional new review questions have been added to most chapters. A significant change has been to the presentation and order of the methods in epidemiology that were previously presented at the end of Section I and more extensively in Section II. Rather than leading with the randomized trial (or the "experimental" design) and then comparing observational study design to the gold standard, we have organized the presentation of epidemiologic methods along a study continuum from clinical observation, to case-series, to the use of ecologic studies, and then to cross-sectional investigations as the foundational approach to epidemiologic hypothesis development. We then follow with case-control and cohort designs, leading up to the randomized trial. This more organically follows the development, in our opinion, of how epidemiologic observations and hypotheses are developed in the daily practice of *doing* epidemiology.

As with the previous edition, the sixth edition consists of three sections. Section I addresses how epidemiology is used to understand health and the development of diseases in populations as well as the basis for interventions to influence the natural history of disease. The first six chapters provide the conceptual framework underlying the discipline of epidemiology and present many of the basic principles of the discipline. Chapter 1 provides an overview of epidemiology, using many historical examples to illustrate how the field developed. Chapter 2 is concerned with how disease is transmitted in populations, both directly (in the case of infectious pathogens) and indirectly (for example, through a vector such as a mosquito or contaminated air). The basic terms used in epidemics are presented and illustrated to guide the student in seeing how these principles and terms are used. Chapter 3 addresses disease surveillance and how we measure morbidity in populations, while Chapter 4 is concerned with aspects of mortality and measures of disease impact in populations. Chapter 5 focuses on ways to detect disease in populations, comparing different approaches to differentiate people who have a disease from those who are disease free, articulating how screening tests can be adjusted to better diagnose those with or those without the disease in question. The issues of the reliability and validity of screening tests are of critical interest to both clinicians and to those planning for health services. Finally, Chapter 6 presents how the natural history of disease can be used to best express disease prognosis, using examples of case-fatality and survivorship.

Section II details the methods used by epidemiologists primarily to ascribe associations between a hypothesized exposure (risk) and a health outcome. Chapter 7 discusses the initial observations made in clinical practice (the case report) leading to a recognition of an accumulation of cases that appear to have some commonalities (the case series). This is followed by an introduction to the ecologic design and its analysis, with cautions as to its interpretation. Finally, cross-sectional (snapshot) studies are presented as the groundwork for hypothesis development. Chapter 8 then provides an introduction to observational studies as commonly used in epidemiology, addressing case-control and cohort studies, which are then compared in Chapter 9. To this point, we are addressing exposures as they occur in populations, where we are observers of exposures and their putative impacts on health outcomes. In Chapter 10 we then move to the "experimental" approach (randomized trial) in which the investigator "assigns" exposure or health intervention—generally randomly—to study participants to address how this influences the health outcome. In this case the exposure is under the control of the investigator, not the study participant, a crucial difference in the randomized trial as compared to the cohort or other observational study design. Chapter 11 discusses a series of issues involved in the conduct of randomized trials, including sample size, power, and generalizability; determining efficacy (vs. effectiveness); ethical considerations; and the US Federal Drug Administration phases for evaluating new drugs. In Chapter 12 we present issues on estimating risk, including absolute and relative risk and their interpretation, calculating and interpreting an odds ratio in a case-control study and in a cohort study, and doing so in a matched-pairs case-control study. In Chapter 13 the

concept of risk is expanded to include the calculation and interpretation of the attributable risk, the population attributable risks, and their use in evaluating the success of prevention programs. Causal inference is introduced in Chapter 14 and focuses on how to derive inferences in epidemiologic investigations. Chapter 15 presents issues of bias, confounding, and interaction in epidemiologic studies and discusses how they influence causal inference. Finally, Chapter 16 addresses the role of genetic and environmental contributions to the etiology of disease, and presents new methods of genetic research commonly used in epidemiologic studies today.

Section III addresses the uses of epidemiology in everyday public health. The final four chapters address some of the critical issues facing the field today. Chapter 17 illustrates how epidemiologic principles and designs described in Sections I and II are used in the evaluation of health services. Chapter 18 addresses the use of epidemiology to evaluate screening programs, while Chapter 19 details how epidemiology can be used to address major areas of public health policy. The final chapter summarizes ethical issues confronted in the practice of epidemiology and reviews some of the important professional issues confronted by the field today.

We have continued in Professor Gordis' use of illustrations and examples to demonstrate how epidemiologic issues and principles are put into practice. We have updated examples extensively and added new examples throughout the text. Many of the prior chapters have been extensively edited and updated, with some chapters being greatly expanded. The genetic epidemiology presentation has been heavily edited and updated, reflecting the amazing growth in genomics research in the past 5 years. In Chapter 16 we have added a glossary of genetic epidemiology terms to provide the student with some guidance for this somewhat complex field. Finally, new review questions have been added at the end of most chapters.

Our aim for this book is to allow the reader to appreciate how epidemiology can be used to respond to population health problems confronting society today. Our expectation is not that the reader will be able to conduct an epidemiologic investigation. Rather, we hope that there will be an appreciation of what epidemiology is, what the basic research and evaluation designs are, and how to interpret the basic findings in an epidemiologic study. We hope that the excitement we feel about the uses of epidemiology will come across to the reader of this text.

The cover illustration selected for this edition of *Gordis Epidemiology* has special meaning. This original watercolor by Haroutune Armenian, MD, DrPH, created in August 2017, is titled "Remembering Baltimore." Professor Armenian was a professor of epidemiology, deputy chair to Professor Gordis for many years, and interim chair from 1993–94, until Jon Samet became chair. "Remembering Baltimore" truly captures the urban landscape of Baltimore, Dr. Gordis' adopted home for some 60 years. The distinctive rowhomes on the harbor are quintessential Baltimore, much as the "Painted Ladies" are identified with San Francisco. Much of Dr. Gordis' research centered on pediatric and childhood disease in Baltimore, as illustrated in many of the examples in this text. We are particularly proud to include this tribute by Dr. Armenian to Dr. Gordis and to our first revision of his world-renowned text. This sixth edition has kept our mind on our friend and mentor.

David D. Celentano
Moyses Szklo
August 2018

Acknowledgments

This book reflects the contributions of several generations of teachers of epidemiology at Johns Hopkins, first as the School of Hygiene and Public Health, and more recently as the Bloomberg School of Public Health. The course was developed by the Department of Epidemiology faculty and was first taught as Principles of Epidemiology by Dr. Abraham Lilienfeld, the chair of the department from 1970–75. Dr. Leon Gordis became the course instructor following an acute illness experienced by Dr. Lilienfeld in the midst of teaching the subject in 1974. Dr. Gordis then was the primary lecturer for the following 30 years. In addition, Dr. Gordis taught epidemiology to many cohorts of School of Medicine students for a similar period of time. This book was developed from these experiences, and Dr. Gordis was the author of the first five editions of this very popular text.

The current authors were trained in public health at Johns Hopkins and were actively engaged as members of the epidemiology teaching team for many years when they were junior faculty. Dr. Szklo taught the second course in the epidemiology sequence, Intermediate Epidemiology. Upon Dr. Gordis' retirement, Dr. Celentano became the director of Principles of Epidemiology, which has recently been revised in content and renamed Epidemiologic Inference in Public Health 1. Its content reflects this sixth edition of *Gordis Epidemiology*.

Many colleagues have made invaluable contributions to this revision of *Gordis Epidemiology*. Chief among them was the late Dr. George W. Comstock, mentor, adviser, and sage scientist to both of us. We also acknowledge the assistance of many past and current colleagues, including Haroutune Armenian, Dr. Gordis' deputy chair and acting chair when Dr. Gordis stepped down as department chair, who contributed the original cover art, "Remembering Baltimore," for this book. We also acknowledge our former chair, Jonathan Samet, and Michel Ibrahim, who joined us as professor following his 2002 retirement as dean at the University of North Carolina–Chapel Hill. Others who have had major impacts on the teaching program in the department include Javier Nieto, Rosa Crum, Paul Whelton, Stephen Gange, Shruti Mehta, and Alvaro Munoz. To past co-instructors of the introductory course, we acknowledge Bill Moss, Elizabeth Platz, and Jennifer Deal for their dedication to educating scores of public health students in the "art" of epidemiology. In particular, Dr. Deal has made outstanding contributions to our introductory course, and many of the examples introduced in this edition come from her suggestions, for which we are particularly appreciative. The support of many deans of the school is also appreciated, including D.A. Henderson, Al Sommer, Mike Klag, and most recently Ellen MacKenzie. The course on which this book is based would not exist without the long-term dedication and knowledge of our colleague Allyn Arnold who has served as the bridge from the Gordis years to the present.

Preparing the sixth edition of this book was a significant undertaking for us. Our goal was to preserve Dr. Gordis' voice—and humor—and to retain the style of the text as much as possible. We also sought to update examples and to intersperse new illustrations of the epidemiologic principles we are presenting along with time-honored classics that were included in earlier editions.

Youssef Farag, MBBCh, MPH, PhD, was invaluable in preparing the sixth edition. He is a bright, talented, and hardworking young physician-epidemiologist whom we recruited to help us in this extraordinary endeavor. While completing his PhD in epidemiology at Johns Hopkins Bloomberg School of Public Health, Youssef took on the minutia of preparing this text—from updating CDC figures on morbidity and mortality, to working closely with the National Cancer Institute to run new data analyses to illustrate key epidemiologic points, and to finding references vaguely suggested by us. He led the significant reorganization of the chapters in the sixth edition, including rewriting entire new sections from scratch in several chapters. He also took on the initiative to update outdated examples from his knowledge of current medical and public health issues, and his firm grasp of the relevant literature. His creative contributions facilitated simplifying and clarifying conventionally challenging concepts in epidemiology.

During a period of over one year, from our in-depth discussions during weekly meetings, numerous emails in between, and multiple revisions for each chapter, this project would never have run so smoothly without his commitment and calm and determined nature, for which we are very grateful. We firmly believe that he will be a future leader in epidemiology.

The chapter on the role of genetics in contemporary epidemiology was heavily influenced by our genetic epidemiology colleagues Priya Duggal and Terri Beaty. This field has been changing so rapidly—and is technologically complicated to the naïve—that they assisted us in doing a major revision in this sixth edition. We cannot thank them enough for their contributions to this chapter.

Charlotte Gerczak was invaluable in copy-editing this volume. Charlotte worked for many years with Jonathan Samet and is very experienced in working with practicing epidemiologists. Her gifted eye for grammar, sentence structure, and meaning has made this a far better book than would have occurred without her careful review.

Preparing the sixth edition of *Gordis Epidemiology* has brought us many memories of Leon and his legacy at Johns Hopkins. The department has certainly changed since he stepped down as chair in 1993. Today we are a significantly larger faculty, covering many more areas of epidemiology in greater depth, and using tools unimaginable even a decade ago. At the same time, the discipline remains grounded in the ideas first set forth by Wade Hampton Frost at the dawn of our school in 1919. This book is a testament to the thought-leaders and giants of epidemiology who have studied and taught epidemiology at Johns Hopkins over the past 100 years and hopefully will guide us into our second century of practice, education, research, and service.

David D. Celentano
Moyses Szklo

Contents

THE EPIDEMIOLOGIC APPROACH TO DISEASE AND INTERVENTION

This section begins with an overview of the objectives of epidemiology, some of the approaches used in epidemiology, and examples of the applications of epidemiology to human health problems (Chapter 1). It then discusses how diseases are transmitted (Chapter 2). Diseases do not arise in a vacuum; they result from an interaction of human beings with their environment, including other people. An understanding of the concepts and mechanisms underlying the transmission and acquisition of disease is critical to exploring the epidemiology of human disease and to preventing and controlling many infectious diseases.

To discuss the epidemiologic concepts presented in this book, we need to develop a common language, particularly for describing and comparing morbidity and mortality. Chapter 3 therefore discusses morbidity and the important role of epidemiology in disease surveillance. The chapter then presents how measures of morbidity are used in both clinical medicine and public health. Chapter 4 presents the methodology and approaches for using mortality data in investigations relating to public health and clinical practice. Other issues relating to the impact of disease, including quality of life and projecting the future burden of disease, are also discussed in Chapter 4.

Armed with knowledge of how to describe morbidity and mortality in quantitative terms, we then turn to the question of how to assess the quality of diagnostic and screening tests that are used to determine which people in the population have a certain disease (Chapter 5). After we identify people with the disease, we need ways to describe the natural history of disease in quantitative terms; this is essential for assessing the severity of an illness and for evaluating the possible effects on survival of new therapeutic and preventive interventions (Chapter 6).

This first section, then, introduces the student to the nomenclature of epidemiology, surveillance and its ramifications for determining the health of populations, and then focuses on screening and the natural history of disease.

Chapter 1

Introduction

I hate definitions.
—Benjamin Disraeli (1804–1881, British Prime Minister 1868 and 1874–1880)

What Is Epidemiology?

Epidemiology is the study of how disease is distributed in populations and the factors that influence or determine this distribution. Why does a disease develop in some people and not in others? The premise underlying epidemiology is that disease, illness, ill health, and excellent health status are not randomly distributed in human populations. Rather, each of us has certain characteristics that predispose us to, or protect us against, a variety of different diseases. These characteristics may be primarily genetic in origin, the result of exposure to certain environmental hazards, or the behaviors (good and bad) that we engage in. Perhaps most often, we are dealing with an interaction of genetic, environmental, and behavioral and social factors in the development of disease.

A broader definition of epidemiology than that given previously has been widely accepted. It defines epidemiology as "the study of the distribution and determinants of health-related states or events in specified populations and the application of this study to control of health problems."[1] What is noteworthy about this definition is that it includes both a description of the content of the discipline and why epidemiologic investigations are carried out.

Objectives of Epidemiology

What are the specific objectives of epidemiology? First, to identify the *etiology,* or *cause,* of a disease and its relevant risk factors (i.e., factors that increase a person's risk for a disease). We want to know how the disease is transmitted from one person to another or from a nonhuman reservoir to a human population or why it arises due to risk behaviors the person engages in. Our ultimate aim is to intervene to reduce morbidity and mortality from the disease. We want to develop a rational basis for prevention programs. If we can identify the etiologic or causal factors for disease and reduce or eliminate exposure to those factors, we can develop a basis for prevention programs. In addition, we can develop appropriate vaccines and treatments, which can prevent the transmission of the disease to others.

The second objective of epidemiology is to determine the *extent of disease* found in the community. What is the burden of disease in the community? This question is critical for planning health services and facilities and for estimating how many future health care providers should be trained.

A third objective is to study the *natural history and prognosis of disease*. Clearly, certain diseases are more severe than others; some may be rapidly lethal, whereas others may have extended durations of survival. Many diseases are not fatal but may affect quality of life or be associated with disability. We want to define the baseline natural history of a disease in quantitative terms so that as we develop new modes of intervention, either through treatments or through new ways of preventing complications, we can compare the results of using these new modalities with the baseline data to determine whether our new approaches have truly been effective.

Fourth, we use epidemiology to evaluate both *existing and newly developed preventive and therapeutic measures and modes of health care delivery*. For example, does screening men for prostate cancer using the prostate-specific antigen (PSA) test improve survival in people found to have prostate cancer? Has the growth of managed care and other new systems of health care delivery and health care insurance had an impact on the health outcomes of the patients involved and on their quality of life? If so, what has been the nature of this impact and how can it be measured?

Finally, epidemiology can provide the foundation for *developing public policy* relating to environmental problems, genetic issues, and other social and behavioral considerations regarding disease prevention and health promotion. For example, is the electromagnetic radiation that is emitted by cell phones, electric blankets and heating pads, and other household appliances a hazard to human health? Are high levels of atmospheric ozone or particulate matter a cause of adverse acute or chronic health effects in human populations? Is radon in homes a significant risk to human beings? Which occupations are associated with increased risks of disease in workers, and what types of regulation are required to reduce these risks?

CHANGING PATTERNS OF COMMUNITY HEALTH PROBLEMS

A major role of epidemiology is to provide clues to changes that take place over time in the health problems presenting in the community. Fig. 1.1 shows a sign in a cemetery in Dudley, England, in 1839. At that time, cholera was the major cause of death in England; the churchyard was so full that no burials of persons who died of cholera would henceforth be permitted. The sign conveys an idea of the importance of cholera in the public's consciousness and in the spectrum of public health problems in the early 19th century. Clearly, cholera is no longer a major problem in the United States today, but in many low-income and war-torn countries of the world it remains a serious threat, with many countries periodically reporting outbreaks of cholera that are characterized by high death rates, often as a result of inadequate or inaccessible medical care.

Let us compare the major causes of death in the United States in 1900 and 2014 (Fig. 1.2). The categories of causes have been color coded as described in the caption for this figure. In 1900 the leading causes of death were pneumonia and influenza, followed by tuberculosis and diarrhea and enteritis. In 2014 the leading causes of death were heart disease, cancer, chronic lower respiratory diseases, and unintentional injuries. What change has occurred? During the 20th century there was a dramatic shift in the causes of death in the United States. In 1900 the three leading causes of death were infectious diseases; however, now we are dealing with chronic diseases that in most situations are not communicable or infectious in origin. Consequently, the kinds of research, intervention, and services we need today differ from those that were needed in the United States in 1900.

The pattern of disease occurrence currently seen in developing countries is often similar to that which was

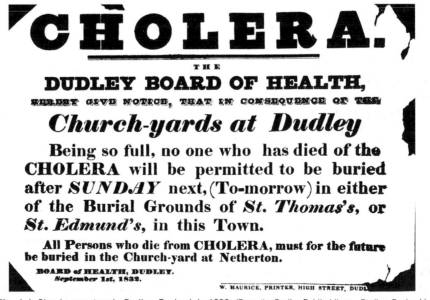

Fig. 1.1 Sign in cemetery in Dudley, England, in 1839. (From the Dudley Public Library, Dudley, England.)

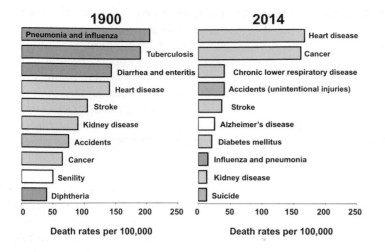

Fig. 1.2 Ten leading causes of death in the United States, 1900 and 2014. Although the definitions of the diseases in this figure are not exactly comparable in 1900 and 2014, the bars in the graphs are color coded to show chronic diseases *(pink)*, infectious diseases *(purple)*, injuries *(aqua)*, and diseases of aging *(white)*. (Redrawn from Grove RD, Hetzel AM. *Vital Statistics Rates of the United States, 1940–1960.* Washington, DC: US Government Printing Office; 1968; and Kochanek KD, Murphy SL, Xu JQ, Tejada-Vera B. Deaths: Final data for 2014. *Natl Vital Stat Rep.* 2016;65(4):1–122. [Hyattsville, MD: National Center for Health Statistics.])

TABLE 1.1 Ten Leading Causes of Death and Their Percentages of All Deaths, United States, 2014

Rank	Cause of Death	No. of Deaths	Percent (%) of Total Deaths	Age-Adjusted Death Rate[a]
	All Causes	2,626,418	100.0	724.6
1	Diseases of the heart	614,348	23.4	167.0
2	Malignant neoplasms (cancer)	591,699	22.5	161.2
3	Chronic lower respiratory diseases	147,101	5.6	40.5
4	Accidents (unintentional injuries)	136,053	5.2	40.5
5	Cerebrovascular diseases	133,103	5.1	36.5
6	Alzheimer disease	93,541	3.6	25.4
7	Diabetes mellitus	76,488	2.9	20.9
8	Influenza and pneumonia	55,227	2.1	15.1
9	Nephritis, nephrotic syndrome, and nephrosis	48,146	1.8	13.2
10	Intentional self-harm (suicide)	42,773	1.6	13.0
	All other causes	687,939	26.2	

[a]Rates are per 100,000 population and age-adjusted for the 2010 US standard population.
Note: Percentages may not total 100 due to rounding.
Data from Centers for Disease Control and Prevention, Xu JQ, Murphy SL, Kochanek KD, Arias E. *Mortality in the United States, 2015.* NCHS data brief, no 267. Hyattsville, MD: National Center for Health Statistics; 2016. https://www.cdc.gov/nchs/data/databriefs/db267_table.pdf. Accessed April 17, 2017.

seen in the United States in 1900: infectious diseases remain the leading causes of death. However, as countries become industrialized they increasingly manifest the mortality patterns currently seen in developed countries, with mortality from chronic diseases becoming the major challenge (this is commonly referred to as the "epidemiologic transition"). However, even in industrialized countries, as human immunodeficiency virus (HIV) infection has emerged and the incidence of tuberculosis has increased, infectious diseases are again becoming major public health problems. Table 1.1 shows the 10 leading causes of death in the United States in 2014. The three leading causes—heart disease, cancer, and chronic lower respiratory diseases—account for almost 55% of all deaths, an observation that suggests specific targets for prevention if a significant reduction in mortality is to be achieved.

Another demonstration of changes that have taken place over time is seen in Fig. 1.3, which shows the remaining years of expected life in the United States at birth and at age 65 years for the years 1900, 1950, and 2014, by race and sex.

The number of years of life remaining after birth has dramatically increased in all of these groups, with most of the improvement having occurred from 1900 to 1950 and much less having occurred since 1950. If we look at the remaining years of life at age 65 years, very little improvement is seen from 1900 to 2014. What primarily accounts for the increase in remaining years of life at birth are the decreases in infant mortality and in mortality from childhood diseases. In terms of diseases that afflict adults, especially those 65 years and older, we have been much less successful in extending the span of life, and this remains a major challenge.

Epidemiology and Prevention

A major use of epidemiologic evidence is to identify subgroups in the population who are at high risk for disease. Why should we identify such high-risk groups? First, if we can identify these high-risk groups, we can direct preventive efforts, such as screening programs for early disease detection, to populations who may not have been screened before and are most likely to benefit from any interventions that are developed for the disease. In sub-Saharan Africa, targeted HIV counseling and testing to men who are not aware of their status can effectively reduce epidemics if they are linked to care, started on antiretroviral therapy, and continued in care.

Second, if we can identify such groups, we may be able to identify the specific factors or characteristics that put them at high risk and then try to modify those factors. It is important to keep in mind that such risk factors may be of two types. Characteristics such as age, sex, and race, for example, are not modifiable, although they may permit us to identify high-risk groups. On the other hand, characteristics such as obesity, smoking, diet, sexual practices, and other lifestyle factors may be potentially modifiable and may thus provide an opportunity to develop and introduce new prevention programs aimed at reducing or changing specific exposures or risk factors.

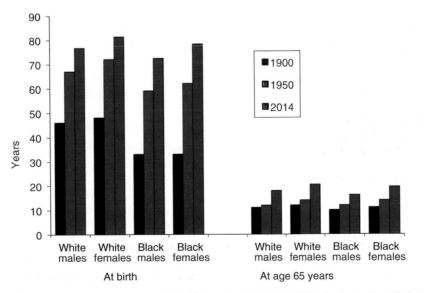

Fig. 1.3 Life expectancy at birth and at 65 years of age, by race and sex, United States, 1900, 1950, and 2014. (Redrawn from National Center for Health Statistics. *Health, United States, 1987 DHHS Publication No. 88–1232.* Washington, DC: Public Health Service; March 1988; National Center for Health Statistics. Health, United States, 2015: with special feature on racial and ethnic health disparities; 2016. https://www.cdc.gov/nchs/hus/contents2015.htm#015. Accessed May 2, 2017.)

PRIMARY, SECONDARY, AND TERTIARY PREVENTION

In discussing prevention, it is helpful to distinguish among primary, secondary, and tertiary prevention (Table 1.2).

Primary prevention denotes an action taken to prevent the development of a disease in a person who is well and does not (yet) have the disease in question. For example, we can immunize a person against certain diseases so that the disease never develops or, if a disease is environmentally induced, we can prevent a person's exposure to the environmental factor involved and thereby prevent the development of the disease. Primary prevention is our ultimate goal. For example, we know that most lung cancers are preventable. If we can help to stop people from ever smoking, we can eliminate 80% to 90% of lung cancer in human beings. However, although our aim is to prevent diseases from occurring in human populations, for many diseases, such as prostate cancer and Alzheimer disease, we do not yet have the biologic, clinical, or epidemiologic data on which to base effective primary prevention programs.

Secondary prevention involves identifying people in whom a disease process has already begun but who have not yet developed clinical signs and symptoms of the illness. This period in the natural history of a disease is called the *preclinical phase* of the illness and is discussed in Chapter 18. Once a person develops clinical signs or symptoms it is generally assumed that under ideal conditions the person will seek and obtain medical advice. Our objective with secondary prevention is to detect the disease earlier than it would have been detected with usual care. By detecting the disease at an early stage in its natural history, often through screening, it is hoped that treatment will be easier and/or more effective. For example, most cases of breast cancer in older women can be detected through mammography. Several recent studies indicate that routine testing of the stool for occult blood can detect treatable colon cancer early in its natural history but colonoscopy is a better test, although far more expensive and invasive. The rationale for secondary prevention is that if we can identify disease earlier in its natural history than would ordinarily occur, intervention measures may be more effective and life prolonged. Perhaps we can prevent mortality or complications of the disease and use less invasive or less costly treatment to do so. Evaluating screening for disease and the place of such intervention in the framework of disease prevention are discussed in Chapter 18.

Tertiary prevention denotes preventing complications in those who have already developed signs and symptoms of an illness and have been diagnosed (i.e., people who are in the clinical phase of their illness). This is generally achieved through prompt and appropriate treatment of the illness combined with ancillary approaches such as physical therapy that are designed to prevent complications such as joint contractures.

TWO APPROACHES TO PREVENTION: A DIFFERENT VIEW

Two possible approaches to prevention are a population-based approach and a high-risk approach.[2] In the population-based approach, a preventive measure is widely applied to an entire population. For example, prudent dietary advice for preventing coronary disease or advice against smoking may be provided to an entire population using mass media and other health education approaches. An alternate approach is to target a high-risk group with the preventive measure. Thus screening for cholesterol in children might be restricted to children from high-risk families. Clearly, a measure applied to an entire population must be relatively inexpensive and noninvasive. A measure that is to be applied to a high-risk subgroup of the population may be more expensive and may be more invasive or inconvenient but also has to be able to correctly identify individuals

TABLE 1.2	**Three Types of Prevention**	
Type of Prevention	**Definition**	**Examples**
Primary	Preventing the *initial development* of a disease	Immunization, reducing exposure to a risk factor
Secondary	Early detection of *existing disease* to reduce severity and complications	Screening for cancer
Tertiary	Reducing the *impact of the disease*	Rehabilitation for stroke

with the disease. More on screening tests is discussed in Chapter 18. Population-based approaches can be considered public health approaches, whereas high-risk approaches more often require a clinical action to identify the high-risk group to be targeted. In most situations, a combination of both approaches is ideal. Often a high-risk approach, such as prevention counseling, is limited to brief encounters with physicians. These approaches are discussed further in Chapter 19.

Epidemiology and Clinical Practice

Epidemiology is critical not only to public health but also to clinical practice. The practice of medicine is dependent on population data. For example, if a physician hears an apical systolic murmur, a heart sound produced when blood flows across the heart valves, how does he or she know whether it represents mitral regurgitation? Where did this knowledge originate? The diagnosis is based on correlation of the clinical findings (such as the auscultatory findings—sounds heard using a stethoscope) with the findings of surgical pathology or autopsy and with the results of echocardiography, magnetic resonance, or catheterization studies in a large group of patients. Thus the process of diagnosis is population based (see Chapter 5). The same holds for prognosis. For example, a patient asks his physician, "How long do I have to live, doctor?" and the doctor replies, "Six months to a year." On what basis does the physician prognosticate? He or she does so on the basis of experience with large groups of patients who have had the same disease, were observed at the same stage of disease, and received the same treatment. Again, prognostication is based on population data (see Chapter 6). Finally, selection of appropriate therapy is also population based. Randomized clinical trials that study the effects of a treatment in large groups of patients are the ideal means (the so-called gold standard) for identifying appropriate therapy (see Chapters 10 and 11). Thus population-based concepts and data underlie the critical processes of clinical practice, including diagnosis, prognostication, and selection of therapy. In effect, the physician applies a population-based probability model to the patient on the examining table.

Fig. 1.4 shows a physician demonstrating that the practice of clinical medicine relies heavily on population

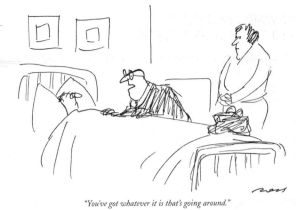

"You've got whatever it is that's going around."

Fig. 1.4 "You've got whatever it is that's going around." (Al Ross/The New Yorker Collection/The Cartoon Bank.)

concepts. What is portrayed humorously here is a true commentary on one aspect of pediatric practice—a pediatrician often makes a diagnosis based on what the parent tells him or her over the telephone and on what he or she knows about which illnesses, such as viral and bacterial infections, are "going around" in the community. Thus the data available about illness in the community can be very helpful in suggesting a diagnosis, even if they are not conclusive. Data regarding the etiology of sore throats according to a child's age are particularly relevant (Fig. 1.5). If the infection occurs early in life, it is likely to be viral in origin. If it occurs at ages 4 to 7 years, it is likely to be streptococcal in origin. In an older child, *Mycoplasma* becomes more typical. Although these data do not make the diagnosis, they do provide the physician or other health care provider with a good clue as to what agent or agents to suspect.

Epidemiologic Approach

How does the epidemiologist proceed to identify the cause of a disease? Epidemiologic reasoning is a multistep process. The first step is to determine whether an association exists between exposure to a factor (e.g., an environmental agent) or a characteristic of a person (e.g., an increased serum cholesterol level) and the presence of the disease in question. We do this by studying the characteristics of groups and the characteristics of individuals.

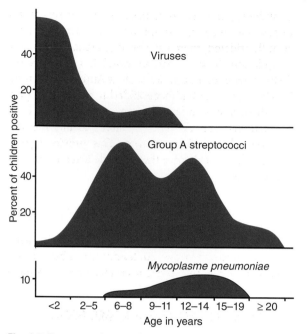

Fig. 1.5 Frequency of agents by age of children with pharyngitis, 1964–1965. (From Denny FW. The replete pediatrician and the etiology of lower respiratory tract infections. *Pediatr Res.* 1969;3:464–470.)

If we find there is indeed an association between an exposure and a disease, is it necessarily a causal relationship? No, not all associations are causal. The second step therefore is to try to derive appropriate inferences about a possible causal relationship from the patterns of the associations that have been previously found. These steps are discussed in detail Chapter 14.

Epidemiology often begins with descriptive data. For example, Fig. 1.6 shows rates of gonorrhea in the United States in 2015 by state. Clearly, there are marked regional variations in reported cases of gonorrhea. The first question to ask when we see such differences between two groups or two regions or at two different times is, "Are these differences real?" In other words, are the data from each area of comparable quality? Before we try to interpret the data, we should be satisfied that the data are valid. If the differences are real, then we ask, "Why have these differences occurred?" Are there differences in potential exposures between high-risk and low-risk areas, or are there differences in the people who live in those areas? This is where epidemiology begins its investigation.

Many years ago, it was observed that communities in which the natural level of fluoride in the drinking

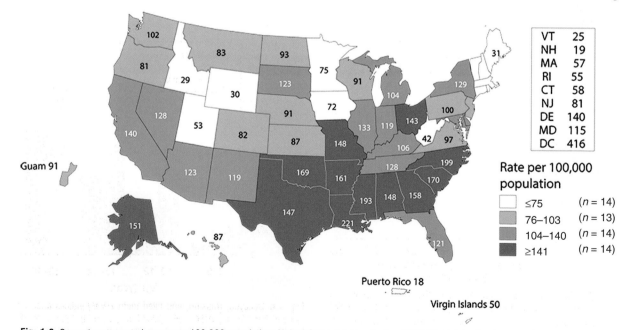

Fig. 1.6 Gonorrhea: reported cases per 100,000 population, United States and territories, 2015. The total rate of reported cases of gonorrhea for the United States and outlying areas (Guam, Puerto Rico, and Virgin Islands) was 122.7 per 100,000 population. (From Gonorrhea—rates by state, United States and outlying areas; 2015. https://www.cdc.gov/std/stats15/figures/15.htm. Accessed April 19, 2015.)

water varied also differed in the frequency of dental caries in the permanent teeth of residents. Communities that had low natural fluoride levels had high levels of caries, and communities that had higher levels of fluoride in their drinking water had low levels of caries (Fig. 1.7). This finding suggested that fluoride might be an effective prevention intervention if it were artificially added to the drinking water supply. A trial was therefore carried out to test the hypothesis. Although, ideally, we would like to randomize a group of people either to receive fluoride or to receive no fluoride, this was not possible to do with drinking water because each community generally shares a common water supply. Consequently, two similar communities in upstate New York, Kingston and Newburgh, were chosen for the trial. The DMF index, a count of decayed, missing, and filled teeth, was used. Baseline data were collected in both cities, and at the start of the study, the DMF indices were comparable in each age group in the two communities. The water in Newburgh was then fluoridated, and the children were reexamined a decade later. Fig. 1.8 shows that, in each age group, the DMF index in Newburgh had dropped significantly 10 years or so later, whereas in Kingston, there was no change. This is strongly suggestive evidence that fluoride was preventing caries.

It was possible to go one step further in trying to demonstrate a causal relationship between fluoride ingestion and low rates of caries. The issue of

fluoridating water supplies has been extremely controversial, and in certain communities in which water has been fluoridated, there have been referenda to stop the fluoridation. It was therefore possible to look at the DMF index in communities such as Antigo, Wisconsin, in which fluoride had been added to its water supply and then, after a referendum, fluoridation had been stopped. As seen in Fig. 1.9, after the fluoride was removed, the DMF index rose. This provided yet a further piece of evidence that fluoride acted to prevent dental caries.

From Observations to Preventive Actions

In this section, three examples from history are discussed that demonstrate how epidemiologic observations have led to effective preventive measures in human populations.

IGNÁZ SEMMELWEIS AND CHILDBED FEVER

Ignáz Semmelweis (Fig. 1.10) was born in 1818 and began as a student of law until he left his studies to pursue medical training. He specialized in obstetrics

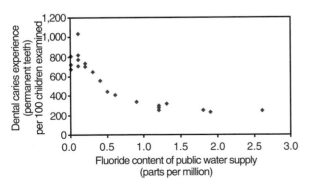

Fig. 1.7 Relationship between rate of dental caries in children's permanent teeth and fluoride content of public water supply. (Modified from Dean HT, Arnold Jr FA, Elvove E. Domestic water and dental caries: V. Additional studies of the relation of fluoride in domestic waters to dental caries experience in 4,425 white children aged 12 to 14 years of 13 cities in 4 states. *Public Health Rep.* 1942;57:1155–1179.)

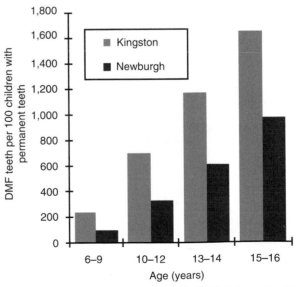

Fig. 1.8 Decayed, missing, and filled teeth *(DMF)* indices after 10 years of fluoridation, 1954–1955. (Modified from Ast DB, Schlesinger ER. The conclusion of a 10-year study of water fluoridation. *Am J Public Health.* 1956;46:265–271. Copyright 1956 by the American Public Health Association. Modified with permission.)

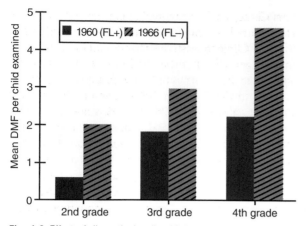

Fig. 1.9 Effect of discontinuing fluoridation in Antigo, Wisconsin, November 1960. *DMF,* Decayed, missing, and filled teeth; *FL+,* during fluoridation; *FL–,* after fluoridation was discontinued. (Modified from Lemke CW, Doherty JM, Arra MC. Controlled fluoridation: the dental effects of discontinuation in Antigo, Wisconsin. *J Am Dent Assoc.* 1970;80:782–786. Reprinted by permission of ADA Publishing Co., Inc.)

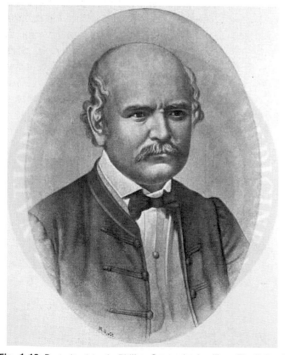

Fig. 1.10 Portrait of Ignáz Philipp Semmelweis. (From The National Library of Medicine.)

and became interested in a major clinical and public health problem of the day: childbed fever, also known as puerperal fever (the word "puerperal" means related to childbirth or to the period after the birth).

In the early 19th century, childbed fever was a major cause of death among women shortly after childbirth, with mortality rates from childbed fever as high as 25%. Many theories of the cause of childbed fever were popular at the time, including atmospheric toxins, "epidemic constitutions" of some women, putrid air, or solar and magnetic influences. This period was a time of growing interest in pathologic anatomy. Because the cause of childbed fever remained a mystery, great interest arose in associating the findings at autopsies of women who had died of the disease with the clinical manifestations that characterized them while ill after childbirth.

Semmelweis was placed in charge of the First Obstetrical Clinic of the Allgemeine Krankenhaus (General Hospital) in Vienna in July 1846. At that time there were two obstetrical clinics, the First and the Second. Pregnant women were admitted for childbirth to the First Clinic or to the Second Clinic on an alternating 24-hour basis. The First Clinic was staffed by physicians and medical students and the Second Clinic by midwives. Physicians and medical students began their days performing autopsies on women who had died from childbed fever; they then proceeded to provide clinical care for women hospitalized in the First Clinic for childbirth. The midwives staffing the Second Clinic did not perform autopsies. Semmelweis had been impressed by mortality rates in the two clinics in 1842 (Fig. 1.11). Mortality in the First Clinic was more than twice as high as in the Second Clinic—16% compared with 7%.

Semmelweis surmised that mortality was higher in the First Clinic than in the Second because the physicians and medical students went directly from the autopsies to their patients. Many of the women in labor had multiple examinations by physicians and by medical students learning obstetrics. Often these manual examinations traumatized the tissues of the vagina and uterus. Semmelweis suggested that the hands of physicians and medical students were transmitting disease-causing particles from the cadavers to the women who were about to deliver. His suspicions were confirmed in 1847 when his friend and colleague Jakob Kolletschka died from an infection contracted when he was accidentally punctured with a medical student's knife while performing an autopsy. The autopsy on Kolletschka showed pathology very similar to that of the women who were dying from childbed fever. Semmelweis concluded that physicians and medical students were carrying the infection from the autopsy room to the patients in the First Clinic and that this accounted for the high mortality rates from childbed fever in the First Clinic. Mortality rates in the Second Clinic remained low because the midwives who staffed the Second Clinic had no contact with the autopsy room.

Semmelweis then developed and implemented a policy for the physicians and medical students in the First Clinic, a policy designed to prevent childbed fever. He required the physicians and medical students in the First Clinic to wash their hands and to brush under their fingernails after they had finished the autopsies and before they came in contact with any of the patients. As seen in Fig. 1.12, in 1848, mortality in the First Clinic dropped from 12.2% to 2.4%, a rate comparable to that seen in the Second Clinic for the same year. When Semmelweis was later replaced by an obstetrician who did not subscribe to Semmelweis's theories, and who therefore eliminated the policy of required handwashing, mortality rates from childbed fever rose again in the First Clinic—further evidence supporting a causal relationship.

Unfortunately, for many years Semmelweis refused to present his findings at major meetings or to submit written reports of his studies to medical journals. His failure to provide supporting scientific evidence was at least partially responsible for the failure of the medical community to accept his hypothesis of causation of childbed fever and his further proposed intervention of handwashing before examining each patient. Among other factors that fostered resistance to his proposal was the reluctance of physicians to accept the conclusion that by transmitting the agent responsible for childbed fever, they had been inadvertently responsible for the deaths of large numbers of women. In addition, physicians claimed that washing their hands before seeing each patient would be too time consuming. Another major factor is that Semmelweis was, to say the least, undiplomatic and had alienated many senior figures in medicine. As a consequence of all of these factors,

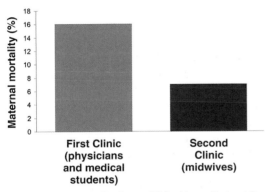

Fig. 1.11 Maternal mortality due to childbed fever, First and Second Clinics, General Hospital, Vienna, Austria, 1842. (Modified from the Centers for Disease Control and Prevention: Hand hygiene in health care settings—supplemental. www.cdc.gov/handhygiene/download/hand_hygiene_supplement.ppt. Accessed April 11, 2013.)

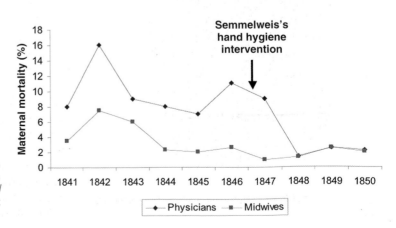

Fig. 1.12 Maternal mortality due to childbed fever, by type of care provider, General Hospital, Vienna, Austria, 1841–1850. (Modified from Mayhall GC. *Hospital Epidemiology and Infection Control.* 2nd ed. Philadelphia: Lippincott Williams & Wilkins; 1999.)

many years passed before a policy of handwashing was broadly adopted. An excellent biography of Semmelweis by Sherwin Nuland was published in 2003.[3]

The lessons of this story for successful policy making are still relevant today to the challenge of enhancing both public and professional acceptance of evidence-based prevention policies. These lessons include the need for clearly presenting supporting scientific evidence for a proposed intervention, the need for implementation of the proposed intervention to be perceived as feasible and cost-effective, and the need to lay the necessary groundwork for the policy, including garnering professional as well as community and political support.

Years later, the major cause of childbed fever was recognized to be a streptococcal infection. Semmelweis's major findings and recommendations ultimately had worldwide effects on the practice of medicine. Amazingly, his observations and suggested interventions preceded any knowledge of germ theory and thus proved that it is possible to implement a prevention strategy even when the exact cause of the disease is not known. However, it is also of interest that, although the need for handwashing has now been universally accepted, recent studies have reported that many physicians in hospitals in the United States and in other developed countries still fail to wash their hands as prescribed (Table 1.3).

EDWARD JENNER AND SMALLPOX

Edward Jenner (Fig. 1.13) was born in 1749 and became very interested in the problem of smallpox, which was a worldwide scourge. For example, in the late 18th century, 400,000 people died from smallpox each year and one-third of survivors were blinded as a result of corneal infections. It was known that those who survived smallpox were subsequently immune to the disease, and consequently it became a common preventive practice to infect healthy individuals with smallpox by administering to them material taken from smallpox patients, a procedure called *variolation*. However, this was not the optimal method: some variolated individuals died from the resulting smallpox, infected others with smallpox, or developed other infections.

Jenner was interested in finding a better, safer approach to preventing smallpox. He observed, as had other people before him, that dairy maids, the young women whose occupation was milking cows, developed a mild disease called cowpox. Later, during smallpox outbreaks, smallpox appeared not to develop in these young women. In 1768 Jenner heard a claim from a dairy maid, "I can't take the smallpox for I have already had the cowpox." These data were observations and were not based on any rigorous study, but Jenner became

TABLE 1.3 **Compliance With Hand Hygiene Among Physicians, by Specialty, at University of Geneva Hospitals**		
Physician Specialty	**No. of Physicians**	**Compliance With Hand Hygiene (% of Observations)**
Internal medicine	32	87.3
Surgery	25	36.4
Intensive care unit	22	62.6
Pediatrics	21	82.6
Geriatrics	10	71.2
Anesthesiology	15	23.3
Emergency medicine	16	50.0
Other	22	57.2

Data from Pittet D. Hand hygiene among physicians: performance, beliefs, and perceptions. *Ann Intern Med.* 2004;141:1–8.

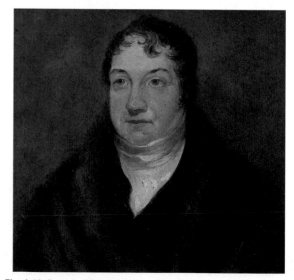

Fig. 1.13 Portrait of Edward Jenner. (From the Wellcome Historical Medical Museum and Library, London.)

convinced that cowpox could protect against smallpox and decided to test his hypothesis.

Fig. 1.14 shows a painting by Gaston Melingue of Edward Jenner performing the first vaccination in 1796. (The term "vaccination" is derived from *vacca*, the Latin word for "cow.") In this painting, a dairy maid, Sarah Nelmes, is bandaging her hand after just having had some cowpox material removed. The cowpox material is being administered by Jenner to an 8-year-old "volunteer," James Phipps. Jenner was so convinced that cowpox would be protective that 6 weeks later, to test his conviction, he inoculated the child with material that had just been taken from a smallpox pustule. The child did not contract the disease. We shall not deal in this chapter with the ethical issues and implications of this experiment. (Clearly, Jenner did not have to justify his study before an institutional review board!) In any event, the results of the first vaccination and of what followed eventually saved literally millions of human beings throughout the world from disability and death caused by the scourge of smallpox. The important point is that Jenner knew nothing about viruses and nothing about the biology of the disease. He operated purely on observational data that provided him with the basis for a preventive intervention.

In 1967 the World Health Organization (WHO) began international efforts to eradicate smallpox using vaccinations with vaccinia virus (cowpox). It has been estimated that, until that time, smallpox afflicted 15 million people annually throughout the world, of whom 2 million died and millions of others were left blind or disfigured. In 1980 the WHO certified that smallpox had been eradicated. The smallpox eradication program,[4] directed at the time by Dr. D.A. Henderson (Fig. 1.15), is one of the greatest disease prevention achievements in human history. The WHO estimated that 350 million new cases had been prevented over a 20-year period. However, after the terrorist attacks that killed nearly 3,000 people in the World Trade Center in New York City on September 11, 2001, worldwide concern developed about potential bioterrorism in the wake of the 2001 anthrax attacks. Ironically, the possibility that smallpox virus might be used for such a purpose

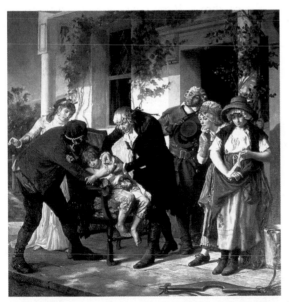

Fig. 1.14 *Une des premières vaccinations d'Edward Jenner* ("One of the first vaccinations by Edward Jenner"), by Gaston Melingue. (Reproduced by permission of the Bibliothèque de l'Académie Nationale de Médecine, Paris, 2007.)

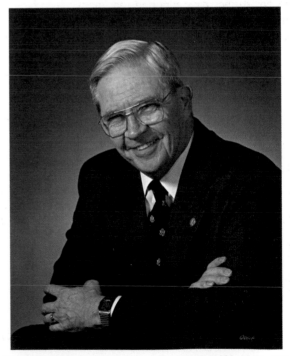

Fig. 1.15 Photograph of Dr. D.A. Henderson (1928–2016), who directed the World Health Organization Smallpox Eradication Program.

reopened issues regarding smallpox and vaccination that many thought had been permanently relegated to history by the successful efforts at eradication of the disease. The magnitude of the smallpox bioterrorism threat, together with issues of vaccinia risk—both to those vaccinated and to those coming in contact with vaccinees, especially in hospital environments—are among many that have had to be addressed. However, often only limited or equivocal data are available on these issues to guide the development of relevant public health prevention policy relating to a potential bioterrorism threat of using smallpox as a weapon.

JOHN SNOW AND CHOLERA

Another example of the translation of epidemiologic observations into public policy immortalized John Snow, whose portrait is seen in Fig. 1.16. Snow lived in the 19th century and was well known as the anesthesiologist who administered chloroform to Queen Victoria during childbirth. Snow's true love, however, was the

epidemiology of cholera, a disease that was a major problem in England in the middle of the 19th century. In the first week of September 1854, approximately 600 people living within a few blocks of the Broad Street pump in London died of cholera. At that time, the Registrar General was William Farr. Snow and Farr had a major disagreement about the cause of cholera. Farr adhered to what was called the *miasmatic* theory of disease. According to this theory, which was commonly held at the time, disease was transmitted by a *miasm*, or cloud, that clung low on the surface of the earth. If this were so, we would expect that people who lived at lower altitudes would be at greater risk of contracting a disease transmitted by this cloud than those living at higher elevations.

Farr collected data to support his hypothesis (Table 1.4). The data are quite consistent with his hypothesis: the lower the elevation, the higher the mortality rate from cholera. Snow did not agree; he believed that cholera was transmitted through contaminated water (Fig. 1.17). In London at that time, water was obtained by signing up with one of the water supply companies. The intakes for the water companies were in a very polluted part of the Thames River. At one point in time, one of the companies, the Lambeth Company, for technical, non–health-related reasons, shifted its water intake upstream in the Thames to a less polluted part of the river; the other companies did not move the locations of their water intakes. Snow reasoned therefore that based on his hypothesis that contaminated

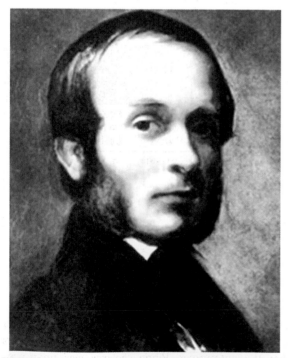

Fig. 1.16 Portrait of John Snow. (Portrait in oil by Thomas Jones Barker, 1847, in Zuck D. Snow, Empson and the Barkers of Bath. *Anaesthesia.* 2001;56:227–230.)

TABLE 1.4 **Deaths From Cholera in 10,000 Inhabitants by Elevation of Residence Above Sea Level, London, 1848–1849**	
Elevation Above Sea Level (ft)	**No. of Deaths**
<20	102
20–40	65
40–60	34
60–80	27
80–100	22
100–120	17
340–360	8

Data from Farr W. *Vital Statistics: A Memorial Volume of Selections from the Reports and Writings of William Farr* (edited for the Sanitary Institute of Great Britain by Noel A. Humphreys). London: The Sanitary Institute; 1885.

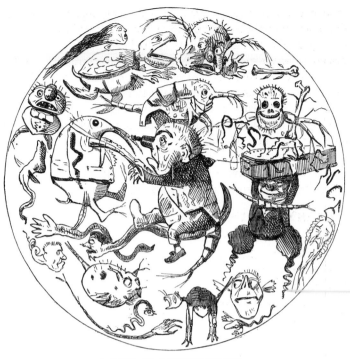

A DROP OF LONDON WATER.

Fig. 1.17 A drop of Thames water, as depicted by *Punch* in 1850. (From The wonders of a London water drop. *Punch Magazine.* May 11, 1850;461:188.)

water caused cholera, the mortality rate from cholera would be lower in people getting their water from the Lambeth Company than in those obtaining their water from the other companies. He carried out what we currently call "shoe-leather epidemiology"—going from house to house, counting all deaths from cholera in each house, and determining which company supplied water to each house.

Snow's findings are shown in Table 1.5. The table shows the number of houses, the number of deaths from cholera, and the deaths per 10,000 houses. Although this is not an ideal way to rate, because a house can contain different numbers of people, it is not a bad approximation. We see that in houses served by the Southwark and Vauxhall Company, which obtained its water from a polluted part of the Thames, the death rate was 315 deaths per 10,000 houses. In homes supplied by the Lambeth Company, which had relocated its water intake upstream, the rate was only 38 deaths per 10,000 houses. His data were so convincing that they led Farr, the Registrar General, to require the registrar of each district in south London to record

TABLE 1.5 **Deaths From Cholera per 10,000 Houses, by Source of Water Supply, London, 1854**			
Water Supply	**No. of Houses**	**Deaths from Cholera**	**Deaths per 10,000 Houses**
Southwark and Vauxhall Co.	40,046	1,263	315
Lambeth Co.	26,107	98	38
Other districts in London	256,423	1,422	56

Data modified from Snow J. On the mode of communication of cholera. In: *Snow on Cholera: A Reprint of Two Papers by John Snow, M.D.* New York: The Commonwealth Fund; 1936.

which water company supplied each house in which a person died of cholera. Remember that, in Snow's day, the enterotoxic *Vibrio cholerae* was unknown. Nothing was known about the biology of the disease. Snow's conclusion that contaminated water was associated with cholera was based entirely on observational data.[5]

The point is that, although it is extremely important for us to maximize our knowledge of the biology and pathogenesis of disease, it is not always necessary to know every detail of the possible pathogenic mechanisms to prevent disease. For example, we know that virtually every case of rheumatic fever and rheumatic heart disease followed a streptococcal infection. Though *Streptococcus* has been studied and analyzed extensively, we still do not know how and why it causes rheumatic fever. We do know that after a severe streptococcal infection, as seen in military recruits, rheumatic fever does not develop in 97 of every 100 infected persons. In civilian populations, such as schoolchildren, in whom the infection is less severe, rheumatic fever develops in only 3 of every 1,000 infected schoolchildren but not in the remaining 997.[6] Why does the disease not develop in those 97 recruits and 997 schoolchildren if they are exposed to the same organism? We do not know. Is the illness the result of an undetected difference in the organism, or is it caused by a cofactor that may facilitate the adherence of streptococci to epithelial cells? What we do know is that, even without fully understanding the chain of pathogenesis from infection with *Streptococcus* to rheumatic fever, we can prevent virtually every case of rheumatic fever if we either prevent or promptly and adequately treat streptococcal infections, as has been the case in the United States. The absence of biologic knowledge about pathogenesis should not be a hindrance or an excuse for not implementing effective preventive services.

Consider cigarette smoking and lung cancer. We do not know what specific carcinogenic agents in cigarettes cause cancer, but we do know that more than 80% of cases of lung cancer are caused by smoking. That does not mean that we should not be conducting laboratory research to better understand how cigarettes cause cancer. But again, in parallel with that research, we should be mounting effective community and public health programs to discourage smoking based on available observational data.

Fig. 1.18 shows mortality data for breast cancer and lung cancer in women in the United States. Breast cancer mortality rates remained relatively constant over several decades but showed evidence of decline in the early years of the 21st century. However, mortality from

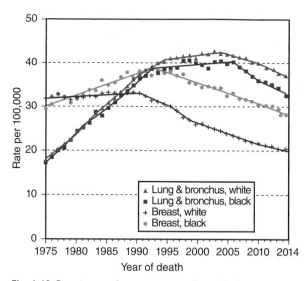

Fig. 1.18 Breast versus lung cancer mortality: white females versus black females, United States, 1975–2014, age-adjusted to 2000 standard. (From Howlader N, Noone AM, Krapcho M, et al, eds. *SEER Cancer Statistics Review, 1975–2014, National Cancer Institute.* Bethesda, MD, https://seer.cancer.gov/csr/1975_2014/, based on November 2016 SEER data submission, posted to the SEER website, April 2017. https://seer.cancer.gov/csr/1975_2014/browse_csr.php; *Figure 4.9.* Accessed April 14, 2017.)

lung cancer in women has been increasing steadily, although it may have begun to stabilize, and even decrease slightly, in recent years. Since 1987, more women in the United States have died each year from lung cancer than from breast cancer. Thus we are faced with the tragic picture of a largely preventable form of cancer, lung cancer, which results from a personal habit, smoking, as the current leading cause of cancer death in American women.

Furthermore, in 1993, environmental tobacco smoke (secondhand smoke from other people's smoking) was classified as a known human carcinogen by the Environmental Protection Agency, which attributed about 3,000 lung cancer deaths in nonsmoking individuals each year to environmental tobacco smoke.

When the Frequency of a Disease Declines, Who Deserves the Credit?

Over the past hundred or so years, mortality rates from a number of common infectious diseases have declined

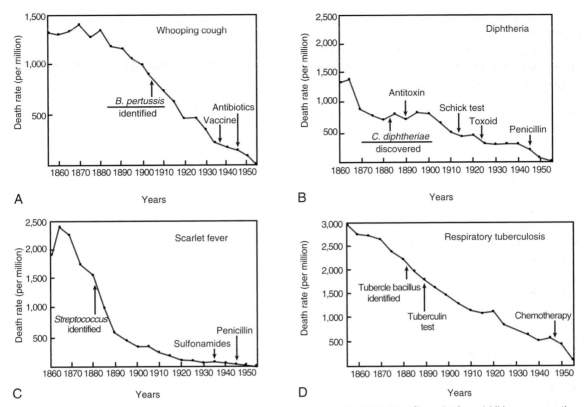

Fig. 1.19 Decline in death rates in England and Wales for (A) whooping cough, (B) diphtheria, (C) scarlet fever (children younger than 15 years of age), and (D) respiratory tuberculosis. (From Kass EH. Infectious diseases and social change. *J Infect Dis*. 1971;123:110–114.)

in the United States. For example, deaths from childhood infections such as diphtheria, pertussis (whooping cough), and scarlet fever (a streptococcal infection) have declined dramatically. In addition, US deaths from tuberculosis have dropped significantly.

It would be tempting to link these declines to improvements in treatments or vaccines that became available for these diseases during this time. However, in 1971 Edward Kass published the graphs shown in Fig. 1.19.[7] These graphs demonstrate that for each of these diseases, the major decline in mortality occurred many years before any effective treatment or vaccine became available. Fig. 1.20 shows a similar presentation of mortality trends over time for rheumatic fever in the 20th century.[8] Clearly, most of the decline in rheumatic fever mortality occurred well before penicillin and other antistreptococcal treatments became available.

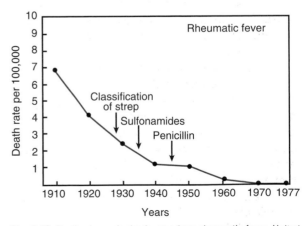

Fig. 1.20 Decline in crude death rates from rheumatic fever, United States, 1910–1977. (From Gordis L. The virtual disappearance of rheumatic fever in the United States: lessons in the rise and fall of disease. T. Duckett Jones Memorial Lecture. *Circulation*. 1985;72:1155–1162.)

What can explain these dramatic declines even before any vaccine or treatment became available? Theoretically, it is possible that when we observe a decline in mortality from an infectious disease, human exposure to the organisms involved may have declined, or the virulence of the organism may have diminished. However, a more likely explanation for the decline in mortality in these and other examples is that they primarily result from improvements in social conditions, safer water, and reduced exposures to pollutants and were not related to any medical intervention. In fact, Kass titled his 1971 paper, in which the graphs in Fig. 1.19 appeared, "Infectious Diseases and Social Change." Although the specific factors that were probably involved are not always clear, improved housing, including sanitation and improved nutrition, in addition to simultaneous lifestyle changes, are major factors that are likely to have contributed significantly to the decline.

We are often eager to attribute temporal declines in mortality to medical interventions. However, the lesson illustrated by the examples in these graphs is that we should be cautious before we conclude that observed declines in mortality are a result of medical intervention. In view of difficulties in deriving inferences about the effectiveness of medical care solely from population-wide declines in mortality, rigorous epidemiologic studies are clearly essential to assess the effectiveness of different medical interventions. Some of the approaches used and the design of such studies for evaluating health services are discussed in Chapter 17.

Integrating Prevention and Treatment

Prevention and therapy all too often are viewed as mutually exclusive activities, as is shown in Fig. 1.21. However, it is clear that prevention is integral to public health, but it is also integral to clinical practice. The physician's role is to maintain health, as well as to treat disease, but even treatment of disease includes a major component of prevention. Whenever we treat illness, we are preventing death, preventing complications in the patient, or preventing the impact on the patient's family. Thus much of the dichotomy between therapy and prevention is an illusion. Therapy involves secondary and tertiary prevention, the latter denoting the prevention of complications such as disability. At times it also involves primary prevention. Thus the entire

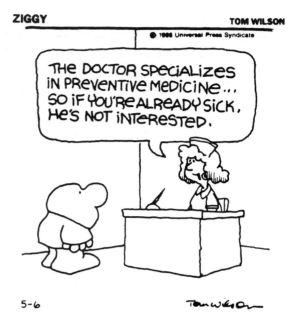

Fig. 1.21 Prevention and therapy viewed as mutually exclusive activities. (ZIGGY © 1986 ZIGGY AND FRIENDS, INC. Reprinted with permission of ANDREWS MCMEEL SYNDICATION. All rights reserved.)

spectrum of prevention should be viewed as integral to both public health and clinical practice.

Two very different decisions in 2012 placed further emphasis on the link between prevention and treatment. In July 2012 the US Food and Drug Administration (FDA) approved the use of a drug, Truvada (combination tenofovir and emtricitabine [antiviral medication]; Gilead Sciences, Foster City, CA, United States), for preventing HIV infection in people who are at high risk of acquiring HIV infection (so-called preexposure prophylaxis [PrEP]). Since 2004 the drug had been marketed only for treatment of individuals already infected with HIV—both for those chronically infected and those exposed to a needle-stick or other traumatic risk (so-called postexposure prophylaxis [PEP]).

The second decision, which was announced in May 2012, was that a 5-year clinical trial for preventing a genetically determined form of Alzheimer disease would be conducted by the National Institutes of Health. Investigators will study 300 people who are cognitively normal but are at very high risk for developing Alzheimer disease. The study was initiated in 2013 and is expected to be completed in 2020. Most of the study participants will be from a large family in Medellin,

Colombia, which is at high risk for a genetically determined form of Alzheimer disease, characterized by early onset of cognitive impairment followed by full dementia at approximately age 53. The drug being studied, crenezumab (antibodies against two types of human beta amyloid; Genentech, South San Francisco, CA, United States) is currently being evaluated in two other clinical trials in people who already have mild to moderate dementia, to determine whether formation of amyloid accumulation or cognitive decline can be slowed. Thus both in the study of HIV discussed in the previous paragraph and in this study of Alzheimer disease, drugs that have been used for patients with clear diagnoses of the diseases in question are now being evaluated as drugs that could prevent these diseases in high-risk patients. Both studies emphasize the need to bridge treatment and prevention in our developing views of other diseases as well.

Conclusion

Epidemiology is an invaluable tool for providing a rational basis on which effective prevention programs can be planned and implemented. Epidemiology is valuable when conducting clinical investigations to evaluate both new therapies and those that have been in use for some time, as well as newly developed interventions for disease prevention. The ultimate goal is to improve the control of disease through both prevention and treatment that will prevent deaths from the disease and will enhance the quality of life of those who have developed serious illness. The study designs used in epidemiology are discussed in later chapters.

REFERENCES

1. Porta M. *A Dictionary of Epidemiology*. 5th ed. New York: Oxford University Press; 2008.
2. Rose G. Sick individuals and sick populations. *Int J Epidemiol*. 1985;14:32–38.
3. Nuland SB. *The Doctors' Plague: Germs, Childbed Fever and the Strange Story of Ignáz Semmelweis*. New York: WW Norton/Atlas Books; 2003.
4. Fenner F, Henderson DA, Arita I, et al. *Smallpox and Its Eradication*. Geneva, Switzerland: World Health Organization; 1988.
5. Johnson S. *The Ghost Map: The Story of London's Most Terrifying Epidemic—and How It Changed Science, Cities, and the Modern World*. New York: Riverhead Books; 2006.
6. Markowitz M, Gordis L. *Rheumatic Fever*. 2nd ed. Philadelphia: WB Saunders; 1972.
7. Kass EH. Infectious diseases and social change. *J Infect Dis*. 1971;123:110–114.
8. Gordis L. The virtual disappearance of rheumatic fever in the United States: lessons in the rise and fall of disease. *Circulation*. 1985;72:1155–1162.

Chapter 2

The Dynamics of Disease Transmission

I keep six honest serving-men
(They taught me all I knew);
Their names are What and Why and When
And How and Where and Who.

—Rudyard Kipling[1] (1865–1936)

Learning Objectives

- To introduce concepts related to disease transmission using the epidemiologic approach to communicable diseases as a model.
- To define important terms related to the occurrence of disease in a population.
- To calculate an attack rate and illustrate how it may be used to measure person-to-person transmission of a disease.
- To describe the steps in an outbreak investigation and introduce how cross-tabulation may be used to identify the source.

Human disease does not arise in a vacuum. It results from an interaction of the host (a person), the agent (e.g., a bacterium), and the environment (e.g., polluted air). Although some diseases are largely genetic in origin, virtually all disease results from an interaction of genetic, behavioral, and environmental factors, with the proportions differing for different diseases. Many of the underlying principles governing the transmission of disease are most clearly demonstrated using communicable diseases as a model. Hence this chapter primarily uses such diseases as examples in reviewing these principles. However, the concepts discussed are also applicable to diseases that are not infectious in origin (e.g., second-hand smoke causing cancer).

Disease has been classically described as the result of the epidemiologic triad shown in Fig. 2.1. According to this diagram, it is the product of an interaction of the human host, an infectious or other type of agent, and the environment that promotes the exposure. A

vector, such as the mosquito or the deer tick, may be involved. For such an interaction to take place, the host must be susceptible. Human susceptibility is determined by a variety of factors including genetic background and behavioral, nutritional, and immunologic characteristics. The immune status of an individual is determined by many factors including prior experience both with natural infection and with immunization.

The factors that can cause human disease include biologic, physical, and chemical factors as well as other types, such as stress or behavioral risks, which may be harder to classify (Table 2.1).

Modes of Transmission

Diseases can be transmitted *directly* or *indirectly*. For example, a disease can be transmitted from person to person (direct transmission) by means of direct contact (as in the case of sexually transmitted infections). Indirect transmission can occur through a common vehicle such as a contaminated air or water supply or by a vector such as the mosquito. Some of the modes of transmission are shown in Box 2.1.

Fig. 2.2 is a classic photograph showing droplet dispersal after a sneeze. It vividly demonstrates the potential for an individual to infect a large number of people in a brief period of time. As Mims has pointed out:

An infected individual can transmit influenza or the common cold to a score of others in the course of an innocent hour in a crowded room. A venereal infection also must spread progressively from person to person if it is to maintain itself in nature, but it would be a formidable task to transmit venereal infection on such a scale.[2]

Thus different organisms spread in different ways, and the potential of a given organism for spreading

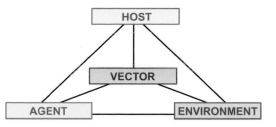

Fig. 2.1 The epidemiologic triad of a disease.

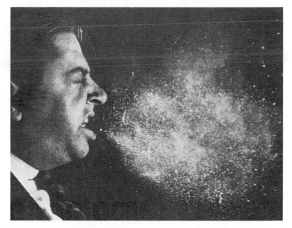

Fig. 2.2 Droplet dispersal following a violent sneeze. (Reprinted with permission from Jennison MW. *Aerobiology.* 17:102, 1947. Copyright 1947 American Association for the Advancement of Science.)

TABLE 2.1 Factors That May Be Associated With Increased Risk of Human Disease		
Host Characteristics	Types of Agents and Examples	Environmental Factors
Age	Biologic	Temperature
Sex	Bacteria,	Humidity
Race	viruses	Altitude
Religion	Chemical	Crowding
Customs	Heavy metals,	Housing
Occupation	alcohol,	Neighborhood
Genetic profile	smoke	Water
Marital status	Physical	Milk
Family	Trauma,	Food
background	radiation,	Radiation
Previous	fire	Air pollution
diseases	Nutritional	Noise
Immune status	Lack, excess	

BOX 2.1 MODES OF DISEASE TRANSMISSION

1. Direct
   a. Person-to-person contact
2. Indirect
   a. Common vehicle
      1) Single exposure
      2) Multiple exposures
      3) Continuous exposure
   b. Vector

and producing outbreaks depends on the characteristics of the organism, such as its rate of growth, the route by which it is transmitted from one person to another, and the number of susceptible persons in the community.

Fig. 2.3 is a schematic diagram of human body surfaces as sites of microbial infection and shedding. The alimentary tract can be considered as an open tube that crosses the body, and the respiratory and urogenital systems are shown as blind pockets. Each offers an opportunity for infection. The skin is another important portal of entry for infectious agents, primarily through scratches, bites, or injury. Agents that often enter through the skin include streptococci or staphylococci and fungi such as tinea (ringworm). Two points should be made in this regard: First, the skin is not the exclusive portal of entry for many of these agents, and second, infections can be acquired through more than one route. The same routes also serve as points of entry for noninfectious disease-causing agents. For example, environmental toxins can be ingested, inspired during respiration, or absorbed directly through the skin. The clinical and epidemiologic characteristics of many infectious and noninfectious conditions often relate to the site of the exposure to an organism or to an environmental substance and to its portal of entry into the body.

Clinical and Subclinical Disease

It is important to recognize the broad spectrum of disease severity. Fig. 2.4 shows the iceberg concept of disease. Just as most of an iceberg is under water and

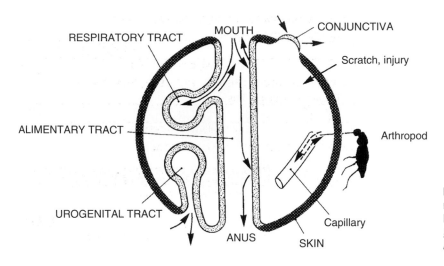

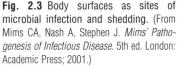

RESPIRATORY TRACT

MOUTH

CONJUNCTIVA

Scratch, injury

ALIMENTARY TRACT

Arthropod

UROGENITAL TRACT

Capillary

ANUS

SKIN

Fig. 2.3 Body surfaces as sites of microbial infection and shedding. (From Mims CA, Nash A, Stephen J. *Mims' Pathogenesis of Infectious Disease.* 5th ed. London: Academic Press; 2001.)

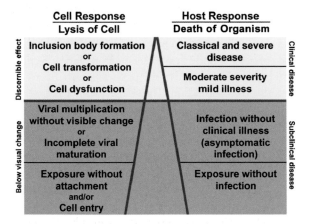

Fig. 2.4 The "iceberg" concept of infectious diseases at the level of the cell and of the host. (Modified from Evans AS, Kaslow RA, eds. *Viral Infections of Humans: Epidemiology and Control.* 4th ed. New York: Plenum; 1997.)

hidden from view with only its tip visible, so it is with disease: only clinical illness is readily apparent (as seen under *Host Response* on the right of Fig. 2.4). However, infections without clinical illness are important, particularly in the web of disease transmission, although they are not clinically apparent. In Fig. 2.4, the corresponding biologic stages of pathogenesis (biologic mechanisms) and disease at the cellular level are seen on the *left*. The iceberg concept is important because

it is not sufficient to count only the clinically apparent cases we see; for example, most cases of polio in prevaccine days were subclinical—that is, many people who contracted polio infection were not clinically ill. Nevertheless, they were still capable of spreading the virus to others. As a result, we cannot understand and explain the spread of polio unless the pool of inapparent cases (subclinical) is recognized. From the viewpoint of inapparent disease, this situation is not any different in many noncommunicable diseases. Although these diseases are not spread from person to person, many individuals, for example, can live a long time with inapparent chronic kidney disease, and it is only when they experience a clinical complication that a diagnosis of chronic kidney disease is made.

Fig. 2.5 shows the spectrum of severity for several diseases. Most cases of tuberculosis, for example, are inapparent. However, because inapparent cases can transmit the disease, such cases must be identified and treated to control the further spread of the disease. In measles, many cases are of moderate severity and only a few are inapparent. At the other extreme, without intervention, rabies has no inapparent cases, and most untreated cases are fatal. Thus we have a spectrum of severity patterns that vary with the disease. Severity appears to be related to the virulence of the organism (how efficient the organism is at producing disease) and to the site in the body where the organism

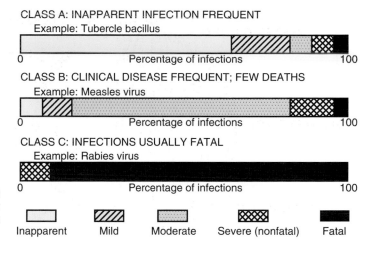

CLASS A: INAPPARENT INFECTION FREQUENT
Example: Tubercle bacillus

CLASS B: CLINICAL DISEASE FREQUENT; FEW DEATHS
Example: Measles virus

CLASS C: INFECTIONS USUALLY FATAL
Example: Rabies virus

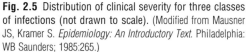

Inapparent   Mild   Moderate   Severe (nonfatal)   Fatal

Fig. 2.5 Distribution of clinical severity for three classes of infections (not drawn to scale). (Modified from Mausner JS, Kramer S. *Epidemiology: An Introductory Text.* Philadelphia: WB Saunders; 1985:265.)

multiplies. All of these factors, as well as such host characteristics as the immune response, must be appreciated to understand how disease spreads from one individual to another.

As clinical and biologic knowledge has increased over the years, so has our ability to distinguish different stages of disease. These include clinical and nonclinical disease.

CLINICAL DISEASE

Clinical disease is characterized by signs and symptoms.

NONCLINICAL (INAPPARENT) DISEASE

Nonclinical disease may include the following:

1. *Preclinical disease:* Disease that is not yet clinically apparent but is destined to progress to clinical disease.
2. *Subclinical disease:* Disease that is not clinically apparent and is not destined to become clinically apparent. This type of disease is often diagnosed by serologic (antibody) response or culture of the organism.
3. *Persistent (chronic) disease:* A person fails to "shake off" the infection, and it persists for years, at times for life. In recent years, an interesting phenomenon has been the manifestation of symptoms many years after an infection was thought to have been resolved. Some adults who recovered from poliomyelitis in childhood report severe chronic fatigue and weakness; this has been called postpolio syndrome in adult life.

These have thus become cases of clinical disease, albeit somewhat different from the initial illness.

4. *Latent disease:* An infection with no active multiplication of the agent, as when viral nucleic acid is incorporated into the nucleus of a cell as a provirus. In contrast to persistent infection, only the genetic message is present in the host, not the viable organism.

Carrier Status

A carrier is an individual who harbors the organism but is not infected as measured by serologic studies (no evidence of an antibody response) or shows no evidence of clinical illness. This person can still infect others, although the infectivity is generally lower than with other infections. Carrier status may be of limited duration or may be chronic, lasting for months or years. One of the best-known examples of a long-term carrier was Mary Mallon, better known as Typhoid Mary, who carried *Salmonella typhi* and died in 1938. Over a period of many years, she worked as a cook in the New York City area, moving from household to household under different names. She was considered to have caused at least 10 typhoid fever outbreaks that included 51 cases and 3 deaths.

Endemic, Epidemic, and Pandemic

Three other terms must be defined: *endemic, epidemic,* and *pandemic. Endemic* is defined as the habitual

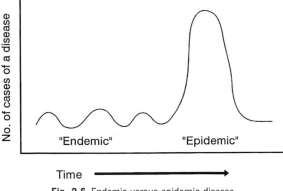

Fig. 2.6 Endemic versus epidemic disease.

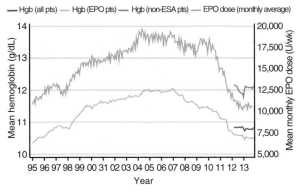

Fig. 2.7 Mean monthly hemoglobin *(Hgb)* level and mean monthly epoetin *(EPO)* dose (expressed as units per week) in adult hemodialysis patients on dialysis ≥90 days, Medicare claims, 1995–2013. (From US Renal Data System. 2015 USRDS annual data report volume 2: ESRD in the United States. https://www.usrds.org/2015/download/vol2_USRDS_ESRD_15.pdf. Accessed June 5, 2017.)

presence of a disease within a given geographic area. It may also refer to the usual occurrence of a given disease within such an area (sometimes referred to as the "background rate of disease"). *Epidemic* is defined as the occurrence in a community or region of a group of illnesses of similar nature, clearly in excess of normal expectancy and derived from a common or a propagated source (Fig. 2.6). *Pandemic* refers to a worldwide epidemic.

How do we know when we have an excess over what is expected? Indeed, how do we know how much to expect? There is no precise answer to either question. Through ongoing surveillance, we may determine what the usual or expected level may be. With regard to excess, sometimes an "interocular test" may be convincing: the difference is so clear that it hits you between the eyes.

Two examples will show how pandemics and fear of pandemics relate to the development of public policy. Patients with chronic kidney disease are often anemic, which is commonly corrected by injection of erythropoiesis-stimulating agents (ESAs); these are genetically engineered forms of the human erythropoietin hormone. The drug manufacturers pay doctors millions of dollars every year in return for prescribing this anemia medication, which led to extensive off-label use and the overutilization of ESAs in the United States (Fig. 2.7). In 2006, two clinical trials were published in the *New England Journal of Medicine* that raised concerns about the safety of using ESAs for anemia correction to optimal levels in patients with chronic kidney disease, as neither study anticipated these results.

The first clinical trial, Cardiovascular Risk Reduction by Early Anemia Treatment with Epoetin Beta (CREATE),[3] showed that early and complete correction of anemia (to a target hemoglobin level in the normal range) failed to reduce the incidence of cardiovascular events as compared with the partial correction of anemia. The second trial, Correction of Hemoglobin and Outcomes in Renal Insufficiency (CHOIR),[4] showed that a higher target hemoglobin value of 13.5 g/dL was associated with increased risk of death, myocardial infarction, hospitalization for congestive heart failure, and stroke, all without an improvement in quality of life as compared with a lower hemoglobin target of 11.3 g/dL (Fig. 2.8). As a result, in 2007, the US Food and Drug Administration issued a black box warning adding significant restrictions on the use of ESAs.[5] The black box warning includes the following: (1) prescribers should use the lowest dose of ESA that will gradually increase the hemoglobin concentration to the lowest level sufficient to avoid the need for red blood cell transfusion and (2) ESAs increase the risk for death and for serious cardiovascular events when administered to target a hemoglobin of greater than 12 g/dL.

The second example involves an issue that arose in 2011 related to laboratory research into the H5N1, or "bird flu," virus (Fig. 2.9). Although transmission of naturally occurring H5N1 has been primarily limited to persons having direct contact with infected animals, in the unusual cases where people do acquire the

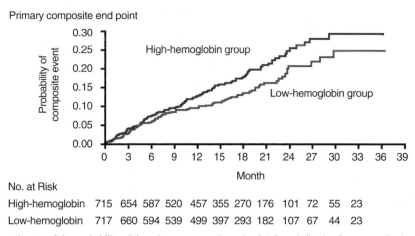

Primary composite end point

Fig. 2.8 Kaplan-Meier estimates of the probability of the primary composite end point (hospitalization for congestive heart failure without renal replacement therapy, myocardial infarction, stroke, and death). (From Singh AK, Szczech L, Tang KL, et al. Correction of anemia with epoetin alfa in chronic kidney disease. *N Engl J Med*. 2006;355:2085–2098.)

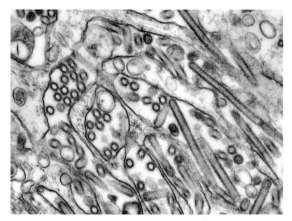

Fig. 2.9 Colorized transmission electron micrograph of avian influenza A H5N1 viruses (seen in *gold*) grown in MDCK cells (seen in *green*). (From Centers for Disease Control and Prevention, Courtesy Cynthia Goldsmith, Jacqueline Katz, and Sherif R. Zaki.)

infection from animals the disease is often very severe with a high mortality. There has therefore been serious concern that certain mutations in the virus might increase transmissibility of the virus to humans and could therefore result in a human pandemic. In order to understand fully the possibility of such a mutation and the potential for preventing it, two government-funded laboratories, one at Erasmus Medical Center in the Netherlands and a second at the University of

Wisconsin-Madison in the United States, created genetically altered H5N1 strains that could be transmitted between mammals (ferrets) through the air.

After reviewing the two studies, the US National Science Advisory Board for Biosecurity, for the first time in its history, recommended against publishing the details of the methodologies used in these studies. The board cited potential misuse by "those who would seek to do harm" by participating in bioterrorist activity. Other scientists, however, including members of an expert panel assembled by the World Health Organization (WHO), disagreed, stating that the work was important to public health efforts to prevent a possible pandemic in humans. In January 2012, a moratorium on some types of H5N1 research was self-imposed by the researchers to allow time for discussion of these concerns by experts and by the public. The results of the two studies were subsequently published in May and June of 2012.[4,6,7]

The major unresolved issue is whether the potential benefits to society from the results of these types of studies outweigh the risks from the uncontrolled spread of mutated virus, resulting from either lapses in biosafety in the laboratory (accidental release of the virus) or bioterrorist activity (intentional release of the virus). Scientists and policy makers are obliged to develop methods for assessing the risks and benefits of conducting different types of experimental research. In addition, these events illustrate that censorship and academic freedom in science remain highly relevant issues today.

Disease Outbreaks

Let us assume that a food becomes contaminated with a microorganism. If an outbreak occurs in the group of people who have eaten the food, it is called a *common-vehicle exposure*, because all the cases that occurred were in persons exposed to the suspected contaminated food. The food may be served only once—for example, at a catered luncheon—resulting in a *single exposure* to the people who eat it, or the food may be served more than once, resulting in *multiple exposures* to people who eat it more than once. When a water supply is contaminated with sewage because of leaky pipes, the contamination can be either *periodic*, causing multiple exposures as a result of changing pressures in the water supply system, which may cause intermittent contamination, or *continuous*, in which case a constant leak leads to persistent contamination. The epidemiologic picture that is manifested depends on whether the exposure is single, multiple, or continuous.

For purposes of this discussion, we will focus on the *single-exposure, common-vehicle outbreak* because the issues discussed are most clearly seen in this type of outbreak. What are the characteristics of such an outbreak? First, such outbreaks are generally explosive—that is, there is a sudden and rapid increase in the number of cases of the disease or condition in a population. (Interestingly, single-exposure common-vehicle epidemics of noncommunicable diseases, such as the epidemic of leukemia following the explosion of an atomic bomb in Hiroshima and Nagasaki, also seem to follow the same pattern.) Second, the cases are limited to people who share the common exposure. This is self-evident, because in the first wave of cases we would not expect the disease to develop in people who were not exposed unless there was another independent source of the disease in the community. Third, in a food-borne outbreak, cases rarely occur in persons who did not eat the food—that is, those who acquire the disease from a primary case who ate the food. The reason for the relative rarity of such secondary cases in this type of outbreak is not well understood.

In the United States, the leading cause of food-borne–related illness is contamination with norovirus (from the Norwalk virus family). Globally, norovirus results in a total of \$4.2 billion in direct health care system costs and \$60.3 billion in societal costs per year.[8]

Over recent decades, a growing number of outbreaks of acute gastroenteritis (AGE) have occurred aboard cruise ships. The Centers for Disease Control and Prevention (CDC) has reported that rates of AGE among passengers on cruise ships have decreased from 27.2 cases per 100,000 travel days in 2008 to 22.3 in 2014, while the rate among crew members was essentially unchanged.[9] This could potentially be attributed to the production of operational manuals or specific guidelines providing hygiene standards, increasing awareness among passengers and crew members, communicable disease surveillance programs, and preventive procedures in addition to regulatory enforcement and strict inspections through the CDC's Vessel Sanitation Program (VSP), which monitors outbreaks on cruise ships and works to prevent and control transmission of illness aboard these ships. (Data from each outbreak are available on their website, http://www.cdc.gov/nceh/vsp/.) In areas with a high prevalence of norovirus, particularly the recombinant GII.2 type, such as in the provinces of Guangdong and Jiangsu, China, outbreaks of AGE continue to occur frequently.[10] For example, on December 14, 2014, a student in third grade vomited in the classroom and washroom several times and was considered the earliest suspected case of norovirus. Over the following 3 days, 27 more cases were reported, which were mainly located on the fourth floor (12 cases) and third floor (9 cases) of the school building. Fig. 2.10 shows the epidemic curve with the number of cases each day. The first peak of the outbreak was on December 17, which was starting to taper off when implementation of control measures such as quarantine and disinfection were followed. However, a few days later, on December 25, the attack rate peaked again, with cases occurring mainly on the second floor (12 cases) and third floor (5 cases). In order to aggressively contain the outbreak, the school was closed temporarily and the outbreak came to an end on December 31.

Immunity and Susceptibility

The amount of disease in a population depends on a balance between the number of people in that population

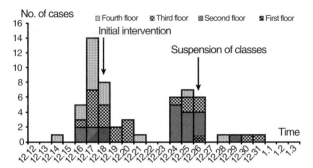

Fig. 2.10 Distribution of cases grouped by floor and by date of outbreak onset in a school in the province of in Jiangsu Province, China, in 2014. (From Shi C, Feng W-H, Shi P et al. An acute gastroenteritis outbreak caused by GII.17 norovirus in Jiangsu Province, China. *Int J Infect Dis.* 2016;49:30–32.)

who are susceptible and therefore at risk for the disease and the number of people who are not susceptible or immune and therefore not at risk. They may be immune because they have had the disease previously (and have antibodies) or because they have been immunized. They also may not be susceptible on a genetic basis. Clearly if the entire population is immune, no epidemic can develop. But the balance is usually struck somewhere in between immunity and susceptibility, and when it moves toward susceptibility, the likelihood of an outbreak increases. This has been observed particularly in formerly isolated populations who were later exposed to disease. For example, in the 19th century, Panum observed that measles occurred in the Faroe Islands in epidemic form when infected individuals entered the isolated and susceptible population.[11] In another example, severe outbreaks of streptococcal sore throats developed when new susceptible recruits arrived at the Great Lakes Naval Station.[12]

Herd Immunity

Herd immunity is defined as the resistance of a group of people to an attack by a disease to which a large proportion of the members of the group are immune. If a large percentage of the population is immune, the entire population is likely to be protected, not just those who are immune. Why does herd immunity occur? It happens because disease spreads from one person to another in any community. Once a certain proportion of people in the community are immune, the likelihood

is small that an infected person will encounter a susceptible person to whom he can transmit the infection; more of his encounters will be with people who are immune. The presence of a large proportion of immune persons in the population lessens the likelihood that a person with the disease will come into contact with a susceptible individual.

Why is the concept of herd immunity so important? When we carry out immunization programs, it may not be necessary to achieve 100% immunization rates to immunize the population successfully. We can achieve highly effective protection by immunizing a large part of the population; the remaining part will be protected because of herd immunity.

For herd immunity to exist, certain conditions must be met. The disease agent must be restricted to a single host species within which transmission occurs, and that transmission must be relatively direct from one member of the host species to another. If we have a reservoir in which the organism can exist outside the human host, herd immunity will not operate because other means of transmission may be available. In addition, infections must induce solid immunity. If immunity is only partial, we will not build up a large proportion of immune people in the community.

What does this mean? Herd immunity operates if the probability of an infected person encountering every *other individual* in the population ("random mixing") is the same. But if a person is infected and all of his or her interactions are with people who are susceptible (i.e., there is no random mixing of the population), he or she is likely to transmit the disease to other susceptible people. Herd immunity operates optimally when populations are constantly mixing together. This is a theoretical concept because, obviously, populations are never completely randomly mixed. All of us associate with family and friends, for example, more than we do with strangers. However, the degree to which herd immunity is achieved depends on the extent to which the population approaches a random mixing. Thus we can interrupt the transmission of disease even if not everyone in the population is immune as long as a critical percentage of the population is immune.

What percentage of a population must be immune for herd immunity to operate? This percentage varies from disease to disease. For example, in the case of measles, which is highly communicable, it has been

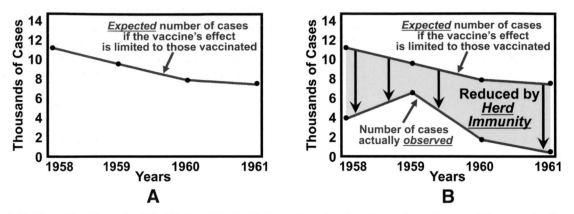

Fig. 2.11 Effect of herd immunity, United States, 1958–61. (A) Expected number of paralytic poliomyelitis cases if the vaccine's effect was limited to vaccinated people. (B) Number of cases observed as a result of herd immunity. (Modified from American Academy of Pediatrics News. Copyright 1998. From Stickle G. Observed and expected poliomyelitis in the United States, 1958–1961. *Am J Public Health.* 1964;54:1222–1229.)

estimated that 94% of the population must be immune before the chain of transmission is interrupted. With decreasing childhood immunization rates in the United States associated with parental concerns regarding the risk of autism spectrum disorder, measles outbreaks are becoming more common. A total of 125 measles cases with rash occurred in a 6-week period; among these cases 110 were California residents (45% unvaccinated), of whom 35% had visited one or both Disney theme parks between December 17 and 20, 2014, the suspected source of exposure. Of the secondary cases, most (26/34) were close contacts. An additional 15 cases associated with the Disney theme parks were reported in seven additional states.[13]

Let us consider poliomyelitis immunization and herd immunity. From 1951 to 1954, an average of 24,220 cases of paralytic poliomyelitis occurred in the United States each year. Two types of vaccine are available. The oral polio vaccine (OPV) protects not only those who are vaccinated but also others in the community through secondary immunity, produced when the vaccinated individual spreads the active vaccine virus to contacts. In effect, the contacts are immunized by the spread of virus from the vaccinated person. If enough people in the community are protected in this way, the chain of transmission is interrupted. However, even inactivated poliovirus vaccine (IPV), which does not produce secondary immunity (does not spread the virus to susceptibles), can produce herd immunity if enough of the population is immunized. Even those who are

not immunized will be protected because the chain of transmission in the community has been interrupted.

From 1958 to 1961, only IPV was available in the United States. Fig. 2.11A shows the expected number of cases each year if the vaccine had protected only those who received the vaccine. Fig. 2.11B shows the number of polio cases actually observed. Clearly far fewer cases occurred than would have been expected from the direct effects of the vaccine alone. The difference between the two curves represents the effect of herd immunity from the vaccine. Thus nonimmunized individuals can gain some protection from either the OPV or IPV.

Incubation Period

The incubation period is defined as the *interval from receipt of infection to the time of onset of clinical illness* (the onset of recognizable symptoms). If you become infected today, the disease with which you are infected may not develop for a number of days or weeks. During this time, the *incubation period*, you feel completely well and show no signs of the disease.

Why does disease not develop immediately at the time of infection? What accounts for the incubation period? It may reflect the time needed for the organism to replicate sufficiently until it reaches the critical mass needed for clinical disease to result. It probably also relates to the site in the body at which the organism replicates—whether it replicates superficially, near the skin surface, or deeper in the body (e.g., in the gut). The dose of the infectious agent received at the time of infection may also influence the length of the incubation period. With a large dose, the incubation period may be shorter.

The incubation period is also of historical interest because it is related to what may have been the only medical advance associated with the Black Death (plague) in Europe. In 1374, when people were terribly frightened of the Black Death, the Venetian Republic appointed three officials who were responsible for inspecting all ships entering the port and for excluding ships that had sick people on board. It was hoped that this intervention would protect the community. In 1377, in the Italian seaport of Ragusa, travelers were detained in an isolated area for 30 days (*trentini giorni*) after arrival to see whether infection developed. This period was found to be insufficient, and the period of detention was lengthened to 40 days (*quarante giorni*). This is the origin of the word *quarantine*.

How long would we want to isolate a person? We would want to isolate a person until he or she is no longer infectious to others (having passed through the suspected incubation period). When a person is clinically ill, we generally have a clear sign of potential infectiousness. An important problem arises *before* the person becomes clinically ill—that is, during the incubation period. If we knew when he or she became infected and also knew the general length of the incubation period for the disease, we would want to isolate the infected person during this period (and perhaps a few days extra to be especially cautious) to prevent transmission of the disease to others. In most situations, however, we do not know that a person has been infected, and we may not know until signs of clinical disease become manifest. In addition, we may not know the distribution of the incubation period.

This leads to an important question: Is it worthwhile to quarantine—isolate—a patient, such as a child with chickenpox? The problem is that, during at least part of the incubation period, when the person is still free of clinical illness, he or she can transmit the disease to others. Thus we have people who are not (yet) clinically ill but who have been infected; they are unaware of their infection status and are able to transmit their disease. For many common childhood diseases, by the time clinical disease develops in the child, he

or she has already transmitted the disease to others. Therefore isolating such a person at the point at which he or she becomes clinically ill will not necessarily be effective. On the other hand, isolation can be very valuable. In September 2012, health officials in Saudi Arabia first reported a severe acute respiratory illness with symptoms of fever, cough, and shortness of breath. The causative organism was shown to be the Middle East Respiratory Syndrome Coronavirus (MERS-CoV), which has an incubation period of about 5 or 6 days. MERS-CoV likely came from infected camels in the Arabian Peninsula and spread through person-to-person close contact, with health care personnel at higher risk of infection if universal precautions were not adhered to. All MERS-CoV cases that have been identified had a positive history of someone living in or traveling to countries in or near the Arabian Peninsula. Another outbreak of MERS-CoV occurred in the Republic of Korea in 2015 and was also linked to a returning traveler from the Arabian Peninsula. As of May 2017, WHO has reported that there had been 1952 laboratory-confirmed cases of infection with MERS-CoV from 27 countries, of whom 693 (36%) had died.

Fig. 2.12 shows the epidemic curve of the confirmed global cases of MERS-CoV reported to WHO as of May 5, 2017. (Note that, unlike the epidemic curve for common vehicle epidemics, the curve for person-to-person spread is multimodal.) An outbreak of MERS-CoV in the Republic of Korea was seen in 2015 but was rather contained, whereas the epidemic remains active in Saudi Arabia. A major contributor to the Korean control of the epidemic was probably the strong infection control measures implemented early on for diagnosing and isolating probable MERS-CoV cases and for reducing interpersonal contacts of travelers with a history of travel to highly affected areas.

Different diseases have different incubation periods. A precise incubation period does not exist for a given disease; rather, a range of incubation periods is characteristic of that disease. Fig. 2.13 shows the range of incubation periods for several diseases. In general the length of the incubation period is characteristic of the infective organism.

The incubation period for infectious diseases has its analogue in noninfectious diseases. Thus, even when an individual is exposed to a carcinogen or other environmental toxin, the disease is often manifest only

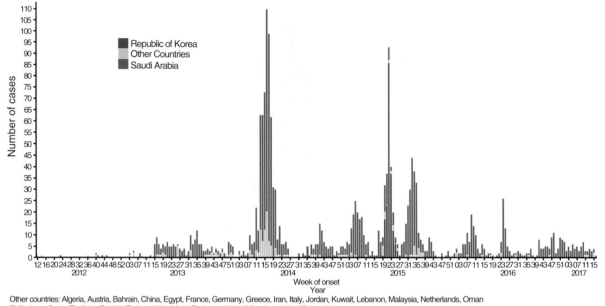

Other countries: Algeria, Austria, Bahrain, China, Egypt, France, Germany, Greece, Iran, Italy, Jordan, Kuwait, Lebanon, Malaysia, Netherlands, Oman
Philippines, Qatar, Thailand, Tunisia, Turkey, United Arab Emirates, United Kingdom, United States, Yemen
Please note that the underlying data are subject to change as the investigations around cases are ongoing. Onset date estimated if not available.

Fig. 2.12 Epidemic curve of all confirmed global cases of Middle East Respiratory Syndrome Coronavirus *(MERS-CoV)* from 2012 to April 2017. (World Health Organization. http://www.who.int/emergencies/mers-cov/mers-epi-5-may-2017.png?ua=1. Accessed May 14, 2017.)

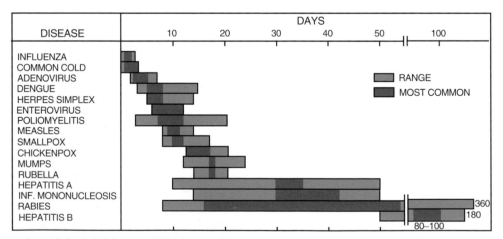

Fig. 2.13 Incubation periods of viral diseases. *INF.,* Infectious. (From Evans AS, Kaslow RA, eds. *Viral Infections of Humans: Epidemiology and Control.* 4th ed. New York: Plenum; 1997.)

after months or even years. For example, mesothelioma resulting from asbestos exposure may occur 20 to 30 years after the exposure. The incubation period for noninfectious diseases is often referred to as the latency period.

Fig. 2.14 is a graphic representation of an outbreak of *Salmonella typhimurium* at a medical conference in Wales in 1986. Each bar represents the number of cases of disease developing at a certain point in time after the exposure; the number of hours since

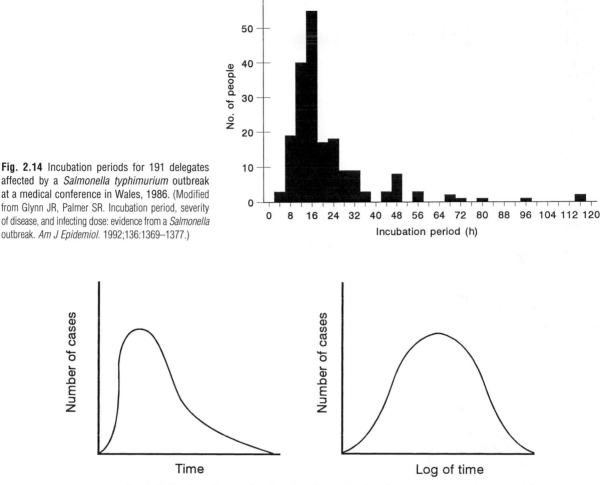

Fig. 2.14 Incubation periods for 191 delegates affected by a *Salmonella typhimurium* outbreak at a medical conference in Wales, 1986. (Modified from Glynn JR, Palmer SR. Incubation period, severity of disease, and infecting dose: evidence from a *Salmonella* outbreak. *Am J Epidemiol.* 1992;136:1369–1377.)

Fig. 2.15 Number of cases plotted against time and against the logarithm of time.

exposure is shown along the horizontal axis. If we draw a line connecting the tops of the bars, it is called the *epidemic curve,* which is defined as the distribution of the times of onset of the disease. In a *single-exposure, common-vehicle epidemic,* the epidemic curve represents the distribution of the incubation periods. This should be intuitively apparent: if the infection took place at one point in time, the interval from that point to the onset of each case is the incubation period in that person.

As seen in Fig. 2.14, involving *Salmonella typhimurium,* there was a rapid, explosive rise in the number of cases within the first 16 hours, which suggests a single-exposure, common-vehicle epidemic. In fact, this pattern is the classic epidemic curve for a single-exposure common-vehicle outbreak (Fig. 2.15, *left*). The reason for this configuration is not known, but it has an interesting property: if the curve is plotted against the logarithm of time rather than against time itself, the curve becomes a normal curve, which has useful statistical properties (see Fig. 2.15, *right*). If plotted on log-normal graph paper, we obtain a straight line, and estimation of the median incubation period is facilitated. Armenian and Lilienfeld[14] showed that a log-normal curve is also typical of single-exposure common-vehicle epidemics of noninfectious diseases.

The three critical variables in investigating an outbreak or epidemic are as follows:

1. When did the exposure take place?
2. When did the disease begin?
3. What was the incubation period for the disease?

If we know any two of these, we can calculate the third.

Attack Rate

An attack rate is defined as:

$$\frac{\text{Number of people at risk in whom}}{\text{Total number of people at risk}}$$

The attack rate is useful for comparing the risk of disease in groups with different exposures. The attack rate can be specific for a given exposure. For example, the attack rate in people who ate a certain food is called a *food-specific attack rate*. It is calculated by:

$$\frac{\text{Number of people who ate a certain food}}{\text{Total number of people who ate that food}}$$

In general, *time* is not explicitly specified in an attack rate because the exposure is common and the illness is acute; given what is usually known about how long after an exposure most cases develop, the time period is implicit in the attack rate.

A person who acquires the disease from that exposure (e.g., from a contaminated food) is called a *primary case*. A person who acquires the disease from exposure to a primary case is called a *secondary case*. The *secondary attack rate* is therefore defined as the attack rate in susceptible people who were not exposed to the suspected agent who have been exposed to a primary case. It is a good measure of person-to-person spread of disease after the disease has been introduced into a population, and it can be thought of as a ripple moving out from the primary case. We often calculate the secondary attack rate in family members of the index case.

The secondary attack rate also has application in noninfectious diseases when family members are examined to determine the extent to which a disease

clusters among first-degree relatives of an index case (heritability or clustering within families), which may yield a clue regarding the relative contributions of genetic and environmental factors to the cause of a disease.

Exploring Occurrence of Disease

The concepts outlined in this chapter form the basis for exploring the occurrence of disease. When a disease appears to have occurred at more than an endemic (usual) level and we wish to investigate its occurrence, we ask:

Who was attacked by the disease?
When did the disease occur?
Where did the cases arise?

It is well known that disease risk is affected by all of these factors.

WHO

The characteristics of the human host are clearly related to disease risk. Factors such as sex, age, and race as well as behavioral risk factors (e.g., smoking) may have major effects.

Gonorrhea

As shown in Fig. 2.16, rates of gonorrhea have historically been higher in men than in women, and this sex difference is observed at least as far back as 1960 (not shown in this graph). Because women are more likely to be asymptomatic, the disease in women has probably been underreported. Rates had been leveling off in both men and women over the past few decades, but since 2013, higher rates of gonorrhea have been observed in men than in women. Such increases in rates among men could be either attributed to increased transmission or increased case ascertainment (e.g., through increased extragenital screening) among gay, bisexual, and other men who have sex with men.

Pertussis

The incidence of pertussis ("whooping cough") in the United States peaked in 2004; the rate reached 8.9 cases per 100,000 population, more than twice that reported in 2003. In 1994, the rate was 1.8. The number of cases in 2004 was the highest reported since 1959. Although childhood pertussis vaccine coverage

Rate (per 100,000 population)

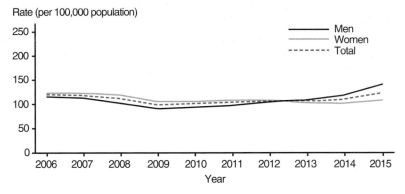

Fig. 2.16 Gonorrhea—rates of reported cases by sex, United States, 2006–15. (From Centers for Disease Control and Prevention. *Sexually Transmitted Disease Surveillance 2010.* Atlanta: US Department of Health and Human Services; 2016. https://www.cdc.gov/std/stats15/figures/13.htm. Accessed May 8, 2017.)

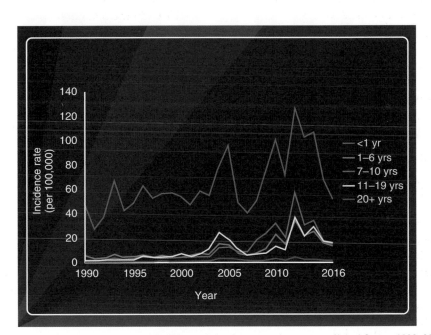

Fig. 2.17 Pertussis (whooping cough) incidence per 100,000 population by year and age group, United States, 1990–2016. (From Centers for Disease Control and Prevention. https://www.cdc.gov/pertussis/images/incidence-graph-age.png. Accessed June 13, 2018.)

is high in the United States, pertussis continues to cause morbidity. Some of this increase may result from improved diagnostics as well as recognition and reporting of cases. As seen in Fig. 2.17, the lowest rates for pertussis in the United States were observed in 1991. Although incidence rates showed two more peaks in 2008 and 2009, they subsequently declined until 2016. Of note, infants aged less than 1 year, who are at the greatest risk for death, continue to have the highest reported rate of pertussis.

Pertussis occurrence is clearly related to age (Fig. 2.18). Although the highest *rate* of pertussis was in infants less than 6 months of age (99 per 100,000 population), the *number* of reported cases was highest in children ages 11 to 19. Approximately half of reported pertussis cases in 2014 and 2015 occurred in 10- to 19-year-olds and in adults over the age of 20 years. Although the specific cause of this phenomenon is unknown, it could result from a waning of protection 5 to 10 years after pertussis immunization.

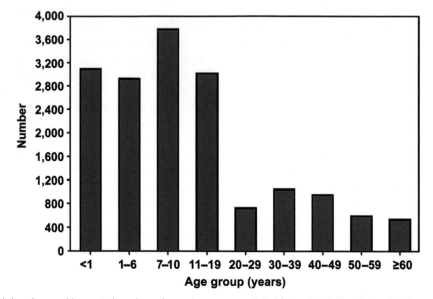

Fig. 2.18 Pertussis (whooping cough), reported numbers of cases by age group, United States, 2009. (From Centers for Disease Control and Prevention. Summary of notifiable diseases, United States, 2009. *Morb Mortal Wkly Rep.* 2011;58:1–100.)

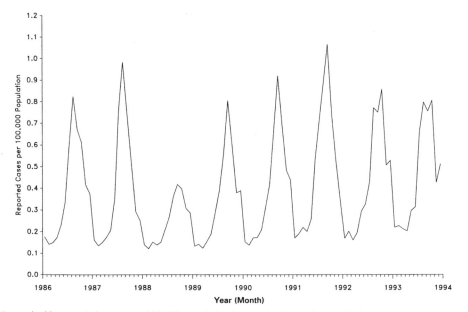

Fig. 2.19 Aseptic meningitis, reported cases per 100,000 population by month, United States, 1986–93. (From Centers for Disease Control and Prevention. Summary of notifiable diseases, United States, 1993. *Morb Mortal Wkly Rep.* 1994;42:22.)

WHEN

Certain diseases occur with a certain periodicity. For example, aseptic meningitis peaks at consistent yearly rates (Fig. 2.19). Often, there is a seasonal pattern to the temporal variation. For example, diarrheal disease is most common during the summer months, and respiratory disease is most common during the winter months. The question of *when* is also addressed by examining trends in disease incidence over time. For example, in the United States, both the incidence of and deaths from acquired immunodeficiency syndrome (AIDS) increased for many years, but it began to decline in 1996, largely as a result of new therapy and health education efforts.

WHERE

Disease is not randomly distributed in time or place. For example, Fig. 2.20 shows the geographic distribution of Lyme disease in the United States in 2015, with each dot representing one case of Lyme disease. There is a clear clustering of cases along the Northeast coast, in the north-central part of the country, and in the Pacific Coast region. The states in which established enzootic cycles of *Borrelia burgdorferi*, the causative agent, have been reported accounted for 95% of the cases. The distribution of the disease closely parallels that of the deer tick vector.

A dramatic example of spread of disease is seen with West Nile virus (WNV) in the United States.[15] WNV was first isolated and identified in 1937 in the West Nile region of Uganda, and for many years it was found only in the Eastern Hemisphere. The basic cycle of the disease is bird-mosquito-bird. Mosquitoes become infected when they bite infected birds. When mosquitoes that bite both birds and humans become infected, they pose a threat to people. Most human infections are subclinical, but approximately 1 of 150 infections in recent years has resulted in meningitis or encephalitis. The risk of neurologic disease is significantly increased in people older than 50 years of age. Other symptoms include fever, nausea and vomiting, rash, headache,

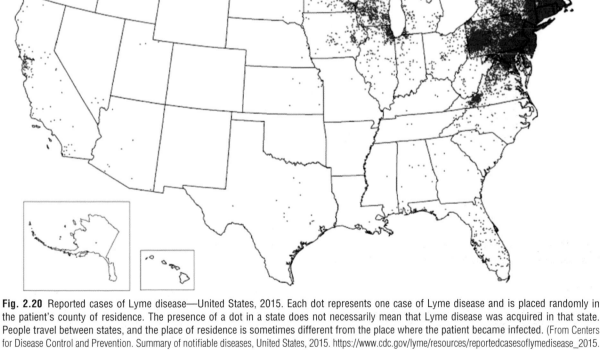

Fig. 2.20 Reported cases of Lyme disease—United States, 2015. Each dot represents one case of Lyme disease and is placed randomly in the patient's county of residence. The presence of a dot in a state does not necessarily mean that Lyme disease was acquired in that state. People travel between states, and the place of residence is sometimes different from the place where the patient became infected. (From Centers for Disease Control and Prevention. Summary of notifiable diseases, United States, 2015. https://www.cdc.gov/lyme/resources/reportedcasesoflymedisease_2015.pdf. Accessed May 8, 2017.)

and muscle weakness. The case-fatality rate, or the proportion of people who develop the disease (cases) who then die of the disease, can be as high as 14%. Advancing age is a major risk factor for death from WNV, with one study reporting death nine times as frequently in older compared with younger patients. Treatment is supportive, and prevention is largely addressed through mosquito control and the use of insect repellents and bed nets. Tracking the distribution of the disease depends on surveillance for human cases and on monitoring birds and animals for the disease and deaths from the disease. Surveillance is discussed in further detail in Chapter 3.

WNV was first identified in New York City in 1999. Fig. 2.21 shows average annual incidence of WNV neuroinvasive disease reported to the CDC by states from 1999 to 2015. During the same reporting period, the WNV disease epidemic peaked during the month of September every year (Fig. 2.22). Much remains to be learned about this disease to facilitate treatment, prevention, and control.

Outbreak Investigation

The characteristics just discussed are the central issues in virtually all outbreak investigations. The steps for investigating an outbreak generally follow this pattern (Box 2.2).

CROSS-TABULATION

When confronted with several possible causal agents, as is often the case in a food-borne disease outbreak,

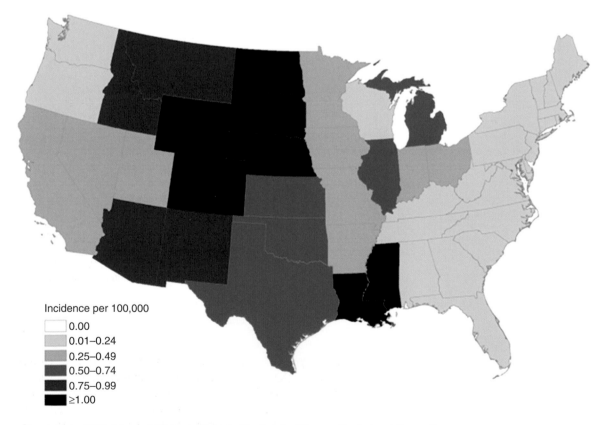

Incidence per 100,000
- 0.00
- 0.01–0.24
- 0.25–0.49
- 0.50–0.74
- 0.75–0.99
- ≥1.00

Source: ArboNET, Arboviral Diseases Branch, Centers for Disease Control and Prevention

Fig. 2.21 Average annual incidence of West Nile virus neuroinvasive disease reported to the Centers for Disease Control and Prevention by state, 1999–2015. (From Centers for Disease Control and Prevention. https://www.cdc.gov/westnile/resources/pdfs/data/6-WNV-Neuro-Incidence-by-State-Map_1999-2015_07072016.pdf. Accessed May 8, 2017.)

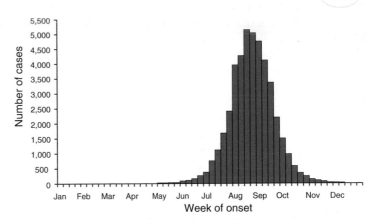

Fig. 2.22 Number of West Nile virus disease cases reported to the Centers for Disease Control and Prevention by week of illness onset, 1999–2015. (From Centers for Disease Control and Prevention. https://www.cdc.gov/westnile/resources/pdfs/data/4-WNV-Week-Onset_for-PDF_1999-2015_07072016.pdf. Accessed May 8, 2017.)

BOX 2.2 STEPS IN INVESTIGATING AN ACUTE OUTBREAK

Investigating an acute outbreak may be primarily deductive (i.e., reasoning from premises or propositions proved previously) or inductive (i.e., reasoning from particular facts to a general conclusion), or it may be a combination of both.

Important considerations in investigating an acute outbreak of infectious diseases include determining that an outbreak has in fact occurred and defining the extent of the population at risk, determining the measure of spread and reservoir, and characterizing the agent.

Steps commonly used are listed below, but depending on the outbreak, the exact order may differ.

1. Define the outbreak and validate the existence of an outbreak
   a. Define the "numerator" (cases)
      1) Clinical features: Is the disease known?
      2) What are its serologic or cultural aspects?
      3) Are the causes partially understood?
   b. Define the "denominator": What is the population at risk of developing disease (i.e., susceptible)?
   c. Determine whether the observed number of cases clearly exceeds the expected number
   d. Calculate the attack rates

2. Examine the distribution of cases by the following:
   a. Time ⎫ Look for time–place interactions
   b. Place ⎭
3. Look for combinations (interactions) of relevant variables
4. Develop hypotheses based on the following:
   a. Existing knowledge (if any) of the disease
   b. Analogy to diseases of known etiology
   c. Findings from investigation of the outbreak
5. Test hypotheses
   a. Further analyze existing data (case-control studies)
   b. Refine hypotheses and collect additional data that may be needed
6. Recommend control measures
   a. Control of current outbreak
   b. Prevention of future similar outbreaks
7. Prepare a written report of the investigation and the findings
8. Communicate findings to those involved in policy development and implementation and to the public

---

a very helpful method for determining which of the possible agents is suspected to be the cause is called *cross-tabulation*. This is illustrated by an outbreak of food-borne streptococcal disease in a Florida jail reported some years ago by the CDC.[16]

In August 1974, an outbreak of group A β-hemolytic streptococcal pharyngitis (sore throat) affected 325 of 690 inmates. On a questionnaire administered to 185 randomly selected inmates, 47% reported a sore throat between August 16 and August 22. Based on a second questionnaire, food-specific attack rates for items that were served to randomly selected inmates showed an association between two food items and the risk of developing a sore throat: a beverage and an egg salad served at lunch on August 16 (Table 2.2).

TABLE 2.2   **Food-Specific Attack Rates for Items Consumed August 16, 1974, Dade County Jail, Miami**

Item Consumed	ATE			DID NOT EAT			
	Sick	Total	% Sick (Attack Rate)	Sick	Total	% Sick (Attack Rate)	P
Beverage	179	264	67.8	22	50	44.0	<.010
Egg salad sandwiches	176	226	77.9	27	73	37.0	<.001

From Centers for Disease Control and Prevention. Outbreak of foodborne streptococcal disease. *MMWR*. 1974;23:365.

TABLE 2.3   **Cross-Table Analysis for Egg Salad and Beverage Consumed August 16, 1974, Dade County Jail, Miami**

	ATE EGG SALAD				DID NOT EAT EGG SALAD			
	Sick	Well	Total	% Sick (Attack Rate)	Sick	Well	Total	% Sick (Attack Rate)
Drank beverage	152	49	201	75.6	19	53	72	26.4
Did not drink beverage	12	3	15	80.0	7	21	28	25.0

From Centers for Disease Control and Prevention. Outbreak of foodborne streptococcal disease. *MMWR*. 1974;23:365.

In Table 2.2, for each of the suspected exposures (beverage and egg salad), the attack rate was calculated for those who ate or drank the item (were exposed) and those who did not eat or drink the item (were not exposed). For both the beverage and the egg salad, attack rates are clearly higher among those who ate or drank the item than among those who did not. However, this table does not permit us to determine whether the beverage or the egg salad accounted for the outbreak.

In order to answer this question, we use the technique of cross-tabulation. In Table 2.3, we again examine the attack rates in those who ate egg salad compared with those who did not, but this time we look separately at those who drank the beverage and those who did not.

Looking at the data by columns, we see that both among those who ate egg salad and among those who did not, drinking the beverage did not increase the incidence of streptococcal illness (75.6% vs. 80% and 26.4% vs. 25%, respectively). However, looking at the data in the table rows, we see that eating the egg salad increased the attack rate of the illness, both in those who drank the beverage (75.6% vs. 26.4%) and in those who did not (80% vs. 25%). Thus, the egg salad is clearly implicated as the source of the infections. Further discussion of the analysis and interpretation of cross-tabulation can be found in Chapter 15.

This example demonstrates the use of cross-tabulation in a food-borne outbreak of an infectious disease, but the method has broad applicability to any condition in which multiple etiologic factors are suspected. It is discussed further in Chapter 15.

Sometimes multiple agents are responsible for an outbreak. An example is a cruise-ship outbreak of gastrointestinal illness that occurred on the same day as a rainstorm, resulting in billions of liters of storm runoff being contaminated with sewage that had been released on the lake where the cruise took place. The cross-tabulation showed that passengers consuming ice had an attack rate more than twice as high as the rate among those who did not consume ice. Stool specimens were positive for multiple agents, including *Shigella sonnei* and *Giardia*.[17]

Conclusion

This chapter reviewed some basic concepts that underlie the epidemiologic approach to acute communicable diseases. Many of these concepts apply equally well to noncommunicable diseases that at this time do not appear to be primarily infectious in origin. Moreover, for an increasing number of chronic diseases originally thought to be noninfectious, infection seems to play some role. Thus hepatitis B infection is a major cause of primary liver cancer. Papillomaviruses and *Helicobacter pylori* infections are necessary for the development of cervical and gastric cancers, respectively. Epstein-Barr virus has been implicated in Hodgkin disease. The boundary between the epidemiology of infectious and noninfectious diseases has blurred in many areas. In addition, even for diseases that are not infectious in origin, inflammation may be involved, the patterns of spread share many of the same dynamics, and the methodologic issues in studying them are similar. Many of these issues are discussed in detail in Section II.

REFERENCES

1. Kipling R. *Just-So Stories: The Elephant's Child, 1902*. Reprinted by Everyman's Library Children's Classics. New York: Alfred A Knopf; 1992:79.
2. Mims CA. *The Pathogenesis of Infectious Disease*. 3rd ed. London: Academic Press; 1987.
3. Drüeke TB, Locatelli F, Clyne N, et al. CREATE Investigators. Normalization of hemoglobin level in patients with chronic kidney disease and anemia. *N Engl J Med*. 2006;355(20):2071–2084.
4. Singh AK, Szczech L, Tang KL, et al. CHOIR Investigators. Correction of anemia with epoetin alfa in chronic kidney disease. *N Engl J Med*. 2006;355(20):2085–2098.
5. Hearing on ensuring kidney patients receive safe and appropriate anemia management care. Hearing before the Subcommittee on Health of the Committee on Ways and Means, U.S. House of Representatives, 110th Congress, First Session, June 26, 2007, Serial No. 110-51. https://www.gpo.gov/fdsys/pkg/CHRG-110hhrg 49981/html/CHRG-110hhrg49981.htm. Accessed May 6, 2017.
6. Imai M, Watanabe T, Hatta M, et al. Experimental adaptation of an influenza H5 HA confers respiratory droplet transmission to a reassortant H5 HA/H1N1 virus in ferrets. *Nature*. 2012;486:420–428.
7. Herfst S, Schrauwen EJ, Linster M, et al. Airborne transmission of influenza A/H5N1 virus between ferrets. *Science*. 2012;336:1534–1541.
8. Bartsch SM, Lopman BA, Ozawa S, et al. Global economic burden of norovirus gastroenteritis. *PLoS ONE*. 2016;11(4):e0151219.
9. Centers for Disease Control and Prevention. Outbreaks of gastroenteritis associated with noroviruses on cruise ships—United States, 2002. *MMWR Morb Mortal Wkly Rep*. 2002;51:1112–1115.
10. Lu J, Fang L, Sun L, et al. Association of GII.P16-GII.2 recombinant norovirus strain with increased norovirus outbreaks, Guangdong, China, 2016. *Emerg Infect Dis*. 2017;23(7):1188–1190.
11. Panum PL. *Observations Made During the Epidemic of Measles on the Faroe Islands in the Year 1846*. New York: Delta Omega Society, Distributed by the American Public Health Association; 1940.
12. Frank PF, Stollerman GH, Miller LF. Protection of a military population from rheumatic fever. *JAMA*. 1965;193:775.
13. Centers for Disease Control and Prevention. *U.S. Multi-State Measles Outbreak, December 2014–January 2015*. Atlanta, GA: US Department of Health and Human Services; 2015. http://emergency.cdc.gov/han/han00376.asp.
14. Armenian HK, Lilienfeld AM. The distribution of incubation periods of neoplastic diseases. *Am J Epidemiol*. 1974;99(2):92–100.
15. Petersen LR, Marfin AA. West Nile virus: a primer for the clinician. *Ann Intern Med*. 2002;137:173–179.
16. Outbreak of foodborne streptococcal disease. *MMWR*. 1974;23:365.
17. Serdarevic F, Jones RC, Weaver KN, et al. Multi-pathogen waterborne disease outbreak associated with a dinner cruise on Lake Michigan. *Epidemiol Infec*. 2012;140:621–625.

REVIEW QUESTIONS FOR CHAPTER 2

1 *Endemic means that a disease:*
   a. Occurs clearly in excess of normal expectancy
   b. Is habitually present in human populations
   c. Affects a large number of countries simultaneously
   d. Exhibits a seasonal pattern
   e. Is prevalent among animals

Questions 2 and 3 are based on the information given below:

The first table shows the total number of persons who ate each of two specified food items that were possibly infective with group A streptococci. The second table shows the number of sick persons (with acute sore throat) who ate each of the various specified combinations of the food items.

Total Number of Persons Who Ate Each Specified Combination of Food Items		
	Ate Tuna	**Did Not Eat Tuna**
Ate egg salad	75	100
Did not eat egg salad	200	50

Total Number of Persons Who Ate Each Specified Combination of Food Items and Who Later Became Sick (With Acute Sore Throats)		
	Ate Tuna	**Did Not Eat Tuna**
Ate egg salad	60	75
Did not eat egg salad	70	15

2 *What is the sore throat attack rate in persons who ate both egg salad and tuna?*
a. 60/75
b. 70/200
c. 60/135
d. 60/275
e. None of the above

3 *According to the results shown in the preceding tables, which of the following food items (or combination of food items) is most likely to be infective?*
a. Tuna only
b. Egg salad only
c. Neither tuna nor egg salad
d. Both tuna and egg salad
e. Cannot be calculated from the data given

4 *In the study of an outbreak of an infectious disease, plotting an epidemic curve is useful because:*
a. It helps to determine what type of outbreak (e.g., single-source, person-to-person) has occurred
b. It shows whether herd immunity has occurred
c. It helps to determine the median incubation period
d. *a* and *c*
e. *a, b,* and *c*

5 *Which of the following is characteristic of a single-exposure, common-vehicle outbreak?*
a. Frequent secondary cases
b. Increasing severity with increasing age
c. Explosive
d. Cases include both people who have been exposed and those who were not exposed
e. All of the above

6 *Which of the following recent widespread disease is considered pandemic?*
a. Ebola virus disease
b. Middle East respiratory syndrome coronavirus (MERS-CoV)
c. H1N1 flu virus (swine flu)
d. Measles

The Occurrence of Disease: I. Disease Surveillance and Measures of Morbidity

We owe all the great advances in knowledge to those who endeavor to find out how much there is of anything.

—James Maxwell, physicist (1831–79)

If you can measure that of which you speak, and can express it by a number, you know something of your subject, but if you cannot measure it, your knowledge is meager and unsatisfactory.

—William Thomson, Lord Kelvin, engineer, mathematician, and physicist (1824–1907)

Learning Objectives

- To describe the important role of epidemiology in disease surveillance.
- To compare different measures of morbidity, including incidence rates, cumulative incidence, attack rates, prevalence, and person-time at risk.
- To illustrate why incidence data are necessary for measuring risk.
- To discuss the interrelationship between incidence and prevalence.
- To describe limitations in defining the numerators and denominators of incidence and prevalence measurements.

In Chapter 2, we discussed how diseases are transmitted. It is clear from that discussion that in order to examine the transmission of disease in human populations, we need to be able to measure the frequency of both disease occurrence and deaths from the disease. In this chapter, we will describe disease surveillance in human populations and its importance in providing information about morbidity from disease. We will then discuss how we use rates and proportions to express the extent of morbidity resulting from a disease, and in Chapter 4 we will turn to expressing the extent of mortality in quantitative terms.

Surveillance

Surveillance is a fundamental role of public health. The Centers for Disease Control and Prevention (CDC) defined epidemiologic surveillance as the "ongoing systematic collection, analysis, and interpretation of health data essential to the planning, implementation, and evaluation of public health practice closely integrated with the timely dissemination of these data to those who need to know."[1] Surveillance may be carried out to monitor changes in disease frequency or to monitor changes in the levels of risks for specific diseases. Much of our information about morbidity and mortality from disease comes from programs of systematic disease surveillance. Surveillance was commonly conducted for infectious diseases, but in recent years it has become increasingly important in monitoring changes in other types of conditions such as congenital malformations, noncommunicable diseases, and environmental toxins, and for injuries and illnesses after natural disasters such as hurricanes or earthquakes. It is the primary method through which federal agencies in the United States, such as the Environmental Protection Agency (EPA), identify contaminants of emerging concern (CEC). Surveillance is also used to monitor for completeness of vaccination coverage and protection of a population and for the prevalence of drug-resistant organisms such as drug-resistant tuberculosis (TB) and malaria.

An important element of this as well as other definitions of surveillance is providing policy makers with guidance for developing and implementing the best strategies for programs for disease prevention and control. In order to enable countries or states to develop coordinated public health approaches, mechanisms for information exchange are essential. Consequently, standardized case definitions of disease and diagnostic criteria are needed that can be applied in different countries or for the purpose of public health surveillance within a country. The CDC defines the surveillance case definition as "a set of uniform criteria used to define a disease for public health," which is intended to aid public health officials in recording and reporting cases.[2] This is different from a clinical definition that is used by clinicians to make a clinical diagnosis to initiate treatment and meet individual patients' needs. The forms used for collecting and reporting data on different diseases must also be standardized.

PASSIVE AND ACTIVE SURVEILLANCE

Passive surveillance denotes surveillance in which available data on reportable diseases are used, or in which disease reporting is mandated or requested by the government or the local health authority, with the responsibility for the reporting often falling on the health care provider or district health officer. This type of reporting is also called *passive reporting*. The completeness and quality of the data reported thus largely depend on this individual and his or her staff, who often take on this role without additional funds or resources. As a result, underreporting and lack of completeness of reporting are likely; to minimize this problem, the reporting instruments must be simple and brief. Examples of reportable diseases include common sexually transmitted infections (syphilis, gonorrhea, human immunodeficiency virus/acquired immune deficiency syndrome [HIV/AIDS]). When passive reporting is used, local outbreaks may be missed because the relatively small number of cases often ascertained becomes diluted within a large denominator of a total population of a province or country. However, a passive reporting system is relatively inexpensive and relatively easy to develop initially. Monitoring flu outbreaks by assessing Google searches or social media are examples of how this may take place in communities. In addition, as many countries have systems of passive reporting for a number of reportable diseases that are generally infectious, passive reporting allows for international comparisons that can identify areas that urgently need assistance in confirming new cases and

in providing appropriate interventions for control and treatment.

Active surveillance denotes a system in which project staff are specifically recruited to carry out a surveillance program. They are recruited to make periodic field visits to health care facilities such as clinics, primary health care centers, and hospitals in order to identify new cases of a disease or diseases or deaths from the disease that have occurred (*case finding*). Active surveillance may involve interviewing physicians and patients, reviewing medical records, and, in developing countries and rural areas, surveying villages and towns to detect cases either periodically on a routine basis or after an index case has been reported. Reporting is generally more accurate when surveillance is active than when it is passive because active surveillance is conducted by individuals who have been specifically employed and trained to carry out this responsibility.

When passive surveillance is used, existing staff members (commonly physicians) are often asked to report new cases. However, they are often overburdened by their primary responsibilities of providing health care and administering health services. For them, filing reports of new cases is an additional burden that they often view as peripheral to their main responsibilities. Furthermore, with active reporting, local outbreaks are generally more easily identified. But active reporting is more expensive to maintain than passive reporting and is often more difficult to develop initially.

Surveillance in developing countries may present additional problems. For example, areas in need of surveillance may be difficult to reach, and it may be difficult to maintain communication from such areas to the central authorities who must make policy decisions and allocate the resources necessary for follow-up and disease control and prevention. Furthermore, definitions of disease used in developed countries may at times be inappropriate or unusable in developing countries because of a lack of the laboratory and other sophisticated resources needed for full diagnostic evaluation of suspected cases. The result may therefore be an underreporting of observed clinical cases. In cases of disease epidemics, the World Health Organization (WHO) and several developed countries, including the United States, mobilize resources to the developing countries to aid local public health officials in case finding and data collection. This was evident in the

2014 West Africa Ebola outbreak and the 2015 Zika virus epidemic in Latin America and the Caribbean.

One example of the challenges in disease surveillance using mortality data is the problem of differing estimates of mortality from malaria, one of the major killers today, especially in poor, developing countries. In 2004, there was a worldwide peak in malaria deaths. Since then, deaths due to malaria have decreased substantially, particularly in sub-Saharan Africa. This has been attributed to the successful expansion of vector control activities, such as insecticide-treated bed nets to prevent infection and improved treatment of those already infected. Murray et al. published an analysis in 2014 in which they reported the global burden from malaria mortality to be approximately 854,000 deaths. This is about 46% higher than what is estimated in the 2014 World Malaria Report of WHO, which was approximately 584,000.[3] This disparity in estimates highlights the difficulties in obtaining reliable data in the absence of a standardized surveillance system, vital registration, and diagnostic testing.

Surveillance may also be carried out to assess changes in levels of environmental risk factors for disease. For example, monitoring levels of particulate air pollution or atmospheric radiation may be conducted, particularly after an accident has been reported. A unique example of this is the explosion of the Fukushima Daiichi nuclear power plant in Fukushima, Japan in 2011. A magnitude 9.0 earthquake, followed by a tsunami, disabled emergency generators necessary for continued cooling that ultimately ended in nuclear meltdown, hydrogen-air chemical explosion, and massive release of radioactive materials into the environment.[4] Such monitoring may give an early warning about a possible rise in rates of disease associated with that environmental agent. Thus surveillance for changes in either disease rates or levels of environmental risk factors may serve as a measure of the severity of the accident and point to possible directions for reducing such hazards in the future.

Stages of Disease in an Individual and in a Population

Let us now consider the levels of a disease in a population over a period of time and how individuals move from one level of disease to another in the population.

Fig. 3.1 shows the timeline for the development of a disease in an individual. An individual is healthy (i.e., without disease), and at some point, biologic onset of a disease occurs. The person is often unaware of the point in time when the disease begins. Later, symptoms develop and lead the patient to seek medical attention. In certain situations, hospitalization may be required, either for diagnosis or for treatment, or for both. In any case, at some point a diagnosis is made and treatment may then follow. One of several outcomes can then result: cure, control of the disease, disability, or death. (This will be examined in further detail in Chapter 18 under "Natural History of Disease.")

Fig. 3.2A–D shows the progression of disease in a population as reflected by the levels of illness and medical care. The outside rectangle represents the total population (see Fig. 3.2A), and the smaller rectangle represents the smaller subset of sick people (see Fig. 3.2B). As a person becomes ill, he or she moves within the sick group to those who seek care and to the subset of those who are hospitalized, from the outside rectangle to the progressively smaller rectangles in the diagram as shown by the curved arrows (see Fig. 3.2C). As seen in Fig. 3.2D, deaths occur in all of these rectangles, as shown by the small straight arrows, but the death rate

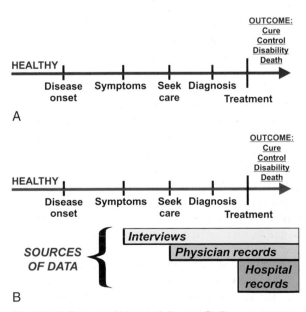

Fig. 3.1 (A) The natural history of disease. (B) The natural history of disease and some sources of data relating to each interval.

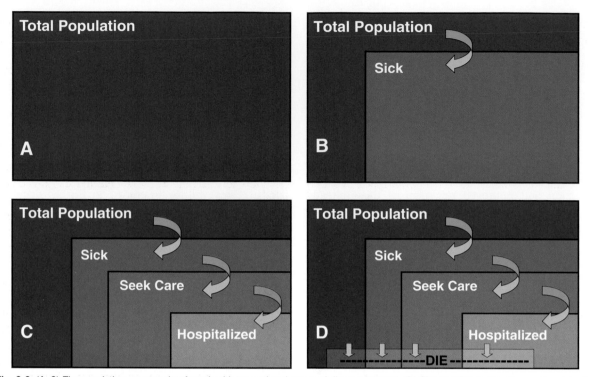

Fig. 3.2 (A–C) The population: progression from health to varying degrees of disease severity. (D) The population: the occurrence of deaths in each group. (Modified from White KL, Williams TF, Greenberg BG. The ecology of medical care. *N Engl J Med.* 1961;265:885–892.)

is proportionately greater in groups with more severe illness such as in those who are hospitalized.

Which sources of data can be used to obtain information about the person's illness? For the period of the illness that necessitates hospitalization, medical and hospital records are useful (see Fig. 3.1B). If hospitalization is not required, primary care providers' records may be the best source. If we want information about the illness before medical care was sought, we may obtain this information from the patient using a questionnaire or an interview. If the patient cannot provide this information, we may obtain it from a family member or someone else who is familiar with the patient's health status. Not shown in this figure are the records of health insurers, which at times can provide very useful information.

The source of data from which cases are identified clearly influences the rates that we calculate for expressing the frequency of disease. For example, hospital records will not include data about patients who obtained care only in physicians' offices. Consequently,

when we see rates for the frequency of occurrence of a certain disease, we must identify the sources of the cases and determine how the cases were identified. When we interpret the rates and compare them to rates reported in other populations and at other times, we must take into consideration the characteristics of the sources from which the data were obtained.

Occurrence of disease can be measured using rates or proportions. *Rates* tell us how fast the disease is occurring in a population; *proportions* tell us what fraction of the population is affected. Let us turn to how we use rates and proportions for expressing the extent of disease in a community or other population. In this chapter, we discuss measures of illness or morbidity; measures of mortality are discussed in Chapter 4.

Measures of Morbidity

INCIDENCE RATE

The incidence rate of a disease is defined as the number of *new* cases of a disease that occur during a specified period of time in a population *at risk* for developing the disease.

Incidence rate per 1,000 =

$$\frac{\begin{array}{c}\text{No. of } new \text{ cases of a disease occurring}\\\text{in the population during}\\\text{a specified period of time}\end{array}}{\begin{array}{c}\text{No. of persons who are at risk of}\\\text{developing the disease during}\\\text{that period of time}\end{array}}\times 1{,}000$$

In this rate, the result has been multiplied by 1,000 so that we can express the incidence per 1,000 persons. The choice of 1,000 is more or less arbitrary—we could have used 10,000, 1 million, or any other figure. However, this choice is generally influenced by the frequency of the disease; for example, for a common disease, such as the common cold, incidence is usually defined as a percentage; for rare diseases, such as aplastic anemia, it is multiplied by 100,000 or even 1,000,000.

The critical element in defining incidence rate is *NEW* cases of disease. Incidence rate is a measure of events—the disease is identified in a person who develops the disease and did not have the disease previously. Because the incidence rate is a measure of events (i.e., transition from a nondiseased to a diseased state), the incidence rate is a measure of risk. This risk can be looked at in any population group, such as a particular age group, among males or females, in an occupational group, or a group that has been exposed to a certain environmental agent, such as radiation or a chemical toxin. For example, Fig. 3.3 shows trends

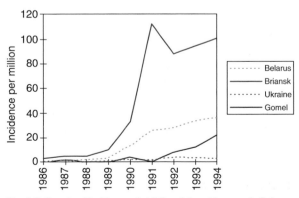

Fig. 3.3 Trends of incidence of childhood thyroid cancer in Belarus, Ukraine, and Russia, 1986–94. (From Bard D, Verger P, Hubert P. Chernobyl, 10 years after: health consequences. *Epidemiol Rev.* 1997;19:187–204.)

in incidence of thyroid cancer in children in Belarus, Ukraine, and Russia from 1986 to 1994, obtained from surveillance data following an explosion in the Chernobyl reactor.[5] The highest incidence rates were found in the most contaminated areas—Gomel in southern Belarus and parts of northern Ukraine. However, a problem in interpreting such data is the possibility that the observed increase could be due to more intensive screening that was initiated following the accident. Such screening could have identified thyroid tumors that might otherwise not have been detected and thus might not have been attributed to the common exposure (the reactor). Nevertheless, there is now general agreement that the observed increase in thyroid cancer in children and adolescents in areas exposed to Chernobyl fallout was, in fact, real.

The denominator of an incidence rate represents the number of people who are at risk for developing the disease. For an incidence rate to be meaningful, any individual who is included in the denominator must have the potential to become part of the group that is counted in the numerator. Thus, if we are calculating incidence of uterine cancer, the denominator must include only women with no history of hysterectomy, because women with a history of hysterectomy and men would never have the potential to become part of the group that is counted by the numerator, that is, both are not at risk for developing uterine cancer. Although this point seems obvious, it is not always so clear, and we shall return to this issue later in the discussion.

Another important issue regarding the denominator is the issue of time. Incidence measures can use two types of denominators: people at risk who are observed throughout a defined time period; or, when all people are not observed for the full time period, person-time (or units of time when each person is observed). Let us consider each of these approaches.

People at Risk Who Are Observed Throughout a Defined Time Period

In the first type of denominator for incidence rate, we specify a period of time, and we must know that all of the individuals in the group represented by the denominator have been followed up for *that entire period*. The choice of time period is arbitrary: We could calculate incidence in 1 week, incidence in 1 month, incidence in 1 year, incidence in 5 years, and so on. The important point is that whatever time period is used in the calculation must be clearly specified, and all individuals included in the calculation must have been observed, and, of course, at risk of developing the outcome of interest, for the entire period. The incidence is calculated using a period of time during which all of the individuals in the population are considered to be at risk for the outcome, also called the *cumulative incidence proportion*, which is a measure of risk.

When All People Are Not Observed for the Full Time Period, Person-Time, or Units of Time When Each Person Is Observed

Often, every individual in the denominator cannot be followed for the full time specified for a variety of reasons, including loss to follow-up or death from a cause other than that being studied. When different individuals are observed for different lengths of time, we calculate an incidence rate (also called an *incidence density*), in which the denominator consists of the sum of the *units of time* that each individual was at risk and was observed. This is called *person-time* and is often expressed in terms of person-months or person-years (py) of observation.

Let us consider py: One person at risk who is observed for 1 year = 1 py. One person at risk observed for 5 years = 5 py. But 5 people at risk, each of whom is observed for only 1 year, also = 5 py.

Let us assume we have a 5-year study and five people have been observed for the entire period (as indicated by the arrow for each person in Fig. 3.4). In each of

the 5 years of the study, all five participants are observed, so that we have 5 py of observation in each of the 5 years, for a total of 25 py of observation in the entire study.

Now let us consider the situation where all five people at risk are not observed for the entire 5 years of the study but are observed for different lengths of time (Fig. 3.5A). In this diagram, the two arrows represent two people who were observed for all 5 years. The timelines for the three other people end with a red "**x**," which indicates the point at which the observation of each individual ended, either because the event of interest occurred or because the person was lost to follow-up, or other problems.

How do we calculate the total number of py observed in this study? Let us look at the first year of the study (see Fig. 3.5B). All five people were observed during the first year, so we have 5 py of observation in the first year (see Fig. 3.5C).

Now look at the second year of the study (see Fig. 3.5D). Note that participant No. 2 was only observed for the first year, so that in the second year we have only four participants, each of whom contributed 1 year of follow-up to the study for a total of 4 py (see Fig. 3.5E).

Looking at the third year of the study, we see that participant No. 3 was only observed for the first 2 years of the study (see Fig. 3.5F). Therefore only three participants were observed in the third year generating 3 py of observation during the third year (see Fig. 3.5G). These participants were also all observed for the fourth year of the study (see Fig. 3.5H) and they again contributed 3 py of observation during the fourth year of the study (see Fig. 3.5I).

Finally, let us look at the fifth year of the study (see Fig. 3.5J). We see that participant No. 5 was only observed for the first 4 years of the study. As a result, only two participants remained and were observed in the fifth year of the study. They contributed 2 py of observation during the fifth year (see Fig. 3.5K). As seen in Fig. 3.5L, we therefore had 5 + 4 + 3 + 3 + 2 py of observation during the entire 5-year study, yielding a total of 17 py of observation. (This compares with 25 py of observation if all five participants had been observed throughout the entire 5 years of the study, as seen in Fig. 3.4.) Thus, *if people at risk are*

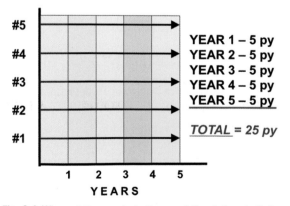

Fig. 3.4 When all the people in the population being studied are observed for the entire period: person-years *(py)* of observation.

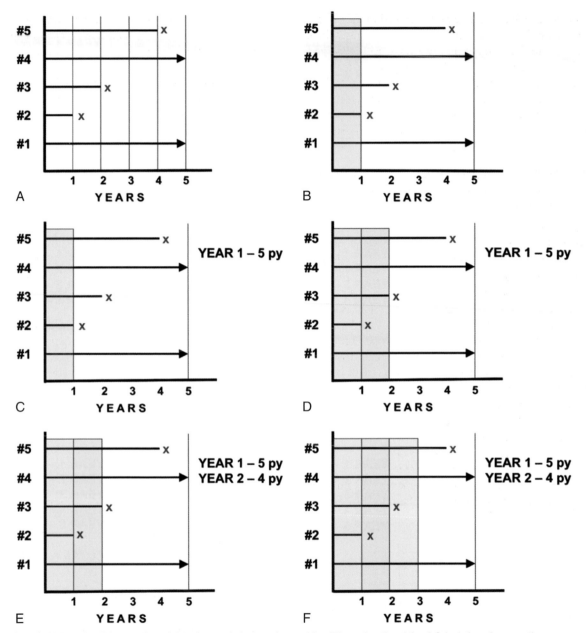

Fig. 3.5 (A–L) But what if the people at risk in the population are observed for different lengths of time? Calculation of person-time as person-years *(py)* observed. (See page 47 for explanation in text.)

Continued

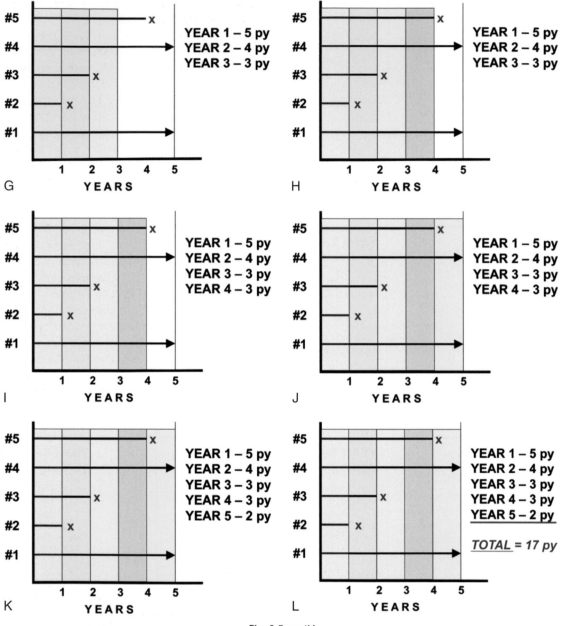

Fig. 3.5 cont'd

observed for different periods of time, the incidence rate is:

Incidence rate per 1,000 =

$$\frac{\begin{array}{c}\text{Number of NEW cases of a disease}\\\text{occurring in a population during a}\\\text{specified period of time}\end{array}}{\begin{array}{c}\text{Total person-time (the sum of the}\\\text{time periods of observation of each}\\\text{person who has been observed for all or}\\\text{part of the entire time period)}\end{array}} \times 1{,}000$$

Person-time is discussed further in Chapter 6.

IDENTIFYING NEW CASES IN ORDER TO CALCULATE INCIDENCE

Practically speaking, when we wish to calculate incidence, how do we identify all new cases in a population during a specified time period? In certain situations, it may be possible to monitor an entire population over time with tests that can detect newly developed cases of a disease. However, often this is not possible and instead a population is identified and screened for the disease at baseline (prevalent cases defined in the next section) (Fig. 3.6). Those who do not have the disease at baseline are followed for the specified time, such as 1 year. They are then rescreened to see if they have developed the disease of interest (Fig. 3.7). Any cases that are identified clearly developed disease during the 1-year period since those followed were free of disease at the beginning of the year. Thus these cases

are new or incident cases and serve as the numerator for the incidence rate.

Although in most situations it is necessary to express incidence by specifying a denominator, at times, the number of cases alone may be informative. For example, Fig. 3.8 shows the number of reported TB cases, United States, 1982–2015. The number of cases reported in a year in the United States (since reporting began) reached an all-time low in 2015. Despite a small decline from 1980 to 1985, the reported number of cases of TB increased by approximately 20% between 1985 and 1992. Much of the increase in TB seen here was associated with the rapidly expanding identification of infections with HIV. However, even before AIDS and HIV were recognized as major public health problems, TB had remained a serious, but often neglected, problem, particularly in certain urban areas of the United States. From 1992 until 2008, the total number of TB cases decreased 2% to 7% annually. This is an example in which a graph that just plots numbers of cases without a denominator can be very helpful when there is no reason to suspect a significant change in the denominator during a given time period.

In general, however, our goal in calculating incidence is to be able to do so with the information needed for both the numerator and denominator so that valid comparisons can be made. Fig. 3.9 presents trends in incidence rates for selected cancers by sex in the United States for males (*left*) and females (*right*) from 1975 to 2013. As seen there, lung cancer incidence has been

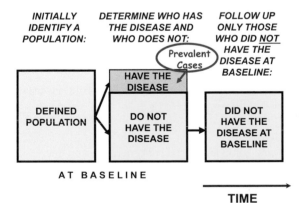

Fig. 3.6 Identifying newly detected cases of a disease. Step 1: screening for prevalent cases at baseline. See page 50 for explanation in text.

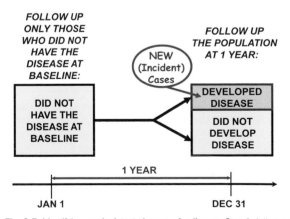

Fig. 3.7 Identifying newly detected cases of a disease. Step 2: follow-up and rescreening at 1 year to identify cases that developed during the year.

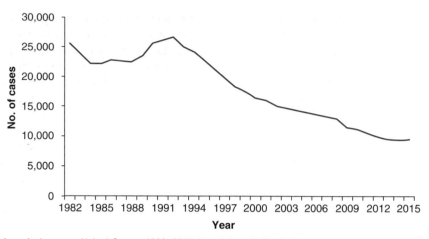

Fig. 3.8 Reported tuberculosis cases, United States, 1982–2015 (as of June 9, 2016). (From Centers for Disease Control and Prevention [CDC]. *Reported Tuberculosis in the United States, 2015.* Atlanta, GA: US Department of Health and Human Services, CDC; 2016. https://www.cdc.gov/tb/statistics/reports/2015/pdfs/2015_surveillance_report_fullreport.pdf. Accessed May 15, 2017.)

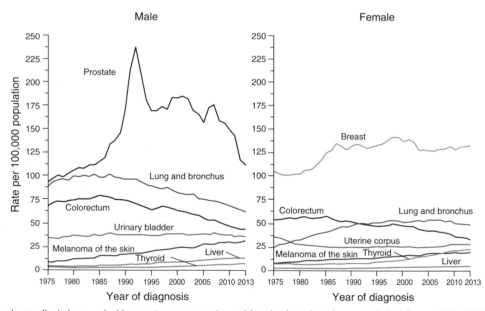

Fig. 3.9 Annual age-adjusted cancer incidence rates among males and females for selected cancers, United States, 1975–2013 (age-adjusted to the 2000 US standard population). (From Siegel R, Miller K, Jemal A. Cancer statistics, 2017. *CA Cancer J Clin.* 2017;67:7–30.)

declining in men and leveling off in women. After marked rises in incidence for many years, prostate cancer in men has been declining since 2001. Breast cancer in women in the United States has declined between 1998 and 2003, followed by a slight increase from 2004 to 2013. After having been level for a number of years, colon and rectal cancers have been decreasing in both men and women.

ATTACK RATE

Occasionally, time associated with the denominator may be specified implicitly rather than explicitly. For example, in Chapter 2 we discussed investigating a food-borne disease outbreak, in which we speak of an *attack rate*, which is defined as the number of people exposed to a suspect food who became ill, divided by the number of people who were exposed to that food. The attack rate does not explicitly specify the time interval because for many food-borne disease outbreaks we know that most cases occur within a few hours or a few days after the exposure. Consequently, cases that develop months later are not considered part of the same common-source outbreak. However, in many situations, current knowledge of the biology and natural history of the disease does not clearly define a time frame, and so the time must be stated explicitly. A further consideration is that attack rate is not truly a rate but a proportion. Since the term *rate* should include a time unit in the calculation, a food-borne *attack rate* is not an accurate term because it actually tells us the *proportion* of all people who ate a certain food who became ill. However, the term *attack rate* has been traditionally used for a long time. We will go on to discuss the use of proportions in measuring the occurrence of disease below.

PREVALENCE

Prevalence is defined as the number of affected persons present in the population at a specific time divided by the number of persons in the population at that time; that is, what proportion of the population is affected by the disease at that time?

$$\text{Prevalence per } 1{,}000 = \frac{\substack{\text{No. of cases of a disease present} \\ \text{in the population at a specified time}}}{\substack{\text{No. of persons in the population} \\ \text{at that specified time}}} \times 1{,}000$$

For example, if we are interested in knowing the prevalence of arthritis in a certain community on a certain date, we might visit every household in that community and, using interviews or physical examinations, determine how many people have arthritis on that day. This number becomes the numerator for prevalence. The denominator is the population in the community on that date.

What is the difference between *incidence* and *prevalence*? Prevalence can be viewed as a snapshot or a slice

through the population at a point in time at which we determine who has the disease and who does not. But in so doing, we are not determining when the disease developed. Some individuals may have developed arthritis yesterday, some last week, some last year, and some 10 or 20 years ago. Thus, when we survey a community to estimate the prevalence of a disease, we generally do not take into account the duration of the disease. Consequently, the numerator of prevalence includes a mix of people with different durations of disease, and as a result we do not have a measure of risk. If we wish to measure risk, we must use incidence, because in contrast to prevalence, it includes only new cases or events and a specified time period during which those events occurred.

In the medical and public health literature, the word *prevalence* is often used in two ways:

- *Point prevalence:* Prevalence of the disease at a certain point in time—this is the use of the term *prevalence* that we have just discussed.
- *Period prevalence:* How many people have had the disease at any point during a certain time period? The time period referred to may be arbitrarily selected, such as a month, a single calendar year, or a 5-year period. Some people may have developed the disease during that period, and others may have had the disease before and died or been cured during that period. The important point is that every person represented by the numerator had the disease at some time during the period specified.

The two types of prevalence, as well as cumulative incidence, are illustrated in Table 3.1 using questions regarding asthma.

Returning to *point prevalence*, practically speaking, it is virtually impossible to survey an entire city on

TABLE 3.1 Examples of Point and Period Prevalence and Cumulative Incidence in Interview Studies of Asthma

Interview Question	Type of Measure
"Do you currently have asthma?"	Point prevalence
"Have you had asthma during the last [n] years?"	Period prevalence
"Have you ever had asthma?"	Cumulative incidence

a single day. Therefore although conceptually we are thinking in terms of a single point in time, in reality, the survey would take much longer. When we see the word *prevalence* used without any modifier, it generally refers to point prevalence, and for the rest of this chapter, we will use *prevalence* to mean point prevalence.

Let us consider incidence and prevalence. Fig. 3.10 shows five cases of a disease in a community in 2017. The first case of the disease occurred in 2016, and the patient died in 2017.

The second case developed in 2017 and continued into 2018. The third case was a person who became ill in 2017 and was cured in 2017. The fourth case occurred in 2016, and the patient was cured in 2017. The fifth case occurred in 2016 and continued through 2017 and into 2018.

For this example, we will consider only the cases (numerators) and will ignore the denominators. In this example, what is the numerator for incidence in 2017? We know that incidence counts only new cases, and because two of the five cases developed in 2017, the numerator for incidence in 2017 is 2.

What about the numerator for point prevalence in 2017? This depends on when we do our prevalence survey (Fig. 3.11). If we do the survey in May, the numerator will be 5. If we do the survey in July, the numerator will be 4. If we do the survey in September, however, the numerator will be 3, and if we do it in December, the numerator will be 2. Thus the prevalence

will depend on the point during the year at which the survey is performed.

Fig. 3.12A–D shows the dynamic relationship between incidence and prevalence. A flask is shown that represents a community (see Fig. 3.12A), and the beads in the flask represent the prevalent cases of a disease in the community. How can we add to or increase the *prevalence*? As seen in Fig. 3.12B, we can do so through *incidence*—by the addition of new cases. What if we could drain beads from the flask and lower the prevalence? How might this be accomplished? As seen in Fig. 3.12C, it could occur through either death or cure. Clearly, these two outcomes represent a major difference to a patient, but with regard to prevalence, cure and death have the same effect: they reduce the number of diseased persons in the population and thus lower prevalence. Therefore what exists is the dynamic situation shown in Fig. 3.12D. A continual addition of new cases (incidence) increases the prevalence, while death and/or cure decrease the prevalence.

This effect of lowering prevalence through either death or cure underlies an important issue in public health and clinical medicine. For example, when insulin first became available, what happened to the prevalence of diabetes? The prevalence increased because diabetes was not cured, but was only controlled. Many patients with diabetes who formerly would have died now survived; therefore the prevalence increased. This seeming paradox is often the case with public health

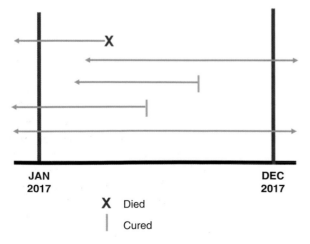

Fig. 3.10 Example of incidence and prevalence: I.

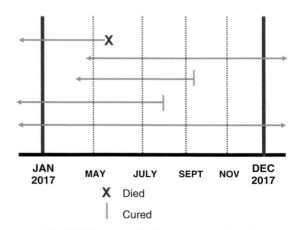

Fig. 3.11 Example of incidence and prevalence: II.

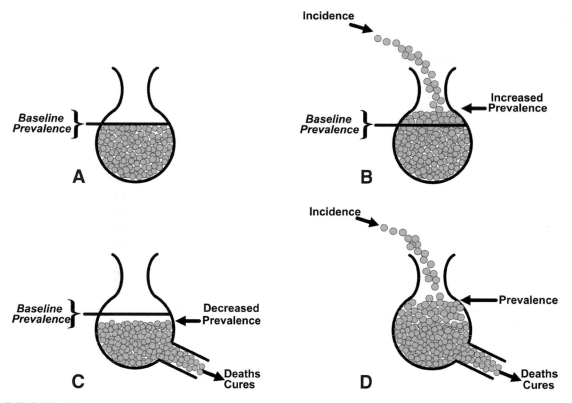

Fig. 3.12 Relationship between incidence and prevalence. (A) Level of prevalence in the population. (B) Increased prevalence resulting from incidence. (C) Decreased prevalence resulting from deaths and/or cures. (D) Overall impact on prevalence of incidence, deaths, and/or cures.

programs: a new health care intervention (e.g., highly active antiretroviral therapy for HIV infection) is introduced that enhances survival (fewer then die of HIV/AIDS) or it may work by early detection of disease in more people, and the net effect is an apparent increase in prevalence. It may be difficult to convince some people that a program is successful if the prevalence of the disease that is the target of the program actually increases. However, this clearly occurs when death is prevented and the disease is not cured or eradicated.

We have said that prevalence is not a measure of risk. If so, why bother to estimate prevalence? Prevalence is an important and useful measure of the burden of disease in a community to inform resource allocation by decision-makers. For example, how many people in the community have osteoarthritis? This information might help us to determine, for example, how many clinics are needed, what types of rehabilitation services are needed, and how many and which types of health professionals are needed. Prevalence is therefore valuable for planning health services. When we use prevalence, we also want to make future projections and anticipate the changes that are likely to take place in the disease burden. However, if we want to look at the cause, or etiology, of disease, we must explore the relationship between an exposure and the risk of disease, and to do this, we need data on incidence.

Nevertheless, prevalence data may at times be very useful—they may be suggestive if not confirmatory in studies of the etiology of certain diseases. For example, asthma is a disease of children for which incidence is difficult to measure because the exact time of the beginning of the disease (its inception) is often hard to determine, given the difficulties in defining the disease and ascertaining the initial symptoms. For this reason, when we are interested in time trends and geographic distribution of asthma, prevalence is the measure most frequently used. Information on prevalence of asthma is often obtained from self-reports such as interviews or questionnaires.

Fig. 3.13 shows the adjusted prevalence of stages 3 and 4 chronic kidney disease (CKD) in US adults, by presence or absence of diabetes, from the National Health and Nutrition Examination Survey (NHANES) 1988–94 through 2011–12; NHANES conducts yearly cross-sectional studies with samples that are representative of the US general population. CKD was defined as an estimated glomerular filtration rate (eGFR) of 15 to 59 mL/min/1.73 m^2, estimated with the Chronic Kidney Disease Epidemiology Collaboration (CKD-EPI) equation from calibrated single serum creatinine measurements. We can observe an initial increase in adjusted prevalence of stages 3 and 4 CKD, which stopped around the 2000s among nondiabetic individuals, whereas the prevalence continued to increase for diabetic individuals. This could be partly explained by the longer survival of diabetic CKD patients.

Another example of the value of prevalence data is seen in Fig. 3.14. One of the most significant and challenging public health problems today in the United States and in other developed countries is the

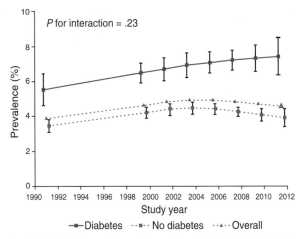

Fig. 3.13 Adjusted prevalence of stages 3 and 4 chronic kidney disease (estimated glomerular filtration rate of 15 to 59 mL/min/1.73 m^2 calculated with **Chronic Kidney Disease Epidemiology Collaboration** equation) in US adults, by age, **1990–2012.** (From Murphy D, McCulloch CE, Lin F, et al. Centers for Disease Control and Prevention Chronic Kidney Disease Surveillance Team. Trends in prevalence of chronic kidney disease in the United States. *Ann Intern Med.* 2016;165:473–481.)

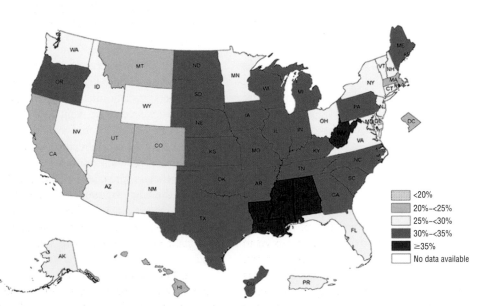

Fig. 3.14 Prevalence of self-reported obesity among US adults by state and territory, Behavioral Risk Factor Surveillance System, 2015. Obesity was defined by body mass index ≥30, or ~30 lb overweight for a 5′4″ person. (Modified from Centers for Disease Control and Prevention. https://www.cdc-gov.ezp.welch.jhmi.edu/obesity/data/prevalence-maps.html. Accessed May 16, 2017.)

BOX 3.1 SOME SOURCES OF MORBIDITY STATISTICS

1. Disease reporting—communicable diseases, cancer registries
2. Data accumulated as a by-product of insurance and prepaid medical care plans
   a. Group health and accident insurance
   b. Prepaid medical care plans
   c. State disability insurance plans
   d. Life insurance companies
   e. Hospital insurance plans—Blue Cross
   f. Railroad Retirement Board
3. Tax-financed public assistance and medical care plans
   a. Public assistance, aid to the blind, aid to the disabled
   b. State or federal medical care plans
4. Hospitals and clinics
5. Absenteeism records—industry and schools
6. Pre-employment and periodic physical examinations in industry and schools
7. Case-finding programs
8. Records of military personnel
   a. Armed Forces
   b. Veterans Administration
9. Morbidity surveys on population samples (e.g., National Health Survey, National Cancer Surveys)

dramatically increasing prevalence of obesity. Obesity is associated with significant morbidity and mortality and is a risk factor for diseases such as arthritis, hypertension, type 2 diabetes, coronary disease, and stroke. In this figure, in which self-reported prevalence of obesity by state is shown for 2015, no state reported a prevalence of obesity of less than 20%, and 44 had a prevalence equal to or greater than 25%. We can also observe that the highest prevalence of obesity is in the Southern states.

One limitation of these data is that they are based on self-reported heights and weights given by respondents by telephone. Survey respondents, especially in telephone surveys of obesity, generally understate their weights, overstate their heights, or both. In this study, the participants were classified according to their body mass index (BMI), which is defined as a person's weight in kilograms divided by the square of the person's height in meters (BMI = weight [kg]/height^2 [meters^2]). A BMI of 25 or greater is categorized as *overweight* and a BMI of 30 or greater as *obese*. The result is likely an underestimation of obesity prevalence based on BMI so that the true prevalence of obesity by state is probably higher than that seen in Fig. 3.14. Given the trends described above and seen in Fig. 3.14, an enormous public health effort and commitment will be needed to reverse this steadily worsening public health problem. In addition, the use of BMI itself to define obesity has its own limitations. BMI does not distinguish between excess fat, muscle, or bone mass, and does not provide any information on the fat distribution within each individual.

Box 3.1 lists some possible sources of morbidity statistics. Each has its limitations, primarily because most of these sources are not established for research purposes but rather for administrative or billing purposes. Therefore they may be characterized by incomplete or ambiguous data and, at times, may only refer to a highly selected population that may not be representative of the population to which we would like to generalize the findings.

PROBLEMS WITH INCIDENCE AND PREVALENCE MEASUREMENTS

Problems With Numerators

The first problem is defining who has the disease. Some diseases are difficult to diagnose, and when such a diagnostic difficulty arises, expert groups are often convened to develop sets of diagnostic criteria. There are five sets of diagnostic criteria for health care–associated (HCA) *Staphylococcus aureus* bacteremia, each with different level of stringency (Table 3.2). Fig. 3.15 shows the proportion of patients classified as having HCA *S. aureus* bacteremia (SAB) according to the five different definitions in 2,638 patients using data from Northern Denmark. We see that the prevalence estimate is significantly affected by the set of criteria that is used.

Another example is given by a cohort of 1,879 men and women 65 years of age and older who were enrolled in the Canadian Study of Health and Aging (CSHA).[6] The proportion who were given a diagnosis of dementia using six commonly used classification systems was

TABLE 3.2	Definitions 1–5 of Health Care–Associated *Staphylococcus aureus* Bacteremia	
Highest level of stringency	Definition	Criteria:
		Blood culture performed within 2 days of admission and the following:
	1.	• Any hospital inpatient admission within the previous 30 days
	2.	• Any hospital inpatient admission within the previous 30 days or
		• Hospital outpatient clinic contact including surgery or contact to clinics of oncology, hematology, or nephrology within the previous 30 days
Lowest level of stringency	3.	• Any hospital inpatient admission within the previous 30 days or
		• Any type of hospital outpatient clinic contact within the previous 30 days
	4.	• Any hospital inpatient admission within the past 90 days or
		• Any type of hospital outpatient clinic contact within the previous 30 days
	5.	• Any hospital inpatient admission within the past 90 days or
		• Any type of hospital outpatient clinic contact within the previous 30 days or
		• Antibiotic or immunosuppressive therapy 30 days prior to admission

Modified from Smit J, Søgaard M, Schønheyder HC, et al. Classification of healthcare-associated *Staphylococcus aureus* bacteremia: influence of different definitions on prevalence, patient characteristics, and outcome. *Infect Control Hosp Epidemiol.* 2016;37(2):208–211.

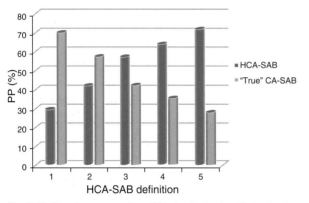

Fig. 3.15 Prevalence proportion *(PP)* of patients classified as health care–associated *Staphylococcus aureus* bacteremia *(HCA-SAB)* and true community-acquired *(CA)* SAB according to the five different definitions. (Modified from Smit J, Søgaard M, Schønheyder HC, et al. Classification of healthcare-associated *Staphylococcus aureus* bacteremia: influence of different definitions on prevalence, patient characteristics, and outcome. *Infect Control Hosp Epidemiol.* 2016;37:208–211.)

calculated. Depending on which diagnostic system was used, the proportion of subjects with dementia varied from 3.1% to 29.1% (Fig. 3.16). This marked variation in prevalence estimates has important potential implications both for research and for the provision of appropriate health services. When the results of any morbidity survey are reported, it is essential that the precise definition used for a case be clearly specified. The decision as to which definition to use is not always simple. Often it will largely depend on the specific purpose for which a given survey has been conducted.

The next issue relating to numerators is that of ascertaining which persons should be included in the numerator. How do we find the cases? We can use regularly available data or, as discussed earlier in this chapter, we can conduct a study specifically designed to gather data for estimating incidence or prevalence. In many such studies the data are obtained from interviews, and some of the potential limitations with interview data are listed in Box 3.2. Ideally, we would have laboratory or other confirmatory evidence. However, often such evidence is not available, and despite these limitations, interview data are extremely valuable in providing information about new cases.

Problems With Denominators

Many factors affect the denominators used. Of these, selective undercounting of certain groups in the population may occur. For example, young men in ethnic minority groups and recent immigrants have been missed in many counts of the population. Frequently, we wish to determine whether a certain group has a higher-than-expected risk of disease so that appropriate preventive measures can be directed to that group. We are therefore interested in the rates of disease for different ethnic groups rather than just for the population as a whole. However, there are different ways to classify

Fig. 3.16 Number of people with and prevalence (%) of dementia in the Canadian Study of Health and Aging cohort (*n* = 1,879) as diagnosed by different classification systems. The various abbreviations refer to commonly used diagnostic manuals for medical conditions. *CAMDEX,* Cambridge Mental Disorders of the Elderly Examination; *CLIN CONS,* Clinical Consensus; *DSM,* Diagnostic and Statistical Manual of Mental Disorders; *ICD,* International Classification of Diseases. (Data from Erkinjuntti T, Østbye T, Steenhuis R, Hachinski V. The effect of different diagnostic criteria on the prevalence of dementia. *N Engl J Med.* 1997;337:1667–1674.)

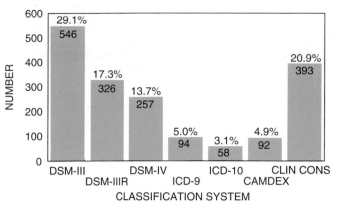

BOX 3.2 SOME POSSIBLE SOURCES OF ERROR IN INTERVIEW SURVEYS

1. Problems due to difficulties in diagnosis:
   a. The participant may have the disease, but may have no symptoms and may not be aware of the disease.
   b. The participant may have the disease and may have had symptoms, but may not have had medical attention and therefore may not know the name of the disease.
   c. The participant may have the disease and may have had medical attention, but the diagnosis may not have been made or conveyed to the person or the person may have misunderstood.
   d. The participant may not accurately recall an episode of illness or events and exposures related to the illness.
2. Problems associated with the study participant:
   a. The participant may be involved in litigation about the illness and may choose not to respond or may alter his or her response.
   b. The participant may be reluctant to provide accurate information if he or she has concerns that certain responses may not please the interviewer or may elicit a possible stigma.
   c. The participant is too ill to respond. As a result, either that participant is not included in the study or a surrogate, such as a family member or friend, is interviewed. Surrogates, however, often have incomplete information about the participant's past exposures.
3. Problems associated with the interviewer:
   a. The participant may provide the information, but the interviewer may not record it or may record it incorrectly.
   b. The interviewer may not ask the question he or she is supposed to ask or may ask it incorrectly.
   c. The interviewer may be biased by knowing the hypothesis being tested and may probe more intensively in one group of participants than in another.

people by ethnic group, such as by language, country of origin, heritage, or parental ethnic group. When different studies use different definitions, comparison of the results is difficult. What is most important in any study is that the working definition be clearly stated so that the reader can judge whether the results are truly comparable.

In an earlier section, we stated that for a rate to make sense, everyone in the group represented by the denominator must have the potential to enter the group that is represented by the numerator. The issue is not a simple one. For example, hysterectomy is one of the most commonly performed surgical procedures in the United States. This raises a question about cervical or endometrial cancer mortality rates. If we include women who have had hysterectomies in the denominator, clearly, they are not at risk for developing cervical or endometrial cancer. Fig. 3.17 shows cervical cancer mortality rates from the United States; both uncorrected rates and rates corrected for hysterectomy are presented. We see that the corrected rates are higher. Why? Because in the corrected rates women who have had

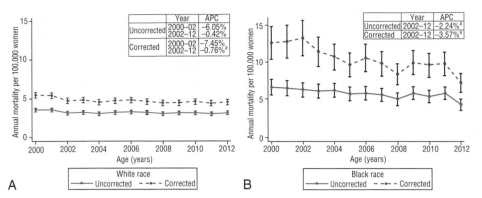

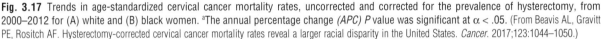

Fig. 3.17 Trends in age-standardized cervical cancer mortality rates, uncorrected and corrected for the prevalence of hysterectomy, from 2000–2012 for (A) white and (B) black women. [a]The annual percentage change *(APC) P* value was significant at $\alpha < .05$. (From Beavis AL, Gravitt PE, Rositch AF. Hysterectomy-corrected cervical cancer mortality rates reveal a larger racial disparity in the United States. *Cancer.* 2017;123:1044–1050.)

BOX 3.3 SOME LIMITATIONS OF HOSPITAL DATA

1. Hospital admissions are selective in relation to:
   a. Personal characteristics
   b. Severity of disease
   c. Associated conditions
   d. Admission policies
2. Hospital records are not designed for research. They may be:
   a. Incomplete, illegible, or missing
   b. Variable in diagnostic quality
3. Population(s) at risk (denominator) is (are) generally not defined

BOX 3.4 SOME NOTES DICTATED BY PHYSICIANS FOR INCLUSION IN PATIENTS' MEDICAL RECORDS

"Patient has two teenage children, but no other abnormalities."
"On the second day the knee was better and on the third day it had completely disappeared."
"Patient was alert and unresponsive."
"When she fainted, her eyes rolled around the room."
"Rectal examination revealed a normal size thyroid."
"By the time he was admitted, his rapid heart had stopped, and he was feeling better."

---

hysterectomies are removed from the denominator. Consequently, the denominator gets smaller and the rate increases. However, in this case the trend over time is not significantly changed whether we use corrected or uncorrected rates.

Problems With Hospital Data

Data from hospital records (now often electronic medical records) are one of the most important sources of information for epidemiologic studies. However, Box 3.3 lists some of the problems that arise in using hospital data for research purposes. First, hospital admissions are selective. They may be selective on the basis of personal characteristics, severity of disease, associated medical conditions, and admissions policies that vary from hospital to hospital. Second, hospital records are

not designed for research but rather for patient care. Records may be incomplete, illegible, or missing. The diagnostic quality of the records of hospitals, physicians, and clinical services may differ. Thus, if we want to combine patients from different hospitals, we may have problems of comparability. Third, if we wish to calculate rates, we have a problem defining denominators, because most hospitals in the United States do not have defined catchment areas—that is, areas that require that all persons in those areas who are hospitalized be admitted to a particular hospital, and that none from outside the catchment area be admitted to that hospital.

On a lighter note, Box 3.4 lists some notes that were dictated by physicians for inclusion in their patients' medical records.

RELATIONSHIP BETWEEN INCIDENCE AND PREVALENCE

We have said that incidence is a measure of risk and that prevalence is not, because it does not take into account the duration of the disease. However, there is an important relationship between incidence and prevalence: in a steady-state situation, in which the rates are not changing and in-migration equals out-migration, and when the prevalence is not too high, the following equation applies:

$$\text{Prevalence} = \text{Incidence} \times \text{Duration of Disease}$$

This is demonstrated in the following hypothetical example. Using chest x-rays, 2,000 persons are screened for TB: 1,000 are upper-income individuals from Hitown and 1,000 are lower-income individuals from Lotown (Table 3.3). X-ray findings are positive in 100 of the Hitown people and in 60 of the Lotown people. Can we therefore conclude that the risk of TB is higher in Hitown people than in Lotown people? Clearly, we cannot, for what we are measuring with a chest x-ray is the point prevalence of disease—we do not know how long any of the people with positive x-rays have had their disease (Table 3.4). We could in fact consider a hypothetical scenario that might explain the higher prevalence in Hitown people that is not related to any higher risk in Hitown people (Table 3.5). We have said

that prevalence = incidence × duration. Let us assume that Lotown people have a much higher risk (incidence) of TB than Hitown people—20 cases/year in Lotown people compared with 4 cases/year in Hitown people. But for a variety of reasons, such as poorer access to medical care and poorer nutritional status, Lotown people survive with their disease, on average, for only 3 years, whereas Hitown people survive, on average, for 25 years. In this example, therefore, there is a higher prevalence in Hitown people than in Lotown people not because the risk of disease is higher in Hitown people, but because affected Hitown people survive longer; the prevalence of disease (incidence × duration) is therefore higher in Hitown people than in Lotown people.

Fig. 3.18 shows the percentage of all births in New Zealand that were extramarital from 1962 to

TABLE 3.5 **Hypothetical Example of Chest X-Ray Screening: III. Prevalence, Incidence, and Duration**			
Screened Population	Point Prevalence per 1,000	Incidence (Occurrences/ Year)	Duration (Years)
Hitown	100	4	25
Lotown	60	20	3
	Prevalence = Incidence × Duration		

TABLE 3.3 **Hypothetical Example of Chest X-Ray Screening: I. Populations Screened and Numbers With Positive X-Rays**	
Screened Population	No. With Positive X-Ray
1,000 Hitown	100
1,000 Lotown	60

TABLE 3.4 **Hypothetical Example of Chest X-Ray Screening: II. Point Prevalence**		
Screened Population	No. With Positive X-Ray	Point Prevalence per 1,000 Population
1,000 Hitown	100	100
1,000 Lotown	60	60

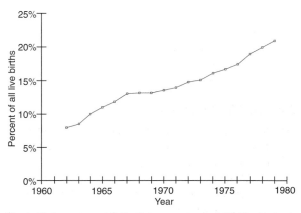

Fig. 3.18 Percentage of births that were extramarital in New Zealand, 1962–79, based on data from the Department of Statistics. (Modified from Benfield J, Kjellstrom T. New Zealand ex-nuptial births and domestic purposes benefits in a different perspective. *N Z Nurs J.* 1981;74:28–31.)

1979. Much concern was expressed because of the apparent steady rise in extramarital births. However, as seen in Fig. 3.19, there had really been no increase in the rate of extramarital births; there had been a decline in total births that was largely accounted for by a decline in births to married women. The extramarital births, as a result, accounted for a greater percentage of all births, even though the rate of extramarital births had not increased over the 17-year period.

This example makes two points: First, a proportion is *not* a rate, and we shall return to this point in our discussion of mortality. Second, birth can be viewed as an *event*, just as the development of disease is an event, and appropriate rates can be computed. In discussing babies born with malformations, some people prefer to speak of the prevalence of malformations at birth rather than the incidence of malformations at birth, because the malformation was clearly present (but often unrecognized), even before birth. Furthermore, because some proportion of cases with malformations abort before birth, any estimate of the frequency of malformations at birth is probably a significant underestimate of the true incidence. Hence, the term "prevalence at birth" is often used.

Fig. 3.20 shows breast cancer incidence rates in women by age and the distribution of breast cancer in women by age. Ignore the bar graph for the moment, and consider the line curve. The pattern is one of continually increasing incidence with age, with a change in the slope of the curve between ages 45 and 50 years. This change is observed in many countries. It has been suggested that something happens near the time of menopause, and that premenopausal and postmenopausal breast cancer may be different diseases. Note that, even in old age, the incidence or risk of breast cancer continues to rise.

Now let us look at the bar chart—the distribution of breast cancer cases by age. If the incidence is increasing so dramatically with age, why are only fewer than 5% of the cases occurring in the oldest age group of women? The answer is that there are very few women alive in that age group, so that even though they have a very high risk of breast cancer, the group is so small that they contribute only a small proportion of the total number of breast cancer cases seen at all ages. The fact that so few cases of breast cancer are seen in the older age groups has contributed to a false public impression that the risk of breast cancer is low in these groups and that mammography is therefore not important in the elderly. This is a serious misperception. The need to change public thinking on this issue is a major public health challenge. We therefore see the importance of recognizing the distinction between the distribution of disease or the proportion of cases, and the incidence rate or risk of the disease.

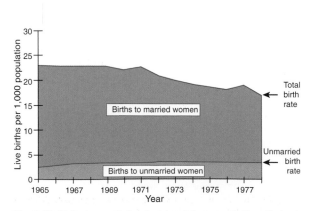

Fig. 3.19 Births to married and unmarried women in New Zealand, 1965–78, based on data from the Department of Statistics. (Modified from Benfield J, Kjellstrom T. New Zealand ex-nuptial births and domestic purposes benefits in a different perspective. *N Z Nurs J.* 1981;74:28–31.)

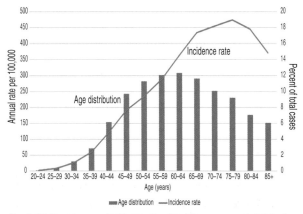

Fig. 3.20 Breast cancer incidence rates in white women and distribution of cases by age, 2000–13. (Data from Surveillance, Epidemiology, and End Results [SEER] Program [www.seer.cancer.gov] SEER*Stat Database: Incidence—SEER 18 Regs Research. Courtesy Dr. Louise Brinton and Mr. Jake Thistle.)

Geographic Information System

One approach to examining geographic or spatial differences in the distribution of cases, whether incidence or prevalence, is to plot the cases on a map. Mapping the geographic distribution of the cases dates back to the work of Dr. John Snow, an English physician, in the midst of the cholera outbreak in Soho district of London, England, in 1854. Fig. 3.21 shows the map on which Snow plotted the cholera-related deaths and the city's water pumps. Snow used the map to show that the cholera cases were centered on a water pump on Broad Street, which was operated by a company that took water from a sewage-polluted part of the Thames River. When the pump was shut off, the incidence of cholera cases sharply decreased, proving Snow's theory that the source of the epidemic was the contaminated water.

The science of using maps continued to evolve. The Geographic Information System (GIS) uses a variety of information on the geographic distribution of disease and how it is related to the environment that the people live in, and subsequently identifies *clusters* of diseases.

This aids policy makers in identifying and prioritizing health problems and resource allocation. However, many apparent clusters are due only to chance, and an important epidemiologic challenge is to investigate such groups of cases and rule out an environmental etiology for what appears to be a greater-than-expected proximity of cases of a disease in time and space, and that is where the role of modern spatial epidemiologic and statistical methods come to work.

Fig. 3.22 shows a map of Baltimore city displaying the violent crimes per 100 residents (color gradient) per census tract between 2006 and 2010, and the number of alcohol outlets (circles). Using geospatial modeling, the researchers found that the increased numbers of alcohol outlets was associated with increased violent crime in Baltimore. Such findings have very important public health and policy implications.

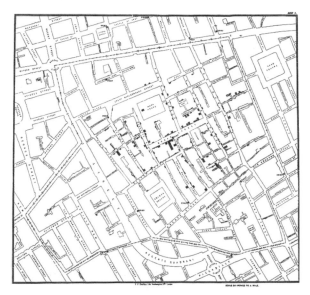

Fig. 3.21 Map of Soho district in London, England, showing clusters of cholera deaths around the Broad Street pump. (Published by C.F. Cheffins, Lith, Southhampton Buildings, London, England, 1854 in Snow J. *On the Mode of Communication of Cholera.* 2nd ed. New Burlington Street, London: John Churchill; 1855. https://en.wikipedia.org/wiki/File:Snow-cholera-map-1.jpg.)

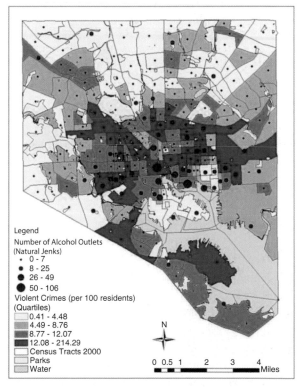

Fig. 3.22 Violent crimes (per 100 residents) per census tract, Baltimore City, 2006–10. (Modified from Jennings JM, Milam AJ, Greiner A, Furr-Holden CD, Curriero FC, Thornton RJ. Neighborhood alcohol outlets and the association with violent crime in one mid-Atlantic City: the implications for zoning policy. *J Urban Health.* 2014;91:62–71.)

Zoning code policies should take into account how alcohol outlets in residential areas could impact violent crimes.

Conclusion

In this chapter, we have emphasized the important role that epidemiology plays in surveillance of diseases in human populations and the importance of surveillance of morbidity for the planning and development of health services. This is especially challenging in developing countries, many of which lack the infrastructure for gathering vital statistics and other routine data on large (representative) populations. We have reviewed different approaches to measuring morbidity, and we have seen that a rate involves specification of a numerator, a denominator of people at risk, and time—either explicitly or implicitly. In the next chapter, we will turn to measuring mortality. In Chapter 5, we will discuss how we use screening and diagnostic tests to identify individuals who are ill (who are included in the numerator) and distinguish them from those in the population who are not ill. In Chapter 18, we will discuss how epidemiology is used for evaluating screening programs.

REFERENCES

1. Thacker S, Berkelman RL. Public health surveillance in the United States. *Epidemiol Rev*. 1988;10:164–190.
2. Centers for Disease Control and Prevention. National Notifiable Diseases Surveillance System (NNDSS). https://wwwn.cdc.gov/nndss/case-definitions.html. Accessed June 1, 2017.
3. Murray CJL, Ortblad KF, Guinovart C, et al. Global, regional, and national incidence and mortality for HIV, tuberculosis, and malaria during 1990–2013: a systematic analysis for the Global Burden of Disease Study 2013. *Lancet*. 2014;384(9947):1005–1070.
4. International Atomic Energy Agency. The Fukushima Daiichi accident; 2015. http://www.pub.iaea.org/books/IAEABooks/10962/The-Fukushima-Daiichi-Accident. Accessed May 15, 2017.
5. Bard D, Verger P, Hubert P. Chernobyl, 10 years after: health consequences. *Epidemiol Rev*. 1997;19:187–204.
6. Erkinjuntti T, Østbye T, Steenhuis R, et al. The effect of different diagnostic criteria on the prevalence of dementia. *N Engl J Med*. 1997;337:1667–1674.

REVIEW QUESTIONS FOR CHAPTER 3

1 *At an initial examination in Oxford, Massachusetts, migraine headache was found in 5 of 1,000 men aged 30 to 35 years and in 10 of 1,000 women aged 30 to 35 years. The inference that women have a two times greater risk of developing migraine headache than do men in this age group is:*
a. Correct
b. Incorrect, because a ratio has been used to compare male and female rates
c. Incorrect, because of failure to recognize the effect of age in the two groups
d. Incorrect, because no data for a comparison or control group are given
e. Incorrect, because of failure to distinguish between incidence and prevalence

2 *A prevalence survey conducted from January 1 through December 31, 2012, identified 1,000 cases of schizophrenia in a city of 2 million persons. The incidence rate of schizophrenia in this population is 5/100,000 persons each year. What percentage of the 1,000 cases were newly diagnosed in 2012? _____*

3 *Which of the following is an advantage of active surveillance?*
a. Requires less project staff
b. Is relatively inexpensive to employ
c. More accurate due to reduced reporting burden for health care providers
d. Relies on different disease definitions to account for all cases
e. Reporting systems can be developed quickly

4 *What would be the effect on age-specific incidence rates of uterine cancer if women with hysterectomies were excluded from the denominator of the calculations, assuming that there are some women in each age group who have had hysterectomies?*

a. The rates would remain the same

b. The rates would tend to decrease

c. The rates would tend to increase

d. The rates would increase in older groups and decrease in younger groups

e. It cannot be determined whether the rates would increase or decrease

5 *A survey was conducted among the nonhospitalized adult population of the United States during 2008 through 2011. The results from this survey are shown below.*

Age Group	Persons With Hypertension (%)
18–29 years	4
30–39 years	10
40–49 years	22
50–59 years	43
60–69 years	54
70 and older	64

The researchers stated that there was an age-related increase in the risk of hypertension in this population. You conclude that the researchers' interpretation:

a. Is correct

b. Is incorrect because it was not based on rates

c. Is incorrect because incidence rates do not describe risk

d. Is incorrect because prevalence is used

e. Is incorrect because the calculations are not age-adjusted

Questions 6 and 7 use the information below:

Population of the city of Atlantis on March 30, 2012 = 183,000

No. of new active cases of TB occurring between January 1 and June 30, 2012 = 26

No. of active TB cases according to the city register on June 30, 2012 = 264

6 *The incidence rate of active cases of TB for the 6-month period was:*

a. 7 per 100,000 population

b. 14 per 100,000 population

c. 26 per 100,000 population

d. 28 per 100,000 population

e. 130 per 100,000 population

7 *The prevalence rate of active TB as of June 30, 2012, was:*

a. 14 per 100,000 population

b. 130 per 100,000 population

c. 144 per 100,000 population

d. 264 per 100,000 population

e. None of the above

8 *Disease X has a duration of 15 years and a low incidence (5 per 100,000 person-years). Disease Y has a duration of 5 years and a low incidence (5 per 100,000 person-years). Comparing Disease X to Y in the same population, we would expect Disease X to have a:*

a. Better cure rate

b. Lower prevalence

c. Higher prevalence

d. Higher incidence

e. Shorter average duration

9 *The following health statistics are available on the Internet for country Z about two disease outcomes. Disease A has an annual incidence of 225 per 100,000 population and an annual mortality rate of 150 per 100,000. Disease B has an annual incidence of 500 per 100,000 population and the same annual mortality rate as disease A. Neither disease A or B has a cure. What would you conclude regarding the burden of these diseases in country Z?*

a. The proportionate mortality is higher for disease A than disease B

b. The case fatality ratio is higher for disease B than disease A

c. Disease A has a higher prevalence than disease B

d. Disease B has a higher prevalence than disease A

e. Years of potential life lost (YPLL) is greater for disease B than disease A

10 *Chikungunya virus infection was recently introduced into the Dominican Republic. During the first year after introduction, the virus has infected a total of 251,880 people in the Dominican Republic, which has a population size of 10.4 million people. Infection by the chikungunya virus is rarely fatal. Which of the following is correct?*

a. The incidence of chikungunya infection is 251,880 per year

b. The prevalence of chikungunya infections is 251,880

c. The mortality rate of chikungunya is 24.2 per 1,000 person

d. The 1-year cumulative incidence of chikungunya is 24.2 per 1,000 persons

e. The cumulative survival from chikungunya infections is 24.2 per 1,000 persons

The Occurrence of Disease: II. Mortality and Other Measures of Disease Impact

You do not die from being born, nor from having lived, nor from old age. You die from something. ... There is no such thing as a natural death: Nothing that happens to a man is ever natural, since his presence calls the world into question. All men must die: but for every man his death is an accident and, even if he knows it and consents to it, an unjustifiable violation.

—Simone de Beauvoir, writing of her mother's death, in *A Very Easy Death*[1]

Learning Objectives

- To compare different measures of mortality, including mortality rates, case-fatality, proportionate mortality, and years of potential life lost.
- To show when mortality can approximate the risk of disease.
- To introduce issues that arise in comparing mortality across two or more populations.
- To define, calculate, and interpret direct and indirect age-adjusted mortality rates.
- To introduce other measures of disease impact.

Mortality is of great interest for several reasons. First of all, death is the ultimate experience that every human being is destined to have. Death is clearly of tremendous importance to each person including questions of when and how death will occur and whether there is any way to delay it. From the standpoint of studying disease occurrence, expressing mortality in quantitative terms can pinpoint differences in the risk of dying from a disease between people in different geographic areas and subgroups in the population. Mortality rates can serve as measures of disease severity and can help us determine whether the treatment for a disease has become more effective over time. In addition, given the problem that often arises in identifying new cases of a disease, mortality rates may serve as surrogates for incidence rates when the disease being studied is a severe and lethal one. This chapter will address the quantitative expression of mortality and the uses of such measures in epidemiologic studies.

Measures of Mortality

Fig. 4.1 shows the number of cancer deaths from 1969 to 2014 in the United States. Clearly, the absolute *number* of people dying from cancer is seen increasing significantly through the year 2014, but from this graph, we cannot say that the *risk* of dying from cancer is increasing, because the only data that we have in this graph are numbers of deaths (numerators); we do not have denominators (populations at risk). If, for example, the size of the US population is also increasing at the same rate, the risk of dying from cancer does not change.

For this reason, if we wish to address the risk of dying, we must deal with rates. Fig. 4.2 shows mortality rates for several types of cancer in men from 1930 to 2014. The most dramatic increase is in deaths from lung cancer. This increase is clearly of epidemic proportions and, tragically, lung cancer is a preventable cause of death. Fortunately, since the mid-1990s, lung cancer mortality has declined, paralleling earlier decreases in rates of smoking among men. Other cancers are also of interest. Age-adjusted mortality from prostate cancer also peaked in the mid-1990s and has declined since. Cancers of the colon and rectum have declined over many years. The rate of death from stomach cancer has declined dramatically since 1930, although the precise explanation is not known. It has been suggested that the decline may be the result of the increased availability of refrigeration, which decreased the need to smoke foods and thereby decreased human exposure to carcinogens produced in the smoking process. Another possible cause is improved hygiene, which may have reduced the incidence of *Helicobacter pylori* infections that have been implicated in the etiology (or cause) of stomach cancer.

Fig. 4.3 shows a similar presentation for cancer mortality in women for the period 1930 to 2014.

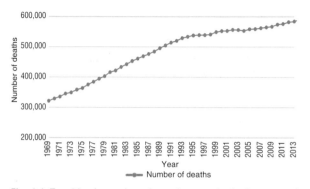

Fig. 4.1 Trend in observed numbers of cancer deaths for men and women in the United States 1969–2014. (Data from Weir HK, Anderson RN, Coleman King SM, et al. Heart disease and cancer deaths—trends and projections in the United States, 1969–2020. *Prev Chronic Dis.* 2016;13:160211.)

Breast cancer mortality remained at essentially the same level for many years but has declined since the early 1990s until 2014. It would be desirable to study changes in the incidence of breast cancer. Such a study is difficult, however, because with aggressive public education campaigns encouraging women to have mammograms and perform breast self-examination, many breast cancers may be detected today at much earlier stages that might have gone undetected years ago. Nevertheless, available evidence suggests that the true incidence of breast cancer in women may have increased for many years but then decreased from 2001 to 2014.

Uterine cancer mortality has declined, perhaps because of earlier detection and diagnosis. Lung cancer mortality in women has increased, and lung cancer has exceeded breast cancer as a cause of death in women. Lung cancer is almost completely preventable, being mostly due to a lifestyle habit, cigarette smoking, which has been voluntarily adopted by many women; today it is the leading cause of cancer death in women in the United States.

We may be particularly interested in mortality relating to age. Fig. 4.4 shows death rates from cancer and

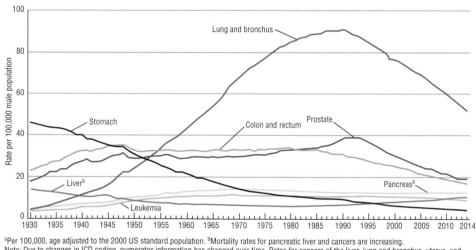

aPer 100,000, age adjusted to the 2000 US standard population. bMortality rates for pancreatic liver and cancers are increasing.
Note: Due to changes in ICD coding, numerator information has changed over time. Rates for cancers of the liver, lung and bronchus, uterus, and colon and rectum are affected by these coding changes.

©2017, American Cancer Society, Inc., Surveillance Research

Fig. 4.2 Cancer death rates for males, United States, 1930–2014 (age-adjusted to the 2000 US standard population). *ICD,* International Classification of Diseases. (From American Cancer Society, Cancer Facts & Figures 2017. Based on US Mortality Volumes 1930 to 1959, US Mortality Data, 1960 to 2014. National Center for Health Statistics, Centers for Disease Control and Prevention.)

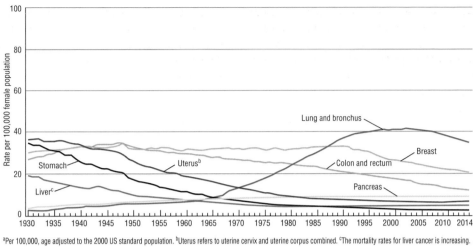

aPer 100,000, age adjusted to the 2000 US standard population. bUterus refers to uterine cervix and uterine corpus combined. cThe mortality rates for liver cancer is increasing.
Note: Due to changes in ICD coding, numerator information has changed over time. Rates for cancers of the liver, lung and bronchus, uterus, and colon and rectum are affected by these coding changes.

©2017, American Cancer Society, Inc., Surveillance Research

Fig. 4.3 Cancer death rates for females, United States, 1930–2014 (age-adjusted to the 2000 US standard population). *ICD,* International Classification of Diseases. (From American Cancer Society, Cancer Facts & Figures 2017. Based on US Mortality Vol. 1930 to 1959, US Mortality Data, 1960 to 2007. National Center for Health Statistics, Centers for Disease Control and Prevention.)

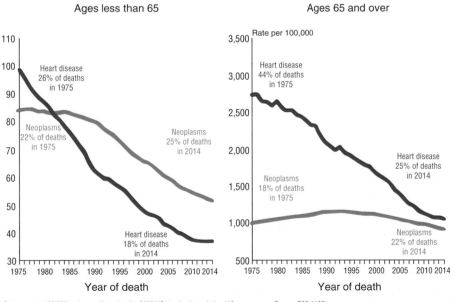

Rates are per 100,000 and age-adjusted to the 2000 US standard population (19 age groups - Census P25-1103).

Fig. 4.4 Death rates from cancer and heart disease for ages younger than 65 and 65 or older (age-adjusted to the 2000 US standard population). (From Howlader N, Noone AM, Krapcho M, et al, eds. *SEER Cancer Statistics Review, 1975–2014.* Bethesda, MD: National Cancer Institute; https://seer.cancer .gov/csr/1975_2014/, based on November 2016 SEER data submission, posted to the SEER website, April 2017. Using data from US Mortality Files, National Center for Health Statistics, Centers for Disease Control and Prevention.)

from heart disease for people younger than 65 and for those 65 or older. Cancer is the leading cause of death in men and women younger than 65 years, but above age 65, heart disease clearly exceeds cancer as a cause of death.

Fig. 4.5 shows the causes of death worldwide for children younger than 5 years in 2015. The leading causes of death among children under 5 years of age in 2015 were preterm birth complications, pneumonia, intrapartum-related complications, diarrhea, and congenital abnormalities. Neonatal deaths accounted for 45% of under-5 deaths in 2015. Infectious diseases accounted for over half of the 5.9 million deaths of children under age 5, with the largest percentages due to pneumonia, diarrhea, and malaria.

MORTALITY RATES

How is mortality expressed in quantitative terms? Let us examine some types of mortality rates. The first is the annual death rate, or mortality rate, from all causes:

Annual mortality rate for all causes
(per 100,000 population) =

$$\frac{\text{Total no. of deaths from all causes in 1 year}}{\text{No. of persons in the population at midyear}} \times 100,000$$

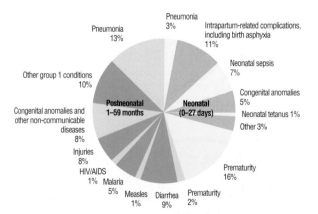

Fig. 4.5 Major causes of death in children under 5 years in 2015. *AIDS,* Acquired immunodeficiency syndrome; *HIV,* human immunodeficiency virus. (From World Health Organization. *MCEE Methods and Data Sources for Child Causes of Death 2000–2015. Global Health Estimates Technical Paper WHO/HIS/IER/GHE/2016.1.*)

Note that because the population changes over time, the number of persons in the population at midyear is generally used as an approximation of average population.

The same principles mentioned in the discussion of morbidity apply to mortality; for a mortality rate to make sense, anyone in the group represented by the denominator must have the potential to enter the group represented by the numerator.

We may not always be interested in a rate for the entire population; perhaps we are interested only in a certain age group, in men or in women, or in one ethnic group. Thus, if we are interested in mortality in children younger than 10 years, we can calculate a rate specifically for that group:

Annual mortality rate from all causes
for children younger than 10 years of age
(per 1,000 population) =

$$\frac{\begin{array}{c}\text{No. of deaths from all causes in 1 year}\\\text{in children younger than 10 years of age}\end{array}}{\begin{array}{c}\text{No. of children in the population}\\\text{younger than 10 years of age at midyear}\end{array}} \times 1,000$$

In putting a restriction on age, for example, the same restriction must apply to *both* the numerator and the denominator, so that every person in the denominator group will be at risk for entering the numerator group. When such a restriction is placed on a rate, it is called a *specific rate*. The above rate, then, is an *age-specific mortality rate*.

We could also place a restriction on a rate by specifying a diagnosis, and thus limit the rate to deaths from a certain disease, that is, a *disease-specific* or a *cause-specific rate*. For example, if we are interested in mortality from lung cancer, we would calculate it in the following manner:

Annual mortality rate from lung cancer
(per 1,000 population) =

$$\frac{\text{No. of deaths from lung cancer in 1 year}}{\text{No. of persons in the population at midyear}} \times 1,000$$

We can also place restrictions on more than one characteristic simultaneously, for example, age and cause of death, as follows:

Annual mortality rate from leukemia in children
<10 years of age (per 1,000 population) =

$$\frac{\text{No. of deaths from leukemia in 1 year}}{\text{No. of children in the population}} \times 1,000$$
$$\frac{\text{in children} <10 \text{ years of age}}{\text{No. of children in the population} <10 \text{ years of age at midyear}} \times 1,000$$

Time must also be specified in any mortality rate. Mortality can be calculated over 1 year, 5 years, or longer. The period selected is arbitrary, but it must be specified precisely.

CASE-FATALITY

We must distinguish between a *mortality rate* and *case-fatality*. Case-fatality is calculated as follows:

Case-fatality (%) =

$$\frac{\text{No. of individuals dying during a specified period of time after disease onset or diagnosis}}{\text{No. of individuals with the specified disease}} \times 100$$

In other words, what percentage of people *who have a certain disease* die within a certain time after their disease was diagnosed? Ideally, we would like to use the date of disease onset as the beginning of the time period specified in the numerator. However, date of disease onset is often hard to standardize since many diseases develop insidiously (without symptoms) over a long period of time. As a result, in many chronic diseases, it may be difficult to determine precisely when the disease process began. For example, many patients with arthritis cannot recall when their joint pain first began. In practice therefore we often use date of diagnosis as a surrogate measure for date of disease onset, because the exact date of diagnosis can generally be documented from available medical records. If the information is to be obtained from respondents, it is worth noting that if the disease in question is a serious one, the date on which the diagnosis was given may well have been a life-changing date for the patient and not easily forgotten.

What is the difference between case-fatality and a mortality rate? In a mortality rate, the denominator represents the entire population at risk of dying from the disease, including both those who have the disease and those who do not have the disease

(but who are *at risk* of developing the disease). In case-fatality, however, the denominator is limited to those who *already have the disease*. Thus, case-fatality is a measure of the *severity* of the disease. It can also be used to measure any benefits of a new therapy; as therapy improves, case-fatality would be expected to decline.

The numerator of case-fatality should ideally be restricted to deaths *from that disease*. However, it is not always easy to distinguish between deaths from that disease and deaths from other causes. For example, an alcoholic person may die in a car accident; however, the death may or may not be related to alcohol intake.

Let us look at a hypothetical example to clarify the difference between mortality and case-fatality (Box 4.1).

Assume that in a population of 100,000 persons, 20 have disease X. In 1 year, 18 people die from that disease. The mortality is very low (0.018%) because the disease is rare; however, once a person has the disease, the chances of his or her dying are great (90%).

PROPORTIONATE MORTALITY

Another measure of mortality is proportionate mortality, which is not a rate. The proportionate mortality from cardiovascular disease in the United States in 2015 is defined as follows:

Proportionate mortality from cardiovascular diseases in the US in 2015 (%) =

$$\frac{\text{No. of deaths from cardiovascular diseases in the US in 2015}}{\text{Total deaths in the US in 2015}} \times 100$$

In other words, of all deaths in the United States, what *proportion* was caused by cardiovascular disease?

BOX 4.1 COMPARISON OF MORTALITY RATE WITH CASE-FATALITY IN THE SAME YEAR

Assume a population of 100,000 people of whom 20 are sick with disease X, and in 1 year, 18 of the 20 die from disease X

Mortality rate from disease $X = \dfrac{18}{100,000} = 0.00018$, or 0.018%

Case-fatality from disease $X = \dfrac{18}{20} = 0.9$, or 90%

Fig. 4.6 shows proportionate mortality from heart disease by age group. In each age group, the full bar represents all deaths (100%), and deaths from heart disease are indicated by the dark blue portion. We see that the *proportion* of deaths from heart disease increases with age. However, this does not tell us that the *risk* of death from heart disease is also increasing. This is demonstrated in the following examples.

Table 4.1 shows all deaths and deaths from heart disease in two communities, A and B. All-cause mortality in community A is twice that in community B. When we look at proportionate mortality, we find that 10% of the deaths in community A and 20% of the deaths in community B are due to heart disease. Does this tell us that the risk of dying from heart disease is twice as high in community B as it is in A? The answer is no. When the mortality rates from heart disease are calculated for the two communities (10% of 30/1,000 and

20% of 15/1,000), we find that the mortality rates are identical.

If we observe a change in proportionate mortality from a certain disease over time, the change may be due not to changes in mortality from that disease, but to changes in the mortality of some other disease. Let us consider a hypothetical example: in Table 4.2, we see mortality rates from heart disease, cancer, and other causes in a population in an early period and a later period. First, compare the mortality rates in the two time periods: mortality from heart disease doubled over time (from 40/1,000 to 80/1,000), but mortality rates from cancer and from all other causes (20/1,000) did not change. However, if we now examine the proportionate mortality from each cause, we see that the proportionate mortality from cancer and from other causes has decreased in the population, but only because the proportionate mortality from heart disease has increased. Thus, if the proportion of one segment of the mortality "pie" increases, there will necessarily be a decrease in the proportion of some other segment (Fig. 4.7). Another view of this is seen in Fig. 4.8.

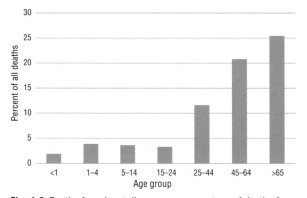

Fig. 4.6 Deaths from heart disease as a percentage of deaths from all causes, by age group, United States, 2014. (From National Center for Health Statistics [NCHS]. *Data from Health, United States, 2015, With Special Feature on Racial and Ethnic Health Disparities.* Hyattsville, MD: NCHS; 2016.)

TABLE 4.1 **Comparison of Mortality Rate and Proportionate Mortality: I. Deaths From Heart Disease in Two Communities**		
	Community A	**Community B**
Mortality rate from all causes	30/1,000	15/1,000
Proportionate mortality from heart disease	10%	20%
Mortality rate from heart disease	3/1,000	3/1,000

TABLE 4.2 **Hypothetical Example of Mortality Rates and Proportionate Mortality in Two Periods**				
	EARLY PERIOD		**LATER PERIOD**	
Cause of Death	**Mortality Rate**	**Proportionate Mortality**	**Mortality Rate**	**Proportionate Mortality**
Heart disease	40/1,000	50%	80/1,000	66.7%
Cancer	20/1,000	25%	20/1,000	16.7%
All other causes	20/1,000	25%	20/1,000	16.7%
All deaths	80/1,000	100%	120/1,000	100.0%

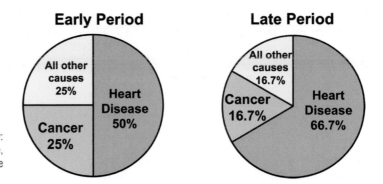

Fig. 4.7 Hypothetical example of proportionate mortality: changes in proportionate mortality from heart disease, cancer, and other causes from the early period to the late period.

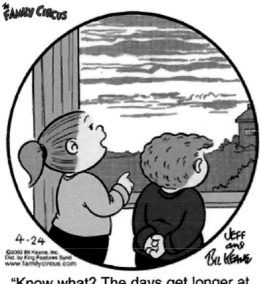

"Know what? The days get longer at the same time the nights get shorter."

Fig. 4.8 Understanding proportionate mortality. (Family Circus © 2002 Bill Keane, Inc. Distributed by King Features Syndicate, Inc.)

TABLE 4.3 **Comparison of Mortality Rate and Proportionate Mortality: II. Deaths From Heart Disease in Two Communities**		
	Community A	**Community B**
Mortality rate from all causes	20/1,000	10/1,000
Proportionate mortality from heart disease	30%	30%
Mortality rate from heart disease	6/1,000	3/1,000

As seen in the example in Table 4.3, if all-cause mortality rates differ, cause-specific mortality rates can differ significantly, even when the proportionate mortality is the same. Thus, these examples show that, although proportionate mortality can give us a quick look at the major causes of death, it cannot tell us the risk of dying from a disease. For that, we need a mortality rate.

YEARS OF POTENTIAL LIFE LOST

In recent years, another mortality index, years of potential life lost (YPLL), has been increasingly used for setting health priorities. YPLL is a measure of premature mortality, or early death. YPLL recognizes that death occurring in a person at a younger age clearly involves a greater loss of future productive years than death occurring at an older age. Two steps are involved in this calculation: in the first step, for each cause, each deceased person's age at death is subtracted from a predetermined (or "average") age at death. In the United States, this predetermined "standard" age is usually 75 years. Thus, an infant dying at 1 year of age has lost 74 years of life (75 to 1), but a person dying at 50 years of age has lost 25 years of life (75 to 50). Thus, the younger the age at which death occurs, the more years of potential life are lost. In the second step, the "years of potential life lost" for each individual are then added together to yield the total YPLL for the specific cause of death. When looking at reports that use YPLL, it is important to note what assumptions the author has made, including what predetermined standard age has been selected.

Fig. 4.9 shows the YPLL in the United States before age 75 years in 2015. The top bar shows the total

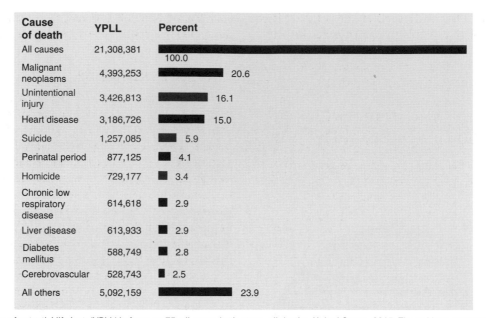

Fig. 4.9 Years of potential life lost *(YPLL)* before age 75, all races, both sexes, all deaths, United States, 2015. The red bars represent nondisease-related causes of death. (Modified from Centers for Disease Control and Prevention, National Center for Injury Prevention and Control. Years of potential life lost [YPLL] reports, 1999–2015. https://webappa.cdc.gov/sasweb/ncipc/ypll10.html. Accessed June 6, 2017.)

YPLL from all causes (100%), and the bars below show the individual YPLL from each leading cause of death, with the percentage of YPLL from all causes for which it accounts. We see that the greatest single source of YPLL was malignant neoplasms, which, in the same year, was the second leading cause of death by its mortality rate (see Fig. 1.2 and Table 1.1). In 2015, the ranking of unintentional injury by its mortality rate was fourth, while its ranking by YPLL was second. This discrepancy results from the fact that injury is the leading cause of death up to age 34 years, and therefore it accounts for a large proportion of YPLL.

Fig. 4.10 shows YPLL from unintentional injuries before age 75 years among persons aged 0 to 19 years. We see that the YPLL from motor vehicle accidents accounts for over half of the YPLL in this group. Thus, if we want to have an impact on YPLL in children and young adults, we should address this specific cause of injury related to motor vehicles.

Table 4.4 shows a ranking of causes of death in the United States for 2014 by YPLL, together with cause-specific age-adjusted mortality rates. By cause-specific mortality, suicide is ranked seventh, but by

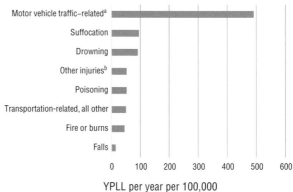

[a]Categorized by injured person and includes motor vehicle traffic occupant, motorcyclist, pedal cyclist, pedestrian, occupant or rider of other modes of transport in a motor vehicle traffic crash, and motor vehicle traffic crashes for which the injured person is unspecified.
[b]Cut or pierced, unintentional firearm-related injury, machinery-related injury, injury via natural and environmental cause, overexertion, struck by or against an object, and other specified and unspecified.

Fig. 4.10 Annualized years of potential life lost *(YPLL)* per 100,000 persons aged 0 to 19 years from unintentional injuries, United States, 2000–09. (Modified from Centers for Disease Control and Prevention. Years of potential life lost from unintentional injuries among persons aged 0–19 years—United States, 2000–2009. *MMWR Morb Mortal Wkly Rep.* 2012;61:830–833. https://www.cdc.gov/mmwr/preview/mmwrhtml/mm6141a2.htm. Accessed June 6, 2017.)

YPLL, it ranked fourth. This reflects the fact that a large proportion of suicide-related deaths occur in young persons.

YPLL can assist in three important public health functions: establishing research and resource priorities,

TABLE 4.4 **Estimated YPLL Before Age 75 Years and Age-Adjusted Mortality Rates per 100,000 Persons, by Cause of Death, United States, 2014**		
Disease	**Age-Adjusted Death Rate**	**YPLL in 2014**
Heart disease	167	3,130,959
Cancer	161.2	4,416,968
Chronic lower respiratory diseases	40.5	596,470
Accidents unintentional injuries	40.5	3,146,798
Diabetes mellitus	20.9	562,659
Influenza and pneumonia	15.1	293,372
Suicide	13	1,206,515
Septicemia	12.2	263,766
Chronic liver disease and cirrhosis	12	581,980
Hypertension	9.5	130,533

YPLL, Years of potential life lost.
Data from Centers for Disease Control and Prevention. Deaths: final data for 2014. *Natl Vital Stat Rep.* 2016; 65(4):1–122.

surveillance of temporal trends in premature mortality, and evaluating the effectiveness of program interventions.[2]

WHY LOOK AT MORTALITY?

Mortality is clearly an index of the severity of a disease from both clinical and public health standpoints, but mortality can also be used as an index of the risk of disease, as shown in Figs. 4.2 and 4.3. In general, mortality data are easier to obtain than incidence data for a given disease, and it therefore may be more feasible to use mortality data as a proxy indicator for incidence. However, when a disease is mild and not fatal, mortality may not be a good index of incidence. A mortality rate is a good reflection of the incidence rate under two conditions: first, when the case-fatality rate is high (as in untreated rabies), and second, when the duration of disease (survival) is short. Under these conditions, mortality is a good measure of incidence, and thus a measure of the risk of disease. For example, cancer of the pancreas is a highly lethal disease: death generally occurs within a few months of diagnosis, and long-term survival is rare. Thus, unfortunately, mortality from pancreatic cancer is a good surrogate for incidence of the disease.

Fig. 4.11 shows mortality trends in the United States from 1980 to 2014 by race. It is evident that the mortality rates for black and white individuals have

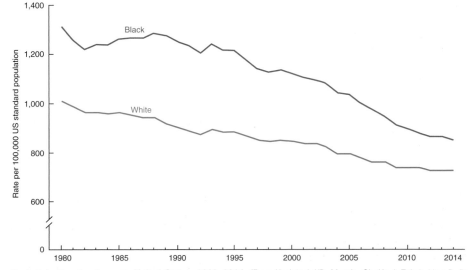

Fig. 4.11 Age-adjusted death rates, by race: United States, 1980–2014. (From Kochanek KD, Murphy SL, Xu J, Tejada-Vera B. Deaths: final data for 2014. *Natl Vital Stat Rep.* 2016;65:1–122.)

gone down, but yet there is a clear disparity between the two races as shown by the consistent gap between the two curves. Fig. 4.12 shows mortality trends in the United States from 1955 to 2014 by gender and age group. In both panels for males and females, we can see that there is a steady decline in the death rate throughout the years, particularly in the age groups less than 14 years. This could be potentially attributed to the widespread coverage of childhood vaccinations. On the other hand, the decline was modest in the age groups 45 to 64 years due to improvements in the early detection of cardiovascular diseases and cancer, and the evolving new effective treatments. If we look at the left panel for males, we see an increase in the mortality rate for age groups 25 to 44 years in the 1980s, followed by a sharp decline in the early 1990s. This can be explained by the then-emerging human immunodeficiency virus (HIV) disease, and followed by the newly introduced, highly active antiretroviral therapy, as well as lifestyle changes resulting from public health education.

A comparison of mortality and incidence is seen in Figs. 4.13 and 4.14. Fig. 4.13 shows breast cancer rates by year in selected European countries from 1975 to 2010. During this period, the age-standardized rates per 100,000 increased in all countries shown in the figure. This increase has been attributed to early detection and improved diagnostic modalities. As seen in Fig. 4.14, however, death rates from breast cancer in selected countries decreased markedly during the 1990s onward, perhaps as a result of earlier detection and increasingly prompt medical and surgical intervention.

Fig. 4.15 presents recent data on time trends in incidence and mortality from breast cancer in black women and white women in the United States. Compare the time trends in incidence and mortality. What do these curves tell us about new cases of breast cancer over time and survival from breast cancer? Compare the experiences of black women and white women in regard to both incidence and mortality. How can we describe the differences, and what could be some of the possible explanations?

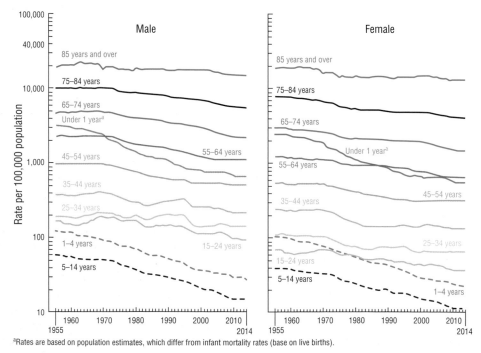

Fig. 4.12 Death rates, by age and sex: United States, 1955–2014. (From Kochanek KD, Murphy SL, Xu J, Tejada-Vera B. Deaths: final data for 2014. *Natl Vital Stat Rep.* 2016;65:1–122.)

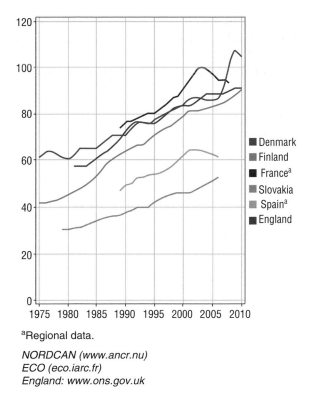

aRegional data.

NORDCAN (www.ancr.nu)
ECO (eco.iarc.fr)
England: www.ons.gov.uk

Fig. 4.13 Trends in incidence of female breast cancer in selected countries: age-standardized rate (W) per 100,000 in selected European countries, 1975–2010. (From International Agency for Research on Cancer, GLOBOCAN; 2012. http://globocan.iarc.fr/old/FactSheets/cancers/breast-new .asp. Accessed June 7, 2017.)

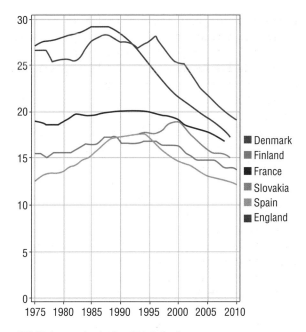

WHO (www.who.int/healthinfo/en/)

Fig. 4.14 Trends in mortality of female breast cancer in selected countries: age-standardized rate per 100,000 in selected European countries, 1975–2010. (From International Agency for Research on Cancer, GLOBOCAN; 2012. http://globocan.iarc.fr/old/FactSheets/cancers/breast-new .asp. Accessed June 7, 2017.)

A final example relates to reports in recent years that the incidence of thyroid cancer in the United States has been increasing. One of two possible explanations is likely. The first explanation is that these reports reflect a true increase in incidence that has resulted from increases in prevalence of risk factors for the disease. The second explanation is that the reported increased incidence is only an increase in *apparent* incidence. It does not reflect any true increase in new cases but rather an increase in the early detection and diagnosis of subclinical cases, because new diagnostic methods permit us to identify small and asymptomatic thyroid cancers that could not be detected previously.

In order to distinguish between these two possible explanations, Lim et al.[3] studied changes in incidence and mortality from thyroid cancer in the United States from 1974 to 2013. Fig. 4.16 shows that during the period of the study, the *incidence rate* (panel A) of thyroid cancer more than doubled but during the same period, *mortality* (panel B) from thyroid cancer remained virtually unchanged.

Thyroid cancer is characterized by different histologic types, as seen in Fig. 4.17; at one extreme, papillary carcinoma has the best prognosis and at the opposite extreme, poorly differentiated types—medullary and anaplastic—are generally the most aggressive with poorest prognoses. The authors found that the increase in incidence of thyroid cancer was almost entirely due to an increase in the incidence of papillary cancer (Fig. 4.18). Within the papillary cancers, most of the increase in this incidence was accounted for by the smallest-sized tumors (Fig. 4.19). Thus, the authors found that 87% of the increase in thyroid cancer incidence over a 30-year period was accounted for by an increase in the smallest-sized papillary cancers, tumors that have the best prognosis. A number of earlier

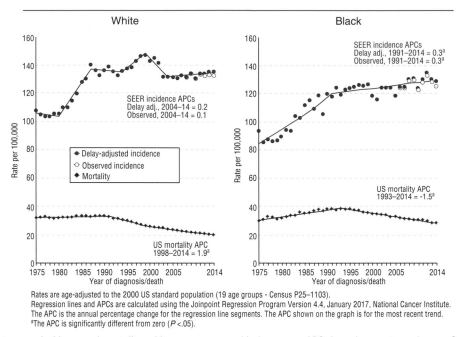

Fig. 4.15 Breast cancer incidence and mortality: white women versus black women. *APC,* Annual percentage change; *SEER,* Surveillance, Epidemiology, and End Results. (From SEER Cancer Statistics Review; 1975–2014. National Cancer Institute, Bethesda, MD. https://seer.cancer.gov/csr/1975_2014/browse_csr.php?sectionSEL=4&pageSEL=sect_04_zfig.01.html. Accessed June 7, 2017.)

studies have shown a high prevalence of previously unrecognized, asymptomatic small papillary cancers at autopsy. If the increased incidence was due to the availability of more refined diagnostic methods, we would expect to see an increase in the incidence of small tumors, which is exactly what the authors found in their study.

PROBLEMS WITH MORTALITY DATA

Most of our information about deaths comes from death certificates. A death certificate is shown in Fig. 4.20. By international agreement, deaths are coded according to the *underlying cause.* The underlying cause of death is defined as "the disease or injury which initiated the train of morbid events leading directly or indirectly to death or the circumstances of the accident or violence which produced the fatal injury."[4] Thus, the death certificate from which Fig. 4.21 is taken would be coded as a death from chronic ischemic heart disease, the underlying cause, which is always found on the lowest line used in part I of item 32 of the certificate. The underlying cause of death therefore "excludes

information pertaining to the immediate cause of death, contributory causes and those causes that intervene between the underlying and immediate causes of death."[5] As pointed out by Savage and coworkers,[6] the total contribution of a given cause of death may not be reflected in the mortality data as generally reported; this may apply to a greater extent in some diseases than in others.

Countries and regions vary greatly in the quality of the data provided on their death certificates. Studies of validity of death certificates compared with hospital and autopsy records generally find higher validity for certain diseases, such as cancers, than for others.

Deaths are coded according to the International Classification of Diseases (ICD), now in its 10th revision. Because coding categories and regulations change from one revision to another, any study of time trends in mortality that spans more than one revision must examine the possibility that observed changes could be due entirely or in part to changes in the ICD. In 1949, mortality rates from diabetes showed a dramatic decline in both men and women (Fig. 4.22). However, any

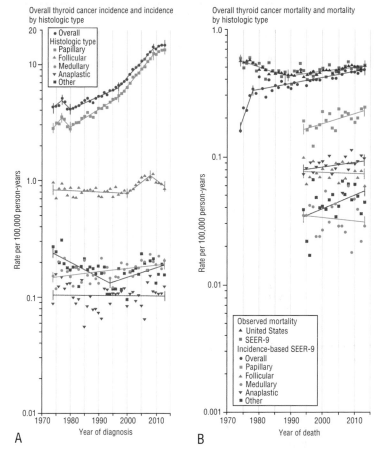

Fig. 4.16 Thyroid cancer incidence (A) and mortality (B), 1974–2013. *SEER,* Surveillance, Epidemiology, and End Results. (From Lim H, Devesa SS, Sosa JA, et al. Trends in thyroid cancer incidence and mortality in the United States, 1974–2013. *JAMA.* 2017;317:1338–1348.)

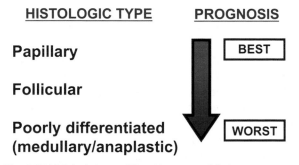

Fig. 4.17 Histologic types of thyroid cancer and their prognoses.

euphoria that these data might have caused was short-lived; analysis of this drop indicated that it occurred at a time of change from the seventh revision to the eighth revision of the ICD. Prior to 1949, the policy was that any death certificate that included mention of diabetes anywhere be coded as a death from diabetes. After 1949, only death certificates on which the underlying cause of death was listed as diabetes were coded as a death from diabetes. Hence, the decline seen in Fig. 4.22 was an artifact of the change in coding. Whenever we see a time trend of an increase or a decrease in mortality, the first question we must ask is, "Is it real?" Specifically, when we look at trends in mortality over time, we must ask whether any changes took place in how death certificates were coded during the period being examined and whether these changes could have contributed to changes observed in mortality during the same period.

Changes in the definition of disease can also have a significant effect on the number of cases of the disease that are reported or that are subsequently classified as meeting the diagnostic criteria for the

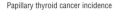

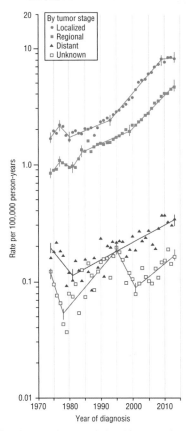

Fig. 4.18 Trends in incidence of thyroid cancer by tumor stage (1974–2013) in the United States. (From Lim H, Devesa SS, Sosa JA, et al. Trends in thyroid cancer incidence and mortality in the United States, 1974–2013. *JAMA.* 2017;317:1338–1348.)

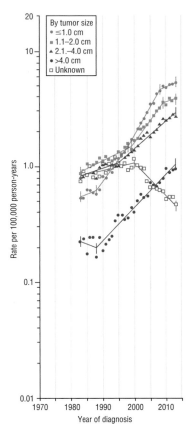

Fig. 4.19 Trends in incidence of papillary tumors of the thyroid, by size, United States, 1983–2013. (From Lim H, Devesa SS, Sosa JA, et al. Trends in thyroid cancer incidence and mortality in the United States, 1974–2013. *JAMA.* 2017;317:1338–1348.)

disease. In early 1993, a new definition of acquired immunodeficiency syndrome (AIDS) was introduced; as shown in Fig. 4.23, this change resulted in a rapid rise in the number of reported cases. With the new definition, even after the initial peak, the number of reported cases remained higher than it had been for several years.

In discussing morbidity in Chapter 3, we said that everyone in the group represented by the denominator must be at risk to enter the group represented by the numerator, and we looked at cervical cancer incidence rates as an example. The same principle regarding numerator and denominator applies to mortality rates. Fig. 4.24 shows a similar set of observations for mortality rates from cervical cancers. Once again, correcting

BOX 4.2 SOME CAUSES OF DEATH THAT WERE REPORTED ON DEATH CERTIFICATES IN THE EARLY 1900S

"Died suddenly without the aid of a physician"
"A mother died in infancy"
"Deceased had never been fatally sick"
"Died suddenly, nothing serious"
"Went to bed feeling well, but woke up dead"

for hysterectomy reduces the number of women in the denominator and thus increases the mortality rate. In a lighter vein, Box 4.2 lists some causes of death that were listed on death certificates early in the 20th century.

U.S. STANDARD CERTIFICATE OF DEATH

LOCAL FILE NO.   STATE FILE NO.

1. DECEDENT'S LEGAL NAME (Include AKA's if any) (First, Middle, Last) | 2. SEX | 3. SOCIAL SECURITY NUMBER

4a. AGE-Last Birthday (Years) | 4b. UNDER 1 YEAR (Months / Days) | 4c. UNDER 1 DAY (Hours / Minutes) | 5. DATE OF BIRTH (Mo/Day/Yr) | 6. BIRTHPLACE (City and State or Foreign Country)

7a. RESIDENCE-STATE | 7b. COUNTY | 7c. CITY OR TOWN

7d. STREET AND NUMBER | 7e. APT. NO. | 7f. ZIP CODE | 7g. INSIDE CITY LIMITS? □ Yes □ No

8. EVER IN US ARMED FORCES? □ Yes □ No | 9. MARITAL STATUS AT TIME OF DEATH □ Married □ Married, but separated □ Widowed □ Divorced □ Never Married □ Unknown | 10. SURVIVING SPOUSE'S NAME (If wife, give name prior to first marriage)

11. FATHER'S NAME (First, Middle, Last) | 12. MOTHER'S NAME PRIOR TO FIRST MARRIAGE (First, Middle, Last)

13a. INFORMANT'S NAME | 13b. RELATIONSHIP TO DECEDENT | 13c. MAILING ADDRESS (Street and Number, City, State, Zip Code)

14. PLACE OF DEATH (Check only one: see instructions)

IF DEATH OCCURRED IN A HOSPITAL: □ Inpatient □ Emergency Room/Outpatient □ Dead on Arrival | IF DEATH OCCURRED SOMEWHERE OTHER THAN A HOSPITAL: □ Hospice facility □ Nursing home/Long term care facility □ Decedent's home □ Other (Specify):

15. FACILITY NAME (If not institution, give street & number) | 16. CITY OR TOWN , STATE, AND ZIP CODE | 17. COUNTY OF DEATH

18. METHOD OF DISPOSITION: □ Burial □ Cremation □ Donation □ Entombment □ Removal from State □ Other (Specify): | 19. PLACE OF DISPOSITION (Name of cemetery, crematory, other place)

20. LOCATION-CITY, TOWN, AND STATE | 21. NAME AND COMPLETE ADDRESS OF FUNERAL FACILITY

22. SIGNATURE OF FUNERAL SERVICE LICENSEE OR OTHER AGENT | 23. LICENSE NUMBER (Of Licensee)

NAME OF DECEDENT For use by physician or institution / To Be Completed/ Verified By: FUNERAL DIRECTOR:

ITEMS 24-28 MUST BE COMPLETED BY PERSON WHO PRONOUNCES OR CERTIFIES DEATH | 24. DATE PRONOUNCED DEAD (Mo/Day/Yr) | 25. TIME PRONOUNCED DEAD

26. SIGNATURE OF PERSON PRONOUNCING DEATH (Only when applicable) | 27. LICENSE NUMBER | 28. DATE SIGNED (Mo/Day/Yr)

29. ACTUAL OR PRESUMED DATE OF DEATH (Mo/Day/Yr) (Spell Month) | 30. ACTUAL OR PRESUMED TIME OF DEATH | 31. WAS MEDICAL EXAMINER OR CORONER CONTACTED? □ Yes □ No

CAUSE OF DEATH (See instructions and examples) | Approximate interval: Onset to death

32. PART I. Enter the chain of events--diseases, injuries, or complications--that directly caused the death. DO NOT enter terminal events such as cardiac arrest, respiratory arrest, or ventricular fibrillation without showing the etiology. DO NOT ABBREVIATE. Enter only one cause on a line. Add additional lines if necessary.

IMMEDIATE CAUSE (Final disease or condition ——→ resulting in death)   a._____   Due to (or as a consequence of):

Sequentially list conditions, if any, leading to the cause listed on line a. Enter the **UNDERLYING CAUSE** (disease or injury that initiated the events resulting in death) **LAST**   b._____   Due to (or as a consequence of):

c._____   Due to (or as a consequence of):

d._____

PART II. Enter other significant conditions contributing to death but not resulting in the underlying cause given in PART I | 33. WAS AN AUTOPSY PERFORMED? □ Yes □ No

34. WERE AUTOPSY FINDINGS AVAILABLE TO COMPLETE THE CAUSE OF DEATH? □ Yes □ No

35. DID TOBACCO USE CONTRIBUTE TO DEATH? □ Yes □ Probably □ No □ Unknown | 36. IF FEMALE: □ Not pregnant within past year □ Pregnant at time of death □ Not pregnant, but pregnant within 42 days of death □ Not pregnant, but pregnant 43 days to 1 year before death □ Unknown if pregnant within the past year | 37. MANNER OF DEATH □ Natural □ Homicide □ Accident □ Pending Investigation □ Suicide □ Could not be determined

38. DATE OF INJURY (Mo/Day/Yr) (Spell Month) | 39. TIME OF INJURY | 40. PLACE OF INJURY (e.g., Decedent's home; construction site; restaurant; wooded area) | 41. INJURY AT WORK? □ Yes □ No

42. LOCATION OF INJURY: State: City or Town:
Street & Number: Apartment No.:   Zip Code:

43. DESCRIBE HOW INJURY OCCURRED: | 44. IF TRANSPORTATION INJURY, SPECIFY: □ Driver/Operator □ Passenger □ Pedestrian □ Other (Specify)

45. CERTIFIER (Check only one):
□ Certifying physician-To the best of my knowledge, death occurred due to the cause(s) and manner stated.
□ Pronouncing & Certifying physician-To the best of my knowledge, death occurred at the time, date, and place, and due to the cause(s) and manner stated.
□ Medical Examiner/Coroner-On the basis of examination, and/or investigation, in my opinion, death occurred at the time, date, a nd place, and due to the cause(s) and manner stated.
Signature of certifier:_____

46. NAME, ADDRESS, AND ZIP CODE OF PERSON COMPLETING CAUSE OF DEATH (Item 32)

47. TITLE OF CERTIFIER | 48. LICENSE NUMBER | 49. DATE CERTIFIED (Mo/Day/Yr) | 50. **FOR REGISTRAR ONLY**- DATE FILED (Mo/Day/Yr)

To Be Completed By: MEDICAL CERTIFIER

51. DECEDENT'S EDUCATION-Check the box that best describes the highest degree or level of school completed at the time of death.
□ 8th grade or less
□ 9th - 12th grade; no diploma
□ High school graduate or GED completed
□ Some college credit, but no degree
□ Associate degree (e.g., AA, AS)
□ Bachelor's degree (e.g., BA, AB, BS)
□ Master's degree (e.g., MA, MS, MEng, MEd, MSW, MBA)
□ Doctorate (e.g., PhD, EdD) or Professional degree (e.g., MD, DDS, DVM, LLB, JD)

52. DECEDENT OF HISPANIC ORIGIN? Check the box that best describes whether the decedent is Spanish/Hispanic/Latino. Check the "No" box if decedent is not Spanish/Hispanic/Latino.
□ No, not Spanish/Hispanic/Latino
□ Yes, Mexican, Mexican American, Chicano
□ Yes, Puerto Rican
□ Yes, Cuban
□ Yes, other Spanish/Hispanic/Latino (Specify) _____

53. DECEDENT'S RACE (Check one or more races to indicate what the decedent considered himself or herself to be)
□ White
□ Black or African American
□ American Indian or Alaska Native (Name of the enrolled or principal tribe) _____
□ Asian Indian
□ Chinese
□ Filipino
□ Japanese
□ Korean
□ Vietnamese
□ Other Asian (Specify)_____
□ Native Hawaiian
□ Guamanian or Chamorro
□ Samoan
□ Other Pacific Islander (Specify)_____
□ Other (Specify)_____

54. DECEDENT'S USUAL OCCUPATION (Indicate type of work done during most of working life. DO NOT USE RETIRED).

55. KIND OF BUSINESS/INDUSTRY

To Be Completed By: FUNERAL DIRECTOR

REV. 11/2003

Fig. 4.20 US standard certificate of death. (From Centers for Disease Control and Prevention. https://www.cdc.gov/nchs/data/dvs/death11-03final-acc.pdf. Accessed June 7, 2017.)

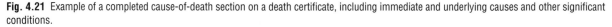

CAUSE OF DEATH (See instructions and examples)		Approximate interval: Onset to death
32. **PART I.** Enter the <u>chain of events</u>--diseases, injuries, or complications--that directly caused the death. DO NOT enter terminal events such as cardiac arrest, respiratory arrest, or ventricular fibrillation without showing the etiology. DO NOT ABBREVIATE. Enter only one cause on a line. Add additional lines if necessary.		
IMMEDIATE CAUSE (Final disease or condition ---------> resulting in death)	a. Rupture of myocardium	Mins
	Due to (or as a consequence of):	
Sequentially list conditions, if any, leading to the cause listed on line a. Enter the **UNDERLYING CAUSE** (disease or injury that initiated the events resulting in death) **LAST**	b. Acute myocardial infarction	6 days
	Due to (or as a consequence of):	
	c. Chronic ischemic heart disease	5 years
	Due to (or as a consequence of):	
	d.	
PART II. Enter other <u>significant conditions contributing to death</u> but not resulting in the underlying cause given in PART I	33. WAS AN AUTOPSY PERFORMED? □ Yes □ No	
Diabetes, Chronic obstructive pulmonary disease, smoking	34. WERE AUTOPSY FINDINGS AVAILABLE TO COMPLETE THE CAUSE OF DEATH? □ Yes □ No	

Fig. 4.21 Example of a completed cause-of-death section on a death certificate, including immediate and underlying causes and other significant conditions.

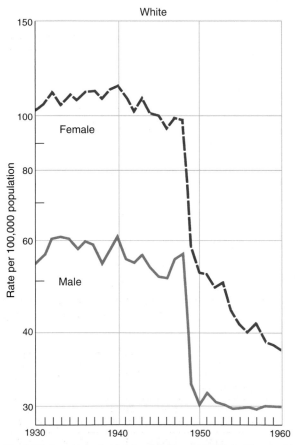

Fig. 4.22 Drop in death rates for diabetes among 55- to 64-year-old men and women, United States, 1930–60, due to changes in International Classification of Diseases coding. (From *US Public Health Service Publication No. 1000, Series 3, No. 1*. Washington, DC: US Government Printing Office; 1964.)

TABLE 4.5 **Crude Mortality Rates by Race, State of Maryland, United States 2015**	
Race	**Mortality per 1,000 Population**
White	9.95
Black	7.35

Comparing Mortality in Different Populations

An important use of mortality data is to compare two or more populations, or one population in different time periods. Such populations may differ with regard to many characteristics that affect mortality, of which the age distribution is the most important. In fact, age is the single most important predictor of mortality. Therefore methods have been developed for comparing mortality in such populations while effectively holding constant characteristics such as age.

Table 4.5 shows data that exemplify this problem. Mortality rates for white and black residents of the State of Maryland in 2015 are given. The data may seem surprising because we would expect rates to have been higher for blacks, given the problems associated with poorer living conditions and less access to medical care. When we look at Table 4.6, we see the data from Table 4.5 on the left, but now we have added data for each age-specific stratum (layer) of the population. Interestingly, although in each age-specific group, mortality is higher in blacks than in whites, the overall mortality (also called *crude* or *unadjusted mortality*) is

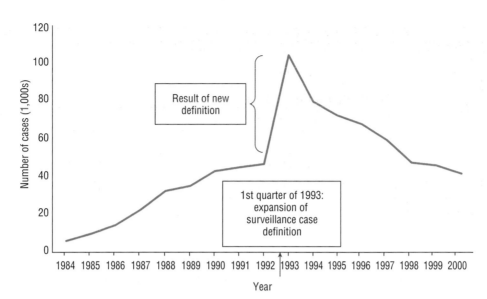

Fig. 4.23 Acquired immunodeficiency syndrome cases by quarter year of report, United States, 1984–2000. (From Centers for Disease Control and Prevention. Summary of notifiable diseases, United States, 2000. *MMWR.* 2000;49:86; and Centers for Disease Control and Prevention. Summary of notifiable diseases, United States, 1993. *MMWR.* 1993;45:68.)

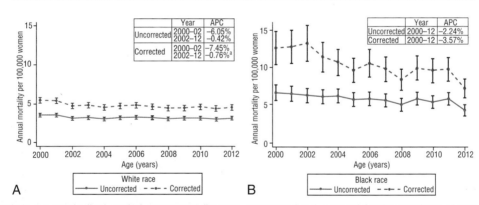

Fig. 4.24 Trends in age-standardized cervical cancer mortality rates, uncorrected and corrected for the prevalence of hysterectomy, from 2000–2012 for (A) white and (B) black women. *APC,* Annual percentage change. (From Beavis AL, Gravitt PE, Rositch AF. Hysterectomy-corrected cervical cancer mortality rates reveal a larger racial disparity in the United States. *Cancer.* 2017;123:1044–1050.)

TABLE 4.6	Death Rates by Age and Race, State of Maryland, 2015											
	DEATH RATES BY AGE PER 1,000 POPULATION[a]											
Race	All Ages	<1 Year	1–4 Years	5–14 Years	15–24 Years	25–34 Years	35–44 Years	45–54 Years	55–64 Years	65–74 Years	75–84 Years	>85 Years
White	9.95	4.06	0.21	0.11	0.64	1.29	1.73	3.62	7.68	16.45	45.39	138.7
Black	7.35	11.25	0.43	0.18	1.14	1.74	2.23	5.09	11.14	21.55	49.49	124.45

[a]Age-adjusted to the 2000 US population.

From Maryland Vital Statistics Annual Report; 2015. https://health.maryland.gov/vsa/Documents/15annual.pdf. Accessed June 8, 2017. Certain data were provided by the Vital Statistics Administration, Maryland Department of Health, Baltimore, Maryland. The Department disclaims responsibility for any analyses, interpretations, or conclusions.

higher in whites than in blacks. Why is this so? This is a reflection of the fact that in both whites and blacks, mortality increases markedly in the oldest age groups; older age is the major contributor to mortality. However, the white population in this example is older than the black population, and in 2015, there were few blacks in the oldest age groups. Thus, in whites, the overall mortality is heavily weighted by high rates in the oldest age groups. The overall (or crude) mortality rate in whites is increased by the greater number of deaths in the large subgroup of older whites, but the overall mortality rate in blacks is not increased as much

because there are so many fewer deaths in the small number of blacks in the older age groups. Clearly, the crude mortality reflects both differences in the force of mortality and differences in the age composition of the population. Let us look at two approaches for dealing with this problem: direct and indirect age adjustment.

DIRECT AGE ADJUSTMENT

Tables 4.7 through 4.9 show a hypothetical example of direct age adjustment. Table 4.7 shows mortality in a population in two different time periods. The mortality

TABLE 4.7   Hypothetical Example of Direct Age Adjustment: I. Comparison of Total Death Rates in a Population at Two Different Times

EARLY PERIOD			LATER PERIOD		
Population	No. of Deaths	Death Rate per 100,000	Population	No. of Deaths	Death Rate per 100,000
900,000	862	96	900,000	1,130	126

TABLE 4.8   Hypothetical Example of Direct Age Adjustment: II. Comparison of Age-Specific Death Rates in Two Different Time Periods

	EARLY PERIOD			LATER PERIOD		
Age Group (years)	Population	No. of Deaths	Death Rates per 100,000	Population	No. of Deaths	Death Rates per 100,000
All ages	900,000	862	96	900,000	1,130	126
30–49	500,000	60	12	300,000	30	10
50–69	300,000	396	132	400,000	400	100
70+	100,000	406	406	200,000	700	350

TABLE 4.9   Hypothetical Example of Direct Age Adjustment: III. Carrying Out an Age Adjustment Using the Total of the Two Populations as the Standard

Age Group (years)	Standard Population	"Early" Age-Specific Mortality Rates per 100,000	Expected No. of Deaths Using "Early" Rates	"Later" Age-Specific Mortality Rates per 100,000	Expected No. of Deaths Using "Later" Rates
All ages	1,800,000				
30–49	800,000	12	96	10	80
50–69	700,000	132	924	100	700
70+	300,000	406	1,218	350	1,050
Total no. of deaths expected in the standard population:			2,238		1,830
Age-adjusted rates:		"Early" $= \dfrac{2,238}{1,800,000} = 124.3$		"Later" $= \dfrac{1,830}{1,800,000} = 101.7$	

rate is considerably higher in the later period. These data are supplemented with age-specific data in Table 4.8. Here, we see three age groups, and age-specific mortality for the later period is lower in each group. How, then, is it possible to account for the higher overall mortality in the later period in this example?

The answer lies in the changing age structure of the population. Mortality is highest in the oldest age groups, and during the later period, the size of the oldest group doubled from 100,000 to 200,000, whereas the number of young people declined substantially, from 500,000 to 300,000. We would like to eliminate this age difference and, in effect, ask: if the age composition of the populations were the same, would there be any differences in mortality between the early period and the later period?

In *direct age adjustment*, a standard population is used in order to eliminate the effects of any differences in age between two or more populations being compared (see Table 4.9). A hypothetical "standard" population is created to which we apply both the age-specific mortality rates from the early period and the age-specific mortality rates from the later period. By applying mortality rates from both periods to a single standard population, we eliminate any possibility that observed differences could be a result of age differences in the population. (In this example, we have created a standard by adding the populations from the early and the later periods, but any population could have been used.)

By applying each age-specific mortality rate to the population in each age group of the standard population, we derive the expected number of deaths that would have occurred had those rates been applied. We can then calculate the total number of deaths expected in the standard population had the age-specific rates of the early period applied and the total number of deaths expected in the standard population had the age-specific rates of the later period applied. Dividing each of these two total expected numbers of deaths by the total standard population, we can calculate an expected mortality rate in the standard population if it had had the mortality experience of the early period and the expected mortality rate for the standard population if it had had the mortality experience for the later period. These are called *age-adjusted rates*, and they appropriately reflect the decline seen in the age-specific rates.

Differences in age-composition of the population are no longer a factor.

In this example the rates have been adjusted for age, but adjustment can be carried out for any characteristic such as sex, socioeconomic status, or race, and techniques are also available to adjust for multiple variables simultaneously.

Although age-adjusted rates can be very useful in making comparisons, the first step in examining and analyzing comparative mortality data should always be to carefully examine the *age-specific* rates for any interesting differences or changes. These differences may be hidden by the *age-adjusted* rates, and may be lost if we proceed immediately to age adjustment without first examining the age-specific rates.

Age-adjusted rates are *hypothetical* because they involve applying actual age-specific rates to a hypothetical standard population. They do not reflect the true mortality risk of a "real" population because the numerical value of an age-adjusted death rate depends on the standard population used. Selection of such a population is somewhat arbitrary because there is no "correct" standard population, but it is generally accepted that the "standard" should not be markedly different from the populations that are being compared with regard to age or whatever the variable is for which the adjustment is being made. In the United States, for more than 50 years, the 1940 US population was regularly used as the standard population for age adjustment for most purposes, but in recent years, this population was increasingly considered outdated and incompatible with the older age structure of the US population. Beginning with 1999 mortality statistics, the US population in the year 2000 replaced the 1940 population as the standard population for adjustment.

The change in standard population to the year 2000 US population has had some significant effects, as illustrated with a comparison of cause-specific mortality rates using data through 1995.[7] These include increases in age-adjusted mortality rates that were observed for causes in which risk increases significantly with age. For example, age-adjusted death from cerebrovascular diseases (stroke) is 26.7 deaths per 100,000 using the 1940 standard, but it is 63.9 per 100,000 using the 2000 standard. Cancer mortality increased using the 2000 population standard compared to when an earlier population was used as a standard because more people are surviving into older ages, when many of the leading types of cancer are more common. Rates for heart disease, chronic obstructive lung disease, diabetes, kidney disease, and Alzheimer's disease were similarly affected because age-specific death rates for all these conditions are higher in older age groups.

Age-adjusted rates of cancer are higher in blacks compared to whites in the United States, but the differential between blacks and whites is less with the 2000 population standard than with the earlier standard population. Thus, the change to the year 2000 US population as the standard complicates comparisons of age-adjusted rates before and after 1999, because many of the rates before 1999 were calculated using the 1940 standard population. However, the rates from 1999 forward are being calculated using the year 2000 population as the new standard.

In summary, the goal of direct adjustment is to compare rates in at least two different populations when we wish to eliminate the possible effect of a given factor, such as age, on the rates we are comparing. It is important to keep in mind that adjusted rates are not "real" rates in the populations being compared, because they depend on the choice of the standard population used in carrying out the adjustment. Nevertheless, direct adjustment is a very useful tool for making such comparisons and in fact, comparison of rates in different populations almost always utilizes direct adjustment, such as adjustment for age. Note that adjustment is based on replacing each population with a common set of weights (the standard population) in order to estimate weighted averages—that is, the adjusted rates.

INDIRECT AGE ADJUSTMENT (STANDARDIZED MORTALITY RATIOS)

Indirect age adjustment is often used when numbers of deaths for each age-specific stratum are not available. It is also used to study mortality in an occupationally exposed population: Do people who work in a certain industry, such as mining or construction, have a higher mortality than people of the same age in the general population? Is an additional risk associated with that occupation?

To answer the question of whether a population of workers has a higher mortality than we would expect in a similar population that is not engaged in the occupation being observed, the age-specific rates for a known population, such as all men of the same age, are applied to each age group in the population of interest. This will yield the number of deaths expected in each age group in the population of interest, if this population had had the mortality experience of the known population. Thus, for each age group, the number of deaths *expected* is calculated, and these numbers are totaled. The numbers of deaths that were actually *observed* in that population are also calculated and totaled. The ratio of the total number of deaths actually observed to the total number of deaths expected, if the population of interest had had the mortality experience of the known population, is then calculated. This ratio is called the *standardized mortality ratio* (*SMR*).

The SMR is defined as follows:

$$\text{SMR} = \frac{\text{Observed no. of deaths per year}}{\text{Expected no. of deaths per year}}$$

Let us look at the example in Table 4.10. In a hypothetical population of 460,463 white male workers, 406 deaths from disease X occurred in 2016. The question we are interested in is whether this mortality experience from disease X is greater than, less than, or about the same as that expected in white men of the same ages in the general population (most of whom are not included in this classification of workers). To help address this question, we may calculate the expected number of deaths for white workers in each age group by applying the known age-specific mortality rate from the general population to the number of workers in each age group. By doing so, we ask, "How many deaths would we expect in these white workers if they had the same mortality experience as white men in the same age group in the general population?" These data are listed in column 3. Column 4 shows the number of deaths observed in the workers.

The SMR is calculated by totaling the observed number of deaths (406) and dividing it by the expected number of deaths (138.8), which yields a result of 2.92. Multiplication by 100 is often done to yield results without decimals. If this were done in this case, the SMR would be 292. An SMR of 100 indicates that the observed number of deaths is the same as the expected

TABLE 4.10 **Hypothetical Computation of a Standardized Mortality Ratio (SMR) for Disease X for White Workers Ages 20–59 Years, 2016**

	Estimated Population for White Workers	Death Rate (per 100,000) for Disease X in Males in the General Population	Expected Deaths From Disease X in White Workers If They Had Same Risk as General Population	Observed Deaths From Disease in White Workers
Age (years)	1	2	$3 = 1 \times 2$	4
20–24	62,253	8.9	5.5	5
25–29	72,732	12.7	9.3	15
30–34	68,500	18.1	12.4	17
35–44	136,525	30.6	41.7	93
45–54	90,304	53.4	48.2	169
55–59	30,149	71.8	21.7	107
Totals	460,463		138.8	406

$$\text{SMR (for 20- to 59-year-olds)} = \frac{406}{138.8} \times 100 = 292$$

TABLE 4.11 **Age-Period Contingency Table for Obesity Prevalence by Age (Rows) and Period (Columns) in the United States, 1971–2006 ($N = 91{,}755$)**

	NHANES I 1971–75	NHANES II 1976–80	NHANES III, Phase 1 1988–91	NHANES III, Phase 2 1991–94	NHANES 99–00 1999–2000	NHANES 01–02 2001–02	NHANES 03–04 2003–04	NHANES 05–06 2005–06
2–4	3.1	3.25	3.48	4.34	7.02	6.29	8.72	8.54
5–9	5.48	7.17	8.75	13.12	17.45	16.92	20.22	16.25
10–14	6.88	7.9	8.93	13.57	18.97	18.72	22.85	21.81
15–19	6.64	5.5	8.31	13.55	18.03	17.8	19.94	18.43
20–24	6.08	7.14	9.87	13.81	20.59	26.67	26.59	24.98
25–29	10.34	10.49	11.97	18.74	27.69	26.55	26.47	35.9
30–34	13.64	13.49	18.02	20.07	31.64	24.82	30.19	36.6
35–39	14.34	14.73	17.24	23.3	29.08	30.19	36.54	33.3
40–44	16.76	15.82	19.27	24.63	32.68	32.85	39.68	42.69
45–49	15.26	18.05	18.85	30.75	31.93	35.83	35.79	38.5
50–54	17.18	17.46	22.37	35.42	40.55	31.69	39.32	38.73
55–59	19.5	19.62	26.55	32.46	35.7	38	38.62	46.9
60–64	18.68	17.57	20.82	30.67	41.37	44.28	34.49	42.67
65–69	16.83	18.51	21.26	27.79	41.23	35.43	38	40.64
70–74	17.15	16.31	18.68	25.03	29.34	34.87	32.48	31.45

NHANES, National Health and Nutrition Examination Survey.
From Keyes KM, Utz RL, Robinson W, Li G. What is a cohort effect? Comparison of three statistical methods for modeling cohort effects in obesity prevalence in the United States, 1971–2006. *Soc Sci Med.* 2010;70(7):1100–1108.

number of deaths. An SMR greater than 100 indicates that the observed number of deaths exceeds the expected number, and an SMR less than 100 indicates that the observed number of deaths is less than the expected number.

THE COHORT EFFECT

Table 4.11 shows age-specific obesity prevalence (%) from 1971 to 2006 in the United States using data from National Center for Health Statistics. (For this discussion, we will ignore the data for age groups 2 to

TABLE 4.12   **Age-Period Contingency Table for Obesity Prevalence by Age (Rows) and Period (Columns) in the United States, 1971–2006 ($N = 91,755$)**

Age (years)	NHANES I 1971–75	NHANES II 1976–80	NHANES III, Phase 1 1988–91	NHANES III, Phase II 1991–94	NHANES 99–00 1999–2000	NHANES 01–02 2001–02	NHANES 03–04 2003–04	NHANES 05–06 2005–06
2–4	3.1	3.25	3.48	4.34	7.02	6.29	8.72	8.54
5–9	5.48	7.17	8.75	13.12	17.45	16.92	20.22	16.25
10–14	6.88	7.9	8.93	13.57	18.97	18.72	22.85	21.81
15–19	6.64	5.5	8.31	13.55	18.03	17.8	19.94	18.43
20–24	**6.08**	7.14	9.87	13.81	20.59	26.67	26.59	24.98
25–29	10.34	**10.49**	11.97	18.74	27.69	26.55	26.47	35.9
30–34	13.64	13.49	**18.02**	20.07	31.64	24.82	30.19	36.6
35–39	14.34	14.73	17.24	**23.3**	29.08	30.19	36.54	33.3
40–44	16.76	15.82	19.27	24.63	**32.68**	32.85	39.68	42.69
45–49	15.26	18.05	18.85	30.75	31.93	**35.83**	35.79	38.5
50–54	17.18	17.46	22.37	35.42	40.55	31.69	**39.32**	38.73
55–59	19.5	19.62	26.55	32.46	35.7	38	38.62	**46.9**
60–64	18.68	17.57	20.82	30.67	41.37	44.28	34.49	42.67
65–69	16.83	18.51	21.26	27.79	41.23	35.43	38	40.64
70–74	17.15	16.31	18.68	25.03	29.34	34.87	32.48	31.45

Bold black boxes denote persons who were 20 to 24 years of age during the 1971–1975 cycle and were followed over time, forming a cohort.

NHANES, National Health and Nutrition Examination Survey.

From Keyes KM, Utz RL, Robinson W, Li G. What is a cohort effect? Comparison of three statistical methods for modeling cohort effects in obesity prevalence in the United States, 1971–2006. *Soc Sci Med.* 2010;70(7):1100–1108.

19 years, since childhood obesity is a somewhat different phenomenon.) If, for example, we then read *down* the column in the table (the data for a given National Health and Nutrition Examination Survey [NHANES] cycle) for 1971–75, it appears that obesity prevalence peaks in the age group 55 to 59 years and then declines with advancing age. Such a view of the data, by year, is called a *cross-sectional view.*

Actually, however, the picture of obesity prevalence is somewhat different (Table 4.12). A person who was 20 to 24 years of age in 1971 was 25 to 29 years of age in 1976. In other words, persons who were born in a certain year are moving through time together. We can now examine the obesity prevalence over time of the same cohort (i.e., a group of people who share the same experience), born in the same 5-year period. Looking at persons who were 20 to 24 years of age in the 1971–75 cycle and following them over time, as indicated by the bold black boxes in the table, it is apparent that obesity prevalence for this *cohort* has been increasing throughout the years and did not decline

later on, as we have seen in the cross-sectional view of the data. When we examine changes in prevalence over time, we should always ask whether any apparent changes that are observed could be the result of such a cohort effect.

INTERPRETING OBSERVED CHANGES IN MORTALITY

If we find a difference in mortality over time or between populations—either an increase or a decrease—it may be an artifact or it may be real. If it is an artifact, the artifact could result from problems with either the numerator or the denominator (Table 4.13). However, if we conclude that the change is real, what could be the possible explanation? Some possibilities are seen in Box 4.3.

Other Measures of the Impact of Disease

QUALITY OF LIFE

Most diseases have a major impact on the afflicted individuals above and beyond mortality. Diseases that

TABLE 4.13 Possible Explanations of Trends or Differences in Mortality: I. Artifactual

1. Numerator	Errors in diagnosis
	Errors in age
	Changes in coding rules
	Changes in classification
2. Denominator	Errors in counting population
	Errors in classifying by demographic characteristics (e.g., age, race, sex)
	Differences in percentages of populations at risk

BOX 4.3 POSSIBLE EXPLANATIONS OF TRENDS OR DIFFERENCES IN MORTALITY: II. REAL

Change in survivorship without change in incidence
Change in incidence
Change in age composition of the population(s)
A combination of the above factors

may not be lethal may be associated with considerable physical and emotional suffering resulting from disability associated with the illness. It is therefore important to consider the total impact of a disease as measured by its effect on a person's quality of life, even though such measures are not, in fact, measures of disease occurrence. For example, it is possible to examine the extent to which patients with arthritis are compromised by the illness in carrying out activities of daily living. Although considerable controversy exists about which quality-of-life measures are most appropriate and valid, there is general agreement that such measures can be reasonably used to plan short-term treatment programs for groups of patients. Such patients can be evaluated over a period of months to determine the effects of the treatment on their self-reported quality of life. Quality-of-life measures have also been used for establishing priorities in situations of scarce health care resources. Although prioritizing health care resources is often primarily based on mortality data, quality of life must also be taken into account for this purpose, because many diseases are chronic and non–life-threatening but may be associated with many years of disability. Patients

may place different weights on different quality-of-life measures depending on differences in their occupations and other activities, personalities, cultural backgrounds, education, and moral and ethical values. As a result, measuring quality of life and developing valid indices that are useful for obtaining comparative data in different patients and in different populations remain major challenges.

PROJECTING THE FUTURE BURDEN OF DISEASE

An interesting and valuable use of current data to predict the future impact of disease was a comprehensive assessment of current mortality and disability from diseases, injuries, and risk factors for all regions of the world in 1990, which was projected to the year 2020. The study, titled the Global Burden of Disease, attempted to quantify not only deaths but also the impact of premature death and disability on a population and to combine these into a single index to express the overall "burden of disease."[8] The index that was developed for this study is the disability-adjusted life year (DALY), which is the number of years of life lost to premature death and years lived with a disability of specified severity and duration. Thus, a DALY is 1 lost year of healthy life.

The results showed that 5 of the 10 leading causes of disability in 1990 were psychiatric conditions; psychiatric and neurologic conditions accounted for 28% of all years lived with disability of known severity and duration, compared with 1.4% of all deaths and 1.1% of years of life lost. Fig. 4.25 shows selected leading causes of disease burden globally in both high-income and low-income countries in 2015.[9] Again, the importance of ischemic heart disease in high-income countries and lower respiratory tract infections in low-income countries is dramatically evident.

In 2015 the disease burden was not equitably distributed. As seen in Table 4.14, the top 20 causes of disease burden were responsible for 55.7% of all DALYs. Five of them primarily affect children younger than 5 years of age. Three of the top 10 (ischemic heart disease, stroke, and depression) are chronic conditions. This table shows the value of using a measure such as DALYs to assess the burden of disease, a measure that is not limited to either morbidity or mortality, but is weighted by both.

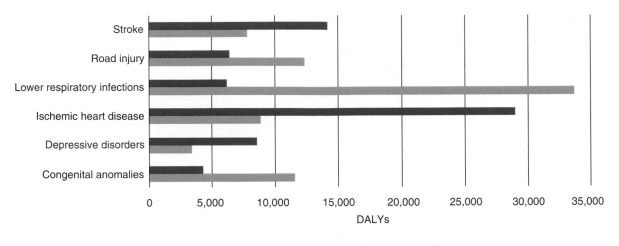

Fig. 4.25 Selected causes of disease burden by low- versus high-income countries, 2015. *DALYs,* Disability-adjusted life years. (From Global Health Estimates 2015. *Disease Burden by Cause, Age, Sex, by Country and by Region, 2000–2015.* Geneva, Switzerland: World Health Organization; 2016.)

Rank	Cause	DALYs (000s)	% DALYs	DALYs per 100,000 Population
TABLE 4.14	**Global Health Estimates 2015: 20 Leading Causes of DALYs Globally, 2015**			
0	**All Causes**	**2,668,296**	**100.0**	**36,331**
1	Ischemic heart disease	192,056	7.2	2,615
2	Lower respiratory infections	142,384	5.3	1,939
3	Stroke	139,874	5.2	1,905
4	Preterm birth complications	102,297	3.8	1,393
5	Diarrheal diseases	84,928	3.2	1,156
6	Road injury	76,020	2.8	1,035
7	Chronic obstructive pulmonary disease	72,815	2.7	991
8	Diabetes mellitus	70,667	2.6	962
9	Birth asphyxia and birth trauma	67,266	2.5	916
10	Congenital anomalies	64,825	2.4	883
11	HIV/AIDS	62,759	2.4	855
12	Tuberculosis	56,037	2.1	763
13	Depressive disorders	54,215	2.0	738
14	Iron-deficiency anemia	52,080	2.0	709
15	Back and neck pain	52,016	1.9	708
16	Cirrhosis of the liver	41,486	1.6	565
17	Trachea, bronchus, lung cancers	41,129	1.5	560
18	Malaria	38,520	1.4	524
19	Kidney diseases	38,104	1.4	519
20	Self-harm	37,672	1.4	513

AIDS, Acquired immunodeficiency syndrome; *DALYs,* disability-adjusted life years; *HIV,* human immunodeficiency virus.
Data from World Health Organization. Health statistics and information systems. http://www.who.int/healthinfo/global_burden_disease/estimates/en/index2.html. Accessed June 9, 2017. From *The Global Burden of Disease: 2004 Update.* Geneva, Switzerland: World Health Organization; 2004.

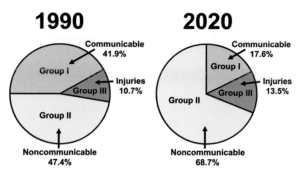

Fig. 4.26 The "epidemiologic transition": distribution of deaths from communicable and noncommunicable causes in developing countries, 1990 and projected into 2020. (From Murray CJL, Lopez AD. *The Global Burden of Disease: a Comprehensive Assessment of Mortality and Disability from Diseases, Injuries, and Risk Factors in 1990 and Projected to 2020.* Cambridge: Harvard University Press on behalf of the World Health Organization and the World Bank; 1996.)

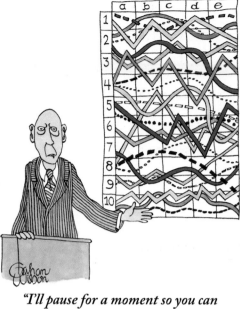

"I'll pause for a moment so you can let this information sink in."

Fig. 4.27 "I'll pause for a moment so you can let this information sink in." (Gahan Wilson/The New Yorker Collection/The Cartoon Bank.)

With the aging of the population worldwide and advances in economic development, particularly in low- and middle-income countries, an "epidemiologic transition" is taking place so that, by 2020, noncommunicable diseases are likely to account for 70% of all deaths in developing countries. As projected in Fig. 4.26, by 2020, the disease burden due to communicable diseases, maternal and perinatal conditions, and nutritional deficiencies (group I) is expected to decrease dramatically. The burden due to noncommunicable diseases (group II) is expected to increase sharply, as will the burden from injuries (group III). Also by 2020, the burden of disease attributable to tobacco is expected to exceed that caused by any single disease—clearly a strong call for public health action. Although there is no universal agreement on the methodology or applicability of a single measure of disease burden such as the DALY, this study is an excellent demonstration of an attempt at worldwide surveillance designed to develop such a measure to permit valid regional comparisons and future projections so that appropriate interventions can be developed.

Conclusion

Chapters 3 and 4 have reviewed important approaches to quantitatively measuring and expressing human morbidity and mortality. The concepts reviewed in these chapters may at first seem overwhelming (Fig. 4.27)

but, as we shall see in later chapters, they are critical to understanding how epidemiology helps us to elucidate the measurement of disease risk, the determination of disease causation, and the evaluation of the effectiveness of intervening to modify the disease process.

In Chapter 5, we will turn to questions about the numerators of morbidity rates: how do we identify those people who have a disease and distinguish them from those who do not, and how do we evaluate the quality of the diagnostic and screening tests that are used to separate these individuals and populations? A discussion of the use of screening tests in public health programs is presented in Chapter 18.

REFERENCES

1. De Beauvoir S. *A Very Easy Death.* Translated by Patrick O'Brian. New York: Pantheon Books; 1965.
2. Centers for Disease Control and Prevention. Premature mortality in the United States: public health issues in the use of years of potential life lost. *MMWR Suppl.* 1986;35:1S–11S.
3. Lim H, Devesa SS, Sosa JA, et al. Trends in thyroid cancer incidence and mortality in the United States, 1974–2013. *JAMA.* 2017;317(13):1338–1348.

4. National Center for Health Statistics (NCHS). *Instructions for Classifying the Underlying Cause of Death.* Hyattsville, MD: NCHS; 1983.

5. Chamblee RF, Evans MC. TRANSAX: *The NCHS System for Producing Multiple Cause-of-Death Statistics, 1968–1978.* Vital and Health Statistics, Series 1, No. 20, DHHS Publication No. (PHS) 86–1322. Washington, DC: Bureau of Vital and Health Statistics; June 1986.

6. Savage G, Rohde FC, Grant B, et al. *Liver Cirrhosis Mortality in the United States, 1970–90: Surveillance Report No. 29.* Bethesda,

MD: Department of Health and Human Services; December 1993.

7. Anderson RN, Rosenberg HM. *Age Standardization of Death Rates: Implementation of the Year 2000 Standard.* National Vital Statistics Reports, Vol. 47, No. 3, pp. 1–16. Hyattsville, MD: National Center for Health Statistics; October 7, 1998.

8. Murray CJL, Lopez AD. *The Global Burden of Disease.* Cambridge, MA: Harvard University Press; 1996.

9. World Health Organization (WHO). *The Global Burden of Disease: 2015 Update.* Geneva, Switzerland: WHO; 2015.

REVIEW QUESTIONS FOR CHAPTER 4

Questions 1 and 2 are based on the information given below:

In an Asian country with a population of 6 million people, 60,000 deaths occurred during the year ending December 31, 2010. These included 30,000 deaths from cholera in 100,000 people who were sick with cholera.

1 *What was the cause-specific mortality rate from cholera in 2010?* _____

2 *What was the case-fatality from cholera in 2010?* _____

3 *Age-adjusted death rates are used to:*
a. Correct death rates for errors in the statement of age
b. Determine the actual number of deaths that occurred in specific age groups in a population
c. Correct death rates for missing age information
d. Compare deaths in persons of the same age group
e. Eliminate the effects of differences in the age distributions of populations in comparing death rates

4 *The mortality rate from disease X in city A is 75/100,000 in persons 65 to 69 years old. The mortality rate from the same disease in city B is 150/100,000 in persons 65 to 69 years old. The inference that disease X is two times more prevalent in persons 65 to 69 years old in city B than it is in persons 65 to 69 years old in city A is:*
a. Correct
b. Incorrect, because of failure to distinguish between prevalence and mortality
c. Incorrect, because of failure to adjust for differences in age distributions
d. Incorrect, because of failure to distinguish between period and point prevalence
e. Incorrect, because a proportion is used when a rate is required to support the inference

5 *The incidence rate of a disease is five times greater in women than in men, but the prevalence rates show no sex difference. The best explanation is that:*
a. The crude all-cause mortality rate is greater in women
b. The case-fatality from this disease is greater in women
c. The case-fatality from this disease is lower in women
d. The duration of this disease is shorter in men
e. Risk factors for the disease are more common in women

6 *For a disease such as pancreatic cancer, which is highly fatal and of short duration:*
a. Incidence rates and mortality rates will be similar
b. Mortality rates will be much higher than incidence rates
c. Incidence rates will be much higher than mortality rates
d. Incidence rates will be unrelated to mortality rates
e. None of the above

7 *In 1990, there were 4,500 deaths due to lung diseases in miners aged 20 to 64 years. The expected number of deaths in this occupational group, based on age-specific death rates from lung diseases in all males aged 20 to 64 years, was 1,800 during 1990. What was the standardized mortality ratio (SMR) for lung diseases in miners? _____*

Question 8 is based on the information given below:

Annual Cancer Deaths in White Male Workers in Two Industries				
	INDUSTRY A		INDUSTRY B	
Cancer Site	No. of Deaths	% of All Cancer Deaths	No. of Deaths	% of All Cancer Deaths
Respiratory system	180	33	248	45
Digestive system	160	29	160	29
Genitourinary	80	15	82	15
All other sites	130	23	60	11
Totals	550	100	550	100

Based on the preceding information, it was concluded that workers in industry B are at higher risk of death from respiratory system cancer than workers in industry A. (Assume that the age distributions of the workers in the two industries are nearly identical.)

8 *Which of the following statements is true?*
  a. The conclusion reached is correct
  b. The conclusion reached may be incorrect because proportionate mortality rates were used when age-specific mortality rates were needed
  c. The conclusion reached may be incorrect because there was no comparison group
  d. The conclusion reached may be incorrect because proportionate mortality was used when cause-specific mortality rates were needed
  e. None of the above

9 *A program manager from an international health funding agency needs to identify regions that would benefit from an intervention aimed at reducing premature disability. The program manager asks a health care consultant to develop a proposal using an index that would help her make this decision. Which of the following would best serve this purpose?*
  a. Case-fatality
  b. Crude mortality rate
  c. Disability-adjusted life-years
  d. Standardized mortality ratio

10 *The following are standardized mortality ratios (SMRs) for lung cancer in England:*

	STANDARDIZED MORTALITY RATIOS	
Occupation	1949–60	1968–79
Carpenters	209	135
Bricklayers	142	118

Based on these SMRs alone, it is possible to conclude that:
  a. The number of deaths from lung cancer in carpenters in 1949–60 was greater than the number of deaths from lung cancer in bricklayers during the same period
  b. The proportionate mortality from lung cancer in bricklayers in 1949–60 was greater than the proportionate mortality from lung cancer in the same occupational group in 1968–79

c. The age-adjusted rate of death from lung cancer in bricklayers was greater in 1949–60 than it was in 1968–79

d. The rate of death from lung cancer in carpenters in 1968–79 was greater than would have been expected for a group of men of similar ages in all occupations

e. The proportionate mortality rate from lung cancer in carpenters in 1968–79 was 1.35 times greater than would have been expected for a group of men of similar ages in all occupations

Questions 11, 12, and 13 are based on the information given below:

Numbers of People and Deaths from Disease Z by Age Group in Communities X and Y				
	COMMUNITY X		**COMMUNITY Y**	
Age Group	**No. of People**	**No. of Deaths From Disease Z**	**No. of People**	**No. of Deaths From Disease Z**
Young	8,000	69	5,000	48
Old	11,000	115	3,000	60

Calculate the age-adjusted death rate for disease Z in communities X and Y by the direct method, using the total of both communities as the standard population.

11 *The age-adjusted death rate from disease Z for community X is:* _____

12 *The proportionate mortality from disease Z for community Y is:* _____
   a. 9.6/1,000
   b. 13.5/1,000
   c. 20.0/1,000
   d. 10.8/1,000
   e. None of the above

13 *Which of the following statements regarding direct adjustment is TRUE?*
   a. The age-adjusted mortality rate of community X is still higher than the mortality rate of community Y, as compared to the crude mortality rate
   b. Age-adjusted mortality rates for community X should be used to make decisions regarding allocation of funding for hospital care of the dying in community X
   c. For direct age-adjustment, the weight for a given age category is the percentage of deaths for that age group
   d. For direct age-adjustment, the weight for a given age category is the number of individuals in the standard population for that age group
   e. The difference in the adjusted mortality rates between community X and community Y is always attributable to differences in age composition between the two populations

14 *Surveillance data indicate that the prevalence of chronic liver disease in the United States increased 104% between the years 1990 and 2008. While chronic liver disease occurs in persons of all ages, the highest mortality rate occurs in people 65 years old or older. The United States has proportionately more people 65 years or older than Country X. What would happen if crude mortality rates in the United States were age standardized to the population of Country X in order to compare the risk of dying of chronic liver disease in the two populations?*
   a. The age-standardized mortality rate for the United States would be less than the crude mortality rate for the United States
   b. The age-standardized mortality rate for the United States would be greater than the crude mortality rate for the United States

c. The age-standardized mortality rate for the United States would be the same as the crude mortality rate for the United States

d. The age-standardized mortality rate for the United States cannot be used for this comparison

e. The age-standardized mortality rate for the United States would be the same as the proportionate mortality rate

15 *Among workers in a fish processing plant, 30% of all deaths were due to myocardial infarction. Among workers in a brewery, 10% of all deaths were due to myocardial infarction. Investigators concluded that workers in the fish processing plant had a greater risk of death due to myocardial infarction than workers in the brewery. This conclusion:*

a. Is correct

b. May be incorrect because it is based on proportionate mortality

c. May be incorrect because it assumes the same case fatality for myocardial infarction in both work sites

d. May be incorrect because consumed fish oil is protective against death due to myocardial infarction

e. May be incorrect because the prevalence of myocardial infarction in the two groups is not known

Chapter 5

Assessing the Validity and Reliability of Diagnostic and Screening Tests

A normal individual is a person who has not been sufficiently examined.

—Anonymous

Learning Objectives

- To define the validity and reliability of screening and diagnostic tests.
- To compare measures of validity, including sensitivity and specificity.
- To illustrate the use of multiple tests (sequential and simultaneous testing).
- To introduce positive and negative predictive value.
- To address measures of reliability, including percent agreement and kappa.

To understand how a disease is transmitted and develops and to provide appropriate and effective health care, it is necessary to distinguish between people in the population who have the disease and those who do not. This is an important challenge, both clinically, where patient care is the issue, and in the public health arena, where secondary prevention programs involving early disease detection through screening and interventions are fielded and where etiologic studies are conducted to provide a basis for primary prevention, if possible. Thus the quality of screening and diagnostic tests is a critical issue. Regardless of whether the test is a physical examination, a chest x-ray, an electrocardiogram, or a blood or urine assay, the same issue arises: *How good is the test in identifying populations of people with and without the disease in question?* This chapter addresses the question of how we assess the quality of newly available screening and diagnostic tests to make reasonable decisions about their use and interpretation.

Biologic Variation of Human Populations

In using a test to distinguish between individuals with normal and abnormal results, it is important to understand how characteristics are distributed in human populations.

Fig. 5.1 shows the distribution of newly reported confirmed cases of hepatitis C virus infection in Massachusetts for 2009. We can see that there are two peaks of hepatitis C virus infection cases among young adults and middle-aged persons. This type of distribution, in which there are two peaks, is called a *bimodal curve.* The bimodal distribution permits the identification of increased rates of *new cases* among these two distinct age groups, which could be related to different reasons. In this situation, there has been a dramatic increase in hepatitis among injection drug users, a practice associated with sharing of injection equipment that led to this bimodal distribution.

In general, however, most human characteristics are not distributed bimodally. Fig. 5.2 shows the distribution of achieved low-density lipoprotein cholesterol (LDL-C) in participants of a clinical trial to study the safety of intensively reducing LDL-C as compared with less intensive LDL-C level lowering in patients after acute coronary syndrome. In this figure, there is no bimodal curve; what we see is a *unimodal curve*—a single peak. Therefore if we want to separate those in the group who achieved a safe low level of LDL-C, a cutoff level of LDL-C must be set below which people are labeled as achieving the "safe low level" and above which they are not labeled as such. This study shows that there is no obvious level of LDL-C that should be a treatment target. Although we could choose a cutoff based on statistical considerations, as the authors in this study showed, we would ideally like to choose a cutoff

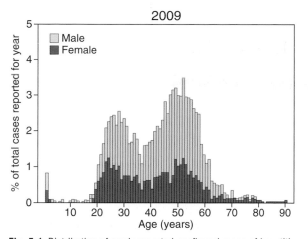

Fig. 5.1 Distribution of newly reported confirmed cases of hepatitis C virus infection in Massachusetts for 2009. (Modified from Centers for Disease Control and Prevention. Hepatitis C virus infection among adolescents and young adults: Massachusetts, 2002–2009. *MMWR Morb Mortal Wkly Rep.* 2011;60:537–541.)

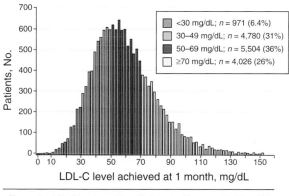

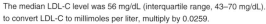

The median LDL-C level was 56 mg/dL (interquartile range, 43–70 mg/dL). to convert LDL-C to millimoles per liter, multiply by 0.0259.

Fig. 5.2 Distribution of achieved calculated low-density lipoprotein cholesterol *(LDL-C)* level at 1 month among patients who did not have a primary efficacy or prespecified safety event prior to the sample. (Data from Giugliano RP, Wiviott SD, Blazing MA, et al. Long-term safety and efficacy of achieving very low levels of low-density lipoprotein cholesterol: a prespecified analysis of the IMPROVE-IT trial. *JAMA Cardiol.* 2017;2:547–555.)

on the basis of some biologic information—that is, we would want to know that an intensive LDL-C lowering strategy below the chosen cutoff level is associated with increased risk of subsequent treatment side effects; adverse muscle, hepatobiliary, and neurocognitive events; or disease complications; hemorrhagic stroke, heart failure, cancer, and noncardiovascular death.

Unfortunately, for many human characteristics, we do not have such information to serve as a guide in setting this level.

In either distribution—unimodal or bimodal—it is usually easy to distinguish between the extreme values of abnormal and normal. With either type of curve, however, uncertainty remains about cases that fall into the gray zone.

Validity of Screening Tests

The *validity* of a test is defined as its ability to distinguish between who has a disease and who does not. Validity has two components: sensitivity and specificity. The *sensitivity* of the test is defined as the ability of the test to identify correctly those who *have* the disease. The *specificity* of the test is defined as the ability of the test to identify correctly those who *do not have* the disease.

TESTS WITH DICHOTOMOUS RESULTS (POSITIVE OR NEGATIVE)

Suppose we have a hypothetical population of 1,000 people, of whom 100 have a certain disease and 900 do not. A test is available that gives either positive or negative results. We want to use this test to distinguish persons who have the disease from those who do not. The results obtained by applying the test to this population of 1,000 people are shown in Table 5.1.

How good was the test? First, how good was the test in correctly identifying those who had the disease? Table 5.1 indicates that of the 100 people with the disease, 80 were correctly identified as "positive" by the test, and a positive identification was missed in 20. Thus the *sensitivity* of the test, which is defined as the proportion of diseased people who were correctly identified as "positive" by the test, is 80/100, or 80%.

Second, how good was the test in correctly identifying those who did not have the disease? Looking again at Table 5.1, of the 900 people who did not have the disease, the test correctly identified 800 as "negative." The *specificity* of the test, which is defined as the proportion of nondiseased people who are correctly identified as "negative," is therefore 800/900, or 89%.

To calculate the sensitivity and specificity of a test, we must know who "really" has the disease and who "does not" from a source other than the test we are using. We are, in fact, comparing our test results with

TABLE 5.1	**Calculation of the Sensitivity and Specificity of Screening Examinations**

Example: Assume a population of 1,000 people, of whom 100 have the disease and 900 do not have the disease. A screening test is used to identify the 100 people who have the disease.

TRUE CHARACTERISTICS
IN THE POPULATION

Results of Screening	Have the Disease	Do Not Have the Disease	Totals
Positive	80	100	180
Negative	20	800	820
Totals	100	900	1,000

Sensitivity: $\dfrac{80}{100} = 80\%$ Specificity: $\dfrac{800}{900} = 89\%$

some gold standard—an external source of "truth" regarding the disease status of each individual in the population. Sometimes this truth may be the result of another test that has been in use, and sometimes it is the result of a more definitive, and often more invasive, test (e.g., tumor biopsy, cardiac catheterization, or tissue biopsy). However, in real life, when we use a test to identify diseased and nondiseased persons in a population, we clearly do not know who has the disease and who does not. (If this were already established, testing would be pointless.) But to quantitatively assess the sensitivity and specificity of a test, we must have another source of truth with which to compare the test results.

Table 5.2 compares the results of a dichotomous test (results are unambiguously either positive or negative) with the actual disease status. Ideally, we would like all of the tested subjects to fall into the two cells shown in the upper left and lower right on the table: people with the disease who are correctly called "positive" by the test (*true positives*) and people without the disease who are correctly called "negative" by the test

(*true negatives*). Unfortunately, such is rarely if ever the case. Some people who do not have the disease are erroneously called "positive" by the test (*false positives*), and some people with the disease are erroneously called "negative" (*false negatives*).

Why are these issues important? When we conduct a screening program, we often have a large group of people who screened positive, including both people who really have the disease (*true positives*) and people who do not have the disease (*false positives*). The issue of *false positives* is important because all people who screened positive are brought back for more sophisticated and more expensive tests or perhaps undergo an invasive procedure that is not necessary. Of the several problems that result, the first is a burden on the health care system. Another is the anxiety and worry induced in persons who have been told that they have tested positive. Considerable evidence indicates that many people who are labeled "positive" by a screening test never have that label completely erased, even if the results of a subsequent evaluation are negative. For example, children labeled "positive" in

TABLE 5.2	**Comparison of the Results of a Dichotomous Test With Disease Status**	
	TRUE CHARACTERISTICS IN THE POPULATION	
Test Results	**Have the Disease**	**Do Not Have the Disease**
Positive	**True Positive (TP):** Have the disease and test positive	**False Positive (FP):** Do not have the disease but test positive
Negative	**False Negative (FN):** Have the disease but test negative	**True Negative (TN):** Do not have the disease and test negative

$$\text{Sensitivity} = \frac{TP}{TP + FN} \qquad \text{Specificity} = \frac{TN}{TN + FP}$$

a screening program for heart disease may be handled as handicapped by parents and school personnel even after being told that subsequent more definitive tests were negative. In addition, such individuals may be limited in regard to employment and insurability by erroneous interpretation of positive screening test results, even if subsequent tests fail to substantiate any positive finding.

Why is the problem of *false negatives* important? If a person has the disease but is erroneously informed that the test result is negative, and if the disease is a serious one for which effective intervention is available, the problem is indeed critical. For example, if the disease is a type of cancer that is curable only in its early stages, a false-negative result could represent a virtual death sentence. Thus the importance of false-negative results depends on the nature and severity of the disease being

screened for, the effectiveness of available intervention measures, and whether the effectiveness is greater if the intervention is administered early in the natural history of the disease.

TESTS OF CONTINUOUS VARIABLES

So far we have discussed a test with only two possible results: positive or negative. But we often test for a continuous variable, such as blood pressure or blood glucose level, for which there is no obvious "positive" or "negative" result. A decision must therefore be made in establishing a cutoff level above which a test result is considered positive and below which a result is considered negative. Let's consider the diagrams shown in Fig. 5.3.

Fig. 5.3A shows a population of 20 diabetics and 20 nondiabetics who are being screened using a blood

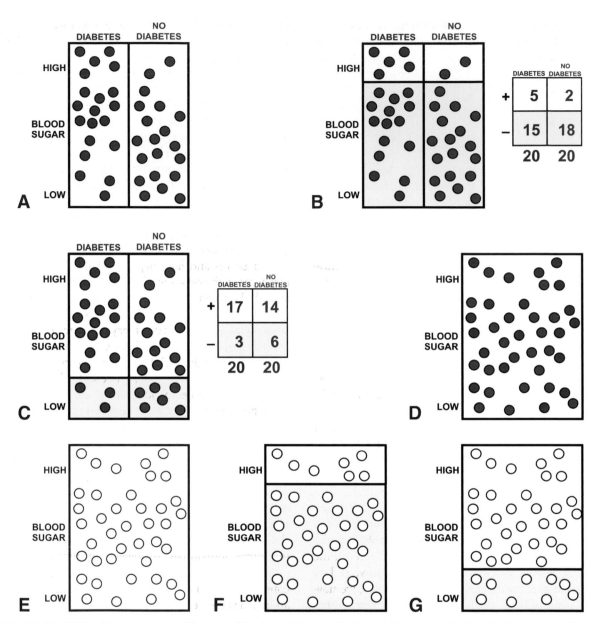

Fig. 5.3 (A to G) The effects of choosing different cutoff levels to define a positive test result when screening for diabetes using a continuous marker, blood sugar, in a hypothetical population. (See discussion in the text under the subheading "Tests of Continuous Variables" on page 97.)

sugar test whose scale is shown along the vertical axis from high to low. The diabetics are represented by blue circles and the nondiabetics by red circles. We see that although blood sugar levels tend to be higher in diabetics than in nondiabetics, no level clearly separates the two groups; there is some overlap of diabetics and

nondiabetics at every blood sugar level. Nevertheless, we must select a cutoff point so that those whose results fall above the cutoff can be called "positive," and can be called back for further testing, and those whose results fall below that point are called "negative," and are not called back for further testing.

Suppose a relatively high cutoff level is chosen (see Fig. 5.3B). Clearly, many of the diabetics will not be identified as positive; on the other hand, most of the nondiabetics will be correctly identified as negative. If these results are distributed on a 2 × 2 table, the sensitivity of the test using this cutoff level will be 25% (5/20) and the specificity will be 90% (18/20). So, most of the diabetics will not be detected, but most of the nondiabetics will be correctly classified.

What if a low cutoff level is chosen (see Fig. 5.3C)? Very few diabetics would be misdiagnosed. What, then, is the problem? A large proportion of the nondiabetics are now identified as positive by the test. As seen in the 2 × 2 table, the sensitivity is now 85% (17/20), but the specificity is only 30% (6/20).

The difficulty is that in the real world, no vertical line separates the diabetics and nondiabetics, and they are indeed mixed together (see Fig. 5.3D); in fact, they are not even distinguishable by red or blue circles (see Fig. 5.3E). So if a high cutoff level is used (see Fig. 5.3F), all those with results below the line will be assured they do not have the disease and will not be followed further; if the low cutoff is used (see Fig. 5.3G), all those with results above the line will be brought back for further testing.

Fig. 5.4A shows actual data from a historical report regarding the distribution of blood sugar levels in diabetics and nondiabetics. Suppose we were to screen this population. If we decide to set the cutoff level so that we identify all of the diabetics (100% sensitivity), we could set the level at 80 mg/dL (see Fig. 5.4B). The problem is, however, that in so doing we will also call many of the nondiabetics positive—that is, the specificity will be very low. On the other hand, if we set the level at 200 mg/dL (see Fig. 5.4C) so that we call all the nondiabetics negative (100% specificity), we now miss many of the true diabetics because the sensitivity will be very low. Thus there is a trade-off between sensitivity and specificity: if we increase the sensitivity by lowering the cutoff level, we decrease the specificity; if we increase the specificity by raising the cutoff level, we decrease the sensitivity. To quote an unknown sage: "There is no such thing as a free lunch."

The dilemma involved in deciding whether to set a high cutoff or a low cutoff rests in the problem of the false positives and the false negatives that result from the testing. It is important to remember that in screening we end up with groups classified only on the basis of the results of their screening tests, either positive or negative. We have no information regarding their true disease status, which, of course, is the reason for carrying out the screening. In effect, the results of the screening test yield not four groups, as seen in Fig. 5.5, but rather two groups: one group of people who tested positive and one group who tested negative. Those who tested positive will be notified of their test result and will be asked to return for additional examinations. The other group, who tested negative, will be notified that their test result was negative and will therefore not be asked to return for further testing (Fig. 5.6).

The choice of a high or a low cutoff level for screening therefore depends on the importance we attach to false positives and false negatives. False positives are associated with costs—emotional and financial—as well as with the difficulty of "delabeling" a person who tests positive and is later found not to have the disease. In addition, false-positive results may pose a major burden to the health care system, in that a large group of people need to be brought back for a retest, when only a few of them may have the disease. Those with false-negative results, on the other hand, will be told they do not have the disease and will not be followed, so a serious disease might possibly be missed at an early treatable stage. Thus the choice of cutoff level relates to the relative importance of false positivity and false negativity for the disease in question.

Use of Multiple Tests

Often more than one screening test may be applied in the same individuals to detect an illness—either sequentially (one after another) or simultaneously (both conducted at the same time). The results of these approaches are described in this section.

SEQUENTIAL (TWO-STAGE) TESTING

In sequential (or two-stage) screening, a less expensive, less invasive, or less uncomfortable test is generally performed first, and those who screen positive are recalled for further testing with a more expensive, more invasive, or more uncomfortable test, which may have greater sensitivity and specificity. It is hoped that bringing back for further testing only those who screen positive will reduce the problem of false positives.

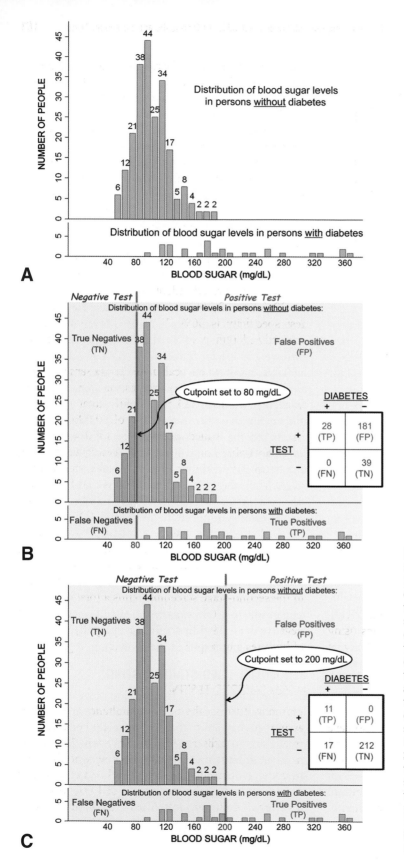

Fig. 5.4 (A) Distribution of blood sugar levels in hospital patients with diabetes and without diabetes. (The number of people with diabetes is shown for each specific blood sugar level in the *[upper]* distribution for persons *without* diabetes. Because of limited space, the number of people for each specific level of blood sugar is not shown in the *[lower]* distribution for persons *with* diabetes.) (B) and (C) show two different blood sugar cutpoints that were used in the study to define diabetes. Data from the graphs are presented to the right of each graph in a 2 × 2 table. (B) When a blood sugar cutpoint of ≥80 mg/dL is used to define diabetes in this population, sensitivity of the screening test is 100%, but specificity is low. (C) When a blood sugar cutpoint of ≥200 mg/dL is used to define diabetes in this population, sensitivity of the screening test is low, but specificity is 100%. (See explanation in the text under the subheading "Tests of Continuous Variables" on page 97.) *FN*, False negatives; *FP*, false positives; *TN*, true negatives; *TP*, true positives. (Modified from Blumberg M. Evaluating health screening procedures. *Oper Res.* 1957;5:351–360.)

DISEASE

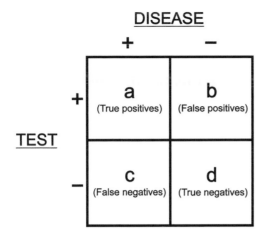

Fig. **5.5** Diagram showing four possible groups resulting from screening with a dichotomous test.

DISEASE (+) and (−)

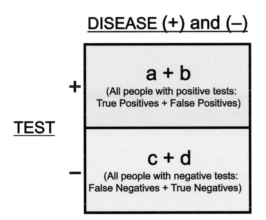

Fig. **5.6** Diagram showing the two groups of people resulting from screening with a dichotomous screening test: all people with positive test results and all people with negative test results.

Consider the hypothetical example in Fig. 5.7A, in which a population is screened for diabetes using a test with a sensitivity of 70% and a specificity of 80%. How are the data shown in this table obtained? The disease prevalence in this population is given as 5%, so that in the population of 10,000, 500 persons have the disease. With a sensitivity of 70%, the test will correctly identify 350 of the 500 people who have the disease. With a specificity of 80%, the test will correctly identify as nondiabetic 7,600 of the 9,500 people who are free of diabetes; however, 1,900 of these 9,500 will have positive results. Thus a total of 2,250 people will test positive and will be brought

back for a second test. (Remember that in real life we do not have the vertical line separating diabetics and nondiabetics, and we do not know that only 350 of the 2,250 have diabetes.)

Now those 2,250 people are brought back and screened using a second test (such as a glucose tolerance test), which, for purposes of this example, is assumed to have a sensitivity of 90% and a specificity of 90%. Fig. 5.7B shows test 1 together with test 2, which deals only with the 2,250 people who tested positive in the first screening test and have been brought back for second-stage screening.

Since 350 people (of the 2,250) have the disease and the test has a sensitivity of 90%, 315 of those 350 will be correctly identified as positive. Because 1,900 (of the 2,250) do not have diabetes and the test specificity is 90%, 1,710 of the 1,900 will be correctly identified as negative and 190 will be false positives.

We are now able to calculate the *net sensitivity* and the *net specificity* of using both tests in sequence. After finishing both tests, 315 people of the total 500 people with diabetes in this population of 10,000 will have been correctly called positive: 315/500 = 63% *net sensitivity* (which can also be calculated by multiplying the sensitivity of the first test times the sensitivity of the second test; i.e., 0.70 × 0.90 = 0.63). Thus there is a loss in net sensitivity by using both tests sequentially. To calculate *net specificity*, note that 7,600 people of the 9,500 in this population who do not have diabetes were correctly called negative in the first-stage screening and were not tested further; an additional 1,710 of those 9,500 nondiabetics were correctly called negative in the second-stage screening. Thus a total of 7,600 + 1,710 of the 9,500 nondiabetics were correctly called negative: 9,310/9,500 = 98% *net specificity*. Thus use of both tests in sequence has resulted in a gain in *net specificity*.

SIMULTANEOUS TESTING

Let's now turn to the use of simultaneous tests. We assume that in a population of 1,000 people, the prevalence of a disease is 20%. Therefore 200 people have the disease, but we do not know who they are. In order to identify the 200 people who have this disease, we screen this population of 1,000 using two tests for this disease, test A and test B, at the same

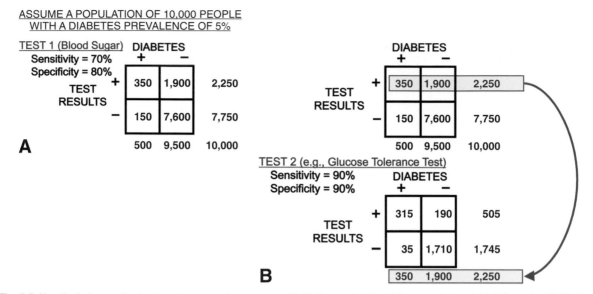

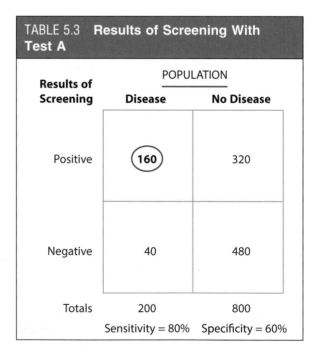

Fig. 5.7 Hypothetical example of a two-stage screening program. (A) Findings using Test 1 in a population of 10,000 people. (B) Findings using Test 2 in participants who tested positive using Test 1. (See explanation in the text under the subheading "Sequential (Two-Stage) Testing" on page 99.)

time. We assume that the sensitivity and specificity of the two tests are as follows:

Test A	Test B
Sensitivity = 80%	Sensitivity = 90%
Specificity = 60%	Specificity = 90%

NET SENSITIVITY USING TWO SIMULTANEOUS TESTS

The first question we ask is, "What is the *net sensitivity* using test A and test B *simultaneously*?" To be considered positive and therefore included in the numerator for net sensitivity for two tests used simultaneously, a person must be identified as positive by test A, test B, or both tests.

To calculate net sensitivity, let's first consider the results of screening with test A whose sensitivity is 80%: of the 200 people who have the disease, 160 test positive (Table 5.3). In Fig. 5.8A, the oval represents the 200 people who have the disease. In Fig. 5.8B the pink circle within the oval represents the 160 who test positive with test A. These 160 are the true positives using test A.

Consider next the results of screening with test B whose sensitivity is 90% (Table 5.4). Of the 200 people

TABLE 5.3 Results of Screening With Test A

Results of Screening	POPULATION	
	Disease	No Disease
Positive	(160)	320
Negative	40	480
Totals	200	800

Sensitivity = 80%   Specificity = 60%

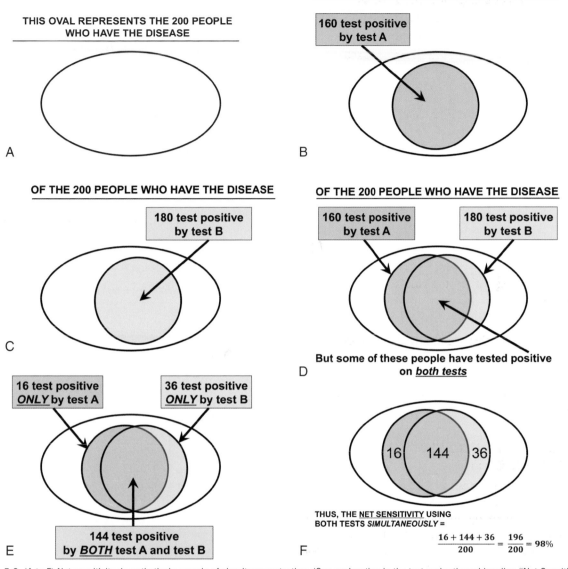

Fig. 5.8 (A to F) Net sensitivity: hypothetical example of simultaneous testing. (See explanation in the text under the subheading "Net Sensitivity Using Two Simultaneous Tests" on page 102.)

who have the disease, 180 test positive by test B. In Fig. 5.8C, the oval again represents the 200 people who have the disease. The blue circle within the oval represents the 180 who test positive with test B. These 180 are the true positives using test B.

In order to calculate the numerator for net sensitivity, we cannot just add the number of persons who tested

positive using test A to those who tested positive using test B because some people tested positive on both tests. These people are shown in lavender by the overlapping area of the two circles, and we do not want to count them twice (see Fig. 5.8D). How do we determine how many people tested positive on both tests?

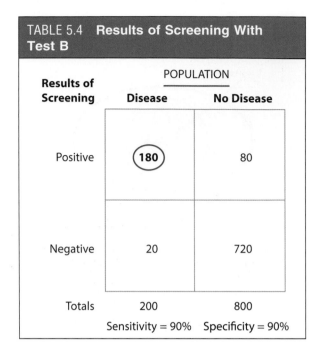

TABLE 5.4 **Results of Screening With Test B**

Results of Screening	POPULATION	
	Disease	No Disease
Positive	180	80
Negative	20	720
Totals	200	800

Sensitivity = 90% Specificity = 90%

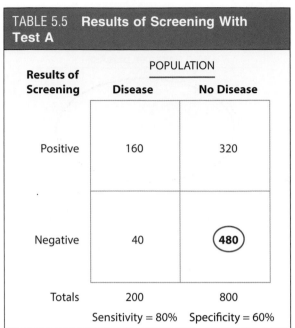

TABLE 5.5 **Results of Screening With Test A**

Results of Screening	POPULATION	
	Disease	No Disease
Positive	160	320
Negative	40	480
Totals	200	800

Sensitivity = 80% Specificity = 60%

Test A has a sensitivity of 80% and thus identifies as positive 80% of the 200 who have the disease (160 people). Test B has a sensitivity of 90%. Therefore it identifies as positive 90% of the same 160 people who are identified by test A (144 people). Thus when tests A and B are used simultaneously, 144 people are identified as positive by both tests (see Fig. 5.8E).

Recall that test A correctly identified 160 people with the disease as positive. Because 144 of them were identified by both tests, 160 − 144, or 16 people, were correctly identified *only* by test A.

Test B correctly identified 180 of the 200 people with the disease as positive. Because 144 of them were identified by both tests, 180 − 144, or 36 people, were correctly identified *only* by test B. Thus as seen in Fig. 5.8F, using tests A and B simultaneously,

$$\text{Net sensitivity} = \frac{16 + 144 + 36}{200} = \frac{196}{200} = 98\%$$

NET SPECIFICITY USING TWO SIMULTANEOUS TESTS

The next question is, "What is the *net specificity* using test A and test B *simultaneously*?" To be included in the numerator for net specificity for two tests used

simultaneously, a person must be identified as *negative by both tests*. In order to calculate the numerator for net specificity, we therefore need to determine how many people had negative results on both tests. How do we do this?

Test A has a specificity of 60% and thus correctly identifies 60% of the 800 who do not have the disease (480 people; Table 5.5). In Fig. 5.9A, the oval represents the 800 people who do not have the disease. The green circle within the oval in Fig. 5.9B represents the 480 people who test negative with test A. These are the true negatives using test A.

Test B has a specificity of 90% and thus identifies as negative 90% of the 800 people who do not have the disease (720 people; Table 5.6 and the yellow circle in Fig. 5.9C). However, to be called negative in simultaneous tests, only people who test negative on both tests are considered to have had negative results (see Fig. 5.9D). These people are shown in light green by the overlapping area of the two circles. Test B also identifies as negative 90% of the same 480 people identified as negative by test A (432 people). Thus, as shown by the overlapping circles, when tests A and B are used simultaneously, 432 people are identified as negative by both tests (see Fig. 5.9E).

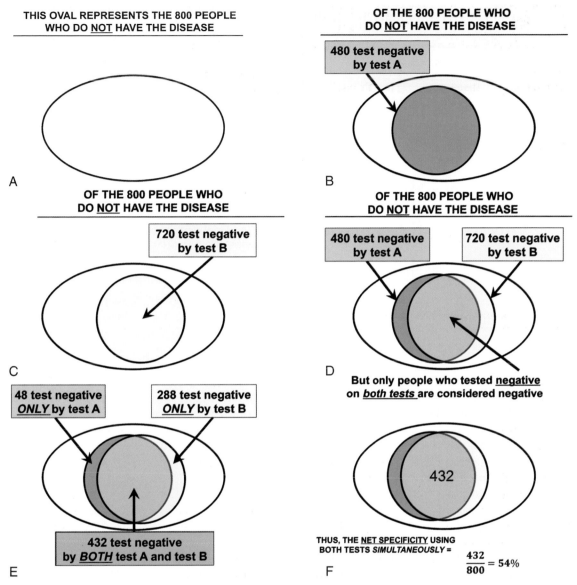

THIS OVAL REPRESENTS THE 800 PEOPLE WHO DO NOT HAVE THE DISEASE

A

OF THE 800 PEOPLE WHO DO NOT HAVE THE DISEASE

480 test negative by test A

B

OF THE 800 PEOPLE WHO DO NOT HAVE THE DISEASE

720 test negative by test B

C

OF THE 800 PEOPLE WHO DO NOT HAVE THE DISEASE

480 test negative by test A

720 test negative by test B

D

But only people who tested **negative** on **both tests** are considered negative

48 test negative **ONLY** by test A

288 test negative **ONLY** by test B

432 test negative by **BOTH** test A and test B

E

432

THUS, THE **NET SPECIFICITY** USING BOTH TESTS *SIMULTANEOUSLY* = $\dfrac{432}{800} = 54\%$

F

Fig. 5.9 (A to F) Net specificity: hypothetical example of simultaneous testing. (See explanation in the text under the subheading "Net Specificity Using Two Simultaneous Tests" on page 104.)

Thus when tests A and B are used simultaneously (see Fig. 5.9F),

$$\text{Net specificity} = \frac{432}{800} = 54\%$$

Therefore when two simultaneous tests are used, there is a net gain in sensitivity (from 80% using test A and 90% using test B to 98% using both tests simultaneously). However, there is a net loss in specificity (net

specificity = 54%) compared with using either test alone (specificity of 60% using test A and 90% using test B).

COMPARISON OF SIMULTANEOUS AND SEQUENTIAL TESTING

In a clinical setting, multiple tests are often used simultaneously. For example, a patient admitted to a hospital may have an array of tests performed at the time of admission. When multiple tests are used simultaneously

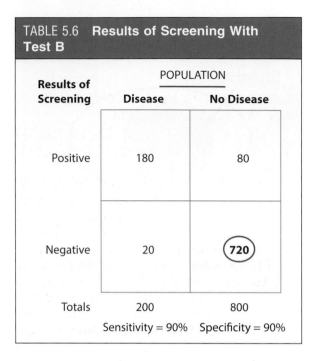

Results of Screening	POPULATION	
	Disease	No Disease
Positive	180	80
Negative	20	(720)
Totals	200	800
	Sensitivity = 90%	Specificity = 90%

TABLE 5.6 **Results of Screening With Test B**

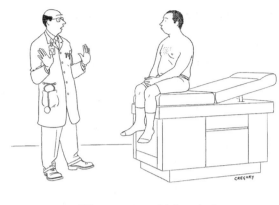

"Whoa—way too much information."

Fig. 5.10 "Whoa—*way* too much information." A physician comments on excessive information. (Alex Gregory/The New Yorker Collection/The Cartoon Bank.)

to detect a specific disease, the individual is generally considered to have tested "positive" if he or she has a positive result on *any* one or more of the tests. The individual is considered to have tested "negative" if he or she tests negative on *all* of the tests. The effects of such a testing approach on sensitivity and specificity differ from those that result from sequential testing. In sequential testing, when we retest those who tested positive on the first test, there is a loss in net sensitivity and a gain in net specificity. In simultaneous testing, because an individual who tests positive on *any* one or multiple tests is considered positive, there is a gain in net sensitivity. However, to be considered negative, a person would have to test negative on *all* the tests performed. As a result, there is a loss in net specificity.

In summary, as we have seen previously, when two sequential tests are used and those who test positive by the first test are brought in for the second test, there is a net loss in sensitivity, but a net gain in specificity, compared with either test alone. However, when two simultaneous tests are used, there is a net gain in sensitivity and a net loss in specificity, compared with either test alone.

Given these results, the decision to use either sequential or simultaneous testing often is based both on the objectives of the testing, including whether testing is being done for screening or diagnostic purposes, and on practical considerations related to the setting in which the testing is being done, including the length of hospital stay, costs, and degree of invasiveness of each of the tests, as well as the extent of third-party insurance coverage. Fig. 5.10 shows a physician dealing with perceived information overload.

Predictive Value of a Test

So far we have asked, "How good is the test at identifying people with the disease and people without the disease?" This is an important issue, particularly in screening free-living populations who have no symptoms of the disease being evaluated. In effect, we are asking, "If we screen a population, what proportion of people who have the disease will be correctly identified?" This is clearly an important public health consideration. In the clinical setting, however, a different question may be important for the clinician: If the test results are positive in this patient, what is the probability that this patient has the disease? This is called the *positive predictive value* (PPV) of the test. In other words, what proportion of patients who test positive actually have the disease in question? To calculate the PPV, we divide the number of true positives by the total number who tested positive (true positives + false positives).

Let's return to the example shown in Table 5.1, in which a population of 1,000 persons is screened. As seen in Table 5.7, a 2 × 2 table shows the results of a dichotomous screening test in that population. Of the 1,000 subjects, 180 have a positive test result; of these 180 subjects, 80 have the disease. Therefore the PPV is 80/180, or 44%.

A parallel question can be asked about negative test results: "If the test result is negative, what is the probability that this patient does not have the disease?" This is called the *negative predictive value* (NPV) of the test. It is calculated by dividing the number of true negatives by all those who tested negative (true negatives + false negatives). Looking again at the example in Table 5.7, 820 people have a negative test result, and of these, 800 do not have the disease. Thus the NPV is 800/820, or 98%.

Every test that a clinician performs—history, physical examination, laboratory tests, x-rays, electrocardiograms, and other procedures—is used to enhance the likelihood of making the correct diagnosis. What he or she wants to know after administering a test to a patient is: "Given this positive test result, what is the likelihood that the patient has the disease?"

Unlike the sensitivity and specificity of the test, which can be considered characteristic of the test being used, the PPV is affected by two factors: the *prevalence* of the disease in the population tested and, when the disease is infrequent, the *specificity* of the test being used. Both of these relationships are discussed in the following sections.

RELATIONSHIP BETWEEN POSITIVE PREDICTIVE VALUE AND DISEASE PREVALENCE

In the discussion of predictive value that follows, the term *predictive value* is used to denote the *positive* predictive value of the test.

The relationship between predictive value and *disease prevalence* can be seen in the example given in Table 5.8. First, let's direct our attention to the upper part of the table. Assume that we are using a test with a sensitivity of 99% and a specificity of 95% in a population of 10,000 people in which the disease prevalence is 1%. Because the prevalence is 1%, 100 of the 10,000 persons have the disease and 9,900 do not. With a sensitivity of 99%, the test correctly identifies 99 of the 100 people who have the disease. With a specificity of 95%, the test correctly identifies as negative 9,405 of the 9,900 people who do not have the disease. Thus, in this population with a 1% prevalence, 594 people are identified as positive by the test (99 + 495). However, of these 594 people, 495 (83%) are false positives and the PPV is therefore 99/594, or only 17%.

Let's now apply the same test—with the same sensitivity and specificity—to a population with a higher disease prevalence, 5%, as seen in the lower part of

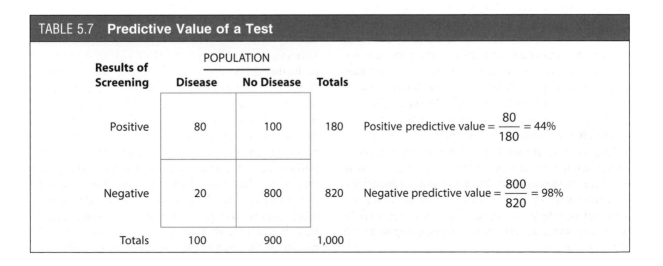

TABLE 5.7   Predictive Value of a Test

Results of Screening	POPULATION			
	Disease	No Disease	Totals	
Positive	80	100	180	Positive predictive value $= \dfrac{80}{180} = 44\%$
Negative	20	800	820	Negative predictive value $= \dfrac{800}{820} = 98\%$
Totals	100	900	1,000	

TABLE 5.8   **Relationship of Disease Prevalence to Positive Predictive Value**

		EXAMPLE: SENSITIVITY = 99%, SPECIFICITY = 95%			
Disease Prevalence	**Test Results**	**Sick**	**Not Sick**	**Totals**	**Positive Predictive Value**
1%	+	99	495	594	$\dfrac{99}{594} = 17\%$
	−	1	9,405	9,406	
	Totals	100	9,900	10,000	
5%	+	495	475	970	$\dfrac{495}{970} = 51\%$
	−	5	9,025	9,030	
	Totals	500	9,500	10,000	

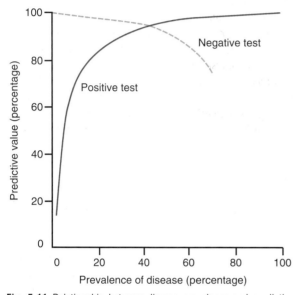

Fig. 5.11 Relationship between disease prevalence and predictive value in a test with 95% sensitivity and 95% specificity. (From Mausner JS, Kramer S. *Mausner and Bahn Epidemiology: An Introductory Text.* Philadelphia: WB Saunders; 1985:221.)

Table 5.8. Using calculations similar to those used in the upper part of the table, the PPV is now 51%. Thus the higher prevalence in the screened population has led to a marked increase in the PPV using the same test. Fig. 5.11 shows the relationship between disease prevalence and predictive value from a classic example. Clearly most of the gain in predictive value occurs with increases in prevalence at the lowest rates of disease prevalence.

Why should we be concerned about the relationship between predictive value and disease prevalence? As we have seen, the higher the prevalence, the higher the predictive value. Therefore a screening program is most productive and more cost-effective if it is directed to a high-risk target population. Screening a total population for a relatively infrequent disease can be a wasteful use of resources and may yield few previously undetected cases relative to the amount of effort involved. However, if a high-risk subset can be identified and screening can be directed to this group, the program is likely to be far more productive. In addition, a high-risk population may be more motivated to participate in such a screening program and more likely to take recommended action if their screening results are positive.

The relationship between predictive value and disease prevalence also shows that the results of any test must be interpreted in the context of the prevalence of the disease in the population from which the subject originates. An interesting example is seen with the measurement of the maternal serum α-fetoprotein (MSAFP) level for prenatal diagnosis of spina bifida. Fig. 5.12 shows the distribution of MSAFP levels in normal unaffected pregnancies and in pregnancies in which the fetus has Down syndrome; spina bifida, which is a neural tube defect; or anencephaly. For the purpose of this example, we will focus on the curves for unaffected pregnancies and spina bifida. Although the distribution of these two curves is bimodal, there is a range in which the curves overlap, and within that range, it may not always be clear to which curve the mother and fetus belong. If MSAFP is in the higher range for an unaffected pregnancy, the true prevalence of spina bifida will be low for the same range. Thus such overlap in the MSAFP in the unaffected pregnancies and those with fetuses with spina bifida has led to the test having a very low PPV, of only 2% to 6%.[1]

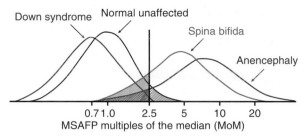

Fig. 5.12 Maternal serum alpha-fetoprotein *(MSAPF)* distribution for singleton pregnancies at 15 to 20 weeks. The screen cutoff value of 2.5 multiples of the median is expected to result in a false-positive rate of up to 5% *(black hatched area)* and false-negative rates of up to 20% for spina bifida *(orange hatched area)* and 10% for anencephaly *(red hatched area)*. (Modified from Prenatal diagnosis. In: Cunningham F, Leveno KJ, Bloom SL, et al, eds. *Williams Obstetrics.* 24th ed. New York: McGraw-Hill; 2013. http://accessmedicine.mhmedical.com.ezp.welch.jhmi.edu/content.aspx?bookid=1057&sectionid=59789152. Accessed June 19, 2017.)

It is possible that the same test can have a very different predictive value when it is administered to a high-risk (high prevalence) population or to a low-risk (low prevalence) population. This has clear clinical implications: A woman may make a decision to terminate a pregnancy, and a physician may formulate advice to such a woman on the basis of the test results. However, the same test result may be interpreted differently, depending on whether the woman comes from a pool of high-risk or low-risk women, which will be reflected in the PPV of the test. Consequently, by itself, the test result may not be sufficient to serve as a guide without taking into account the other considerations just described.

The following true examples highlight the importance of this issue:

The head of a firefighters' union consulted a university cardiologist because the fire department physician had read an article in a leading medical journal reporting that a certain electrocardiographic finding was highly predictive of serious, generally unrecognized, coronary heart disease. On the basis of this article, the fire department physician was disqualifying many young, able-bodied firefighters from active duty. The cardiologist read the paper and found that the study had been carried out in hospitalized patients.

What was the problem? Because hospitalized patients have a much higher prevalence of heart disease than does a group of young, able-bodied firefighters, the fire department physician had erroneously taken the high predictive value obtained in studying a high-prevalence population and inappropriately applied it to a low-prevalence population of healthy firefighters, in whom the same test would actually have a much lower predictive value.

Here is another example:

A physician visited his general internist for a regular annual medical examination, which included a stool examination for occult blood. One of the three stool specimens examined in the test was positive. The internist told his physician-patient that the result was of no significance because he regularly encountered many false-positive test results in his busy practice. The test was repeated on three new stool specimens, and all three of the new specimens were now negative. Nevertheless, sensing his patient's lingering concerns, the internist referred his physician-patient to a gastroenterologist. The gastroenterologist said, "In my experience, the positive stool finding is serious. Such a finding is almost always associated with pathologic gastrointestinal disorders. The subsequent negative test results mean nothing, because you could have a tumor that only bleeds intermittently."

Who was correct in this episode? The answer is that both the general internist and the gastroenterologist were correct. The internist gave his assessment of predictive value based on his experience in his general medical practice—a population with a low prevalence of serious gastrointestinal disease. On the other hand, the gastroenterologist gave his assessment of the predictive value of the test based on his experience in his referral practice—a practice in which most patients are referred because of a likelihood of serious gastrointestinal illness, a high-prevalence population.

RELATIONSHIP BETWEEN POSITIVE PREDICTIVE VALUE AND SPECIFICITY OF THE TEST

In the discussion that follows, the term *predictive value* is used to denote the PPV of the test.

A second factor that affects the predictive value of a test is the *specificity* of the test. Examples of this are shown first in graphical form and then in tabular form. Fig. 5.13A to D diagrams the results of screening a

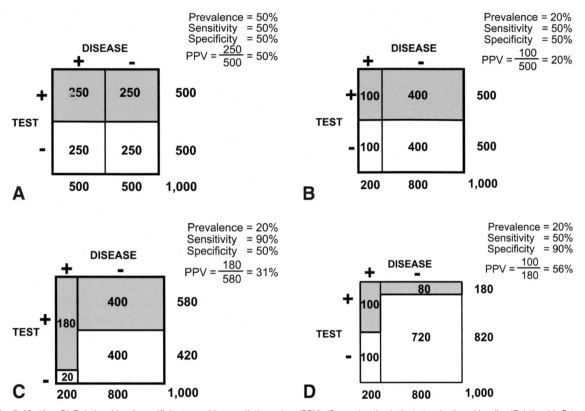

Fig. 5.13 (A to D) Relationship of specificity to positive predictive value *(PPV)*. (See explanation in the text under the subheading "Relationship Between Positive Predictive Value and Specificity of the Test" on page 109.)

population; however, the 2 × 2 tables in these figures differ from those shown in earlier figures. Each cell is drawn with its size proportional to the population it represents. In each figure the cells that represent persons who tested positive are shaded blue; these are the cells that will be used in calculating the PPV.

Fig. 5.13A presents the baseline screened population that is used in our discussion: a population of 1,000 people in whom the prevalence is 50%; thus 500 people have the disease and 500 do not. In analyzing this figure, we also assume that the screening test that was used has a sensitivity of 50% and a specificity of 50%. Because 500 people tested positive, and 250 of these have the disease, the predictive value is 250/500, or 50%.

Fortunately, the prevalence of most diseases is much lower than 50%; we are generally dealing with relatively infrequent diseases. Therefore Fig. 5.13B

assumes a lower prevalence of 20% (although even this would be an unusually high prevalence for most diseases). Both the sensitivity and the specificity remain at 50%. Now only 200 of the 1,000 people have the disease, and the vertical line separating diseased from nondiseased persons is shifted to the left. The predictive value is now calculated as 100/500, or 20%.

Given that we are screening a population with the lower prevalence rate, can we improve the predictive value? What would be the effect on predictive value if we increased the sensitivity of the test? Fig. 5.13C shows the results when we leave the prevalence at 20% and the specificity at 50%, but increase the sensitivity to 90%. The predictive value is now 180/580, or 31%—a modest increase.

What if, instead of increasing the sensitivity of the test, we increase its specificity? Fig. 5.13D shows the results when prevalence remains 20% and sensitivity remains 50%, but specificity is increased to 90%. The predictive value is now 100/180, or 56%. Thus an increase in specificity resulted in a much greater increase in predictive value than the same increase in sensitivity.

Why does specificity have a greater effect than sensitivity on predictive value? The answer becomes clear by examining these figures. Because we are dealing with infrequent diseases, most of the population falls to the right of the vertical line. Consequently, any change to the right of the vertical line affects a greater number of people than would a comparable change to the left of the line. Thus a change in specificity has a greater effect on predictive value than a comparable change in sensitivity. If we were dealing with a high-prevalence disease, the situation would be different.

The effect of changes in specificity on predictive value is also seen in Table 5.9 in a form similar to that used in Table 5.8. As seen in this example, even with 100% sensitivity, a change in specificity from 70% to 95% has a dramatic effect on the PPV.

Reliability (Repeatability) of Tests

Let's consider another aspect of assessing diagnostic and screening tests—the question of whether a test is reliable or repeatable. Can the results obtained be replicated (getting the same result) if the test is repeated? Clearly, regardless of the sensitivity and specificity of a test, if the test results cannot be reproduced, the value and usefulness of the test are minimal. The rest of this chapter focuses on the reliability or repeatability

of diagnostic and screening tests. The factors that contribute to the variation between test results are discussed first: intrasubject variation (variation within individual subjects), intraobserver variation (variation in the reading of test results by the same reader), and interobserver variation (variation between those reading the test results).

INTRASUBJECT VARIATION

The values obtained in measuring many human characteristics often vary over time, even during a short period of 24 hours, or a longer period, such as seasonal variation. Fig. 5.14 shows changes in blood pressure readings over a 24-hour period in 28 normotensive individuals. Variability over time is considerable. This, as well as the conditions under which certain tests are conducted (e.g., shortly after eating or post-exercise, at home or in a physician's office), clearly can lead to different results in the same individual. Therefore in evaluating any test result, it is important to consider the conditions under which the test was performed, including the time of day.

INTRAOBSERVER VARIATION

Sometimes variation occurs between two or more readings of the same test results made by the same observer. For example, a radiologist who reads the same group of x-rays at two different times may read one or more of the x-rays differently the second time. Tests and examinations differ in the degree to which subjective factors enter into the observer's conclusions, and the greater the subjective element in the reading, the greater the intraobserver variation in readings is likely to be (Fig. 5.15).

TABLE 5.9	**Relationship of Specificity to Positive Predictive Value**				
	EXAMPLE: PREVALENCE = 10%, SENSITIVITY = 100%				
Specificity	**Test Results**	**Sick**	**Not Sick**	**Totals**	**Predictive Value**
70%	+	1,000	2,700	3,700	$\frac{1,000}{3,700} = 27\%$
	−	0	6,300	6,300	
	Totals	1,000	9,000	10,000	
95%	+	1,000	450	1,450	$\frac{1,000}{1,450} = 69\%$
	−	0	8,550	8,550	
	Totals	1,000	9,000	10,000	

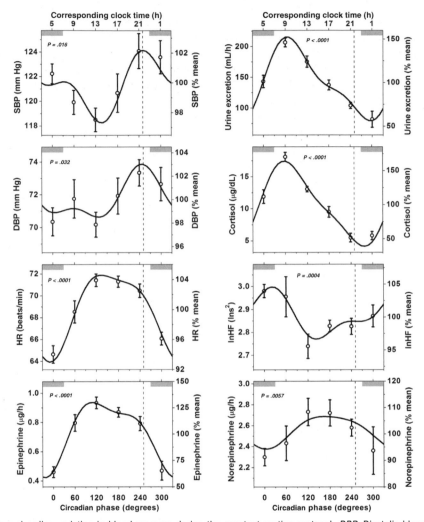

Fig. 5.14 Endogenous circadian variation in blood pressure during the constant routine protocol. *DBP,* Diastolic blood pressure; *HR,* heart rate; *SBP,* systolic blood pressure. (From Shea SA, Hilton MF, Hu K, et al. Existence of an endogenous circadian blood pressure rhythm in humans that peaks in the evening. *Circ Res.* 2011;108:980–984.)

INTEROBSERVER VARIATION

Another important consideration is variation between observers. Two examiners often do not give the same result. The extent to which observers agree or disagree is an important issue, whether we are considering physical examinations, laboratory tests, or other means of assessing human characteristics. We therefore need to be able to express the extent of agreement in quantitative terms.

Percent Agreement

Table 5.10 shows a schema for examining variation between observers. Two observers were instructed to categorize each test result into one of the following four categories: abnormal, suspect, doubtful, and normal. This diagram might refer, for example, to readings performed by two radiologists. In this diagram, the readings of observer 1 are cross-tabulated against those of observer 2. The number of readings in each cell is denoted by a letter of the alphabet. Thus A x-rays were read as abnormal by both radiologists. C x-rays were read as abnormal by radiologist 2 and as doubtful by radiologist 1. M x-rays were read as abnormal by radiologist 1 and as normal by radiologist 2.

As seen in Table 5.10, to calculate the overall percent agreement, we add the numbers in all of the cells in which readings by both radiologists agreed (A + F + K + P), divide that sum by the total number of x-rays read, and multiply the result by 100 to yield a percentage. Fig. 5.16A shows the use of this approach for a test with possible readings of either "positive" or "negative."

In general, most persons who are tested have negative results. This is shown in Fig. 5.16B, in which the size of each cell is drawn in proportion to the number of people in that cell. There is likely to be considerable

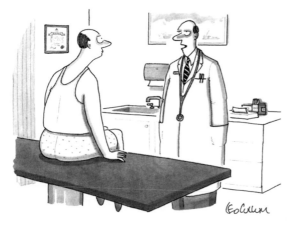

"This is a second opinion. At first, I thought you had something else."

Fig. 5.15 "This *is* a second opinion. At first, I thought you had something else." One view of a second opinion. (Leo Cullum/The New Yorker Collection/The Cartoon Bank.)

agreement between the two observers about these negative, or normal, subjects (cell d). Therefore when percent agreement is calculated for all study subjects, its value may be high only because of the large number of clearly negative findings (cell d) on which the observers agree. Thus the high value may conceal significant disagreement between the observers in identifying subjects who are considered positive by at least one observer.

One approach to this problem, seen in Fig. 5.16C, is to disregard the subjects who were labeled negative by both observers (cell d) and to calculate percent agreement using as a denominator only the subjects who were labeled abnormal by at least one observer (cells a, b, and c; Fig. 5.16D).

Thus in the paired observations in which at least one of the findings in each pair was positive, the following equation is applicable:

$$\text{Percent agreement} = \frac{a}{a+b+c} \times 100$$

Kappa Statistic

Percent agreement between two observers is often of value in assessing the quality of their observations. The extent to which two observers, such as two physicians or two nurses, for example, agree with one another is often an important index of the quality of the health care being provided. However, the percent agreement between two observers does not entirely depend on the quality of their training and practice. The extent of their agreement is also significantly influenced by the fact that even if two observers use completely different criteria to identify subjects as positive or negative, we would expect the observers to agree about the observations

TABLE 5.10	**Observer or Instrument Variation: Percent Agreement**						
	Reading No. 1						
Reading No. 2	Abnormal		Suspect		Doubtful		Normal
Abnormal	A	+	B		C		D
Suspect	E		F	+	G		H
Doubtful	I		J		K	+	L
Normal	M		N		O		P
	Percent agreement = $\dfrac{A + F + K + P}{\text{Total readings}} \times 100$						

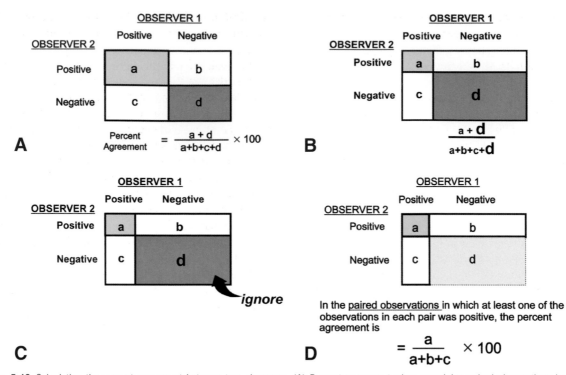

Fig. 5.16 Calculating the percent agreement between two observers. (A) Percent agreement when examining paired observations between observer 1 and observer 2. (B) Percent agreement when examining paired observations between observer 1 and observer 2, considering that cell d (agreement on the negatives) is very high. (C) Percent agreement when examining paired observations between observer 1 and observer 2, ignoring cell d. (D) Percent agreement when examining paired observations between observer 1 and observer 2, using only cells a, b, and c for the calculation.

made, at least in some of the participants, solely as a function of chance. What we really want to know is how much better their level of agreement is than that which results just from chance. The answer to this question will presumably tell us, for example, to what extent the education and training that the observers received improved the quality of their readings so that the percent agreement between them was increased beyond what we would expect from chance alone.

This can be shown intuitively in the following example: you are the director of a radiology department that is understaffed 1 day, and a large number of chest x-rays remain to be read. To solve your problem, you go out to the street and ask a few neighborhood residents, who have no background in biology or medicine, to read the unread x-rays and assess them as either positive or negative. The first person goes through the pile of x-rays, reading them haphazardly as positive, negative, negative, positive, and so on. The second

person does the same, in the same way, but completely independent of the first reader. Given that both readers have no knowledge, criteria, or standards for reading x-rays, would any of their readings on a specific x-ray agree? The answer is clearly yes; they would agree in some cases, purely by chance alone.

However, if we want to know how well two observers read x-rays, we might ask, "To what extent do their readings agree *beyond what we would expect by chance alone?*" In other words, to what extent does the agreement between the two observers exceed the level of agreement that would result just from chance? One approach to answering this question is to calculate the kappa statistic, proposed by Cohen in 1960.[2] In this section, we will first discuss the rationale of the kappa statistic and the questions that the kappa statistic is designed to answer. This will be followed by a detailed calculation of the kappa statistic to serve as an example for intrepid readers. Even if you do not follow through the detailed calculation presented here, it is important to be sure that you understand the rationale of the kappa statistic because it is frequently applied both in clinical medicine and in public health.

Rationale of the Kappa Statistic. In order to understand kappa, we ask two questions. First, how much better is the agreement between the observers' readings than would be expected by chance alone? This can be calculated as the percent agreement observed minus the percent agreement we would expect by chance alone. This is the numerator of kappa:

(Percent agreement observed)

— (Percent agreement expected by chance alone)

Our second question is, "What is the most that the two observers could have improved their agreement over the agreement that would be expected by chance alone?" Clearly the maximum that they could agree would be 100% (full agreement, where the two observers agree completely). Therefore the most that we could expect them to be able to improve (the denominator of kappa) would be:

100% − (Percent agreement expected by chance alone)

Kappa expresses the extent to which the observed agreement exceeds that which would be expected by chance alone (i.e., percent agreement observed − percent agreement expected by chance alone [numerator]) relative to the maximum that the observers could hope to improve their agreement (i.e., 100% − percent agreement expected by chance alone [denominator]).

Thus kappa quantifies the extent to which the observed agreement that the observers achieved exceeds that which would be expected by chance alone, and expresses it as the proportion of the maximum improvement that could occur beyond the agreement expected by chance alone. The kappa statistic can be defined by the equation:

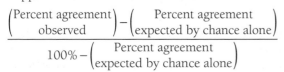

$$\text{Kappa} = \frac{\left(\begin{array}{c}\text{Percent agreement}\\\text{observed}\end{array}\right) - \left(\begin{array}{c}\text{Percent agreement}\\\text{expected by chance alone}\end{array}\right)}{100\% - \left(\begin{array}{c}\text{Percent agreement}\\\text{expected by chance alone}\end{array}\right)}$$

Calculation of the Kappa Statistic: An Example. To calculate the numerator for kappa, we must first calculate the amount of agreement that might be expected on the basis of chance alone. As an example, let's consider data on breast density reported on the radiologic classification of breast density on synthetic 2D images as compared with digital 2D mammograms.[3] Fig. 5.17A shows data comparing the findings of the two methods in classifying 309 such cases.

The first question is, "What is the observed agreement between the two types of mammograms?" Fig. 5.17B shows the classifications using the synthetic 2D mammography along the bottom of the table and those of digital 2D mammography along the right margin. Thus synthetic 2D mammography identified 179 (or 58%) of all of the 309 breast images as nondense and 130 (or 42%) of the images as dense. Digital 2D mammography identified 182 (or 59%) of all of the images as nondense and 127 (or 41%) of the images as dense. As discussed earlier, the percent agreement is calculated by the following equation:

$$\text{Percent agreement observed} = \frac{168 + 116}{309} = 91.9\%$$

That is, the two mammography devices had the same breast image classification on 91.9% of the readings.

The next question is, "If the two types of mammography had used entirely different sets of criteria for classifying a breast image as dense versus nondense, how much agreement would have been expected *solely on the basis of chance*?" Synthetic 2D mammography read 58% of all 309 images (179 images) as being nondense and 42% (130 images) as dense. If these readings had used criteria independent of those used by digital 2D mammography, we would expect that synthetic 2D mammography would read as nondense both 58% of the images that the digital had identified as dense and 58% of the images that digital 2D mammography had identified as dense. Therefore we would expect that 58% (73.44) of the 182 images identified as nondense by digital 2D mammography would be identified as nondense by synthetic 2D mammography, and that 58% (73.44) of the 127 images identified as dense by digital 2D mammography would also be identified as nondense by synthetic 2D mammography (see Fig. 5.16C). Of the 127 images called dense by digital 2D mammography, 42% (53.34)

A

		Synthetic 2D mammography		
		Nondense	Dense	Total by digital 2D mammography
Digital 2D mammography	Nondense	168	14	182 (59%)
	Dense	11	116	127 (41%)
	Total by synthetic 2D mammography	179 (58%)	130 (42%)	309 (100%)

B

		Synthetic 2D mammography		
		Nondense	Dense	Total by digital 2D mammography
Digital 2D mammography	Nondense	168	14	182 (59%)
	Dense	11	116	127 (41%)
	Total by synthetic 2D mammography	179 (58%)	130 (42%)	309 (100%)

Percent agreement observed $= \dfrac{168 + 116}{309} = 91.9\%$

C

		Synthetic 2D mammography		
		Nondense	Dense	Total by digital 2D mammography
Digital 2D mammography	Nondense	105.56	76.66	182 (59%)
	Dense	73.44	53.34	127 (41%)
	Total by synthetic 2D mammography	179 (58%)	130 (42%)	309 (100%)

Percent agreement expected by chance alone $= \dfrac{105.56 + 53.34}{309} = 51.4\%$

Fig. 5.17 (A) Radiologic classification of breast density on synthetic 2D images as compared with digital 2D mammograms. (B) Percent agreement by synthetic and digital 2D mammograms. (C) Percent agreement by synthetic and digital 2D mammograms *expected by chance alone*. (From Alshafeiy TI, Wadih A, Nicholson BT, et al. Comparison between digital and synthetic 2D mammograms in breast density interpretation. *AJR Am J Roentgenol.* 2017;209: W36–W41. Reprinted with permission from the American Journal of Roentgenology.)

would also be classified as dense by synthetic 2D mammography.

Thus the agreement expected by chance alone would be

$$= \frac{105.56}{309} + \frac{53.34}{309} = \frac{158.9}{309} = 51.4\%$$

of all images read.

Having calculated the figures needed for the numerator and denominator, kappa can now be calculated as follows:

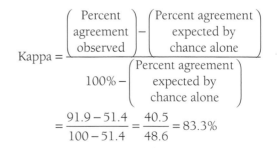

$$Kappa = \frac{\left(\begin{array}{c} \text{Percent} \\ \text{agreement} \\ \text{observed} \end{array} \right) - \left(\begin{array}{c} \text{Percent agreement} \\ \text{expected by} \\ \text{chance alone} \end{array} \right)}{100\% - \left(\begin{array}{c} \text{Percent agreement} \\ \text{expected by} \\ \text{chance alone} \end{array} \right)}$$

$$= \frac{91.9 - 51.4}{100 - 51.4} = \frac{40.5}{48.6} = 83.3\%$$

Landis and Koch[4] suggested that a kappa greater than 0.75 represents excellent agreement beyond chance, a kappa below 0.40 represents poor agreement, and a kappa of 0.40 to 0.75 represents intermediate to good agreement. Testing for the statistical significance of kappa is described by Fleiss.[5] Considerable discussion has arisen about the appropriate use of kappa, a subject addressed by MacLure and Willett.[6]

Validity of Tests With Multicategorical Results. Validity, as a concept, can be applied to any test against a gold standard. As we explained earlier, we use sensitivity/specificity to validate the results of tests with dichotomous results against a gold standard. What about tests with multicategorical results? In this case, we can calculate kappa statistic, which we demonstrated earlier as a tool to assess reliability.

Validity of Self-Reports. Often we obtain information on health and disease status by directly asking patients or study participants about their medical history, their habits, and other factors of interest. Most people today know their date of birth, so the assessment of age is usually without significant error. However, many people underreport their weight, their drinking and smoking practices, and other types of risks. Self-reports of sexual behaviors are considered to be subject to considerable error. To overcome these reporting biases, biomarkers have become commonly used in field studies. For example, Zenilman et al.[7] used a polymerase chain reaction (PCR) assay to detect Y chromosome fragments in self-collected vaginal swabs. This biomarker can detect coitus in women for a 2-week period, and can validate self-reports of condom use.[8]

Relationship Between Validity and Reliability

To conclude this chapter, let's compare validity and reliability using a graphical presentation.

The horizontal line in Fig. 5.18 is a scale of values for a given variable, such as blood glucose level, with the true value indicated. The test results obtained are shown by the curve. The curve is narrow, indicating that the results are quite reliable (repeatable); unfortunately, however, they cluster far from the true value, so they are not valid. Fig. 5.19 shows a curve that is broad and therefore has low reliability. However, the values obtained cluster around the true

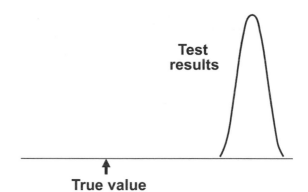

Fig. 5.18 Graph of hypothetical test results that are reliable, but not valid.

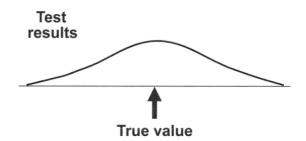

Fig. 5.19 Graph of hypothetical test results that are valid, but not reliable.

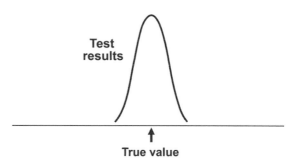

Fig. 5.20 Graph of hypothetical test results that are both valid and reliable.

value and thus are valid. Clearly, what we would like to achieve are results that are both valid and reliable (Fig. 5.20).

It is important to point out that in Fig. 5.20, in which the distribution of the test results is a broad curve centered on the true value, we describe the results as valid. However, the results are valid only for a group (i.e., they tend to cluster around the true value). It is important to remember that what may be valid for a group or a population may not be so for an individual in a clinical setting. When the reliability or repeatability of a test is poor, the validity of the test for a given individual also may be poor. The distinction between group validity and individual validity is therefore important to keep in mind when assessing the quality of diagnostic and screening tests.

Conclusion

This chapter has discussed the validity of diagnostic and screening tests as measured by their sensitivity and specificity, their predictive value, and the reliability or repeatability of these tests. Clearly, regardless of how sensitive and specific a test may be, if its results cannot be replicated, the test is of little use. All these characteristics must therefore be borne in mind when evaluating such tests, together with the purpose for which the test will be used.

REFERENCES

1. Prenatal diagnosis. In: Cunningham F, Leveno KJ, Bloom SL, et al, eds. *Williams Obstetrics*. 24th ed. New York: McGraw-Hill; 2013. http://accessmedicine.mhmedical.com.ezp.welch.jhmi.edu/content.aspx?bookid=1057&sectionid=59789152. Accessed June 19, 2017.
2. Cohen J. A coefficient of agreement for nominal scales. *Educ Psychol Meas*. 1960;20:37.
3. Alshafeiy TI, Wadih A, Nicholson BT, et al. Comparison between digital and synthetic 2D mammograms in breast density interpretation. *AJR Am J Roentgenol*. 2017;209:W36–W41.
4. Landis JR, Koch GG. The measurement of observer agreement for categorical data. *Biometrics*. 1977;33:159–174.
5. Fleiss JL. *Statistical Methods for Rates and Proportions*. 2nd ed. New York: John Wiley & Sons; 1981.
6. MacLure M, Willett WC. Misinterpretation and misuse of the kappa statistic. *Am J Epidemiol*. 1987;126:161–169.
7. Zenilman JM, Yeunger J, Galai N, et al. Polymerase chain reaction detection of Y chromosome sequences in vaginal fluid: preliminary studies of a potential biomarker. *Sex Transm Dis*. 2005;32:90–94.
8. Ghanem KG, Melendez JH, McNeil-Solis C, et al. Condom use and vaginal Y-chromosome detection: the specificity of a potential biomarker. *Sex Transm Dis*. 2007;34:620.

Review questions on pages 121–122.

Appendices to Chapter 5

The text of Chapter 5 focuses on the logic behind the calculation of sensitivity, specificity, and predictive value. Appendix 1 summarizes measures of validity for screening tests to detect the absence or presence of a given disease, the pages in the text where the measures are first introduced, and the interpretation of each measure. For those who prefer to see the formulae for each measure, they are provided in the right-hand column of this table; however, they are not essential for understanding the logic behind the calculation of each measure.

Appendix 1 to Chapter 5: Measures of Test Validity and Their Interpretation

	Measure of Test Validity	Page Numbers	Interpretation	Formula
INDIVIDUAL screening tests	Sensitivity	95	The proportion of those *with* the disease who test *positive*	$\dfrac{TP}{TP+FN}$
	Specificity	95	The proportion of those *without* the disease who test *negative*	$\dfrac{TN}{TN+FP}$
	Positive predictive value	106–107	The proportion of those who test *positive* who do have the disease	$\dfrac{TP}{TP+FP}$
	Negative predictive value	107	The proportion of those who test *negative* who do NOT have the disease	$\dfrac{TN}{TN+FN}$
SEQUENTIAL screening tests	Net sensitivity	99–101	The proportion of those *with* the disease who test *positive* on BOTH Test 1 and Test 2	(Sensitivity of Test 1)×(Sensitivity of Test 2)
	Net specificity	99–101	The proportion of those *without* the disease who test *negative* on EITHER Test 1 or Test 2	$\left(\begin{array}{c}\text{Specificity of Test 1}\\+\\\text{Specificity of Test 2}\end{array}\right) - \left(\begin{array}{c}\text{Specificity of Test 1}\\\times\\\text{Specificity of Test 2}\end{array}\right)$
SIMULTANEOUS screening tests	Net sensitivity	101–104	The proportion of those *with* the disease who test *positive* on EITHER Test 1 or Test 2	$\left(\begin{array}{c}\text{Sensitivity of Test 1}\\+\\\text{Sensitivity of Test 2}\end{array}\right) - \left(\begin{array}{c}\text{Sensitivity of Test 1}\\\times\\\text{Sensitivity of Test 2}\end{array}\right)$
	Net specificity	105–106	The proportion of those *without* the disease who test *negative* on BOTH Test 1 and Test 2	(Specificity of Test 1)×(Specificity of Test 2)

FN, False negatives; *FP*, false positives; *TN*, true negatives; *TP*, true positives.

Appendix 2 summarizes the three steps required to calculate kappa statistic.

Appendix 2 to Chapter 5: The Three Steps Required for Calculating Kappa Statistic (κ)	
Components	**Steps**
NUMERATOR How much better is the observed agreement than the agreement expected by chance alone?	STEP 1: $$\left(\begin{array}{c}\text{Percent agreement}\\\text{observed}\end{array}\right)-\left(\begin{array}{c}\text{Percent agreement}\\\text{expected by chance alone}\end{array}\right)$$
DENOMINATOR What is the maximum the observers could have improved upon the agreement expected by chance alone?	STEP 2: $$100\%-\left(\begin{array}{c}\text{Percent agreement}\\\text{expected by chance alone}\end{array}\right)$$
$\dfrac{\text{NUMERATOR}}{\text{DENOMINATOR}} = \text{KAPPA STATISTIC } (\kappa)$ Of the maximum improvement in agreement expected beyond chance alone that could have occurred, what proportion has in fact occurred?	STEP 3: $$\kappa = \frac{\left(\begin{array}{c}\text{Percent agreement}\\\text{observed}\end{array}\right)-\left(\begin{array}{c}\text{Percent agreement}\\\text{expected by}\\\text{chance alone}\end{array}\right)}{100\%-\left(\begin{array}{c}\text{Percent agreement}\\\text{expected by chance alone}\end{array}\right)}$$

A full discussion of kappa and a sample calculation starts on page 113.

REVIEW QUESTIONS FOR CHAPTER 5

Questions 1, 2, and 3 are based on the information given below:

A physical examination was used to screen for breast cancer in 2,500 women with biopsy-proven adenocarcinoma of the breast and in 5,000 age- and race-matched control women. The results of the physical examination were positive (i.e., a mass was palpated) in 1,800 cases and in 800 control women, all of whom showed no evidence of cancer at biopsy.

1 *The sensitivity of the physical examination was:* _____

2 *The specificity of the physical examination was:* _____

3 *The positive predictive value of the physical examination was:* _____

Question 4 is based on the following information:

A screening test is used in the same way in two similar populations, but the proportion of false-positive results among those who test positive in population A is lower than that among those who test positive in population B.

4 *What is the likely explanation for this finding?*
a. It is impossible to determine what caused the difference
b. The specificity of the test is lower in population A
c. The prevalence of disease is lower in population A
d. The prevalence of disease is higher in population A
e. The specificity of the test is higher in population A

Question 5 is based on the following information:

A physical examination and an audiometric test were given to 500 persons with suspected hearing problems, of whom 300 were actually found to have them. The results of the examinations were as follows:

	HEARING PROBLEMS	
Result	**Present**	**Absent**
Physical Examination		
Positive	240	40
Negative	60	160
Audiometric Test		
Positive	270	60
Negative	30	140

5 *Compared with the physical examination, the audiometric test is:*
a. Equally sensitive and specific
b. Less sensitive and less specific
c. Less sensitive and more specific
d. More sensitive and less specific
e. More sensitive and more specific

Question 6 is based on the following information:

Two pediatricians want to investigate a new laboratory test that identifies streptococcal infections. Dr. Kidd uses the standard culture test, which has a sensitivity of 90% and a specificity of 96%. Dr. Childs uses the new test, which is 96% sensitive and 96% specific.

6 *If 200 patients undergo culture with both tests, which of the following is correct?*

a. Dr. Kidd will correctly identify more people with streptococcal infection than Dr. Childs

b. Dr. Kidd will correctly identify fewer people with streptococcal infection than Dr. Childs

c. Dr. Kidd will correctly identify more people without streptococcal infection than Dr. Childs

d. The prevalence of streptococcal infection is needed to determine which pediatrician will correctly identify the larger number of people with the disease

Questions 7 and 8 are based on the following information:

A colon cancer screening study is being conducted in Nottingham, England. Individuals 50 to 75 years old will be screened with the Hemoccult test. In this test, a stool sample is tested for the presence of blood.

7 *The Hemoccult test has a sensitivity of 70% and a specificity of 75%. If Nottingham has a prevalence of 12/1,000 for colon cancer, what is the positive predictive value of the test? _____*

8 *If the Hemoccult test result is negative, no further testing is done. If the Hemoccult test result is positive, the individual will have a second stool sample tested with the Hemoccult II test. If this second sample also tests positive for blood, the individual will be referred for more extensive evaluation. What is the effect on net sensitivity and net specificity of this method of screening?*

a. Net sensitivity and net specificity are both increased

b. Net sensitivity is decreased and net specificity is increased

c. Net sensitivity remains the same and net specificity is increased

d. Net sensitivity is increased and net specificity is decreased

e. The effect on net sensitivity and net specificity cannot be determined from the data

Questions 9 through 12 are based on the information given below:

Two physicians were asked to classify 100 chest x-rays as abnormal or normal independently. The comparison of their classification is shown in the following table:

Classification of Chest X-Rays by Physician 1 Compared With Physician 2			
	Physician 2		
Physician 1	Abnormal	Normal	Total
Abnormal	40	20	60
Normal	10	30	40
Total	50	50	100

9 *The simple percent agreement between the two physicians out of the total is: _____*

10 *The percent agreement between the two physicians, excluding the x-rays that both physicians classified as normal, is: _____*

11 *The value of kappa is: _____*

12 *This value of kappa represents what level of agreement?*

a. Excellent

b. Intermediate to good

c. Poor

Chapter 6

The Natural History of Disease: Ways of Expressing Prognosis

Learning Objectives

- To compare five different ways of describing the natural history of disease: case-fatality, 5-year survival, observed survival, median survival time, and relative survival.
- To describe two approaches for calculating observed survival over time: the life table approach and the Kaplan-Meier method.
- To illustrate the use of life tables for examining changes in survival.
- To describe how improvements in available diagnostic methods may affect the estimation of prognosis (stage migration).

At this point, we have learned how diagnostic and screening tests permit the categorization of sick and healthy individuals. Once a person is identified as having a disease, the question arises: *How can we characterize the natural history of the disease in quantitative terms?* Such quantification is important for several reasons. First, it is necessary to describe the *severity* of a disease to establish priorities for clinical services and public health programs. Second, patients often ask questions about *prognosis* (Fig. 6.1). Third, such quantification is important to establish a baseline for natural history, so that as new treatments become available, the effects of these treatments can be compared with the expected outcome without them. This is also important to identify different treatments or management strategies for different stages of the disease. Furthermore, if different types of therapy are available for a given disease, such as surgical or medical treatments or two different types of surgical procedures, we want to be able to compare the effectiveness of the various types of therapy. Therefore, to allow such a comparison, we need a quantitative means of expressing the prognosis in groups receiving the different treatments.

This chapter describes some of the ways in which prognosis can be described in quantitative terms for a group of patients. Thus the natural history of disease (and hence its prognosis) is discussed in this chapter; later chapters discuss the issue of how to intervene in the natural history of disease to improve prognosis: Chapters 10 and 11 discuss how randomized trials are used to select the most appropriate intervention (medical, surgical, or lifestyle), and Chapter 18 discusses how, through screening, disease can be detected at an earlier point than usual in its natural history to maximize the effectiveness of treatment. To discuss prognosis, let's begin with a schematic representation of the natural history of disease in a patient, as shown in Fig. 6.2.

Point A marks the biologic onset of disease. Often, this point cannot be identified because it occurs subclinically, perhaps as a subcellular change, such as an alteration in DNA. At some point in the progression of the disease process (point P), pathologic evidence of disease could be obtained if it were sought by population screening or by a physician, probably during a routine screening; this evidence can also be an incidental finding while managing another disease or complaint in the same patient. Subsequently, signs and symptoms of the disease develop in the patient (point S), and at some time after that, the patient may seek medical care (point M). The patient may then receive a diagnosis (point D), after which treatment may be given (point T). The subsequent course of the disease might result in cure or remission, control of the disease (with or without disability), or even death.

At what point do we begin to quantify survival time? Ideally we might prefer to do so from the onset of disease. However, this is not generally possible, because the time of biologic onset in an individual is most often not known. If we were to count from the time at which symptoms begin, we would introduce considerable subjective variability in measuring length of survival because we inadvertently ignored the time between the biologic onset of disease to the first symptoms and signs, which could range from hours or days (for an acute infection) to month or years (e.g., as in prostate cancer). In general, in order to standardize the calculations, duration of survival is counted from the time of diagnosis. However, even with the use of this starting point, variability still occurs, because patients differ in the point at which they seek medical care. In addition, some diseases, such as certain types of arthritis, are indolent (pain-free) and develop slowly, so that patients may not be able to accurately pinpoint the onset of

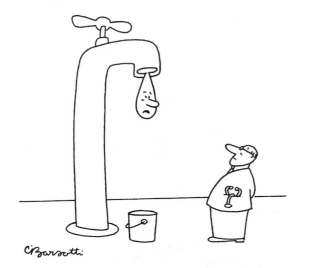

"How much time do I have, Doc?"

Fig. 6.1 "How much time do I have, Doc?" Concern about prognosis. (Charles Barsotti/The New Yorker Collection/The Cartoon Bank.)

symptoms or recall the point in time at which they sought medical care. Furthermore, when survival is counted from the time of diagnosis, any patients who may have died before a diagnosis was made are excluded from the count. What effect would this have on our estimates of prognosis?

An important related question is, "How is the diagnosis made?" Is there a clear *pathognomonic* test for the disease in question? Such a test is often not available. Sometimes a disease may be diagnosed by the isolation of an infectious agent, but because people can be carriers of organisms without actually being infected, we do not always know that the isolated organism is the cause of disease. For some diseases, we might prefer to make a diagnosis by tissue confirmation taken by biopsy, but there is often variability in the interpretation of tissue slides by different pathologists. An additional issue is that with certain health problems, such as headaches, lower back pain, and dysmenorrhea, a specific tissue diagnosis is not possible. Consequently, when we say that survivorship is measured from the time of diagnosis, the time frame is not always clear. These issues should be kept in mind as we proceed to discuss different approaches to estimating prognosis.

Prognosis can be expressed either in terms of deaths from the disease or in terms of survivors with the disease. Although both approaches are used in the following discussion, the final end point used for the purposes of our discussion in this example is death. Because death is inevitable, we are not talking about dying versus not dying, but rather about extending

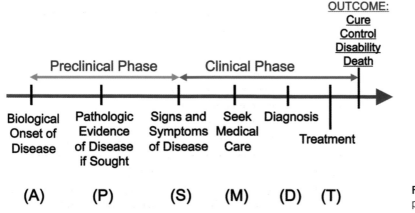

Fig. 6.2 The natural history of disease in a patient.

the interval until death occurs following diagnosis. Other end points might be used, including the interval from diagnosis to recurrence of disease or from diagnosis to the time of functional impairment, disease-specific complication, disability, or changes in the patient's quality of life, all of which may be affected by the invasiveness of the available treatment, when the treatment was initiated, or the extent to which some of the symptoms can be relieved—even if the patient's life span cannot be extended. These are all important measures, but they are not discussed in this chapter.

Case-Fatality

The first way to express prognosis is *case-fatality*, which was discussed in Chapter 4. Case-fatality is defined as the number of people who die of a disease divided by the number of people who have the disease. Given that a person has the disease, what is the likelihood that he or she will die of the disease? Note that the denominator for case-fatality is the number of people who have the disease, which makes it a proportion, while sometimes it is incorrectly referred to as a rate. This differs from a *mortality rate*, in which the denominator includes anyone at risk of dying of the disease—both persons who have the disease and persons who do not (yet) have the disease, but in whom it could develop.

Case-fatality does not include any explicit statement of time. However, time is expressed implicitly, because case-fatality is generally used for acute diseases in which death, if it occurs, occurs relatively soon after diagnosis. Thus if the usual natural history of the disease is known, the term *case-fatality* refers to the period after diagnosis during which death might be expected to occur.

Case-fatality is ideally suited to diseases that are short-term, acute conditions. In chronic diseases, in which death may occur many years after diagnosis and the possibility of death from other causes becomes more likely, case-fatality becomes a less useful measure. For example, in the study of prostate cancer, most men with this diagnosis die from some other cause, due to the very slow progression of this cancer. We therefore use different approaches for expressing prognosis in such diseases.

Person-Years

A useful way of expressing mortality is in terms of the number of deaths divided by the person-years over which a group is observed. Because individuals are often observed for different periods of time, the unit used for counting observation time is the person-year. (Person-years were previously discussed in Chapter 3, pages 47–50.) The number of person-years for two people, each of whom is observed for 5 years, is equal to that of 10 people, each of whom is observed for 1 year—that is, 10 person-years. The numbers of person-years can then be added together and the number of events such as deaths can be calculated per the number of person-years observed.

One problem in using person-years is that each person-year is assumed to be equivalent to every other person-year (i.e., the risk is the same in any person-year observed). However, this may not be true. Consider the situation in Fig. 6.3 showing two examples of 10 person-years: two people each observed for 5 years and five people each observed for 2 years. Are they equivalent?

Suppose the situation is that shown in Fig. 6.4, in which the period of greatest risk of dying is from shortly after diagnosis until about 20 months after diagnosis. Clearly most of the person-years in the first example (i.e., two persons observed for 5 years) will be outside the period of greatest risk (Fig. 6.5), the times from 20 months to 60 months. In contrast, most of the 2-year intervals of the five persons shown in the second example will occur during the period of highest risk

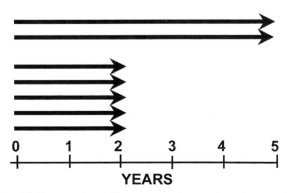

Fig. 6.3 Two examples of 10 person-years: two people, each observed for 5 years, and five people, each observed for 2 years.

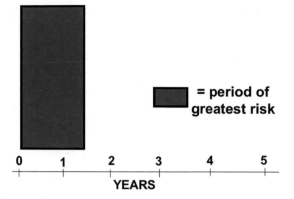

Fig. 6.4 Timing of period of greatest risk is from shortly after diagnosis until about 20 months after diagnosis.

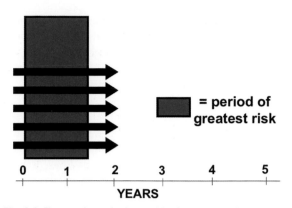

Fig. 6.6 Five people, each observed for 2 years, and the relation to the period of greatest risk.

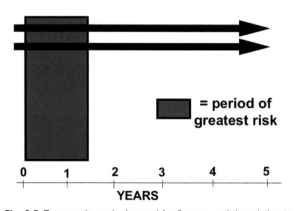

Fig. 6.5 Two people, each observed for 5 years, and the relation to the period of greatest risk.

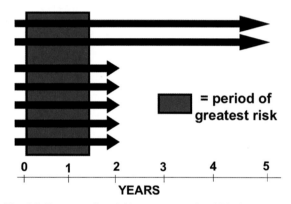

Fig. 6.7 Two examples of 10 person-years in which the period of greatest risk is from shortly after diagnosis until about 20 months after diagnosis.

(Fig. 6.6). Consequently, when we compare the two examples (Fig. 6.7), more deaths would be expected in the example of five persons observed for 2 years than in the example of two persons observed for 5 years. Despite this issue, person-years are useful as denominators of rates of events in many situations, such as randomized trials (see Chapters 10 and 11) and cohort studies (see Chapter 8). Note that, as discussed in other textbooks,[1] a rate per person-years is equivalent to an average yearly rate. Thus a rate per person-years can be compared to a Vital Statistics yearly rate based on the period's midpoint population estimate. This is useful when it is of interest to compare rates of per person-years in a study with population rates.

Five-Year Survival

Another measure used to express prognosis is *5-year survival*. This term is frequently used in clinical medicine, particularly in evaluating treatments for cancer.

The 5-year survival is the percentage of patients who are alive 5 years after treatment begins or 5 years after diagnosis. (Although 5-year survival is often referred to as a rate, it is actually a proportion.) Despite the widespread use of the 5-year interval, it should be pointed out that there is nothing magical about 5 years. Certainly no significant biologic change occurs abruptly at 5 years in the natural history of a disease that would justify its use as an end point. However, most deaths from cancer typically occurred during this period after diagnosis when it was first used in the 1950s, so 5-year survival has been used as an index of success in cancer treatment since. Some literature on chronic diseases, such as cardiovascular diseases, use 10-year survival instead of 5-year survival.

One problem with the use of 5-year survival has become more prominent in recent years with the advent of better screening programs. Let's examine a hypothetical example: Fig. 6.8 shows a timeline for a woman who had biologic onset of breast cancer in 2005. Because the disease was subclinical at that time, she had no symptoms. In 2013, she felt a lump in her breast, which precipitated a visit to her physician, who made the diagnosis. The patient then underwent a mastectomy. In 2015, she died of metastatic cancer. As measured by 5-year survival, which is often used in oncology as a measure of whether therapy has been successful, this patient is not a "success," because she survived for only 2 years after diagnosis.

Let's now imagine that this woman lived in a community in which there was an aggressive breast cancer mammography screening campaign (lower timeline in Fig. 6.9). As before, biologic onset of disease occurred in 2005, but in 2010, she was identified through screening as having a very small mass in her breast. She had surgery in 2010 but died in 2015. Because she survived for 5 years after diagnosis and therapy, she would now be identified as a therapeutic "success" in terms of 5-year survival. However, this apparently longer survival is an artifact. Death still occurred in 2015; the patient's life was not lengthened by early detection and therapy. What has happened is that the interval between her diagnosis (and treatment) and her death was increased through earlier diagnosis, but there was no delay in the time of death. (The interval between the earlier diagnosis in 2010, made possible by the screening test, and the later usual time of diagnosis in 2013 is called the *lead time*. This concept is discussed in detail in Chapter 18 in the context of evaluating screening programs.) It is misleading to conclude that, given the patient's 5-year survival, the outcome of the second scenario is any better than that of the first, because no change in the natural history of the disease has occurred, as reflected by the year of death. Indeed, the only change that has taken place is that when the diagnosis was made 3 years earlier (2010 vs. 2013), the patient received medical care for breast cancer, with all its attendant difficulties, for an additional 3 years. Thus, when screening is performed, a higher 5-year survival may be observed, not because people live longer, but only because an earlier diagnosis has been made. This type of potential bias (known as *lead time bias*) must be taken into account in evaluating any screening program before it can be concluded that the screening is beneficial in extending survival.

Another problem with 5-year survival is that if we want to look at the survival experience of a group of patients who were diagnosed less than 5 years ago, we clearly cannot use this criterion, because 5 years of observation are necessary in these patients to calculate 5-year survival. Therefore if we want to assess a therapy that was introduced less than 5 years ago, 5-year survival is not an appropriate measure.

A final issue relating to 5-year survival is shown in Fig. 6.10. Here we see survival curves for two populations, A and B. Five-year survival is about 10%. However, the curves leading to the same 5-year survival are quite different. Although survival at 5 years is the same in both groups, most of the deaths in group A did not occur until the fifth year, whereas most of the deaths in group B occurred in the first year since they

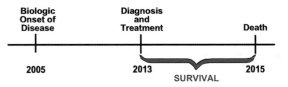

Fig. 6.8 The problem of 5-year survival in a screened population: I. Situation without screening.

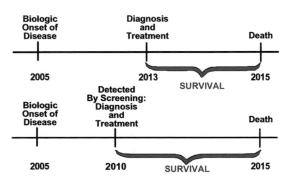

Fig. 6.9 The problem of 5-year survival in a screened population: II. Earlier disease detection by screening.

generally had a shorter time to event (death) compared with group A. Thus despite the identical 5-year survivals, survival during the 5 years is clearly better for those in group A.

Observed Survival

RATIONALE FOR THE LIFE TABLE

Another approach to quantifying prognosis is to use the actual observed survival of patients followed over time, based on knowing the interval within which the event has occurred. For this purpose, we use a *life table*. Life tables have been used by actuaries to estimate risk in populations for centuries when there were no data on individuals. Actuarial methods and models have been applied in a large number of situations, including property/casualty, life insurance, pensions and health insurance, among others. Actuaries are credentialed, with a foundation of statistics and probability, stochastic processes, and actuarial methods and models.

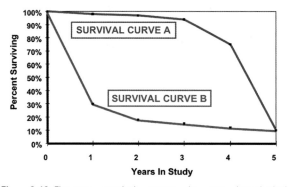

Fig.   6.10 Five-year   survival   curves   in   two   hypothetical populations.

Let's examine the conceptual framework underlying the calculation of survival rates using a life table, especially when the exact event time is not known, but rather we use the interval within which the event took place.

Table 6.1 shows a hypothetical study of treatment results in patients who were treated from 2010 to 2014 and followed to 2015. (By just glancing at this table, you can tell that the example is hypothetical, because the title indicates that no patients were lost to follow-up!)

For each calendar year of treatment, the table shows the number of patients enrolled in treatment and the number of patients alive at each calendar year after the initiation of that treatment. For example, of 84 patients enrolled in treatment in 2010, 44 were alive in 2011, a year after beginning treatment; 21 were alive in 2012; and so on.

The results in Table 6.1 include all the data available for assessing the treatment. If we want to describe the prognosis in these treated patients using all of the data in the table, obviously we cannot use 5-year survival, because the entire group of 375 patients has not been observed for 5 years. We could calculate 5-year survival using only the first 84 patients who were enrolled in 2010 and observed until 2015, because they were the only ones observed for 5 years. However, this would require us to discard the rest of the data, which would be unfortunate, given the effort and expense involved in obtaining the data, and also given the additional light that the survival experience of those patients would cast on the effectiveness of the treatment. The question is: How can we use *all* of the information in Table 6.1 to describe the survival experience of the patients in this study?

TABLE 6.1	**Hypothetical Study of Treatment Results in Patients Treated From 2010–2014 and Followed to 2015 (None Lost to Follow-Up)**					
		NUMBER ALIVE ON ANNIVERSARY OF TREATMENT				
Year of Treatment	**No. of Patients Treated**	**2001**	**2002**	**2003**	**2004**	**2005**
2010	84	44	21	13	10	8
2011	62		31	14	10	6
2012	93			50	20	13
2013	60				29	16
2014	76					43

To use all of the data, we rearrange the data from Table 6.1 as shown in Table 6.2. In this table, the data show the number of patients who started treatment each calendar year and the number of those who remained alive on each anniversary of the initiation of treatment. The patients who started treatment in 2014 were observed for only 1 year, because the study ended in 2015.

With the data in this format, how do we use the table? First we ask, "What is the probability of surviving for 1 year after the beginning of treatment?" To answer this, we divide the total number of patients who were alive 1 year after the initiation of treatment (197) by the total number of patients who started treatment (375; Table 6.3).

The probability of surviving the first year (P_1) is:

$$P_1 = \frac{197}{375} = 0.525$$

Next, we ask, "What is the probability that, having survived the first year after beginning treatment, the patients will survive the second year?" We see in Table 6.4 that 197 people survived the first year, but for 43 of them (the ones who were enrolled in 2014), we have no further information because they were observed for only 1 year. Because 71 survived the second year, we calculate the probability of surviving the second year, if the patient survived the first year (P_2), as:

$$P_2 = \frac{71}{197 - 43} = 0.461$$

In the denominator we subtract the 43 patients for whom we have no data for the second year.

Following this pattern, we ask, "Given that a person has survived to the end of the second year, what is the probability, on average, that he or she will survive to the end of the third year?"

In Table 6.5, we see that 36 survived the third year. Although 71 had survived the second year, we have no further information on survival for 16 of them because they were enrolled late in the study. Therefore we subtract 16 from 71 and calculate the probability

TABLE 6.2 Rearrangement of Data in Table 6.1, Showing Survival Tabulated by Years Since Enrollment in Treatment (None Lost to Follow-Up)

Year of Treatment	No. of Patients Treated	NUMBER ALIVE AT END OF YEAR				
		1st Year	2nd Year	3rd Year	4th Year	5th Year
2010	84	44	21	13	10	8
2011	62	31	14	10	6	
2012	93	50	20	13		
2013	60	29	16			
2014	76	43				

TABLE 6.3 Analysis of Survival in Patients Treated From 2010–2014 and Followed to 2015 (None Lost to Follow-Up): I

Year of Treatment	No. of Patients Treated	NUMBER ALIVE AT END OF YEAR				
		1st Year	2nd Year	3rd Year	4th Year	5th Year
2010	84	44	21	13	10	8
2011	62	31	14	10	6	
2012	93	50	20	13		
2013	60	29	16			
2014	76	43				
Totals	375	197				

P_1 = Probability of surviving the 1st year = $\frac{197}{375}$ = 0.525

TABLE 6.4 Analysis of Survival in Patients Treated From 2010–2014 and Followed to 2015 (None Lost to Follow-Up): II

Year of Treatment	No. of Patients Treated	NUMBER ALIVE AT END OF YEAR				
		1st Year	2nd Year	3rd Year	4th Year	5th Year
2010	84	44	21	13	10	8
2011	62	31	14	10	6	
2012	93	50	20	13		
2013	60	29	16			
2014	76	43				
Totals		197	71			

$$P_2 = \text{Probability of surviving the 2nd year} = \frac{71}{197 - 43} = 0.461$$

TABLE 6.5 Analysis of Survival in Patients Treated From 2010–2014 and Followed to 2015 (None Lost to Follow-Up): III

Year of Treatment	No. of Patients Treated	NUMBER ALIVE AT END OF YEAR				
		1st Year	2nd Year	3rd Year	4th Year	5th Year
2010	84	44	21	13	10	8
2011	62	31	14	10	6	
2012	93	50	20	13		
2013	60	29	16			
2014	76	43				
Totals			71	36		

$$P_3 = \text{Probability of surviving the 3rd year} = \frac{36}{71 - 16} = 0.655$$

of surviving the third year, given survival to the end of the second year (P₃), as:

$$P_3 = \frac{36}{71-16} = 0.655$$

We then ask, "If a person survives to the end of the third year, what is the probability that he or she will survive to the end of the fourth year?"

As seen in Table 6.6, a total of 36 people survived the third year, but we have no further information for 13 of them. Because 16 survived the fourth year, the probability of surviving the fourth year, if the person has survived the third year (P₄), is:

$$P_4 = \frac{16}{36-13} = 0.696$$

Finally, we do the same calculation for the fifth year (Table 6.7). We see that 16 people survived the fourth

year, but that no further information is available for 6 of them.

Because 8 people were alive at the end of the fifth year, the probability of surviving the fifth year, if the person has survived the fourth year (P₅), is:

$$P_5 = \frac{8}{16-6} = 0.800$$

Using all of the data that we have calculated, we ask, "What is the probability of surviving for all 5 years?" Box 6.1 shows all of the probabilities of surviving for each individual year that we have calculated.

Now we can answer the question, "If a person is enrolled in the study, what is the probability that he or she will survive 5 years after beginning treatment?" The probability of surviving for 5 years is the product of each of the probabilities of surviving each year, shown in Box 6.1. So the probability of surviving for 5 years is:

TABLE 6.6 **Analysis of Survival in Patients Treated From 2010–2014 and Followed to 2015 (None Lost to Follow-Up): IV**

Year of Treatment	No. of Patients Treated	NUMBER ALIVE AT END OF YEAR				
		1st Year	2nd Year	3rd Year	4th Year	5th Year
2010	84	44	21	13	10	8
2011	62	31	14	10	6	
2012	93	50	20	13		
2013	60	29	16			
2014	76	43				
Totals					36	16

$$P_4 = \text{Probability of surviving the 4th year} = \frac{16}{36-13} = 0.696$$

TABLE 6.7 **Analysis of Survival in Patients Treated From 2010–2014 and Followed to 2015 (None Lost to Follow-Up): V**

Year of Treatment	No. of Patients Treated	NUMBER ALIVE AT END OF YEAR				
		1st Year	2nd Year	3rd Year	4th Year	5th Year
2010	84	44	21	13	10	8
2011	62	31	14	10	6	
2012	93	50	20	13		
2013	60	29	16			
2014	76	43				
Totals					16	8

$$P_5 = \text{Probability of surviving the 5th year} = \frac{8}{16-6} = 0.800$$

BOX 6.1 PROBABILITY OF SURVIVAL FOR EACH YEAR OF THE STUDY

$P_1 = \text{Probability of surviving the 1st year} = \dfrac{197}{375} = 0.525 = 52.5\%$

$P_2 = \text{Probability of surviving the 2nd year given survival to the end of the 1st year} = \dfrac{71}{197-43} = 0.461 = 46.1\%$

$P_3 = \text{Probability of surviving the 3rd year given survival to the end of the 2nd year} = \dfrac{36}{71-16} = 0.655 = 65.5\%$

$P_4 = \text{Probability of surviving the 4th year given survival to the end of the 3rd year} = \dfrac{16}{36-13} = 0.696 = 69.6\%$

$P_5 = \text{Probability of surviving the 5th year given survival to the end of the 4th year} = \dfrac{8}{16-6} = 0.800 = 80.0\%$

$$= P_1 \times P_2 \times P_3 \times P_4 \times P_5$$
$$= 0.525 \times 0.461 \times 0.655 \times 0.696 \times 0.800$$
$$= 0.088, \text{ or } 8.8\%$$

The probabilities for surviving different lengths of time are shown in Box 6.2. These calculations can be presented graphically in a survival curve, as seen in Fig. 6.11. Note that these calculations use all of the data we have obtained, including the data for patients who were not observed for the full 5 years of the study. As a result, the use of data is economical and efficient.

BOX 6.2 CUMULATIVE PROBABILITIES OF SURVIVING DIFFERENT LENGTHS OF TIME

Probability of surviving 1 year = P_1 = 0.525 = 52.5%
Probability of surviving 2 years = $P_1 \times P_2$ = 0.525 × 0.461 = 0.242 = 24.2%
Probability of surviving 3 years = $P_1 \times P_2 \times P_3$ = 0.525 × 0.461 × 0.655 = 0.159 = 15.9%
Probability of surviving 4 years = $P_1 \times P_2 \times P_3 \times P_4$ = 0.525 × 0.461 × 0.655 × 0.696 = 0.110 = 11.0%
Probability of surviving 5 years = $P_1 \times P_2 \times P_3 \times P_4 \times P_5$ = 0.525 × 0.461 × 0.655 × 0.696 × 0.800 = 0.088 = 8.8%

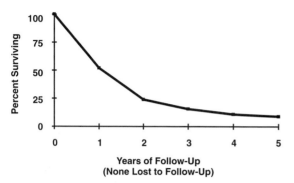

Fig. 6.11 Survival curve for a hypothetical example of patients treated from 2010–2014 and followed until 2015.

TABLE 6.8 **Rearrangement of Data in Standard Format for Life Table Calculations**

(1) Interval Since Beginning Treatment	(2) Alive at Beginning of Interval	(3) Died During Interval	(4) Withdrew During Interval
x	l_x	d_x	w_x
1st year	375	178	0
2nd year	197	83	43
3rd year	71	19	16
4th year	36	7	13
5th year	16	2	6

CALCULATING A LIFE TABLE

Let's now view the data from this example in the standard tabular form in which they are usually presented for calculating a life table. In the example just discussed, the persons for whom data were not available for the full 5 years of the study were those who were enrolled sometime after the study had started, so they were not observed for the full 5-year period. In virtually every survival study, however, subjects are also lost to follow-up. Either they cannot be found or they decline to continue participating in the study. In calculating the life table, persons for whom data are not available for the full period of follow-up—either because follow-up was not possible or because they were enrolled after the study was started—are called *withdrawals* (or *losses to follow-up* or *censored observations*).

Table 6.8 shows the data from this example with information provided about the number of deaths and the number of withdrawals in each interval. The columns are numbered merely for reference (i.e., there is no meaning inherent to the numbering). The row directly under the column labels gives the terms that are often used in life table calculations. The next

five rows of the table give data for the 5 years of the study.

The columns are as follows:

Column (1): The interval since beginning treatment.

Column (2): The number of study subjects who were alive at the beginning of each interval.

Column (3): The number of study subjects who died during that interval.

Column (4): The number who "withdrew" during the interval—that is, the number of study subjects who could not be followed for the full study period, either because they were lost to follow-up or because they were enrolled after the study had started.

Table 6.9 adds four additional columns to Table 6.8. These columns show the calculations. The new columns are as follows:

Column (5): The number of people who are effectively at risk of dying during the interval. Losses to follow-up (withdrawals) during each time interval are assumed to have occurred uniformly during the entire interval. (This assumption is most likely to hold when the interval is short.)

TABLE 6.9	Calculating a Life Table						
(1) Interval Since Beginning Treatment	(2) Alive at Beginning of Interval	(3) Died During Interval	(4) Withdrew During Interval	(5) Effective No. Exposed to Risk of Dying During Interval: Col (2) − $\frac{1}{2}$ [Col (4)]	(6) Proportion Who Died During Interval: $\frac{\text{Col (3)}}{\text{Col (5)}}$	(7) Proportion Who Did Not Die During Interval: 1 − Col (6)	(8) Cumulative Proportion Who Survived From Enrollment to End of Interval: Cumulative Survival
x	l_x	d_x	w_x	l'_x	q_x	p_x	P_x
1st year	375	178	0	375.0	0.475	0.525	0.525
2nd year	197	83	43	175.5	0.473	0.527	0.277
3rd year	71	19	16	63.0	0.302	0.698	0.193
4th year	36	7	13	29.5	0.237	0.763	0.147
5th year	16	2	6	13.0	0.154	0.846	0.124

We therefore assume that, on average, they were at risk for *half* the interval. Consequently, to calculate the number of people at risk during each interval, we subtract half the withdrawals during that interval as indicated in the heading for column 5.

Column (6): The proportion who died during the interval is calculated by dividing:

$$\frac{\text{The number who died during the interval (column 3)}}{\begin{array}{c}\text{The number who were effectively at risk}\\ \text{of dying during the interval (column 5)}\end{array}}$$

Column (7): The proportion who did not die during the interval—that is, the proportion of those who were alive at the beginning of the interval and who survived that entire interval = 1.0 − proportion who died during the interval (column 6).

Column (8): The proportion who survived from the point at which they were enrolled in the study to the end of this interval (cumulative survival). This is obtained by multiplying the proportion who were alive at the beginning of this interval and who survived this interval by the proportion who had survived from enrollment through the end of the previous interval. Thus each of the figures in column 8 gives the proportion of people enrolled in the study who survived to the end of each interval. This will be demonstrated by calculating the first two rows of Table 6.9.

Let's look at the data for the first year. (In these calculations, we will round the results at each step and use the rounded figures in the next calculation. In reality, however, when life tables are calculated, the unrounded figures are used for calculating each subsequent interval, and at the end of all the calculations, all the figures are rounded for purposes of presenting the results.) There were 375 subjects enrolled in the study who were alive at the beginning of the first year after enrollment (column 2). Of these, 178 died during the first year (column 3). All subjects were followed for the first year, so there were no withdrawals (column 4). Consequently 375 people were effectively at risk for dying during this interval (column 5). The proportion who died during this interval was 0.475: 178 (the number who died [column 3]) divided by 375 (the number who were at risk for dying [column 5]). The proportion who did not die during the interval is 1.0 − [the proportion who died (1.0 − 0.475)] = 0.525 (column 7). For the first year after enrollment, this is also the proportion who survived from enrollment to the end of the interval (column 8).

Now let's look at the data for the second year. These calculations are important to understand because they serve as the model for calculating each successive year in the life table.

To calculate the number of subjects alive at the start of the second year, we start with the number alive at the beginning of the *first* year and subtract from that number the number of deaths and withdrawals during that year. At the start of the second year, therefore,

197 subjects were alive at the beginning of the interval (column 2 [375 − 178 − 0]). Of these, 83 died during the second year (column 3). There were 43 withdrawals who had been observed for only 1 year (column 4). As discussed earlier, we subtract half of the withdrawals, 21.5 (43/2), from the 197 who were alive at the start of the interval, yielding 175.5 people who were effectively at risk for dying during this interval (column 5). The proportion who died during this interval (column 6) was 0.473—that is, 83 (the number who died [column 3]) divided by 175.5 (the number who were at risk for dying [column 5]). The proportion who did not die during the interval is 1.0 − the proportion who died (1.0 − 0.473) = 0.527 (column 7). The proportion of subjects who survived from the start of treatment to the end of the second year is the product of 0.525 (the proportion who had survived from the start of treatment to the end of the first year—that is, the beginning of the second year) multiplied by 0.527 (the proportion of people who were alive at the beginning of the second year and survived to the end of the second year) = 0.277 (column 8). Thus 27.7% of the subjects survived from the beginning of treatment to the end of the second year. Looking at the last entry in column 8, we see that 12.4% of all individuals enrolled in the study survived to the end of the fifth year.

Work through the remaining years in Table 6.9 to be sure you understand the concepts and calculations involved.

The Kaplan-Meier Method

In contrast to the life tables approach just demonstrated, in the Kaplan-Meier method,[2] predetermined intervals (such as 1 month or 1 year) are not used. Rather, we identify the exact point in time when each death, or the event of interest, occurred so that each death, or event, terminates the previous interval and a new interval (and a new row in the Kaplan-Meier table) is started. The number of persons who died at that point is used as the numerator, and the number alive up to that point (including those who died at that time point) is used as the denominator, after any withdrawals that occurred before that point are subtracted.

Let's look at the small hypothetical study shown in Fig. 6.12. Six patients were studied, of whom four died and two were lost to follow-up ("withdrawals"). The deaths occurred at 4, 10, 14, and 24 months after enrollment in the study. The data are set up as shown in Table 6.10:

Column (1): The times for each death from the time of enrollment (time that treatment was initiated).

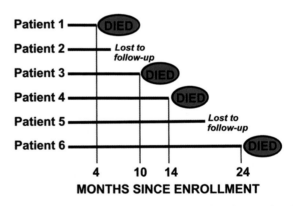

Fig. 6.12 Hypothetical example of a study of six patients analyzed by the Kaplan-Meier method.

TABLE 6.10	Calculating Survival Using the Kaplan-Meier Method[a]				
(1) Times to Deaths From Starting Treatment (Months)	(2) No. Alive at Each Time	(3) No. Who Died at Each Time	(4) Proportion Who Died at That Time: $\frac{Col\ (3)}{Col\ (2)}$	(5) Proportion Who Survived at That Time: 1 − Col (4)	(6) Cumulative Proportion Who Survived to That Time: Cumulative Survival
4	6	1	0.167	0.833	0.833
10	4	1	0.250	0.750	0.625
14	3	1	0.333	0.667	0.417
24	1	1	1.000	0.000	0.000

[a]See text and Fig. 6.12 regarding withdrawals.

Column (2): The number of patients who were alive and followed at the time of that death, including those who died at that time.

Column (3): The number who died at that time.

Column (4): The proportion of those who were alive and followed (column 2) who died at that time (column 3) (column 3/column 2).

Column (5): The proportion of those who were alive and survived (1.0 − column 4).

Column (6): Cumulative survival (the proportion of those who were initially enrolled and survived to that point).

Let's consider the first row of the table. The first death occurred at 4 months, at which time six patients were alive and followed (see Fig. 6.12). One death occurred at this point (column 3), for a proportion of 1/6 = 0.167 (column 4). The proportion who survived at that time is 1.0 − column 4, or 1.0 − 0.167 = 0.833 (column 5), which is also the cumulative survival at this point (column 6).

The next death occurred 10 months after the initial enrollment of the six patients in the study, and data for this time are seen in the next row of the table. Although only one death had occurred before this one, the number alive and followed is only four because there had also been a withdrawal before this point (not shown in the table, but seen in Fig. 6.12). Thus there was one death (column 3), and as seen in Table 6.10, the proportion who died is 1/4, or 0.250 (column 4). The proportion who survived is 1.0 − column 4, or 1.0 − 0.250 = 0.750 (column 5). Finally, the cumulative proportion surviving (column 6) is the product of the proportion who survived to the end of the previous interval (until just before the previous death) seen in column 6 of the first row (0.833) and the proportion who survived from that time until just before the second death (second row in column 5, 0.750). The product = 0.625—that is, 62.5% of the original enrollees survived to this point. Review the next two rows of the table to be sure that you understand the concepts and calculations involved.

The values calculated in column 6 are plotted as seen in Fig. 6.13. Note that the data are plotted in a stepwise fashion rather than in a smoothed slope because, after the drop in survival resulting from each death, survival then remains unchanged until the next death occurs.

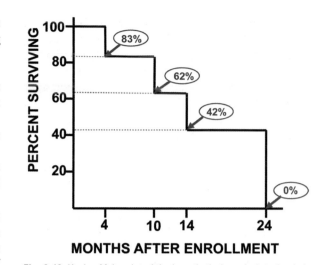

Fig. 6.13 Kaplan-Meier plot of the hypothetical survival study of six patients shown in Fig. 6.12. Percentages in red show cumulative proportions surviving after each of the deaths shown in Fig. 6.12 and are taken from column 6 in Table 6.10. (See discussion of the Kaplan-Meier method on page 134.)

When information on the exact time of death is available, the Kaplan-Meier method clearly makes fullest use of this information because the data are used to define the intervals, instead of predetermined arbitrary intervals used in the life tables method. The use of modern technology to communicate with patients, conducted simultaneously in different study sites, and electronically linking mortality data to research databases allow researchers to identify the examination of time of event. In addition, computer programs are readily available that make the Kaplan-Meier method easily calculated for large data sets as well. The majority of longitudinal studies in the published literature now report data on survival using the Kaplan-Meier method. For example, in 2000, Rosenhek and colleagues reported a study of patients with asymptomatic, but severe, aortic stenosis.[3] An unresolved issue was whether patients with asymptomatic disease should have their aortic valves replaced. The investigators examined the natural history of this condition to assess the overall survival of these patients and to identify predictors of outcome. Gibson and colleagues[4] studied the association between coronary artery calcium (CAC) and incident cerebrovascular events (CVE) in 6,779 participants of the Multi-Ethnic Study of Atherosclerosis (MESA) and then

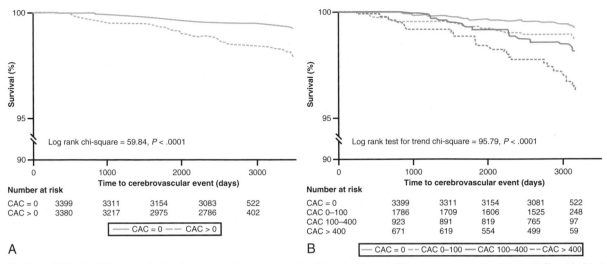

Fig. 6.14 (A) Kaplan-Meier analysis showing the event-free survival of participants with and without coronary artery calcium *(CAC)* and incident cerebrovascular events (CVE) in the MESA (Multi-Ethnic Study of Atherosclerosis) cohort. (B) Kaplan-Meier analysis showing the CVE event-free survival of participants with 0, 0 to 100, >100 to 400, and >400 CAC (Agatston units) and incident CVE in the MESA cohort. (From Gibson AO, Blaha MJ, Arnan MK, et al. Coronary artery calcium and incident cerebrovascular events in an asymptomatic cohort. The MESA Study. *JACC Cardiovasc Imaging.* 2014;7:1108–1115.)

followed for an average of 9.5 years. Fig. 6.14A shows their Kaplan-Meier analysis of CVE-free survival by the presence or absence of CAC at baseline. Participants with CAC present during the baseline examination had a lower CVE-free survival rate as compared with participants with CAC absent at the baseline visit. In Fig. 6.14B, the authors divided the participants into four groups according to their CAC at the baseline visit (CAC: 0, 0 to 100, >100 to 400, and >400 Agatston units), and we can clearly see a separate curve for each group showing a significant graded CVE-free survival.

Assumptions Made in Using Life Tables and Kaplan-Meier Method

Two important assumptions are made in using life tables and Kaplan-Meier methods. The first is that there has been no secular (temporal) change in the effectiveness of treatment or in survivorship over calendar time. That is, we assume that over the period of the study, there has been no improvement in treatment and that survivorship in one calendar year of the study is the same as in another calendar year of the study. Clearly, if a study is conducted over many years, this assumption may not be valid because, fortunately, therapies improve

over time. If we are concerned that the effectiveness of therapy may have changed over the course of the study, we could examine the early data separately from the later data. If they seem to differ, the early and later periods could be analyzed separately and the effects compared.

The second assumption relates to follow-up of persons enrolled in the study. In virtually every real-life study, participants are lost to follow-up. People can be lost to follow-up for many reasons. Some may die and may not be traced. Some may move or seek care elsewhere. Some may be lost because their disease disappears and they feel well. In most studies, we do not know the actual reasons for losses to follow-up. How can we deal with the problem of people lost to follow-up for whom we therefore have no further information on survival? Because we have baseline data on these people, we could compare the characteristics of the persons lost to follow-up with those of persons who remained in the study. If a large proportion of the study population is lost to follow-up, the findings of the study will be less valid. The challenge is to minimize losses to follow-up. In any case, the second assumption made in life table analysis is that the survival experience of people who are lost to follow-up is the same as the experience of those who are followed up. Although this assumption is made for purposes of calculation, in actual fact its validity may often be questionable. For mortality, however, the assumption can be verified by means of linkage with the United States National Death Index, which allows comparing the mortality of those lost to follow up with those who continue to be followed up.

Although the term *life table* might suggest that these methods are useful only for calculating survival, this is not so. Death need not be the end point in these calculations. For example, *survival* can be calculated as time to the development of hypertension, time to the development of a recurrence of cancer, or survival time free of treatment side effects. Furthermore, although we can look at a single survival curve, often the greatest interest lies in comparing two or more survival curves, such as for those who are treated and those who are not treated in a randomized trial. In conducting such comparisons, statistical methods are available to determine whether one curve is significantly different from another.

A third assumption is specific to traditional life tables, but not the Kaplan-Meier method, and deals with the use of predetermined intervals when calculating the life tables. The prime reason to use the life table method over the Kaplan-Meier method is that if we are not able to identify the exact time of event, we must use an arbitrary interval within which the event took place. Subsequently we are not able to identify the exact time of withdrawals from the study. Thus it is important to assume that there is a uniform distribution of risk and withdrawal during each time interval, and that there is no rapid change in the risk or withdrawal within a time interval. A reasonable way to achieve this assumption is to make the interval as short as possible.

EXAMPLE OF USE OF A LIFE TABLE

Life tables are used in virtually every clinical area. However, they are less commonly used nowadays and have been replaced with the Kaplan-Meier method, in which the investigators are able to identify the exact time of event for each study participant. Life tables were the standard means by which survival is expressed and compared for a long time, before the establishment of the Kaplan-Meier method. Let's examine a few examples. One of the great triumphs of pediatrics in

recent decades has been the treatment of leukemia in children. However, the improvement has been much greater for whites than for blacks, and the reasons for this difference are not clear. At a time when survival rates from childhood acute leukemia were increasing rapidly, a study was conducted to explore the racial differences in survivorship. Figs. 6.15 to 6.17 show data from this study.[5] The curves are based on life tables that were constructed using the approach discussed earlier.

Fig. 6.15 shows survival for white and black children with leukemia in Baltimore over a 16-year period. No black children survived longer than 4 years, but some white children survived as long as 11 years in this 16-year period of observation.

What changes took place in survivorship during the 16 years of the study? Fig. 6.16 and Fig. 6.17 show changes in leukemia mortality over time in whites and blacks, respectively. The 16-year period was divided into three periods: 1960 to 1964 (*solid line*), 1965 to 1969 (*dashed line*), and 1970 to 1975 (*dotted line*).

In whites (see Fig. 6.16), survivorship increased in each successive period. For example, if we examine 3-year survival by looking at the 3-year point on each

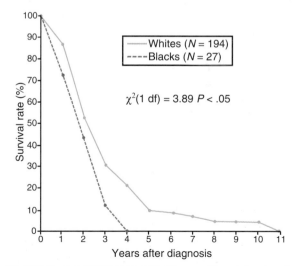

Fig. 6.15 Survival of children aged 0 to 19 years with acute lymphocytic leukemia by race, metropolitan Baltimore, 1960–1975. (From Szklo M, Gordis L, Tonascia J, Kaplan E. The changing survivorship of white and black children with leukemia. *Cancer.* 1978;42:59–66. Copyright 1978 American Cancer Society. Reprinted by permission of Wiley-Liss, Inc., a subsidiary of John Wiley & Sons, Inc.)

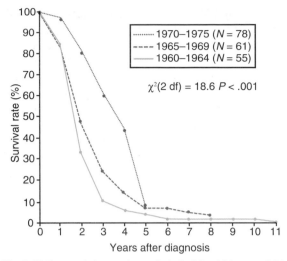

Fig. 6.16 Temporal changes in survival of white children aged 0 to 19 years with acute lymphocytic leukemia, metropolitan Baltimore, 1960–1975. (From Szklo M, Gordis L, Tonascia J, Kaplan E. The changing survivorship of white and black children with leukemia. *Cancer.* 1978;42:59–66. Copyright 1978 American Cancer Society. Reprinted by permission of Wiley-Liss, Inc., a subsidiary of John Wiley & Sons, Inc.)

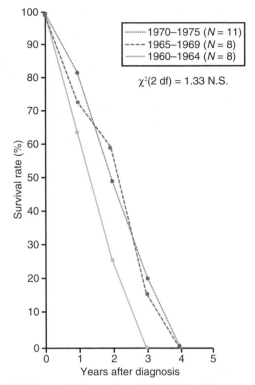

Fig. 6.17 Temporal changes in survival of black children aged 0 to 19 years with acute lymphocytic leukemia, metropolitan Baltimore, 1960–1975. (From Szklo M, Gordis L, Tonascia J, Kaplan E. The changing survivorship of white and black children with leukemia. *Cancer.* 1978;42:59–66. Copyright 1978 American Cancer Society. Reprinted by permission of Wiley-Liss, Inc., a subsidiary of John Wiley & Sons, Inc.)

successive curve, we see that survival improved from 8% to 25% to 58%. In contrast, in blacks (see Fig. 6.17) there was much less improvement in survival over time; the curves for the two later 5-year periods almost overlap.

What accounts for this racial difference? First, we must take account of the small numbers involved and the possibility that the differences could have been due to chance. Let's assume, however, that the differences are real. During the past several decades, tremendous strides have occurred in the treatment of leukemia through combined therapy, including central nervous system radiation added to chemotherapy. Why, then, does a racial difference exist in survivorship? Why is it that the improvement in therapy that has been so effective in white children has not had a comparable benefit in black children? Further analyses of the interval from the time the mother noticed symptoms to the time of diagnosis and treatment indicated that the differences in survival did not appear to be due to a delay in black parents seeking or obtaining medical care. Because acute leukemia is more severe in blacks and more advanced at the time of diagnosis, the racial difference could reflect biologic differences in the disease, such as a

more aggressive and rapidly progressive form of the illness. The definitive explanation is not known.

Apparent Effects on Prognosis of Improvements in Diagnosis

We have discussed the assumption made in using a life table that no improvement in the effectiveness of treatment has occurred over calendar time during the period of the study. Another issue in calculating and interpreting survival rates is the possible effect of improvements in diagnostic methods over calendar time.

An interesting example was reported by Feinstein and colleagues.[6] They compared survival in a cohort of patients with lung cancer first treated in 1977 with survival in a cohort of patients with lung cancer treated from 1953 to 1964. Six-month survival was higher in the latter group for both the total group and for subgroups formed on the basis of stage of disease. The authors found that the apparent improvement in survival was due in part to *stage migration*, a phenomenon shown in Fig. 6.18A to C.

In Fig. 6.18A, patients with cancer are divided into "good" and "bad" stages, on the basis of whether they had detectable metastases in 1980. Some patients who would have been assigned to a "good" stage in 1980 may have had micro-metastases at that time, which would have been unrecognized (see Fig. 6.18B).

However, by 2000, as diagnostic technology improved, many of these patients would have been assigned to a "bad" stage, because their micro-metastases would now have been recognized using improved diagnostic technology that had become available (see Fig. 6.18C). If this had occurred, survival by stage would appear to have improved even if treatment had not become any more effective during this time.

Let's consider a hypothetical example that illustrates this effect of such stage migration. Fig. 6.19A to C show a hypothetical study of cancer case-fatality for 300 patients in two time periods, 1980 and 2000,

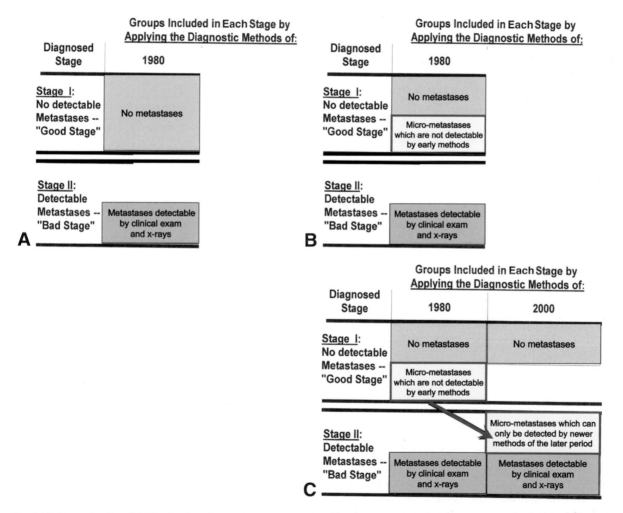

Fig. 6.18 Stage migration. (A) Classification of cases by presence or absence of detectable metastases in 1980. (B) Presence of undetectable micro-metastases in 1980. (C) Impact of improved diagnosis of micro-metastases in 2000 on classification of cases by presence or absence of detectable metastases.

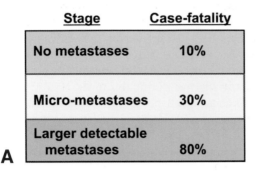

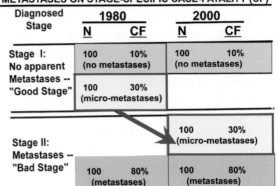

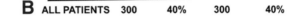

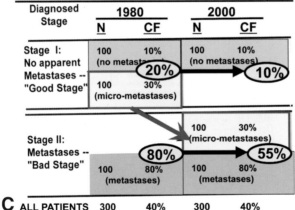

Fig. 6.19 Hypothetical example of stage migration. (A) Assumed case-fatality by stage. (B) Impact of improved diagnosis of micro-metastases on stage-specific case-fatality *(CF)*. (C) Apparent improvements in stage-specific survival as a result of stage migration even without any improvement in effectiveness of treatment.

assuming no improvement in the effectiveness of available therapy between the two periods. We will assume that as shown in Fig. 6.19A, in both time periods, the case-fatality is 10% for patients who have no metastases, 30% for those with micro-metastases, and 80% for those with metastases. Looking at Fig. 6.19B, we see that in 1980, 200 patients were classified as stage I. One hundred of these patients had no metastases, and 100 had unrecognized micro-metastases. Their case-fatalities were thus 10% and 30%, respectively. In 1980, 100 patients had clearly evident metastases and were classified as stage II; their case-fatality was 80%.

As a result of improved diagnostic technology in 2000, micro-metastases were detected in the 100 affected patients, and these patients were classified as stage II (see Fig. 6.19C). Because the prognosis of the patients with micro-metastases is worse than that of the other patients in stage I, and because, in the later study period, patients with micro-metastases are no longer included in the stage I group (because they have migrated to stage II), the case-fatality for stage I patients appears to decline from 20% in the early period to 10% in the later period. However, although the prognosis of the patients who migrated from stage

I to stage II was worse than that of the others in stage I, the prognosis for these patients was still better than that of the other patients in stage II, who had larger, more easily diagnosed metastases and a case-fatality of 80%. Consequently, the case-fatality for patients in stage II also appears to have improved, having declined from 80% in the early period to 55% in the later period, *even in the absence of any improvement in treatment effectiveness.*

The apparent improvements in survival in both stage I and stage II patients result only from the changed classification of patients with micro-metastases in the later period. Looking at the bottom line of the figure, we see that the case-fatality of 40% for all 300 patients has not changed from the early period to the later period. Only the apparent stage-specific case-fatalities have changed. It is therefore important to exclude the possibility of stage migration before attributing any apparent improvement in prognosis to improved effectiveness of medical care.

The authors call stage migration the *Will Rogers phenomenon.* The reference is to Will Rogers, an American humorist during the time of the economic depression of the 1930s. At that time, because of economic hardship, many residents of Oklahoma left the state and migrated to California. Rogers commented, "When the Okies left Oklahoma and moved to California, they raised the average intelligence level in both states."

Median Survival Time

Another approach to expressing prognosis is the median survival time, which is defined as the length of time that half (50%) of the study population survives. Why should we use median survival time rather than mean survival time, which is an average of the survival times? Median survival offers two advantages over mean survival. First, it is less affected by extremes, whereas the mean can be significantly affected by even a single outlier. One or two persons with a very long survival time could significantly affect the mean, even if all of the other survival times were much shorter. Second, if we used mean survival, we would have to observe all of the deaths in the study population before the mean could be calculated. However, to calculate median survival, we would only have to observe the deaths of half of the group under observation.

Relative Survival

Let's consider 5-year survival for a group of 30-year-old men with colorectal cancer. What would we expect their 5-year survival to be if they did not have colorectal cancer? Clearly, it would be nearly 100%. Thus we are comparing the survival observed in young men with colorectal cancer to a survival of almost 100% that is expected in those without colorectal cancer. What if we consider a group of 80-year-old men with colorectal cancer? We would not expect anything near 100% 5-year survival in a population of this age, even if they do not have colorectal cancer. We would want to compare the observed survival in 80-year-old men with colorectal cancer to the expected survival of 80-year-old men without colorectal cancer. So for any group of people with a disease, we want to compare their survival to the survival we would expect in this age group even if they did not have the disease. This is known as the *relative survival.*

Relative survival is thus defined as the ratio of the observed survival to the expected survival:

$$\text{Relative survival} = \frac{\text{Observed survival in people with the disease}}{\text{Expected survival if disease were absent}}$$

Does relative survival really make any difference? Table 6.11 shows data for patients with cancer of

TABLE 6.11 **Five-Year Observed and Relative Survival (%) by Age for Colon and Rectum Cancer, 1990–1998: SEER Program, 1970–2011**		
Age (year)	Observed Survival (%)	Relative Survival (%)
<50	64	65
50–64	61.9	65.4
65–74	54.3	62.9
>75	35.5	55.8

SEER, Surveillance, Epidemiology, and End Results (Study).
Courtesy Dr. Louise Brinton and Mr. Jake Thistle of the National Cancer Institute, using the SEER Program, 1970–2011.

the colon and rectum, both relative survival and observed survival from 1990 to 1998. When we look at the older age groups, which have high rates of mortality from other causes, there is a large difference between the observed and the relative survival. However, in young persons, who generally do not die of other causes, observed and relative survival for cancer of the colon and rectum do not differ significantly.

Another way to view relative survival is by examining the hypothetical 10-year survival curves of 80-year-old men shown in Fig. 6.20A to D. For reference, Fig. 6.20A shows a perfect survival curve of 100% (the horizontal curve at the top) over the 10 years of the study period. Fig. 6.20B adds a curve of observed survival—that is, the actual survival observed in this group of patients with the disease over the 10-year period. As seen in Fig. 6.20C, the expected survival for this group of 80-year-old men is clearly less than 100% because deaths from other causes are significant in this age group. The relative survival is the ratio of observed survival to expected survival. Since expected survival is less than perfect (100%) survival, and expected survival is the denominator for these

calculations, the relative survival will be higher than the observed survival (see Fig. 6.20D).

Generalizability of Survival Data

A final point in connection with the natural history and prognosis of disease is the question of which patients are selected for study. Let's look at one example.

Febrile seizures are common in infants. Children who are otherwise healthy often experience a seizure in association with high fever. The question arises as to whether these children should be treated with a regimen of phenobarbital or another long-term anticonvulsant medication. That is, is a febrile seizure a warning of subsequent epilepsy, or is it simply a phenomenon associated with fever in infants, in which case children are unlikely to have subsequent nonfebrile seizures?

To make a rational decision about treatment, the question we must ask is, "What is the risk that a child who has had a febrile seizure will have a subsequent nonfebrile seizure?" Fig. 6.21 shows the results of an analysis by Ellenberg and Nelson of published studies.[7]

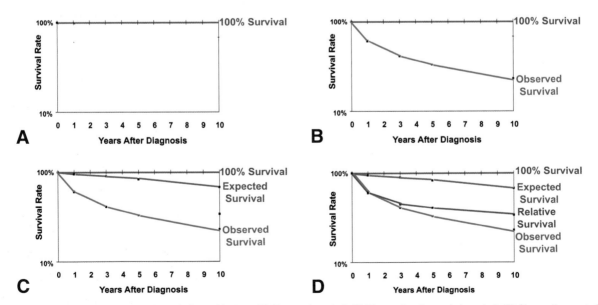

Fig. 6.20 Relative survival. (A) 100% survival over 10 years. (B) Observed survival. (C) Observed and expected survival. (D) Observed, expected, and relative survival.

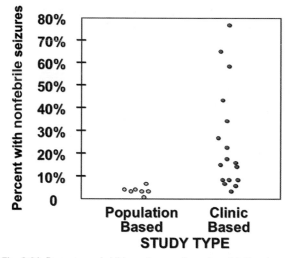

Fig. 6.21 Percentage of children who experienced nonfebrile seizures after one or more febrile seizures, by study design. (Modified from Ellenberg JH, Nelson KB. Sample selection and the natural history of disease: studies on febrile seizures. *JAMA.* 1980;243:1337–1340.)

Each dot shows the percentage of children with febrile seizures who later developed nonfebrile seizures in a different study. The authors divided the studies into two groups: population-based studies and studies based in individual clinics, such as epilepsy or pediatric clinics. The results from different clinic-based studies show a considerable range in the risk of later development of nonfebrile seizures. However, the results of population-based studies show little variation in risk, and the results of all of these studies tend to cluster at a low level of risk.

Why should the two types of studies differ? Which results would you believe? Each of the clinics probably had different selection criteria and different referral patterns. Consequently, the different risks observed in the different clinic-based studies are probably the result of the selection of different populations in each of the clinics. In contrast, in the population-based studies (which may in fact be randomly selected), this type of variation due to selection is reduced or eliminated, which accounts for the close clustering of the data, and for the resultant finding that the risk of nonfebrile seizures is very low. The important point is that it may be very tempting to look at patient records in one hospital and generalize the findings to all patients in

BOX 6.3 FIVE APPROACHES TO EXPRESSING PROGNOSIS

1. Case-fatality
2. 5-year survival
3. Observed survival
4. Median survival time
5. Relative survival

the general population. However, this is not a legitimate approach because patients who come to a certain clinic or hospital often are not representative of all patients in the community. This does not mean that studies conducted at a single hospital or clinic cannot be of value. Indeed, there is much to be learned from conducting studies at single hospitals. However, these studies are particularly prone to *selection bias*, and this possibility must always be kept in mind when the findings from such studies and their potential generalizability are being interpreted.

Conclusion

This chapter has discussed five ways of expressing prognosis (Box 6.3). Which approach is best depends on the type of data that are available, data collection methods, and the purpose of the data analysis.

REFERENCES

1. Szklo M, Nieto FJ. *Epidemiology: Beyond the Basics.* 3rd ed. Burlington, MA: Jones & Bartlett; 2014.
2. Kaplan EL, Meier P. Nonparametric estimation from incomplete observations. *J Am Stat Assoc.* 1958;53:457–481.
3. Rosenhek R, Binder T, Porenta G, et al. Predictors of outcome in severe, asymptomatic aortic stenosis. *N Engl J Med.* 2000;343:611–617.
4. Gibson AO, Blaha MJ, Arnan MK, et al. Coronary artery calcium and incident cerebrovascular events in an asymptomatic cohort. The MESA study. *JACC Cardiovasc Imaging.* 2014;7:1108–1115.
5. Szklo M, Gordis L, Tonascia J, et al. The changing survivorship of white and black children with leukemia. *Cancer.* 1978;42:59–66.
6. Feinstein AR, Sosin DM, Wells CK. The Will Rogers phenomenon: stage migration and new diagnostic techniques as a source of misleading statistics for survival in cancer. *N Engl J Med.* 1985;312:1604–1608.
7. Ellenberg JH, Nelson KB. Sample selection and the natural history of disease: studies on febrile seizures. *JAMA.* 1980;243:1337–1340.

REVIEW QUESTIONS FOR CHAPTER 6 ....

Question 1 is based on the information given in the table below:

Year of Treatment	No. of Patients Treated	NO. OF PATIENTS ALIVE ON EACH ANNIVERSARY OF BEGINNING TREATMENT		
		1st	2nd	3rd
2012	75	60	56	48
2014	63	55	31	
2015	42	37		
Total	180	152	87	48

A total of 180 patients were treated for disease X from 2012 to 2014, and their progress was followed to 2015. The treatment results are given in the table. No patients were lost to follow-up.

1 *What is the probability of surviving for 3 years?* _____

2 *An important assumption in this type of analysis is that:*
   a. Treatment has improved during the period of the study
   b. The quality of record-keeping has improved during the period of the study
   c. No change has occurred in the effectiveness of the treatment during the period of the study
   d. An equal number of men and women were enrolled each year
   e. None of the above

3 *Which of the following is a good index of the severity of a short-term, acute disease?*
   a. Cause-specific death rate
   b. 5-year survival
   c. Case-fatality
   d. Standardized mortality ratio
   e. None of the above

4 *A diagnostic test has been introduced that will detect a certain disease 1 year earlier than it is usually detected. Which of the following is most likely to happen to the disease within the 10 years after the test is introduced? (Assume that early detection has no effect on the natural history of the disease. Also assume that no changes in death certification practices occur during the 10 years.)*
   a. The period prevalence rate will decrease
   b. The apparent 5-year survival will increase
   c. The age-adjusted mortality rate will decrease
   d. The age-adjusted mortality rate will increase
   e. The incidence rate will decrease

5 *Which of the following statements about relative survival is true?*
   a. It refers to survival of first-degree relatives
   b. It is generally closer to observed survival in elderly populations
   c. It is generally closer to observed survival in young populations
   d. It generally differs from observed survival by a constant amount, regardless of age
   e. None of the above

Questions 6 to 8 are based on the data in the table below. The data were obtained from a study of 248 patients with acquired immunodeficiency syndrome (AIDS) who were given a new treatment and followed to determine survival. The study population was followed for 36 months.
Note: Carry your calculations in the table to four decimal places (i.e., 0.1234), but give the final answer to three decimal places (e.g., 0.123 or 12.3%).

6 *For those people who survived the second year, what is the probability of dying in the third year?* _____

7 *What is the probability that a person enrolled in the study will survive to the end of the third year?* _____

Survival of Patients With Acquired Immunodeficiency Syndrome After Diagnosis							
(1) Interval Since Beginning Treatment (Months)	(2) Alive at Beginning of Interval	(3) Died During Interval	(4) Withdrew During Interval	(5) Effective Number Exposed to Risk of Dying During Interval: Col (2) − $\frac{1}{2}$ [Col (4)]	(6) Proportion Who Died During Interval: Col (3) Col (5)	(7) Proportion Who Did Not Die During Interval: 1 − Col (6)	(8) Cumulative Proportion Who Survived From Enrollment to End of Interval: Cumulative Survival
x	l_x	d_x	w_x	l'_x	q_x	p_x	P_x
1–12	248	96	27				
13–24	125	55	13				
25–36	57	55	2				

8 *Before reporting the results of this survival analysis, the investigators compared the baseline characteristics of the 42 persons who withdrew from the study before its end with those of the participants who had complete follow-up. This was done for which of the following reasons:*
   a. To test whether randomization was successful
   b. To check for changes in prognosis over time
   c. To check whether those who remained in the study represent the total study population
   d. To determine whether the outcome of those who remained in the study is the same as the outcome of the underlying population
   e. To check for confounders in the exposed and nonexposed groups

9 *This question is based on a study by Faraday et al. where they examined the association between history of skin infection and surgical site infection (SSI) after elective surgery. They followed 613 patients for about 6 months. The figure below shows the Kaplan-Meier estimates of cumulative incidence of SSI or infectious death by history of skin infection. Using the figure, the median survival time is:*

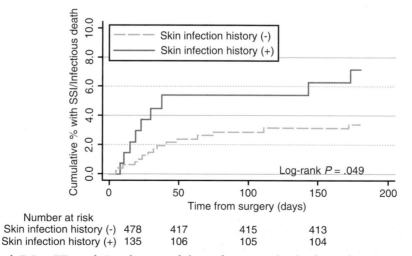

(Faraday N, Rock P, Lin EE, et al. Past history of skin infection and risk of SSI after elective surgery. *Ann Surg.* 2013;257:150–154.)

a. 30–50 days

b. 60–80 days

c. 90–110 days

d. 120–130 days

e. Information cannot be obtained from this figure

10 *In the Faraday study (see question 9), which of the following is/are necessary assumption(s) when using the Kaplan-Meier method to estimate cumulative incidence:*

a. The incidence of SSI events is less than 10% in the study population

b. Those who are lost to follow-up before 6 months have the same survival experience as those who remain in the study

c. Events and loss to follow-up occur at a constant rate during each time interval

d. Those who are censored prior to 6 months are more likely to develop SSI than those who are not censored prior to 6 months

USING EPIDEMIOLOGY TO IDENTIFY THE CAUSE OF DISEASE

In Section I, we addressed the issues of defining and diagnosing disease and describing its transmission, acquisition, and natural history in populations. In Section II, we turn to a different issue: How do we design and conduct studies to elucidate the etiology of and risk factors for human disease? If we mount a preventive intervention, how do we know if it will be effective? Such studies are critically important in both clinical medicine and public health practice.

This section begins with a discussion of the basic study designs that are used in epidemiologic studies (Chapters 7 to 11). We begin with observations that might be made by a practicing physician, where an unusual cluster of disease may occur. We describe the components of observational studies (Chapter 7), first addressing community-level associations and then cross-sectional studies. We then move on to cohort studies (Chapter 8) and the ways in which we measure associations. A brief comparison of cohort and case-control studies follows (Chapter 9). This is followed by two chapters (10 and 11) that present randomized trials, which are true experiments. We then describe how the findings from such studies may be used to estimate the risks of disease associated with specific exposures (Chapters 12 and 13). Finally, we address issues of causal inference (Chapters 15 and 16).

Why should a clinician be concerned with disease etiology? Has not the clinician's traditional role been to treat disease once it has become apparent? To answer this question, several points should be made. First, *prevention* is a major responsibility of the physician and the broader public health community; both prevention and treatment should be viewed by the physician as essential elements of his or her professional role. Indeed, many patients take the initiative and ask their physicians questions about what measures to take to maintain health and prevent certain diseases. "Should I take a baby aspirin to prevent cardiovascular disease?" "Do I really need to get regular mammograms for the early detection of breast cancer?" "What is the highest blood pressure reading you will tolerate before starting me on drugs to lower my blood pressure?" Most opportunities to prevent disease require an understanding of the *etiology* or *causes* of disease, so that exposure to a causative risk factor can be reduced or the pathogenic chain leading from the causal factor to the development of clinical illness can be interrupted.

Second, patients and their families often ask the physician questions about the *risk* of disease. What is the risk that the disease will recur? What is the risk that other family members may develop the disease? For example:

A man who suffers a myocardial infarction at a young age may ask, "Why did it happen to me? Can I prevent having a second infarction? Are my children also at high risk for having an infarction at a young age? If so, can anything be done to lower their risk?"

A woman who delivers a baby with a congenital malformation may ask, "Why did it happen? Is it because of something I did during the pregnancy? If I get pregnant again, is that child also likely to have a malformation?"

Third, in the course of doing clinical work and making bedside observations, a physician often "gets a hunch" regarding a possible relationship between a factor and the risk of a disease that is as yet not understood. For example, Alton Ochsner, the famous surgeon, noted that virtually all the patients on whom he operated for lung cancer were cigarette smokers; this observation led him to suggest that smoking could be causally related to the development of lung cancer and indicated the need to clarify the nature of this relationship by means of rigorously conducted studies in defined human populations.

Whereas clinical practice focuses on individuals, public health practice focuses on populations living in communities. In view of the tremendous potential impact of public health actions, which often affect entire communities, public health practitioners must understand how conclusions regarding health risks to a community are determined and how a foundation for preventive measures and actions is developed on the basis of population-centered data that are properly interpreted in their biologic context. Only in this way can rational policies be adopted for preventing disease and enhancing the health of populations at the lowest possible cost.

Alert and astute physicians and other public health practitioners in academic, clinical, and health department settings have many opportunities to conduct studies of disease etiology or disease risk to confirm or refute preliminary clinical or other impressions regarding the origins of diseases. The findings may be of critical importance in providing the rationale for preventing these diseases, enhancing our understanding of their pathogenesis, and suggesting directions for future laboratory and epidemiologic research. Consequently an understanding of the types of study design that are used for investigating etiology and identifying risk factors, together with an appreciation of the methodologic problems involved in such studies, is fundamental to both clinical medicine and public health practice.

Finally, this section closes with a discussion of how epidemiology can be used to assess the relative contributions of genetic and environmental factors to the causation of human disease—an assessment that has major clinical and public health policy implications (Chapter 16).

Chapter 7

Observational Studies

Learning Objectives

- To describe the motivations for and the design of observational studies.
- To discuss early origins of the research question including case reports, case series, and ecologic studies.
- To describe the cross-sectional study design and its importance.
- To discuss case-control studies, including selection of cases and controls.
- To discuss potential selection biases in case-control studies.
- To discuss information biases in case-control studies, including limitations in recall and recall bias.
- To describe other issues in case-control studies, including matching and the use of multiple controls.
- To introduce the case cross-over study design.

Case Reports and Case Series

Perhaps one of the most common and early origins of medical research questions is through careful observations by physicians and other health care providers of what they see during their clinical practice. Such individual-level observations can be documented in a case report, describing a particular clinical phenomenon in a single patient, or in a case series that describes more than one patient with similar problems. Both case reports and case series are considered the simplest of study designs (although some assert that they are merely "prestudy designs"). The main objective of case reports and case series is to provide a comprehensive and detailed description of the case(s) under observation. This allows other physicians to identify and potentially report similar cases from their practice, especially when they share geographic or specific clinical characteristics. For example, 2015 witnessed an outbreak of

the Zika virus in Latin America. Zika virus is a flavivirus transmitted by *Aedes* mosquitoes, most commonly *Aedes aegypti* and possibly *Aedes albopictus*, and originally isolated from a rhesus monkey in the Zika forest in Uganda in 1947.[1] In early 2016, following increasing numbers of infants born with microcephaly in Zika virus-affected areas, the Centers for Disease Control and Prevention (CDC) published a descriptive case series from Brazil on the possible association between Zika virus infection and microcephaly, a condition in which the baby's head is significantly smaller than expected, potentially due to incomplete brain development.[2] Another case report was published about the offspring of a Slovenian woman who lived and worked in Brazil and became pregnant in February 2015.[3] She got ill with a high fever, followed by severe musculoskeletal and retro-ocular pain and an itching and generalized maculopapular rash. No virologic testing for Zika virus was performed. She returned to Europe in the 28th week of gestation when ultrasonographic imaging showed fetal anomalies. The pregnancy was terminated in the 32nd week of gestation at the mother's request, following the approval of national and institutional ethical committees, and the Zika virus was found in the fetal brain tissue.

Despite the fact that case reports and case series are merely descriptive in nature with no reference group to make a strict comparison, the Brazilian case series was instrumental in the development of the CDC's guidelines[4] (Fig. 7.1) for the evaluation and testing, by health care providers, of infants whose mothers traveled to or resided in an area with ongoing Zika virus transmission during their pregnancies (Fig. 7.2).

Case reports and case series are key hypothesis-generating tools, especially when they are simple, inexpensive, and easy to conduct in the course of busy clinical settings. However, the lack of a comparison group is a major disadvantage. Furthermore, external validity (generalizability) is limited, given the biased selection of cases (all identified in clinical practice).

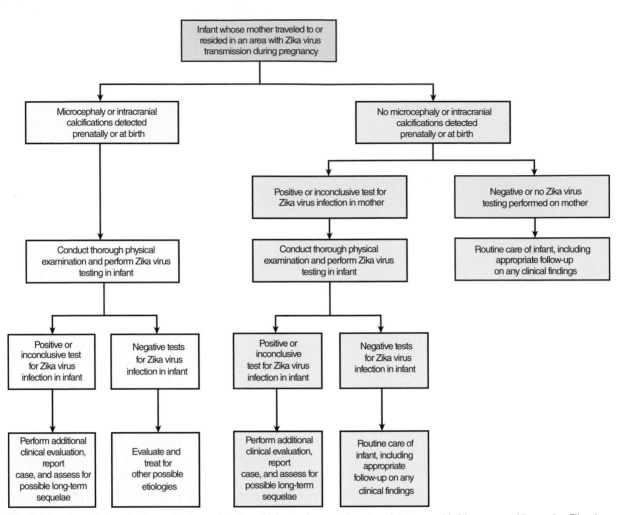

Fig. 7.1 Interim guidelines for the evaluation and testing of infants whose mothers traveled to or resided in an area with ongoing Zika virus transmission during their pregnancies. (Modified from Staples JE, Dziuban EJ, Fischer M, et al. Interim guidelines for the evaluation and testing of infants with possible congenital Zika virus infection—United States, 2016. *MMWR Morb Mortal Wkly Rep.* 2016;65:63–67.)

Finally, any association observed in a case report or a case series is prone to potentially unmeasured confounding unbeknown to the investigators.

Ecologic Studies

The first approach in determining whether an association exists may be a study of group characteristics, the so-called *ecologic studies*. Fig. 7.3 shows the correlation of each country's level of chocolate consumption and its number of Nobel laureates per capita.[5] In this figure, each dot represents a different country. As seen in this

figure, the higher the average chocolate consumption for a country, the higher the number of Nobel laureates per capita. Chocolate, high in dietary flavanols, is thought to improve cognitive function and reduce the risk of dementia. We might therefore be tempted to conclude that chocolate consumption may be a causal factor for being awarded a Nobel Prize. What is the problem with drawing such a conclusion from this type of study? Consider Switzerland, for example, which has the highest number of Nobel laureates per capita and the highest average consumption of chocolate. The problem is that we do not know whether the *individuals*

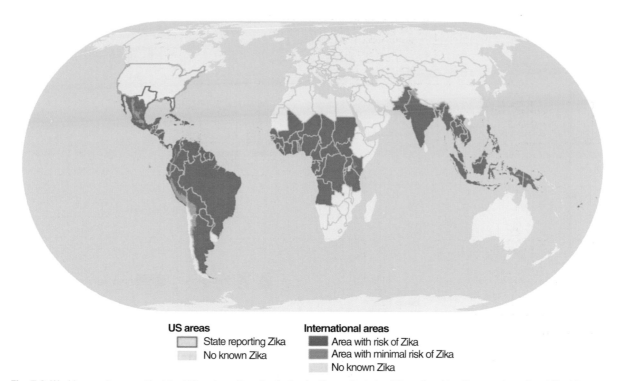

Fig. 7.2 World map of areas with risk of Zika virus. (From the Centers for Disease Control and Prevention. https://wwwnc.cdc.gov/travel/files/zika-areas-of-risk.pdf. Accessed July 24, 2017.)

who won Nobel Prize in that country actually had a high chocolate intake. All we have are *average* values of chocolate consumption and the number of Nobel laureates per capita for each country. In fact, one might argue that, given the same overall picture, it is conceivable that those who won the Nobel Prize ate very little chocolate. Fig. 7.3 alone does not reveal whether this might be true; in effect, individuals in each country are characterized by the average figures (level of consumption and per capita Nobel laureates) for that country. No account is taken of variability between individuals in that country with regard to chocolate consumption. This problem is called the *ecologic fallacy*—we may be ascribing to members of a group some characteristic that they in fact do not possess as individuals. This problem arises in an ecologic study because data are only available for groups; we do not have exposure and outcome data for each individual in the population.

Table 7.1 shows data from a study in Northern California exploring a possible relation between prenatal

TABLE 7.1 Average Annual Crude Incidence Rates and Relative Risks of Acute Lymphocytic Leukemia by Cohort and Trimester of Flu Exposure for Children Younger Than 5 Years, San Francisco/Oakland (1969–1973)

| | No Flu Exposure | FLU EXPOSURE TRIMESTER | | | |
		1st	2nd	3rd	Total
Incidence rates per 100,000	3.19	10.32	8.21	2.99	6.94
Relative risks	1.0	3.2	2.6	0.9	2.2

Modified from Austin DF, Karp S, Dworsky R, et al. Excess leukemia in cohorts of children born following influenza epidemics. *Am J Epidemiol.* 1977;10:77–83.

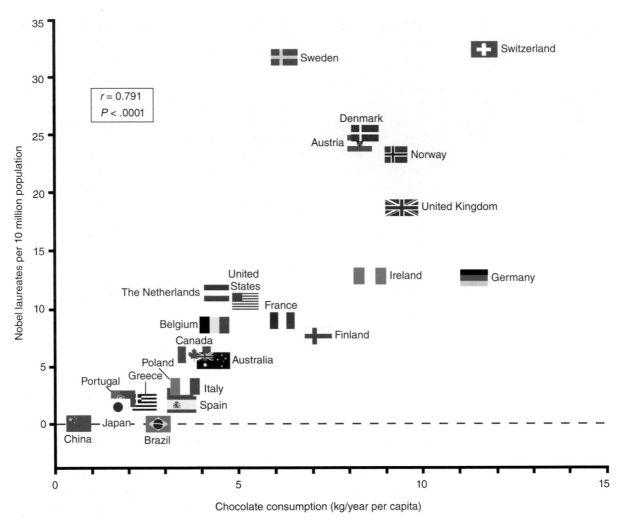

Fig. 7.3 Correlation between countries' annual per capita chocolate consumption and the number of Nobel laureates per 10 million population. (From Messerli FH. Chocolate consumption, cognitive function, and Nobel laureates. *N Engl J Med.* 2012;367:1562–1564.)

exposure to influenza during an influenza outbreak and the later development of acute lymphocytic leukemia in a child.[6] The table shows incidence data for children who were not in utero during a flu outbreak and for children who were in utero in the first, second, or third trimester of the pregnancy during the outbreak. Below these figures, the data are presented as relative risks, with the risk being set at 1.0 for those who were not in utero during the outbreak and the other rates being set relative to this. The data indicate a high relative risk for leukemia in children who were in utero during the flu outbreak in the first trimester.

What is the problem? The authors themselves stated, "The observed association is between pregnancy during an influenza epidemic and subsequent leukemia in the offspring of that pregnancy. It is not known if the mothers of any of these children actually had influenza during their pregnancy."[6] What we are missing are *individual data* on exposure (influenza infection). One might ask, why didn't the investigators obtain the necessary exposure data? The likely reason is that the investigators used birth certificates and data from a cancer registry; both types of data are relatively easy to obtain. This approach did not require follow-up of the children and direct contact with individual subjects. If we are impressed by these ecologic data, we might want to carry out a study specifically designed to explore the possible relationship of prenatal flu and leukemia. However, such a study would probably be considerably more difficult and more expensive to conduct.

In view of these problems, are ecologic studies of value? Yes, they can suggest avenues of research that may be promising in casting light on etiologic relationships. In and of themselves, however, they do not demonstrate conclusively that a true association exists.

For many years, legitimate concerns about the possibility of ecologic fallacy gave ecologic studies a bad name and diverted attention from the importance of studying potentially meaningful relationships that can be only studied ecologically, such as those between the individual and the community in which he or she lives. For example, Rose and associates[7] studied the relationship of socioeconomic and racial characteristics of a neighborhood and the receipt of angiography in a community-based sample who had a myocardial infarction (MI). Among the 9,941 people with MI participating in the Atherosclerosis Risk in Communities Study, compared to whites from high neighborhood-level income areas, blacks from low and medium neighborhood-level income areas as well as whites from low neighborhood-level income areas were less likely to be subjected to an angiographic examination. On the other hand, blacks from high neighborhood-level income areas and whites from medium neighborhood-level income areas were not disadvantaged with respect to receiving angiography. Thus future studies addressing both individual risk factors and ecologic risk factors, such as neighborhood characteristics, and the possible interactions of both types of factors may improve our understanding of access to an angiographic examination.

Another example of the importance of ecologic data is given by shistosomiasis, a disease caused by a freshwater parasite schistosomes that can affect the genitourinary or gastrointestinal tracts as well as the central nervous systems, and that is also a risk factor for bladder and liver cancer. Individuals are exposed from contact with infested water. Those in rural communities are at highest risk for contracting schistosomiasis; exposure may come from agriculture or fishing populations, women washing clothes, or children playing in infested water. Egypt has the highest endemic worldwide prevalence of schistosomiasis, dating back to its dynastic period.[8] Parenteral antischistosomal therapy (PAT) use with potassium antimony tartrate, commonly called tartar emetic, has been used for mass-treatment in Egypt since the 1920s through 12 weekly intravenous injections. These injections are done with reusable glass syringes generally without proper sterilization procedures, which may have been responsible for Egypt having the highest hepatitis C prevalence in the world.[9] (Tartar emetic was the only treatment for schistosomiasis until praziquantel [Biltricide], a highly effective oral treatment, was introduced in the 1980s.) In 2000, Frank et al.[10] studied the ecologic association in Egypt governorate areas between annual PAT use with tartar emetic and seroprevalence of antibodies to hepatitis C virus (HCV) in 8,499 Egyptians aged 10 to 50 years. Overall, age-adjusted prevalence of antibodies to HCV was found to be 21.9%. Fig. 7.4 shows the association between region-specific prevalence of antibodies to HCV with region-specific PAT exposure, which suggests that the variation in seroprevalence of antibodies to HCV between regions may be explained by PAT exposure (odds ratio 1.31 [95% confidence interval {CI}: 1.08–1.59]; $P = .007$). To date, massive HCV transmission through PAT use in Egypt is considered the largest iatrogenic transmission of a blood-borne pathogen ever recorded.

It has been claimed that because epidemiologists generally show tabulated data and refer to characteristics of groups, the data in all epidemiologic studies are group data. This is not true. In cross-sectional, case-control, cohort studies and randomized trials, data on exposure and disease outcome are available for every individual in the study, even though these data are commonly grouped in tables and figures. On the other hand, only grouped data are available in ecologic studies, such as, for example, country-by-country data on average salt consumption and average systolic blood pressure.

Interestingly, when variability of an exposure is limited, ecologic correlations may provide a more valid answer with regard to the presence of an association than studies based on individuals. Wynder and Stellman have summarized this phenomenon as follows: "If cases and controls are drawn from a population in which the range of exposures is narrow, then a study may yield little information about potential health effects."[11]

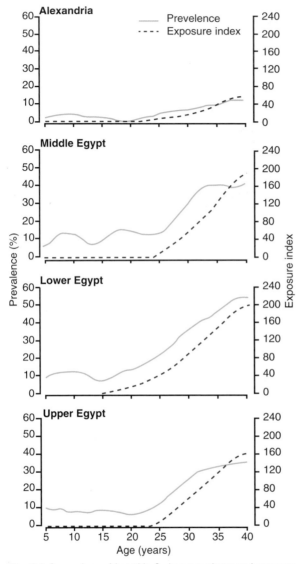

Fig. 7.4 Comparison of hepatitis C virus prevalence and exposure index by cohort and region. (Reprinted with permission from Frank C, Mohamed MK, Strickland GT, et al. The role of parenteral antischistosomal therapy in the spread of hepatitis C virus in Egypt. *Lancet.* 2000;11;355: 887–891.)

An example is the relationship of salt intake and blood pressure, which has not been consistently found in case-control and cohort studies; however, in an ecologic correlation using country populations as the analytic units, a strong and graded correlation has been observed. This phenomenon can be explained by the narrow range of salt intake in individuals within each country, but a fairly large variability of *average* salt intake between countries.

Cross-Sectional Studies

Another common study design used in initially investigating the association between a specific exposure and a disease of interest is the *cross-sectional study.* Let's assume that we are interested in the possible relationship of increased serum cholesterol level (the *exposure*) to electrocardiographic (ECG) evidence of coronary heart disease (CHD, the *disease*). We survey a population, and for each participant we determine the serum cholesterol level and perform an ECG for evidence of CHD. The presence of CHD defines a prevalent case. This type of study design is called a *cross-sectional study* because both exposure and disease outcome are determined *simultaneously* for each study participant; it is as if we were viewing a snapshot of the population at a certain point in time. Another way to describe a cross-sectional study is to imagine that we have sliced through the population, capturing levels of cholesterol *and* evidence of CHD at the same time. Note that in this type of approach, the cases of disease that we identify are *prevalent* cases of the disease in question (which is the reason why a cross-sectional study is also called a "prevalence study"), because we know that they existed at the time of the study, but we do not know their duration (the interval between the onset of the disease and "today"), or whether the exposure happened before the outcome. The impossibility of determining a temporal sequence "exposure-disease" may result in temporal bias when it is the disease that causes the exposure. For example, prevalent cases of CHD may engage in leisure physical activity more often than normal subjects, as the occurrence of an acute episode of CHD may prompt physicians to recommend physical exercise to his or her CHD patients, a phenomenon that is also known as "reverse causality." (Note, however, that when information on exposure is obtained by a questionnaire, it is possible to find out whether a given exposure [e.g., sedentary habits, smoking, or excessive alcohol drinking] was present prior to the disease onset, thus allowing the identification of the temporal sequence between the exposure and the disease.)

In addition to temporal bias, survival/selection bias may also occur in a cross-sectional study when the exposure is related to the duration of the disease; thus, for example, if exposure-induced incident cases have a shorter survival than unexposed incident cases, prevalent cases, which are by definition survivors, may have a lower proportion of past exposure than those that would have been observed if incident cases had been included in the study. In other words, identifying only prevalent cases would exclude those who died sooner after the disease developed but before the study was carried out. For example, we know that a high serum cholesterol level causes CHD. However, when doing a cross-sectional study, the observed association may be a function of both the risk of *developing* CHD and with *survival* after CHD onset.

Another example of survival bias is given by smoking-induced lung emphysema. Smoking not only causes emphysema, but in addition, survival of patients with smoking-induced emphysema is worse than that of patients whose emphysema results from other causes (e.g., asthma or chronic bronchitis). As a result, past smoking will be observed less frequently in prevalent than in incident cases of emphysema. This type of survival bias is also known as *prevalence-incidence bias*.

In view of its biases, results of a cross-sectional study should be used to generate hypotheses that can then be evaluated using a study design that includes incident cases and allows establishing the temporal sequence of the exposure and the outcome. Nevertheless, cross-sectional studies, like political polls and sample surveys, are widely used and are often the first studies conducted before moving on to more valid study designs.

The general design of a cross-sectional (or prevalence) study is seen in Fig. 7.5. We define a population and determine the presence or absence of exposure and the presence or absence of disease for each individual at the same time. Each subject then can be categorized into one of four possible subgroups.

As seen in the 2 × 2 table in the top portion of Fig. 7.6, there will be *a* persons, who have been exposed and have the disease; *b* persons, who have been exposed but do not have the disease; *c* persons, who have the disease but have not been exposed; and *d* persons, who have neither been exposed nor have the disease.

In order to determine whether there is evidence of an association between exposure and disease from a cross-sectional study, we have a choice between two possible approaches, which in Fig. 7.6 are referred to

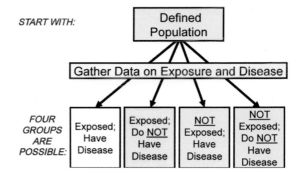

Fig. 7.5 Design of a hypothetical cross-sectional study: I. Identification of four subgroups based on presence or absence of exposure and presence or absence of disease.

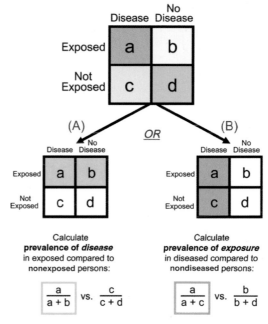

Fig. 7.6 Design of a hypothetical cross-sectional study—II: *(top)* A 2 × 2 table of the findings from the study; *(bottom)* two possible approaches to the analysis of results: (A) Calculate the prevalence of disease in exposed persons compared to the prevalence of disease in nonexposed persons, *or* (B) Calculate the prevalence of exposure in persons with disease compared to the prevalence of exposure in persons without disease.

as (A) and (B). If we use (A), we can calculate the prevalence of disease in persons with the exposure $\left(\dfrac{a}{a+b}\right)$ and compare it with the prevalence of disease in persons without the exposure $\left(\dfrac{c}{c+d}\right)$. If we use

(B), we can compare the prevalence of exposure in persons with the disease $\left(\dfrac{a}{a+c}\right)$ to the prevalence of exposure in persons without the disease $\left(\dfrac{b}{b+d}\right)$. The details of both approaches are shown in the bottom portion of Fig. 7.6.

If we determine in such a study that there appears to be an association between increased cholesterol level and CHD, we are left with several issues we have to consider. First, in this cross-sectional study, we are identifying prevalent (existing) cases of CHD rather than incident (new) cases; such prevalent cases may not be representative of all cases of CHD that have developed in this population. For example, identifying only prevalent cases would exclude those who died after the disease developed but before the study was carried out. Therefore, even if an association of exposure and disease is observed, the association may be with *survival* after CHD rather than with the risk of *developing* CHD. Second, because the presence or absence of both exposure and disease was determined *at the same time* in each participant in the study, it is often not possible to establish a temporal relationship between the exposure and the onset of disease. Thus, in the example given at the beginning of this section, it is not possible to tell whether or not the increased cholesterol level *preceded* the development of CHD. Without information on temporal relationships, it is conceivable that the increased cholesterol level could have occurred as a result of the CHD, in which case we call it "reverse causality," or perhaps both may have occurred as a result of another factor. If it turns out that the exposure did not precede the development of the disease, the association cannot reflect a causal relationship.

Farag et al. used data from the National Health and Nutrition Examination Survey (NHANES), a nationally representative survey of the noninstitutionalized US civilian population, to examine a potential association between vitamin D and erectile dysfunction in men who were free from cardiovascular disease.[12] A dose-response relationship was found between vitamin D deficiency and erectile dysfunction (prevalence ratio 1.30, 95% CI: 1.08–1.57; Fig. 7.7). Notwithstanding the biases inherent to the cross-sectional design, the study's findings suggest the need to perform a randomized trial on the association of vitamin D deficiency and erectile function.

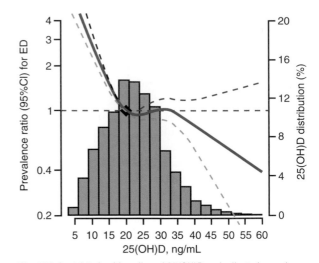

Fig. 7.7 Restricted cubic spline of 25(OH)D and adjusted prevalence ratio of erectile dysfunction *(ED)*, NHANES 2001–2004. Curves represent adjusted prevalence ratio *(solid line)* and the 95% confidence intervals *(dashed lines)* based on restricted cubic splines for 25(OH)D level with knots at 10, 20, 30, and 40 ng/mL. The reference values were set at 20 ng/mL. Model is adjusted for age, race, smoking, alcohol consumption, body mass index, physical activity, hypertension, diabetes, hypercholesterolemia, estimated glomerular filtration rate, C-reactive protein, and the use of antidepressants and beta blockers. (From Farag YM, Guallar E, Zhao D, et al. Vitamin D deficiency is independently associated with greater prevalence of erectile dysfunction: the National Health and Nutrition Examination Survey (NHANES) 2001-2004. *Atherosclerosis.* 2016;252:61–67.)

Serial cross-sectional studies are also useful to evaluate trends in disease prevalence over time in order to inform health care policy and planning. Murphy and colleagues used annual NHANES data, yearly from 1988 to 1994 and every 2 years from 1999 to 2012, to examine trends in chronic kidney disease (CKD) prevalence.[13] Fig. 7.8 shows the temporal trends in adjusted prevalence of stages 3 and 4 CKD from NHANES 1988–1994 through 2011–2012, categorized by the presence or absence of diabetes. As shown in the figure, there was an initial increase in adjusted prevalence of stages 3 and 4 CKD that leveled off in the early 2000s among nondiabetic individuals but continued to increase in diabetic individuals.

To minimize health research costs, researchers often depend on self-reported data. Weight and height are the most common self-reported variables. However, self-reports are prone to under- or overreporting. Cross-sectional data can help validate and correct errors in self-reported weight and height. For example, Jain

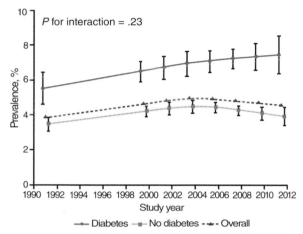

Fig. 7.8 Adjusted prevalence of stage 3 and 4 chronic kidney disease (estimated glomerular filtration rate of 15 to 59 mL/min/1.73 m² calculated with Chronic Kidney Disease Epidemiology Collaboration equation) in US adults, NHANES 1988–1994 through 2011–2012. (From Murphy D, McCulloch CE, Lin F, et al. Trends in prevalence of chronic kidney disease in the United States. *Ann Intern Med.* 2016;165:473–481.)

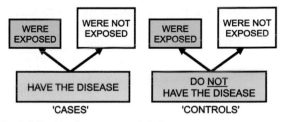

Fig. 7.9 Design of a case-control study.

compared self-reported with measured cross-sectional weight and height data from the NHANES for the period 1999–2006. This comparison allowed him to estimate a correction factor, which was then applied to the prevalence of obesity based on self-reported weight and height obtained from the Behavioral Risk Factor Surveillance System. Jain estimated that the weight/height self-reporting bias resulted in an approximately 5% lower obesity prevalence in both men and women.[14]

Case-Control Studies

Suppose you are a clinician and you have seen a few patients with a certain disease. You observe that many of them have been exposed to a particular agent—biological or chemical. You hypothesize that their exposure is related to their risk of developing this disease. How would you go about confirming or refuting your hypothesis?

Let's consider a real-life example:

It was long thought that hyperacidity is the cause of peptic ulcer disease (PUD). In 1982, Australian physicians Barry Marshall and Robin Warren discovered Helicobacter pylori (H. pylori) *in the stomachs of PUD patients, and showed that* H. pylori *is able to adapt to the acidic environment of the stomach. However,*

their observations were not enough to establish the causal association between H. pylori *and PUD. Subsequently, they suggested that antibiotics, not antacids, are the effective treatments for PUD, a suggestion that was heavily criticized at that time. It wasn't until 1994 when the National Institutes of Health came to a consensus expert opinion based on the available evidence that detection and eradication of* H. pylori *are key in the treatment of PUD. Drs. Marshall and Warren were awarded the Nobel Prize in Physiology or Medicine in 2005.*[15]

To determine the significance of clinical observations in a group of cases reported by physicians, a comparison (sometimes called a control or reference) group is needed. Observations based on case series would have been intriguing, but no firm conclusion would be possible without comparing these observations in cases to those from a series of controls who are similar in most respects to the cases but are free of the disease under study. Comparison is an essential component of epidemiologic investigation and is well exemplified by the case-control study design.

DESIGN OF A CASE-CONTROL STUDY

Fig. 7.9 shows the design of a *case-control study.* To examine the possible relation of an exposure to a certain disease, we identify a group of individuals with that disease (called *cases*) and, for purposes of comparison, a group of people without that disease (called *controls*). We then determine what proportion of the cases was exposed and what proportion was not. We also determine what proportion of the controls was exposed and what proportion was not. In the example of children with cataracts, the cases would consist of children with cataracts, and the controls would consist of children without cataracts. For each child, it would then be necessary to ascertain whether or not the mother was exposed to rubella during her pregnancy with that child. We anticipate that if the exposure (rubella) is in fact related to the disease (cataracts), the prevalence of history of exposure among the cases (children with cataracts) will be greater than that among the controls (children with no cataracts). Thus in a case-control study, if there is an association of an exposure with a disease, the prevalence of history of exposure should be higher in persons who have the disease (cases) than in those who do not have the disease (controls).

Table 7.2 presents a hypothetical schema of how a case-control study is conducted. We begin by selecting cases (with the disease) and controls (without the disease), and then measure past exposure by interview or by review of medical or employee records or of results of chemical or biologic assays of blood, urine, or tissues. If the exposure is dichotomous—that is, exposure has either occurred (yes) or not occurred (no)—breakdown into four groups is possible. There are a cases who were exposed and c cases who were not exposed. Similarly, there are b controls who were exposed and d controls who were not exposed. Thus the total number of cases is $(a + c)$ and the total number of controls is $(b + d)$. If exposure is associated with disease, we would expect the proportion of the cases who were exposed, $\left(\dfrac{a}{a+c}\right)$, to be greater than the proportion of the controls who were not exposed, $\left(\dfrac{b}{b+d}\right)$.

A hypothetical example of a case-control study is seen in Table 7.3. We are conducting a case-control study of whether smoking is related to CHD. We start with 200 people with CHD (cases) and compare them to 400 people without CHD (controls). If there is a relationship between a lifetime history of smoking and CHD, we would anticipate that a greater proportion of the CHD cases than of the controls would have been smokers (exposed). Let's say we find that of the 200 CHD cases, 112 were smokers and 88 were nonsmokers. Of the 400 controls, 176 were smokers and 224 were nonsmokers. Thus 56% of CHD cases were smokers compared to 44% of the controls. This calculation is only a first step. Further calculations to determine whether or not there is an association of the exposure with the disease will be discussed later. This chapter focuses exclusively on issues of design in case-control studies.

Parenthetically, it is of interest to note that if we use only the data from a case-control study, we cannot estimate the prevalence of the disease. In this example we had 200 cases and 400 controls, but this does not imply that the prevalence is 33%, or $\left(\dfrac{200}{200+400}\right)$. The decision as to the number of controls to select per case in a case-control study is in the hands of the investigator and does not reflect the prevalence of disease in the population. In this example, the investigator could have selected 200 cases and 200 controls (1 control per case), or 200 cases and 800 controls (4 controls per case). Because the proportion of the entire study population that consists of cases is determined by the ratio of controls per case, and this proportion is determined by the investigator, it clearly does not reflect the true prevalence of the disease in the population in which the study is carried out.

At this point, we should emphasize that the hallmark of the case-control study is that it begins with people

TABLE 7.2 Design of Case-Control Studies

	FIRST, SELECT:	
	Cases (With Disease)	Controls (Without Disease)
Then, Measure Past Exposure:		
Were exposed	a	b
Were not exposed	c	d
Totals	$a + c$	$b + d$
Proportions who were exposed	$\left(\dfrac{a}{a+c}\right)$	$\left(\dfrac{b}{b+d}\right)$

TABLE 7.3 A Hypothetical Example of a Case-Control Study of CHD and Cigarette Smoking

	CHD Cases	Controls
Smoke cigarettes	112	176
Do not smoke cigarettes	88	224
Totals	200	400
% Smoking cigarettes	56	44

CHD, Coronary heart disease.

with the disease (cases) and compares them to people without the disease (controls). This is in contrast to the design of a cohort study that will be discussed in Chapter 8, which begins with a group of exposed people and compares them to an unexposed group. Some people have the erroneous impression that the distinction between the two types of study design is that cohort studies go forward in time and case-control studies go backward in time. Such a distinction is not correct; in fact, it is unfortunate that the term *retrospective* has been used for case-control studies, because the term incorrectly implies that calendar time is the characteristic that distinguishes case-control from cohort design. As will be shown in an upcoming chapter, a retrospective cohort study also uses data obtained in the past. Thus calendar time is not the characteristic that distinguishes a case-control from a cohort study. What distinguishes the two study designs is whether the study begins with diseased and nondiseased people (case-control study) or with exposed and unexposed people (cohort study). One of the earliest studies of cigarette smoking and lung cancer was conducted by Sir Richard Doll (1912–2005) and Sir Austin Bradford Hill (1897–1991). Doll was an internationally known epidemiologist, and Hill was a well-known statistician and epidemiologist who developed the "Bradford Hill" guidelines for evaluating whether an observed association is causal.[16] Both men were knighted for their scientific work in epidemiology and biostatistics.

Table 7.4 presents data from their frequently cited study of 1,357 males with lung cancer and 1,357 controls according to the average number of cigarettes smoked per day in the 10 years preceding the present illness.[16] We see that there are fewer heavy smokers among the controls and very few nonsmokers among the lung cancer cases, a finding strongly suggestive of an association between smoking and lung cancer. In contrast to the previous example, exposure in this study is not just dichotomized (exposed or not exposed), but the exposure data are further stratified in terms of dose, as measured by the usual number of cigarettes smoked per day. Because many of the environmental exposures about which we are concerned today are not all-or-nothing exposures, the possibility of doing a study and analysis that takes into account the dose of the exposure is very important.

TABLE 7.4 Distribution of 1,357 Male Lung Cancer Patients and a Male Control Group According to Average Number of Cigarettes Smoked Daily Over the 10 Years Preceding Onset of the Current Illness

Average Daily Cigarettes	Lung Cancer Patients	Control Group
0	7	61
1–4	55	129
5–14	489	570
15–24	475	431
25–49	293	154
50+	38	12
Total	1,357	1,357

From Doll R, Hill AB. A study of the aetiology of carcinoma of the lung. *BMJ.* 1952;2:1271–1286.

POTENTIAL BIASES IN CASE-CONTROL STUDIES
Selection Bias

Sources of Cases. In a case-control study, cases can be selected from a variety of sources, including hospital patients, patients in physicians' practices, or clinic patients. Many communities maintain registries of patients with certain diseases, such as cancer, and such registries can serve as valuable sources of cases for such studies.

Several problems must be kept in mind when selecting cases for a case-control study. If cases are selected from a single hospital, any risk factors that are identified may be unique to that hospital as a result of referral patterns or other factors, and the results may not be generalizable to all patients with the disease. Consequently, if hospitalized cases are to be used, it is desirable to select the cases from several hospitals in the community. Furthermore, if the hospital from which the cases are drawn is a tertiary care facility, which selectively admits a large number of severely ill patients, any risk factors identified in the study may be risk factors only in persons with severe forms of the disease. In any event, it is essential that in case-control studies, just as in randomized trials, the criteria for eligibility be carefully specified in writing before the study is begun.

Using Incident or Prevalent Cases. An important consideration in case-control studies is whether to include incident cases of a disease (newly diagnosed cases) or prevalent cases of the disease (people who may have had the disease for some time). The problem with use of incident cases is that we must often wait for new cases to be diagnosed; whereas if we use prevalent cases, which have already been diagnosed, a larger number of cases is often available for study. However, despite this practical advantage of using prevalent cases, it is generally preferable to use incident cases of the disease in case-control studies of disease etiology. The reason is that any risk factors we may identify in a study using prevalent cases may be related more to *survival* with the disease than to the development of the disease (*incidence*). If, for example, most people who develop the disease die soon after diagnosis, they will be underrepresented in a study that uses prevalent cases, and such a study is more likely to include longer-term survivors. This would constitute a highly nonrepresentative group of cases, and any risk factors identified with this nonrepresentative group may not be a general characteristic of all patients with the disease, but only of survivors.

Even if we include only *incident* cases (patients who have been newly diagnosed with the disease) in a case-control study, we will of course be excluding any patients who may have died before the diagnosis was made. There is no easy solution to this problem or to certain other problems in case selection, but it is important that we keep these issues in mind when we finally interpret the data and derive conclusions from the study. At that time, it is critical to take into account possible selection biases that may have been introduced by the study design and by the manner in which the study was conducted.

Selection of Controls

In 1929, Raymond Pearl, professor of biostatistics at Johns Hopkins University in Baltimore, Maryland, conducted a study to test the hypothesis that tuberculosis protected against cancer.[17] From 7,500 consecutive autopsies at Johns Hopkins Hospital, Pearl identified 816 cases of cancer. He then selected a control group of 816 from among the others on whom autopsies had been carried out at Johns Hopkins and determined the percentages of the cases and of the controls who had findings of tuberculosis on autopsy. Pearl's findings are seen in Table 7.5.

TABLE 7.5   Summary of Data From Pearl's Study of Cancer and Tuberculosis

	Cases (With Cancer)	Controls (Without Cancer)
Total no. of autopsies	816	816
No. (%) of autopsies with tuberculosis	54 (6.6)	133 (16.3)

From Pearl R. Cancer and tuberculosis. *Am J Hyg.* 1929;9:97–159.

Of the 816 autopsies of patients with cancer, 54 had tuberculosis (6.6%), whereas of the 816 controls with no cancer, 133 had tuberculosis (16.3%). From the finding that the prevalence of tuberculosis was considerably higher in the control group (no cancer findings) than in the case group (cancer diagnoses), Pearl concluded that tuberculosis had an antagonistic or protective effect against cancer.

Was Pearl's conclusion justified? The answer to this question depends on the adequacy of his control group. If the prevalence of tuberculosis in the *noncancer* patients was similar to that of all people who were free of cancer, his conclusion would be valid. But that was not the case. At the time of the study, tuberculosis was one of the major reasons for hospitalization at Johns Hopkins Hospital. Consequently, what Pearl had inadvertently done in choosing the cancer-free control group was to select a group in which many of the patients had been diagnosed with and hospitalized for tuberculosis. Pearl thought that the control group's rate of tuberculosis would represent the level of tuberculosis expected in the general population, but because of the way he selected the controls, they came from a pool that was heavily weighted with tuberculosis patients, which did not represent the general population. He was, in effect, comparing the prevalence of tuberculosis in a group of patients with cancer with the prevalence of tuberculosis in a group of patients in which many had already been diagnosed with tuberculosis. Clearly his conclusion was not justified on the basis of these data.

How could Pearl have overcome this problem in his study? Instead of comparing his cancer patients with a group selected from all other autopsied patients, he could have compared the patients with cancer to a group of patients admitted for some specific diagnosis other than cancer (and not tuberculosis). In fact, Carlson and Bell[18] repeated Pearl's study but compared the patients who died of cancer with patients who died of heart disease at Johns Hopkins Hospital. They found no difference in the prevalence of tuberculosis at autopsy between the two groups. (It is of interest, however, that despite the methodologic limitations of Pearl's study, bacillus Calmette-Guérin [BCG], a vaccine against tuberculosis, is used today as a form of immunotherapy in several types of cancer.)

The problem with Pearl's study exemplifies the challenge of selecting appropriate controls as the fundamental component in drawing epidemiologically sound conclusions from case-control studies. Yet it remains one of the most difficult problems we confront in the conduct of epidemiologic studies using the case-control approach. The challenge is this: If we conduct a case-control study and find more exposure in the cases than in the controls, we would like to be able to conclude that there is an association between the exposure and the disease in question. The way the controls are selected is a major determinant of whether such a conclusion is valid.

A fundamental conceptual issue relating to selection of controls is whether the controls should be similar to the cases in all respects other than having the disease in question, or whether they should be representative of all persons without the disease in the population from which the cases are selected. This question has stimulated considerable discussion, but in actuality, the characteristics of the nondiseased people in the population from which the cases are selected are often not known, because the reference population may not be well defined.

Consider, for example, a case-control study using hospitalized cases. We want to identify the reference population that is the source of the cases so that we can then sample this reference population to select controls. Unfortunately, it is usually either not easy or not possible to identify such a reference population for hospitalized patients. Patients admitted to a hospital may come from the surrounding neighborhood, may live farther away in the same city, or may, through a referral process, come from another city or another country. Under these circumstances it is virtually impossible to define a specific reference population from which the cases emerged and from which we might select controls. Nevertheless, we want to design our study so that when it is completed, we can be reasonably certain that if we find a difference in exposure history between cases and controls, there are not likely to be any other important differences between them that might limit the inferences we may derive.

Sources of Controls. Controls may be selected from nonhospitalized persons living in the community, from outpatient clinics, or from hospitalized patients admitted for diseases other than that for which the cases were admitted.

Use of Nonhospitalized People as Controls. Nonhospitalized controls may be selected from several sources in the community. Ideally, a probability sample of the total population might be selected, but as a practical matter, this is rarely possible. Other sources include school rosters, registered voters lists, and insurance company lists. Another option is to select, as a control for each case, a resident of a defined area, such as the neighborhood in which the case lives. Such *neighborhood controls* have been used for many years. In this approach, interviewers are instructed to identify the home of a case as a starting point, and from there walk past a specified number of houses in a specified direction and seek the first household that contains an eligible control. Because of increasing problems of security in urban areas of the United States, however, many people will no longer open their doors to interviewers. Nevertheless, in many other countries, particularly in developing countries, the door-to-door approach to obtaining controls may be ideal.

Because of the difficulties in many cities in the United States in obtaining neighborhood controls using the door-to-door approach, an alternative for selecting such controls is to use telephone survey methods. Among these is random-digit dialing. Because telephone exchanges generally match neighborhood boundaries (being in the same area code), a case's seven-digit telephone number, of which the first three digits are the exchange, can be used to select a control telephone number, in which the terminal four digits of the phone number are randomly selected and the same three-digit exchange is used. In many developing countries this approach is impractical, as only government offices and business establishments are likely to have telephones.

With the nearly universal mobile telephone coverage that now exists almost worldwide, the telephone is an intriguing method of control selection. Nevertheless, many persons screen their calls, and response rates are woefully low in many cases.

Another approach to control selection is to use a *best friend control*. In this approach, a person who has been selected as a case is asked for the name of a best friend who may be more likely to participate in the study knowing that his or her best friend is also participating. However, there are also disadvantages to this method of selecting controls. A best friend control obtained in this fashion may be similar to the case in age and in many other demographic and social characteristics. A resulting problem may be that the controls are too similar to the cases in regard to many variables, including the variables that are being investigated in the study. Sometimes, however, it may be useful to select a spouse or sibling control; a sibling may provide some control over genetic differences between cases and controls.

Use of Hospitalized Patients as Controls. Hospital inpatients are often selected as controls because of the extent to which they are a "captive population," easily accessible and clearly identified; it should therefore be relatively more economical to carry out a study using such controls. However, as just discussed, they represent a sample of an ill-defined reference population that usually cannot be characterized and thus to which results cannot be generalized. Moreover, hospital patients differ from people in the community. For example, the prevalence of cigarette smoking is known to be higher in hospitalized patients than in community residents; many of the diagnoses for which people are admitted to the hospital are smoking related.

Given that we generally cannot characterize the reference population from which hospitalized cases come, there is a conceptual attractiveness to comparing hospitalized cases with hospitalized controls from the same institution, who presumably would tend to come from the same reference population[a] (Fig. 7.10). Whatever selection factors in the referral system affected the cases' admission to a particular hospital would also pertain to the controls. However, referral patterns at the

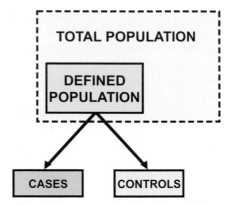

Fig. 7.10 Since both the cases and the hospital controls are selected from the defined population, any factors that affected admission of cases to a certain hospital would also affect the admission of hospital controls.

same hospital may differ for various clinical services; such an assumption may be questionable and generally it is often impossible to know whether it has been met.

When the decision has been made to use hospital controls, the question arises of whether to use a sample of *all* other patients admitted to the hospital (other than those with the cases' diagnosis) or whether to select a *specific* "another diagnosis" or "other diagnoses." If we wish to choose specific diagnostic groups, on what basis do we select those groups, and on what basis do we exclude others? The problem is that although it is attractive to select as hospitalized controls a disease group that is obviously unrelated to the putative causative factor under investigation, such controls are unlikely to be representative of the general reference population of noncases. Taken to its logical end, it will not be clear whether it is the cases or the controls who differ from the general population.

The issue of which diagnostic groups would be eligible for use as controls and which would be ineligible (and therefore excluded) is very important. Let's say we are conducting a case-control study of lung cancer and smoking: we select as cases patients who have been hospitalized with lung cancer, and as controls we select patients who have been hospitalized with emphysema. What problem would this present? Because we know that there is a strong relationship between smoking and emphysema, our controls, the emphysema patients, would include a high number of

_____
[a]In current jargon, the reference population is also known as the "study base."

smokers. Consequently, any relationship of smoking to lung cancer would not be easy to detect in this study, because we would have selected as controls a group of persons in which there is a greater-than-expected prevalence of smoking than exists in the population. We might therefore want to exclude from our control group those persons who have other smoking-related diagnoses, such as CHD, bladder cancer, pancreatic cancer, and emphysema. Such exclusions might yield a control group with a lower-than-expected prevalence of smoking, and the exclusion process becomes overly complex. One alternative is to not exclude any groups from selection as controls in the design of the study, but to analyze the study data separately for different diagnostic subgroups that constitute the control group. This, of course, will drive up the numbers of controls necessary and the expense that accompanies a larger sample size.

Problems in Control Selection. In a classic study published in 1981, the renowned epidemiologist Brian MacMahon and coworkers[19] reported a case-control study of cancer of the pancreas. The cases were patients with a histologically confirmed diagnosis of pancreatic cancer in 11 Boston and Rhode Island hospitals from 1974 to 1979. Controls were selected from patients who were hospitalized at the same time as the cases; they were selected from other inpatients hospitalized by the attending physicians who had hospitalized the cases. Excluded were nonwhites; those older than 79

years; patients with pancreatic, hepatobiliary tract, and smoking-related or alcohol-related diseases; and patients with cardiovascular disease, diabetes, respiratory or bladder cancer, and peptic ulcer. However, the authors did not exclude patients with other kinds of gastrointestinal diseases, such as diaphragmatic hernia, reflux, gastritis, and esophagitis.

One finding in this study was an apparent dose-response relationship between coffee drinking and cancer of the pancreas, particularly in women (Table 7.6). When such a relationship is observed, it is difficult to know whether the disease is *caused* by the coffee drinking or by some factor closely related to the coffee drinking. Because smoking is a known risk factor for cancer of the pancreas, and because coffee drinking was closely related to cigarette smoking at that time (it was rare to find a smoker who did not drink coffee), did MacMahon and others observe an association of coffee drinking with pancreatic cancer because the coffee caused the pancreatic cancer, or because coffee drinking is related to cigarette smoking, and cigarette smoking is known to be a risk factor for cancer of the pancreas? Recognizing this problem, the authors analyzed the data after stratifying for smoking history. The relationship with coffee drinking held both for current smokers and for those who had never smoked (Table 7.7).

This report aroused great interest in both the scientific and lay communities, particularly among coffee manufacturers. Given the widespread exposure of

TABLE 7.6 Distribution of Cases and Controls by Coffee-Drinking Habits and Estimates of Risk Ratios

Sex	Category	0	1–2	3–4	≥5	Total
		COFFEE DRINKING (CUPS/DAY)				
M	No. of cases	9	94	53	60	216
	No. of controls	32	119	74	82	307
	Adjusted relative risk[a]	1.0	2.6	2.3	2.6	2.6
	95% Confidence interval	—	1.2–5.5	1.0–5.3	1.2–5.8	1.2–5.4
F	No. of cases	11	59	53	28	151
	No. of controls	56	152	80	48	336
	Adjusted relative risk[a]	1.0	1.6	3.3	3.1	2.3
	95% Confidence interval	—	0.8–3.4	1.6–7.0	1.4–7.0	1.2–4.6

[a]Chi-square (Mantel extension) with equally spaced scores, adjusted over age in decades: 1.5 for men, 13.7 for women. Mantel-Haenszel estimates of risk ratios, adjusted over categories of age in decades. In all comparisons, the referent category was subjects who never drank coffee.
From MacMahon B, Yen S, Trichopoulos D, et al. Coffee and cancer of the pancreas. *N Engl J Med.* 1981;304:630–633.

TABLE 7.7   **Estimates of Relative Risk[a] of Cancer of the Pancreas Associated With Use of Coffee and Cigarettes**

Cigarette Smoking Status	COFFEE DRINKING (CUPS/DAY)			Total[b]
	0	1–2	≥3	
Never smoked	1.0	2.1	3.1	1.0
Ex-smokers	1.3	4.0	3.0	1.3
Current smokers	1.2	2.2	4.6	1.2 (0.9–1.8)
Total[a]	1.0	1.8 (1.0–3.0)	2.7 (1.6–4.7)	

Values in parentheses are 95% confidence intervals of the adjusted estimates.
[a]The referent category is the group that uses neither cigarettes nor coffee. Estimates are adjusted for sex and age in decades.
[b]Values are adjusted for the other variables, in addition to age and sex, and are expressed in relation to the lowest category of each variable.
From MacMahon B, Yen S, Trichopoulos D, et al. Coffee and cancer of the pancreas. *N Engl J Med.* 1981;304:630–633.

human beings to coffee, if the reported relationship were true, it would have major public health implications.

Let's examine the design of this study. The cases were white patients with cancer of the pancreas at 11 Boston and Rhode Island hospitals. The controls are of particular interest: After some exclusions, they were patients with other diseases who were hospitalized by the same physicians who had admitted the pancreatic cancer cases. That is, when a case had been identified, the attending physician was asked if another of his or her patients who was hospitalized at the same time for another condition could be interviewed as a control. This unusual method of control selection had a practical advantage: One of the major obstacles in obtaining participation of hospital controls in case-control studies is that permission to contact the patient is usually requested of the attending physician. The physicians are often not motivated to have their patients serve as controls, because the patients do not have the disease that is the focus of the study. By asking physicians who had already given permission for patients with pancreatic cancer to participate, the likelihood was increased that permission would be granted for patients with other diseases to participate as controls.

Did that practical decision introduce any problems? The underlying question that the investigators wanted to answer was whether patients with cancer of the pancreas drank more coffee than people without cancer of the pancreas in the same population (Fig. 7.11). What MacMahon and coworkers found was that the

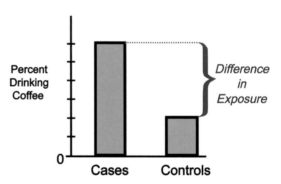

Fig. 7.11 Hypothetical example of a case-control study of coffee drinking and pancreatic cancer: Cases have a higher level of coffee drinking than controls.

level of coffee drinking in cases was greater than the level of coffee drinking in controls.

The investigators would like to be able to establish that the level of coffee drinking observed in the controls is what would be expected in the general population without pancreatic cancer and that cases therefore demonstrate *excessive* coffee drinking (Fig. 7.12A). But the problem is this: Which physicians are most likely to admit patients with cancer of the pancreas to the hospital? Gastroenterologists are often the admitting physicians. Many of their other hospitalized patients (who served as controls) also have gastrointestinal problems, such as esophagitis and gastritis (as mentioned previously, patients with peptic ulcer were excluded from the control group). So, in this study, the persons who served as controls may very well have reduced

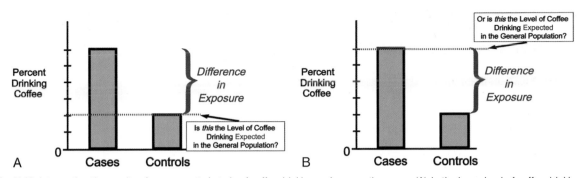

Fig. 7.12 Interpreting the results of a case-control study of coffee drinking and pancreatic cancer. (A) Is the lower level of coffee drinking in the controls the expected level of coffee drinking in the general population? *OR* (B) Is the higher level of coffee drinking in the cases the expected level of coffee drinking in the general population?

their intake of coffee, either because of a physician's instructions or because of their own realization that reducing their coffee intake could relieve their symptoms. We cannot assume that the controls' levels of coffee drinking are representative of the level of coffee drinking expected in the general population; their rate of coffee drinking may be abnormally low. Thus the observed difference in coffee drinking between pancreatic cancer cases and controls may not necessarily have been the result of cases drinking more coffee than expected, but rather of the controls drinking less coffee than expected (see Fig. 7.12B).

MacMahon and his colleagues subsequently repeated their analysis but separated controls with gastrointestinal illness from controls with other conditions. They found that the risk associated with coffee drinking was indeed higher when the comparison was with controls with gastrointestinal illness but that the relationship between coffee drinking and pancreatic cancer persisted, albeit at a lower level, even when the comparison was with controls with other illnesses. This became a classical example for what problematic selection of controls could do to interpreting the results of a case-control study. Several years later, Hsieh and coworkers reported a new study that attempted to replicate these results; it did not support the original findings.[20]

In summary, when a difference in exposure is observed between cases and controls, we must ask whether the level of exposure observed in the controls is really the level expected in the population in which the study was carried out or whether—perhaps given the manner of selection—the controls may have a

particularly high or low level of exposure that might not be representative of the level in the population in which the study was carried out.

Information Bias

Problems of Recall. A major problem in case-control studies is that of recall of a history of past exposure. Recall problems are of two types: limitations in recall and recall bias. Recall bias is the main form of information bias in case-control studies. The problem of recall is not limited to the case-control study design. Most epidemiologic studies inquire about life histories and are thus subject to recall biases. Survey research has identified many ways to mitigate the amount of bias associated with interviewing participants about events in their lives. However, many study participants forget about exposures or other events, tend to bring events that happened long ago forward in time ("telescoping"), and may be reticent to admit to practices that might be considered stigmatizing.

Limitations in Recall. Much of the information relating to exposure in case-control studies often involves collecting data from subjects by interviews. Because virtually all human beings are limited to varying degrees in their ability to recall information, limitations in recall is an important issue in such studies. A related issue that is somewhat different from limitations in recall is that persons being interviewed may simply not have the information being requested.

This was demonstrated years ago in an historic study carried out by Abraham Lilienfeld and Saxon Graham published in 1958.[21] At that time, considerable interest centered on the observation that cancer of the cervix was highly unusual in two groups of women: Jewish women and Catholic nuns. This observation suggested that an important risk factor for cervical cancer could be sexual intercourse with an uncircumcised man, and a number of studies were carried out to confirm this hypothesis. However, the authors were skeptical about the validity of the responses regarding circumcision status. To address this question they asked a group of men whether or not they had been circumcised. The men were then examined by a physician. As seen in Table 7.8, of the 56 men who stated they were circumcised, 19, or 33.9%, were found to be uncircumcised. Of the 136 men who stated they were not circumcised, 47, or 34.6%, were found to be circumcised. These data demonstrate that the findings from studies using interview data may not always be clear-cut.

Table 7.9 shows more recent data (2002) regarding the relationship of self-reported circumcision to actual circumcision status. These data suggest that men have improved in their knowledge and reporting of their circumcision status, or the differences observed may be due to the studies having been conducted in different countries. There may also have been methodological differences, which could have accounted for the different results between the two studies.

If a limitation of recall regarding exposure affects all subjects in a study to the same extent, regardless of whether they are cases or controls, a misclassification of exposure status may result. Some of the cases or controls who were actually exposed will be erroneously classified as unexposed, and some who were actually not exposed will be erroneously classified as exposed. For exposures that have only two categories (e.g., "yes" vs. "no"), this leads to an underestimate of the true risk of the disease associated with the exposure (that is, there will be a tendency to bias the results toward a null finding).

Recall Bias. A more serious potential problem in case-control studies is that of recall bias. Suppose that we are studying the possible relationship of congenital malformations to prenatal infections. We conduct a case-control study and interview mothers of children with congenital malformations (cases) and mothers of children without malformations (controls). Each mother is questioned about infections she may have had during the pregnancy.

A mother who has had a child with a birth defect often tries to identify some unusual event that occurred during her pregnancy with that child. She wants to know whether the abnormality was caused by something she did. Why did it happen? Such a mother may even recall an event, such as a mild respiratory infection, that a mother of a child without a birth defect may not even notice or may have forgotten entirely. This type of bias is known as *recall* bias; Ernst Wynder, a well-known epidemiologist, also called it "rumination bias."

TABLE 7.8 **Comparison of Patients' Statements With Examination Findings Concerning Circumcision Status, Roswell Park Memorial Institute, Buffalo, New York**

| Examination Finding | PATIENTS' STATEMENTS REGARDING CIRCUMCISION | | | |
| | YES | | NO | |
	No.	%	No.	%
Circumcised	37	66.1	47	34.6
Not circumcised	19	33.9	89	65.4
Total	56	100.0	136	100.0

Modified from Lilienfeld AM, Graham S. Validity of determining circumcision status by questionnaire as related to epidemiologic studies of cancer of the cervix. *J Natl Cancer Inst.* 1958;21:713–720.

TABLE 7.9 **Comparison of Patients' Statements With Physicians' Examination Findings Concerning Circumcision Status in the Study of Circumcision, Penile Human Papillomavirus, and Cervical Cancer**

| Physician Examination Findings | PATIENTS' STATEMENTS REGARDING CIRCUMCISION | | | |
| | YES | | NO | |
	No.	%	No.	%
Circumcised	282	98.3	37	7.4
Not circumcised	5	1.7	466	92.6
Total	287	100.0	503	100.0

Modified from Castellsague X, Bosch FX, Munoz N, et al. Male circumcision, penile human papillomavirus infection, and cervical cancer in female partners. *N Engl J Med.* 2002;346:1105–1112.

In the study just mentioned, let's assume that the true infection rate during pregnancy in mothers of malformed infants and in mothers of normal infants is 15%—that is, there is no difference in infection rates. Suppose that mothers of malformed infants recall 60% of any infections they had during pregnancy, and mothers of normal infants recall only 10% of infections they had during pregnancy. As seen in Table 7.10, the *apparent* infection rate estimated from this case-control study using interviews would be 9% for mothers of malformed infants and 1.5% for mothers of control infants. Thus the *differential recall* between cases and controls introduces a recall bias into the study that could artifactually suggest a relation of congenital malformations and prenatal infections. Although a potential for recall bias is self-evident in case-control studies, in point of fact, few actual examples demonstrate that recall bias has been a major problem in case-control studies and has led to erroneous conclusions regarding associations. The small number of examples available could reflect infrequent occurrence of such bias, or the fact that the data needed to clearly demonstrate the existence of such bias in a certain study are frequently not available. Nevertheless, the potential problem cannot be disregarded, and the possibility for such bias must always be kept in mind.

TABLE 7.10 Example of an Artificial Association Resulting From Recall Bias: A Hypothetical Study of Maternal Infections During Pregnancy and Congenital Malformations

	Cases (With Congenital Malformations)	Controls (Without Congenital Malformations)
Assume That:		
True incidence of infection (%)	15	15
Infections recalled (%)	60	10
Result Will Be:		
Infection rate as ascertained by interview (%)	9.0	1.5

OTHER ISSUES IN CASE-CONTROL STUDIES
Matching

A major concern in conducting a case-control study is that cases and controls may differ in characteristics or exposures other than the one that has been targeted for study. If more cases than controls are found to have been exposed, we may be left with the question of whether the observed association could be due to differences between the cases and controls in factors other than the exposure being studied. For example, if more cases than controls are found to have been exposed, and if most of the cases are of low income and most of the controls are of high income, we would not know whether the factor determining development of disease is exposure to the factor being studied or another characteristic associated with having low income. To avoid such a situation, we would like to ensure that the distribution of the cases and controls by socioeconomic status is similar, so that a difference in exposure will likely constitute the critical difference, and the presence or absence of disease is not likely to be attributable to a difference in socioeconomic status.

One approach to dealing with this problem in the design and conduct of the study is to match the cases and controls for factors about which we may be concerned, such as income, as in the preceding example. *Matching* is defined as the process of selecting the controls so that they are similar to the cases in certain characteristics, such as age, race, sex, socioeconomic status, and occupation. Matching may be of two types: (1) group matching and (2) individual matching. It is very important to distinguish between the two types, since each has its own implications for the statistical analysis of the case-control study, which is not discussed in this book.

Group Matching. *Group matching* (or *frequency matching*) consists of selecting the controls in such a manner that the *proportion* of controls with a certain characteristic is *identical* to the proportion of cases with the same characteristic. Thus if 25% of the cases are married, the controls will be selected so that 25% of that group is also married. This type of selection generally requires that all of the cases be selected first. After calculations are made of the proportions of certain characteristics in the group of cases, then a control group, in which the same characteristics occur in the same proportions, is selected. In general, when group matching, we never achieve *exactly* the same proportions of the key characteristic in cases and controls. When group matching is done for age, for example, the distribution that is the same in cases and controls is of the age groups (e.g., 45 to 49, 50 to 54); within each group, however, there may still be differences between cases and controls that must be considered: for example, although 10% of cases and controls are 50 to 54 years old, there may be a higher proportion of cases closer to age 54 than that of controls.

Individual Matching. A second type of matching is *individual matching* (or *matched pairs*). In this approach, for each case selected for the study, a control is selected who is similar to the case in terms of the specific variable or variables of concern. For example, if the first case enrolled in our study is a 45-year-old white woman, we will seek a 45-year-old white female control. If the second case is a 24-year-old black man, we will select a control who is also a 24-year-old black man. This type of control selection yields matched case-control pairs—that is, each case is individually matched to a control. In our hypothetical case, we would absolutely match the cases by gender and race/ethnicity, but we might use a 3- or 5-year bound for age. Thus we might match a 45-year-old white woman with a 42- to 48-year-old white woman control. The implications of this method of control selection for the estimation of excess risk are discussed in Chapter 12.

Individual matching is often used in case-control studies that use hospital controls. The reason for this is more practical than conceptual. Let's say that sex and age are considered important variables, and it is thought to be important that the cases and the controls be comparable in terms of these two characteristics. There is generally no practical way to dip into a pool of hospital patients to select a group with certain sex and age characteristics. Rather, it is easier to identify a case and then choose the next hospital admission that matches the case for sex and age. Thus individual matching is most expedient in studies using hospital controls.

What are the problems with matching? The problems with matching are of two types: practical and conceptual.

Practical Problems With Matching. If an attempt is made to match according to too many characteristics, it may prove difficult or impossible to identify an appropriate control. For example, suppose that it is decided to match each case for race, sex, age, marital status, number of children, ZIP code of residence, and occupation. If the case is a 48-year-old black woman who is married, has four children, lives in ZIP code 21209, and works in a photo-processing plant, it may prove difficult or impossible to find a control who is similar to the case in all of these characteristics. Therefore the more variables on which we choose to match, the more difficult it will be to find a suitable control. Overmatching also leads to an inability to statistically analyze variables used in matching, as we address next.

Conceptual Problems With Matching. Perhaps a more important problem is the conceptual one: Once we have matched controls to cases according to a given characteristic, we cannot study that characteristic. For example, suppose we are interested in studying marital status as a risk factor for breast cancer. If we match the cases (breast cancer) and the controls (no breast cancer) for marital status, we can no longer study whether or not marital status is a risk factor for breast cancer. Why not? Because in matching according to marital status, we have artificially established an identical proportion in cases and controls: if 35% of the cases are married, and through matching we create a control group in which 35% are also married, we have artificially ensured that the proportion of married subjects will be identical in both groups. By using matching to impose comparability for a certain factor, we ensure the same prevalence of that factor in the cases and the controls. Clearly we will not be able to ask whether cases differ from controls in the prevalence of that factor. We would therefore not want to match on the variable of marital status in this study. Indeed, we do not want to match on *any* variable that we may wish to explore in our study.

It is also important to recognize that unplanned matching may inadvertently occur in case-control studies. For example, if we use neighborhood controls, we are in effect matching for socioeconomic status as well as for cultural and other characteristics of a neighborhood. If we use best-friend controls, it is likely that the case and his or her best friend share many lifestyle characteristics, which in effect produces a match for these characteristics. For example, in a study of oral contraceptive use and cervical cancer in which best-friend controls were considered, there was concern that if the case used oral contraceptives it might well be that her best friend would also be likely to be an oral contraceptive user. The result would be an unplanned matching on oral contraceptive use, so that this variable could no longer be investigated in this study. Another and less subtle example would be to match cases and controls on residence when doing a study of the relationship of air pollution to respiratory disease. Unplanned matching on a variable that is strongly related to the exposure being investigated in the study is called *overmatching*.

In carrying out a case-control study, therefore, we match only on variables that we are convinced are risk factors for the disease, which we are therefore not interested in investigating in this study.

Use of Multiple Controls

Early in this chapter, we noted that the investigator can determine how many controls will be used per case in a case-control study and that multiple controls for each case are frequently used. Matching 2:1, 3:1 or 4:1 will increase the statistical power of our study. Therefore many case-control studies will have more controls than cases. These controls may be either (1) *controls of the same type* or (2) *controls of different types*, such as hospital and neighborhood controls or controls with different diseases.

Controls of the Same Type. Multiple controls of the *same type*, such as two controls or three controls for each case, are used to increase the power of the study. Practically speaking, a noticeable increase in power is gained only up to a ratio of about 1 case to 4 controls. One might ask, "Why use multiple controls for each case? Why not keep the ratio of controls to cases at 1:1 and just increase the number of cases?" The answer is that for many of the relatively infrequent diseases we study (which are best studied using case-control designs), there may be a limit to the number of potential cases available for study. A clinic may see only a certain number of patients with a given cancer or with a certain connective tissue disorder each year. Because the number of cases cannot be increased without either extending the study in time to enroll more cases or

developing a collaborative multicenter study, the option of increasing the number of controls per case is often chosen. These controls are of the same type (e.g., neighborhood controls); only the ratio of controls to cases has changed.

Multiple Controls of Different Types. In contrast, we may choose to use *multiple controls of different types*. For example, we may be concerned that the exposure of the hospital controls used in our study may not represent the rate of exposure that is "expected" in a population of nondiseased persons—that is, the controls may be a highly selected subset of nondiseased individuals and may have a different exposure experience. We mentioned earlier that hospitalized patients smoke more than people living in the community, and we are concerned because we do not know what the prevalence level of smoking in hospitalized controls represents or how to interpret a comparison of these rates with those of the cases. To address this problem, we may choose to use an additional control group, such as neighborhood controls. The hope is that the results obtained when cases are compared with hospital controls will be similar to the results obtained when cases are compared with neighborhood controls. If the findings differ, the reason for the discrepancy should be sought. In using multiple controls of different types, the investigator should ideally decide which comparison will be considered the "gold standard of truth" before embarking on the actual study.

In 1979, Ellen Gold and coworkers published a case-control study of brain tumors in children.[22] They used two types of controls: children with no cancer (called *normal controls*) and children with cancers other than brain tumors (called *cancer controls*; Fig. 7.13). What was the rationale for using these two control groups?

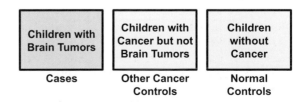

Fig. 7.13 Study groups of Gold et al. for brain tumors in children. (Data from Gold EB, Gordis L, Tonascia J, et al. Risk factors for brain tumors in children. *Am J Epidemiol*. 1979;109:309–319.)

Let's consider the question, "Did mothers of children with brain tumors have more prenatal radiation exposure than control mothers?" Some possible results are seen in Fig. 7.14A.

If the radiation exposure of mothers of children with brain tumors is found to be greater than that of mothers of normal controls, and the radiation exposure of mothers of children with other cancers is also found to be greater than that of mothers of normal children, what are the possible explanations? One conclusion might be that prenatal radiation is a risk factor both for brain tumors and for other cancers—that is, its effect is that of a carcinogen that is not site specific. Another explanation to consider is that the findings could have resulted from recall bias and that mothers of children with any type of cancer recall prenatal radiation exposure better than mothers of normal children.

Consider another possible set of findings, shown in Fig. 7.14B. If mothers of children with brain tumors have a greater radiation exposure history than both mothers of normal controls and mothers of children with other cancers, the findings might suggest that prenatal radiation is a specific carcinogen for the brain. These findings would also reduce the likelihood that recall bias is playing a role, as it would seem implausible that mothers of children with brain tumors would recall prenatal radiation better than mothers of children with other cancers. Thus multiple controls of different types can be valuable for exploring alternate hypotheses and for taking into account possible potential biases, such as recall bias.

Despite the issues raised in this chapter, case-control studies are invaluable in exploring the etiology of disease. Recent reports in the literature demonstrate the utility of the case-control study design in contemporary research.

Kristian Filion and colleagues in Canada addressed the concern that a common antidiabetic class of drugs (incretin-based drugs used in clinical practice) is associated with increased risk of heart failure.[23] Prior reports from clinical trials had been inconsistent. The investigators pooled health care data from four Canadian provinces, the United States, and the United Kingdom and conducted a case-control study in which each patient who was hospitalized for heart failure was matched with 20 controls. Matching criteria included age, sex, time entered into the study, how long diabetes had been treated, and how long patients with diabetes were under observation. Almost 30,000 patients were hospitalized for heart failure from almost 1.5 million total patients. Incretin-based medications were not found to increase hospitalization for heart failure when compared with oral antidiabetic drugs. Another example of the utility of the case-control study is given by Su and colleagues at the University of Michigan, who evaluated the association of occupational and environmental exposures on the risk of developing amyotrophic lateral sclerosis (ALS, commonly known as Lou Gehrig's disease, a progressive neurological disease that affects the neurons in the brain and spinal cord responsible for controlling voluntary muscle movement).[24] Cases were identified

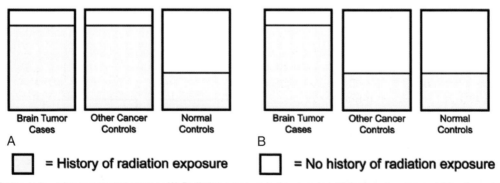

Fig. 7.14 Rationale for using two control groups: (A) Radiation exposure is the same in both brain tumor cases and in other cancer controls, but is higher in both groups than in normal controls: Could this be due to recall bias? (B) Radiation exposure in other cancer controls is the same as in normal controls, but is lower than in brain tumor cases: recall bias is unlikely. (Data from Gold EB, Gordis L, Tonascia J, et al. Risk factors for brain tumors in children. *Am J Epidemiol.* 1979;109:309–319.)

at a tertiary referral center for ALS between 2011 and 2014. Cases consisted of 156 ALS patients; 128 controls were selected from volunteers who responded to online postings. Controls, who were frequency matched to cases by age, gender, and education, self-reported that they were free of neurodegenerative disease and had no first- or second-degree relatives with ALS. A questionnaire ascertained exposure to occupational and environmental exposures. Blood concentrations were assessed for 122 common pollutants. Overall, 101 cases and 110 controls had complete demographic and pollutant data. From the occupational history, military service was associated with ALS. Self-reported pesticide exposure was associated with fivefold increased odds of ALS. When controlling for other possible factors that might be associated with ALS, three exposures measured in the blood were identified: occupational exposures to pesticides and to polychlorinated biphenyls (PCBs) in farming and fishing industries. The authors concluded that persistent environmental pollutants as measured in the blood were significantly associated with ALS and suggested that reducing exposure to these agents might reduce the incidence of ALS at the population level.

A final example of the usefulness of the case-control study relates to its use during a disease outbreak. In a study addressing the association of Guillain-Barré syndrome with Zika virus infection in French Polynesia in 2013–2014, Cao-Lormeau and colleagues noted that during the Zika outbreak, there was an increase in reports of Guillain-Barré syndrome suggestive of a possible relationship.[25] Forty-two patients admitted to the main referral hospital in Papeete, Tahiti, meeting the diagnostic criteria for Guillain-Barré were matched to two types of controls: (1) age-, sex-, and residence-matched patients without fever seen at the facility (n = 98), and (2) age-matched patients with acute Zika free of neurologic symptoms (n = 70). Of the 42 patients with Guillian-Barré syndrome, 98% (41/42) had antibodies against the Zika virus, compared with 56% of controls. All patients in control group 2 had positive confirmation for the Zika virus. The authors concluded that their study provides evidence for Zika virus infection "causing" Guillain-Barré syndrome. This claim seems to go a bit beyond the evidence, as we will see in the next section and is reiterated in subsequent chapters.

WHEN IS A CASE-CONTROL STUDY WARRANTED?

A case-control study is useful as a first step when searching for a cause of an adverse health outcome, as seen in the examples at the beginning of this chapter and those just presented. At an early stage in our search for an etiology, we may suspect any one of several exposures, but we may not have evidence, and certainly no strong evidence, to suggest an association of any one of the suspect exposures with the disease in question. Using the case-control design, we compare people with the disease (cases) and people without the disease (controls; Fig. 7.15A). We can then explore the possible roles of a variety of exposures or characteristics in causing the disease (see Fig. 7.15B). If the exposure is associated with the disease, we would expect the proportion of cases who have been exposed to be greater than

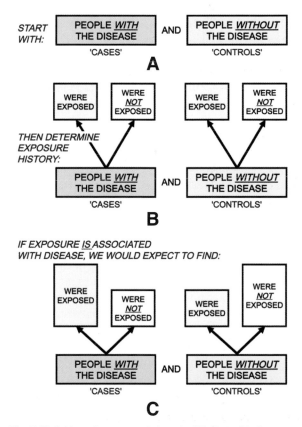

Fig. 7.15 Design of a case-control study. (A) Start with the cases and the controls. (B) Measure past exposure in both groups. (C) Expected findings if the exposure is associated with the disease.

the proportion of controls who have been exposed (see Fig. 7.15C). When such an association is documented in a case-control study, the next step is often to carry out a cohort study to further elucidate the relationship. Because case-control studies are generally less expensive than cohort studies and can be carried out more quickly, they are often the first step in determining whether an exposure is linked to an increased risk of disease.

Case-control studies are also valuable when the disease being investigated is rare. It is often possible to identify cases for study from disease registries, hospital records, or other sources. In contrast, if we conduct a cohort study for a rare disease, an extremely large study population may be needed in order to observe a sufficient number of individuals in the cohort develop the disease in question. In addition, depending on the length of the interval between exposure and development of disease, a cohort design may involve many years of follow-up of the cohort and considerable logistical difficulty and expense in maintaining and following the cohort over the study period.

CASE-CROSSOVER DESIGN

The *case-crossover design* is primarily used for studying the etiology of acute outcomes such as MIs or deaths from acute events in situations where the suspected exposure is transient and its effect occurs over a short time. This type of design has been used in studying exposures such as air pollution characterized by rapid and transient increases in particulate matter. In this type of study, a case is identified (e.g., a person who has suffered an MI) and the level of the environmental exposure, such as level of particulate matter, is ascertained for a short time period preceding the event (the at-risk period). This level is compared with the level of exposure in a control time period that is more remote from the event. Thus each person who is a case serves as his own control, with the period immediately before his adverse outcome being compared with a "control" period at a prior time when no adverse outcome occurred. Importantly, in this type of study, there is inherent matching for variables that do not change (e.g., genetic factors) or variables that only change within a reasonably long period (e.g., height). The question being asked is: Was there any difference in exposure between the time period immediately preceding the outcome and a time period in the more remote

past that was not immediately followed by any adverse health effect?

Let's look at a very small hypothetical 4-month case-crossover study of air pollution and MI (Fig. 7.16A to E).

Fig. 7.16A shows that over a 4-month period, January–April, four cases of MI were identified, symbolized by the small red hearts in the diagrams. The vertical dotted lines delineate 2-week intervals during the 4-month period. For the same 4-month period, levels of air pollution were measured. Three periods of high levels of air pollution of different lengths of time were identified and are shown by the pink areas in Fig. 7.16B.

For each person with an MI in this study, an "at-risk" period (also called a "hazard period") was defined as the 2 weeks immediately prior to the event. These at-risk periods are indicated by the red brackets in Fig. 7.16C. If an exposure has a short-term effect on risk of an MI, we would expect exposure to have occurred during that 2-week at-risk period. The critical element, however, in a case-crossover design is that for each subject in the study, we compare the level of exposure in that at-risk period with a control period (also called a "referent period") that is unlikely to be relevant to occurrence of the event (the MI) because it is too far removed in time from the occurrence. In this example, the control period selected for each subject is a 2-week period beginning 1 month before the at-risk period, and these control periods are indicated by the blue brackets in Fig. 7.16D. Thus, as shown by the yellow arrows in Fig. 7.16E, for each subject, we are comparing the air pollution level in the at-risk period to the air pollution level in the control period. In order to demonstrate an association of MI with air pollution, we would expect to see greater exposure to high levels of air pollution during the at-risk period than during the control period.

In this example, we see that for subject 1 both the at-risk period and the control period were in low pollution times. For subjects 2 and 3, the at-risk periods were in high pollution times and the control periods in low pollution times. For subject 4, both the at-risk and control periods were in high pollution times.

Thus, in the case-crossover design, each subject serves as his or her own control. In this sense the case-crossover design is similar to the planned crossover

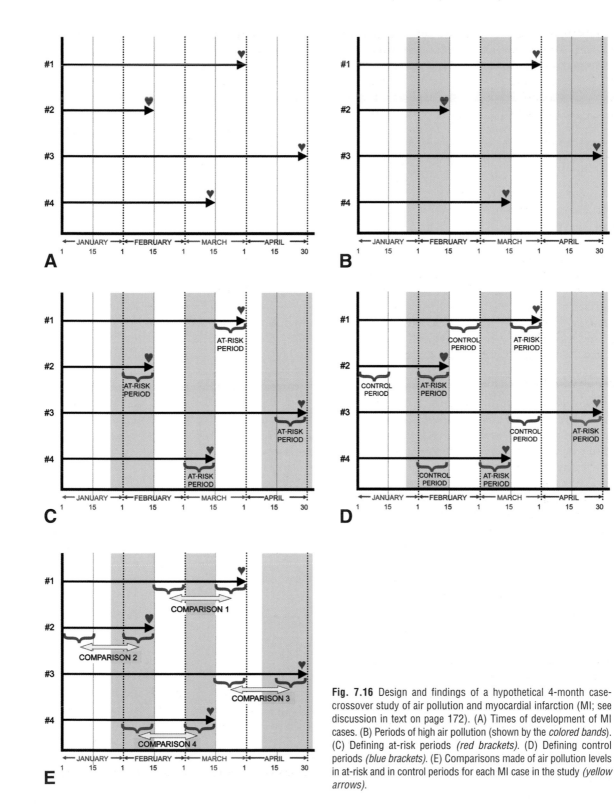

Fig. 7.16 Design and findings of a hypothetical 4-month case-crossover study of air pollution and myocardial infarction (MI; see discussion in text on page 172). (A) Times of development of MI cases. (B) Periods of high air pollution (shown by the *colored bands*). (C) Defining at-risk periods *(red brackets)*. (D) Defining control periods *(blue brackets)*. (E) Comparisons made of air pollution levels in at-risk and in control periods for each MI case in the study *(yellow arrows)*.

TABLE 7.11	**Finding Your Way in the Terminology Jungle**				
Case-control study		=			Retrospective study
Cohort study	=	Longitudinal study	=		Prospective study
Prospective cohort study	=	Concurrent cohort study	=		Concurrent prospective study
Retrospective cohort study	=	Historical cohort study	=		Nonconcurrent prospective study
Randomized trial		=			Experimental study
Cross-sectional study		=			Prevalence survey

design presented in Chapter 10. In this type of design, we are not concerned about other differences between the characteristics of the cases and those of a separate group of controls. This design also eliminates the additional cost that would be associated with identifying and interviewing a separate control population.

Attractive as this design is, unanswered questions remain. For example, the case-crossover design can be used to study people with heart attacks in regard to whether there was an episode of severe grief or anger during the period immediately preceding the attack. In this study design, the frequency of such emotionally charged events during that time interval would be compared, for example, with the frequency of such events during a period a month earlier, which was not associated with any adverse health event. Information on such events in both periods is often obtained by interviewing the subject. The question arises, however, whether there could be recall bias, in that a person may recall an emotionally charged episode that occurred shortly before a coronary event, while a comparable episode a month earlier in the absence of any adverse health event may remain forgotten. Thus recall bias may be a problem not only when we compare cases and controls, as discussed earlier in this chapter, but also when we compare the same individual in two different time periods. Further discussion of case-crossover is provided by Maclure and Mittleman.[26]

Conclusion

We have now reviewed the most basic study observational designs used in epidemiologic investigations and clinical research. Unfortunately, a variety of different terms are used in the literature to describe different study designs, and it is important to be familiar with

them. Table 7.11 is designed to help guide you through the often confusing terminology. The next study design is the "cohort study," which is presented in Chapter 8, and builds upon what we have learned about the initial observational study designs presented in this chapter. We then follow with two chapters on randomized trials, which are not "strictly" observational studies. In observational studies, the investigator merely follows those who are diseased or not diseased, or exposed and not exposed. In the randomized trial study design, the investigator uses a random allocation schedule to determine which participants are exposed or not. Hence the randomized trial is akin to an experiment and is also known as an "experimental study." However, it differs from observational studies only in that the exposure is experimentally (randomly) assigned by the study investigator.

The purpose of all of these types of studies is to identify associations between exposures and diseases. If such associations are found, the next step is to determine whether the associations are likely to be causal. These topics, starting with estimating risk and determining whether exposure to a certain factor is associated with excess risk of the disease, are addressed later.

REFERENCES

1. Dick GW, Kitchen SF, Haddow AJ. Zika virus. I. Isolations and serological specificity. *Trans R Soc Trop Med Hyg*. 1952;46: 509–520.
2. Schuler-Faccini L, Ribeiro EM, Feitosa IM, et al. Possible association between Zika virus infection and microcephaly—Brazil, 2015. *MMWR Morb Mortal Wkly Rep*. 2016;65:59–62.
3. Mlakar J, Korva M, Tul N, et al. Zika virus associated with microcephaly. *N Engl J Med*. 2016;374(10):951–958.
4. Fleming-Dutra KE, Nelson JM, Fischer M, et al. Update: interim guidelines for health care providers caring for infants and children with possible Zika virus infection—United States, February 2016. *MMWR Morb Mortal Wkly Rep*. 2016;65:182–187.

5. Messerli FH. Chocolate consumption, cognitive function, and Nobel laureates. *N Engl J Med.* 2012;367(16):1562–1564.
6. Austin DF, Karp S, Dworsky R, et al. Excess leukemia in cohorts of children born following influenza epidemics. *Am J Epidemiol.* 1975;101:77–83.
7. Rose KM, Suchindran CM, Foraker RE, et al. Neighborhood disparities in incident hospitalized myocardial infarction in four U.S. communities: the ARIC surveillance study. *Ann Epidemiol.* 2009;19(12):867–874.
8. Deelder AM, Miller RL, de Jonge N, et al. Detection of schistosome antigen in mummies. *Lancet.* 1990;335:724–725.
9. El-Sayed NM, Gomatos PJ, et al. Seroprevalence survey of Egyptian tourism workers for hepatitis B virus, hepatitis C virus, HIV and *Treponema pallidum* infections: association of hepatitis C virus infections with specific regions of Egypt. *Am J Trop Med Hyg.* 1996;55:179–184.
10. Frank C, Mohamed MK, Strickland GT, et al. The role of parenteral antischistosomal therapy in the spread of hepatitis C virus in Egypt. *Lancet.* 2000;355(9207):887–891.
11. Wynder EL, Stellman SD. The "over-exposed" control group. *Am J Epidemiol.* 1992;135:459–461.
12. Farag YM, Guallar E, Zhao D, et al. Vitamin D deficiency is independently associated with greater prevalence of erectile dysfunction: the National Health and Nutrition Examination Survey (NHANES) 2001-2004. *Atherosclerosis.* 2016;252: 61–67.
13. Murphy D, McCulloch CE, Lin F, et al. Trends in prevalence of chronic kidney disease in the United States. *Ann Intern Med.* 2016;165(7):473–481.
14. Jain RB. Regression models to predict corrected weight, height and obesity prevalence from self-reported data: data from BRFSS 1999-2007. *Int J Obes (Lond).* 2010;34(11):1655–1664.
15. Barry M. *"Autobiography."* Nobel Foundation; 2005. http://www.nobelprize.org/nobel_prizes/medicine/laureates/2005/marshall-bio.html. Accessed July 25, 2017.
16. Hill AB. The environment and disease: association or causation? *Proc R Soc Med.* 1965;58:295–300.
17. Pearl R. Cancer and tuberculosis. *Am J Hyg.* 1929;9:97–159.
18. Carlson HA, Bell ET. Statistical study of occurrence of cancer and tuberculosis in 11,195 postmortem examinations. *J Cancer Res.* 1929;13:126–135.
19. MacMahon B, Yen S, Trichopoulos D, et al. Coffee and cancer of the pancreas. *N Engl J Med.* 1981;304:630–633.
20. Hsieh CC, MacMahon B, Yen S, et al. Coffee and pancreatic cancer (chapter 2) [letter]. *N Engl J Med.* 1986;315:587–589.
21. Lilienfeld AM, Graham S. Validity of determining circumcision status by questionnaire as related to epidemiologic studies of cancer of the cervix. *J Natl Cancer Inst.* 1958;21:713–720.
22. Gold EB, Gordis L, Tonascia J, et al. Risk factors for brain tumors in children. *Am J Epidemiol.* 1979;109:309–319.
23. Filion KB, Azoulay L, Platt RW, et al. A multicenter observational study of incretin-based drugs and heart failure. *N Engl J Med.* 2016;374:1145.
24. Su F-C, Goutman SA, Chernyak S, et al. Association of environmental toxins with amyotrophic lateral sclerosis. *JAMA Neurol.* 2016;73:803.
25. Cao-Lormeau V-M, Blake A, Mons S, et al. Guillain-Barre syndrome outbreak associated with Zika virus infection in French Polynesia: a case-control study. *Lancet.* 1531;397:2016.
26. Maclure M, Mittleman MA. Should we use a case-crossover design? *Annu Rev Public Health.* 2000;21:193–221.

REVIEW QUESTIONS FOR CHAPTER 7

1 *A case-control study is characterized by all of the following except:*

a. It is relatively inexpensive compared with most other epidemiologic study designs

b. Patients with the disease (cases) are compared with persons without the disease (controls)

c. Incidence rates may be computed directly

d. Assessment of past exposure may be biased

e. Definition of cases may be difficult

2 *Residents of three villages with three different types of water supply were asked to participate in a survey to identify cholera carriers. Because several cholera deaths had occurred recently, virtually everyone present at the time underwent examination. The proportion of residents in each village who were carriers was computed and compared. What is the proper classification for this study?*

a. Cross-sectional study

b. Case-control study

c. Prospective cohort study

d. Retrospective cohort study

e. Experimental study

3 *Which of the following is a case-control study?*

a. Study of past mortality or morbidity trends to permit estimates of the occurrence of disease in the future

b. Analysis of previous research in different places and under different circumstances to permit the establishment of hypotheses based on cumulative knowledge of all known factors

c. Obtaining histories and other information from a group of known cases and from a comparison group to determine the relative

frequency of a characteristic or exposure under study

d. Study of the incidence of cancer in men who have quit smoking

e. Both *a* and *c*

4 *In a study begun in 1965, a group of 3,000 adults in Baltimore were asked about alcohol consumption. The occurrence of cases of cancer between 1981 and 1995 was studied in this group. This is an example of:*
a. A cross-sectional study
b. A prospective cohort study
c. A retrospective cohort study
d. A clinical trial
e. A case-control study

5 *In a small pilot study, 12 women with endometrial cancer (cancer of the uterus) and 12 women with no apparent disease were contacted and asked whether they had ever used estrogen. Each woman with cancer was matched by age, race, weight, and parity to a woman without disease. What kind of study design is this?*
a. Prospective cohort study
b. Retrospective cohort study
c. Case-control study
d. Cross-sectional study
e. Experimental study

6 *The physical examination records of the entire incoming freshman class of 1935 at the University of Minnesota were examined in 1977 to see if their recorded height and weight at the time of admission to the university was related to the development of coronary heart disease (CHD) by 1986. This is an example of:*
a. A cross-sectional study
b. A case-control study
c. A prospective cohort study
d. A retrospective cohort study
e. An experimental study

7 *In a case-control study, which of the following is true?*
a. The proportion of cases with the exposure is compared with the proportion of controls with the exposure
b. Disease rates are compared for people with the factor of interest and for people without the factor of interest
c. The investigator may choose to have multiple comparison groups
d. Recall bias is a potential problem
e. *a, c,* and *d*

8 *In which one of the following types of study designs does a subject serve as his own control?*
a. Prospective cohort study
b. Retrospective cohort study
c. Case-cohort study
d. Case-crossover study
e. Case-control study

9 *Ecologic fallacy refers to:*
a. Assessing exposure in large groups rather than in many small groups
b. Assessing outcome in large groups rather than in many small groups
c. Ascribing the characteristics of a group to every individual in that group
d. Examining correlations of exposure and outcomes rather than time trends
e. Failure to examine temporal relationships between exposures and outcomes

10 *A researcher wants to investigate if tea consumption (assessed by a biomarker for tea metabolism) increases the risk of CHD. He uses a case-control study to answer this question. CHD is rare in younger people. Which two groups are best to enroll and compare for this purpose?*

a. The group of CHD cases and a group of those who do not have CHD individually matched to the cases for tea metabolism biomarker

b. The group of CHD cases and a group of those who do not have CHD frequency matched to the cases for tea metabolism biomarker

c. The group of CHD cases and a group of those who do not develop CHD, matched for age

d. A random sample of those who drink tea and a random sample of those who do not drink tea, matched for age

e. A random sample of those who drink tea and a random sample of those who do not drink tea, unmatched for age

11 *Which of the following is a true conclusion concerning matching?*

a. Once we have matched controls to cases according to a given characteristic, we can only study that characteristic when the prevalence of disease is low

b. If an attempt is made to match on too many characteristics, it may prove difficult or impossible to adjust for all of the characteristics during data analysis

c. Matching on many variables may make it difficult to find an appropriate control

d. Individual matching differs from frequency matching because controls are selected from hospitals instead of from the general population

e. None of the above

Chapter 8

Cohort Studies

Learning Objectives

- To describe the designs of cohort studies and options for the conduct of longitudinal studies.
- To illustrate the cohort study design with two important historical examples.
- To discuss some potential biases in cohort studies.

In this chapter, and in the following chapters in Section II, we turn to the uses of epidemiology to elucidate etiologic or causal relationships. The two steps that underlie the study designs are discussed in this chapter and the chapters on clinical trials. Fig. 8.1 schematically represents these two conceptual steps:

1. First, we determine whether there is an *association* between a factor or a characteristic and the development of a disease. This can be accomplished by studying the characteristics of groups, by studying the characteristics of individuals, or both.
2. Second, we derive appropriate inferences regarding a possible *causal* relationship from the patterns of association that have been found.

Previously, we described the study designs used for step 1. In this chapter, cohort studies are discussed; randomized controlled trials (experiments) are presented in Chapters 10 and 11. Cohort studies, along with ecologic, cross-sectional, and case-control studies, in contrast to randomized controlled trials, are collectively referred to as *observational* studies. That is, there is no experimental manipulation involved; we investigate exposures among study participants (at one point in time or over time) and observe their outcomes either at the same point in time or sometime later on.

Design of a Cohort Study

In a cohort study, the investigator selects a group of exposed individuals and a group of unexposed individuals and follows both groups over time to compare the incidence of disease (or rate of death from disease) in the two groups (Fig. 8.2). The design may include more than two groups (such as no exposure, low exposure, and high exposure levels), although only two groups are shown here for diagrammatic purposes.

If a positive association exists between the exposure and the disease, we would expect that the proportion of the exposed group in whom the disease develops (incidence in the exposed group) would be greater than the proportion of the unexposed group in whom the disease develops (incidence in the unexposed group).

The calculations involved are seen in Table 8.1. We begin with an exposed group and an unexposed group. Of the $(a + b)$ exposed persons, the disease develops in a but not in b. Thus the incidence of the disease among the exposed is $\dfrac{a}{a+b}$. Similarly, in the $(c + d)$ unexposed persons in the study, the disease develops in c but not in d. Thus the incidence of the disease among the unexposed is $\dfrac{c}{c+d}$.

The use of these calculations is seen in a hypothetical example of a cohort study shown in Table 8.2. In this cohort study, the association of smoking with coronary heart disease (CHD) is investigated by selecting for study a group of 3,000 smokers (exposed) and a group of 5,000 nonsmokers (unexposed), all of whom are free of heart disease at baseline. Both groups are followed for the development of CHD, and the *incidence* of CHD in both groups is compared. CHD develops in 84 of the smokers and in 87 of the nonsmokers. The result is an incidence of CHD of 28.0/1,000 in the smokers and 17.4/1,000 in the nonsmokers.

Note that because we are identifying *new* (incident) cases of disease as they occur, we can determine

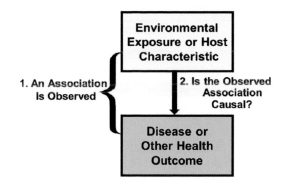

Fig. 8.1 If we observe an association between an exposure and a disease or another outcome *(1),* the question is: Is the association causal *(2)?*

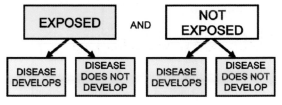

Fig. 8.2 Design of a cohort study.

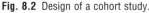

TABLE 8.1	**Design of a Cohort Study**				
First Select {	Exposed	*a*	*b*	*a* + *b*	$\dfrac{a}{a+b}$
	Not exposed	*c*	*d*	*c* + *d*	$\dfrac{a}{a+b}$

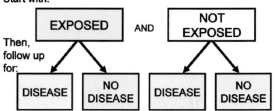

Fig. 8.3 Design of a cohort study beginning with exposed and unexposed groups.

TABLE 8.2	**Results of a Hypothetical Cohort Study of Smoking and Coronary Heart Disease (CHD)**				
		THEN FOLLOW TO SEE WHETHER			
		CHD Develops	**CHD Does Not Develop**	**Totals**	**Incidence per 1,000 per Year**
First Select {	Smoke cigarettes	84	2,916	3,000	28.0
	Do not smoke cigarettes	87	4,913	5,000	17.4

whether a temporal relationship exists between the exposure and the disease (i.e., whether the exposure preceded the onset of the disease). Clearly, such a temporal relationship must be established if we are to consider the exposure a possible cause of the disease in question.

Selection of Study Populations

The essential characteristic in the design of cohort studies is the comparison of outcomes in an exposed group and in an unexposed group (or a group with a certain characteristic and a group without that characteristic, such as older or younger par-

ticipants). There are two basic ways to generate such groups:

1. We can create a study population by selecting groups for inclusion in the study on the basis of whether or not they were exposed (e.g., occupationally exposed cohorts compared with similarly aged community residents who do not work in those occupations) (Fig. 8.3).
2. We can select a defined population before any of its members become exposed or before their exposures are identified. We could select a population on the basis of some factor not related to exposure (such as community of residence) (Fig. 8.4) and take histories of, or perform blood

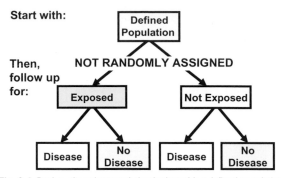

Fig. 8.4 Design of a cohort study beginning with a defined population.

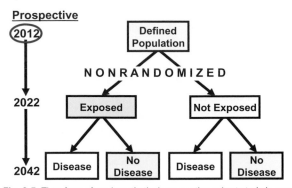

Fig. 8.5 Time frame for a hypothetical prospective cohort study begun in 2012.

tests or other assays on, the entire population. Using the results of the histories or the tests, one can separate the population into *exposed* and *unexposed* groups (or those who have and those who do not have certain biologic characteristics), such as was done in the Framingham Study, described later in this chapter.

Cohort studies, in which we wait for an outcome to develop in a population, often require a long follow-up period, lasting until enough events (outcomes) have occurred. When the second approach is used—in which a population is identified for study based on some characteristic unrelated to the exposure in question—the exposure of interest may not take place for some time, even for many years after the population has been defined. Consequently, the length of follow-up required is even greater with the second approach than it is with the first. Note that with either approach the cohort study design is fundamentally the same: *we compare exposed and unexposed persons.* This comparison is the hallmark of the cohort design.

Types of Cohort Studies

A major issue with the cohort design just described is that the study population often must be followed up for a long period to determine whether the outcome of interest develops. Consider as an example a hypothetical study of the relationship of smoking to lung cancer. We identify a population of elementary school students and follow them; 10 years later, when they are teenagers, we identify those who smoke and those

who do not. We then follow both groups—smokers and nonsmokers—to see who develops lung cancer and who does not. Let us say that we begin our study in 2012 (Fig. 8.5). Let us suppose that many children who will become smokers will do so within 10 years. Exposure status (smoker or nonsmoker) will therefore be ascertained 10 years later, in the year 2022. For purposes of this example, let us assume that the average latent period from beginning smoking to development of lung disease is 20 years. Therefore development of lung cancer will be, on average, ascertained 20 years later, in 2042.

This type of study design is called a *prospective cohort study* (also called by some a *concurrent cohort* or *longitudinal study*). It is *concurrent* (happening or done at the same time) because the investigator identifies the original population at the beginning of the study and, in effect, follows the subjects concurrently through calendar time until the point at which the disease develops or does not develop.

What is the problem with this approach? The difficulty is that, as just described, the study will take at least 30 years to complete. Several problems can result. If one is fortunate enough to obtain a research grant, such funding is generally limited to a maximum of only 5 years. In addition, with a study of this length, there is the risk that the study subjects will outlive the investigator, or at least that the investigator may not survive to the end of the study. Given these issues, the prospective cohort study often proves unattractive to investigators who are contemplating a new research question.

Do these problems mean that the cohort design is not practical? Is there any way to shorten the time period needed to conduct a cohort study? Let us consider an alternate approach using the cohort design (Fig. 8.6). Suppose that we again begin our study in 2012, but now we find that an old roster of elementary schoolchildren from 1982 is available in our community and that they had been surveyed in high school regarding their smoking habits in 1992. Using these data resources in 2012, we can begin to determine who in this population developed lung cancer and who has not. This is called a *retrospective cohort* or *historical cohort study* (also called a *nonconcurrent prospective study*). However, note that the study design does not differ from that of the prospective cohort design—we are still comparing exposed and unexposed groups. What we have done in the retrospective cohort design is to use historical data so that we can telescope (reduce) the frame of calendar time for the study and obtain our results sooner. It is no longer a prospective design, because we are beginning the study with a preexisting population to reduce the duration of the study. However, as shown in Fig. 8.7, the *designs for both the prospective cohort study and the retrospective or historical cohort study are identical: we are comparing exposed and unexposed populations.* The only difference between them is calendar time. In a *prospective cohort design*, exposure and unexposure are ascertained as they occur during the study; the groups are then followed for several years into the future and incidence is measured. In a *retrospective cohort design*, exposure is ascertained from past records and the outcome (development or no

development of disease) is determined when the study is begun.

It is also possible to conduct a study that is a combination of prospective cohort and retrospective cohort designs. With this approach, exposure is ascertained from objective records in the past (as in a historical cohort study) and follow-up and measurement of outcome continue into the future.

Examples of Cohort Studies

EXAMPLE 1: THE FRAMINGHAM STUDY

One of the first, most important, and best-known cohort studies is the Framingham Study of cardiovascular disease, which was begun in 1948.[1] Framingham is a town in Massachusetts, approximately 20 miles west of Boston. It was thought that the characteristics of its population (just less than 30,000 residents) would be appropriate for such a study and would facilitate follow-up of participants because migration out was considered to be low (i.e., the population was stable).

Residents were considered eligible if they were between 30 and 62 years of age at study initiation. The rationale for using this age range was that people younger than 30 years would generally be unlikely to manifest the cardiovascular end points being studied during the proposed 20-year follow-up period. Many persons older than 62 years would already have established coronary disease, and it would therefore not be rewarding to study persons in this age group for identifying the incidence of coronary disease.

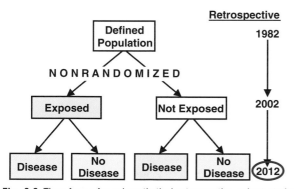

Fig. 8.6 Time frame for a hypothetical retrospective cohort study begun in 2012.

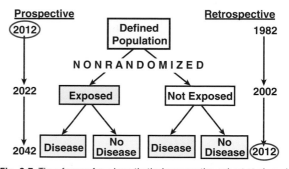

Fig. 8.7 Time frames for a hypothetical prospective cohort study and a hypothetical retrospective cohort study begun in 2012.

The investigators sought a sample size of 5,000. Table 8.3 shows how the final study population was derived. It consisted of 5,127 men and women who were between 30 and 62 years of age at the time of study entry and were free of cardiovascular disease at that time. In this study, many suggested "exposures" were defined, including age and gender, smoking, weight, blood pressure, cholesterol levels, physical activity, and other factors.

New coronary events (incidence) were identified by examining the study population every 2 years and by daily surveillance of hospitalizations at the only hospital in Framingham.

The study was designed to test the following hypotheses:

- The incidence of CHD increases with age. It occurs earlier and more frequently in males.
- Persons with hypertension develop CHD at a greater rate than those who are normotensive.
- Elevated blood cholesterol level is associated with an increased risk of CHD.
- Tobacco smoking and habitual use of alcohol are associated with an increased incidence of CHD.
- Increased physical activity is associated with a decrease in the development of CHD.
- An increase in body weight predisposes a person to the development of CHD.
- An increased rate of development of CHD occurs in patients with diabetes mellitus.

When we examine this list nowadays, we might wonder why such obvious and well-known relationships should have been examined in such an extensive study. The danger of this "hindsight" approach should be kept in mind; it is primarily *because* of the Framingham Study, a classic cohort study that made fundamental contributions to our understanding of the epidemiology of cardiovascular disease, that these relationships are currently well known.

This study used the second method described earlier in the chapter for selecting a study population for a cohort study: A defined population was selected on the basis of location of residence or other factors not related to the exposure(s) in question. The population was then observed over time to determine which individuals developed or already had the "exposure(s)" of interest and, later on, to determine which study participants developed the cardiovascular outcome(s) of interest. This approach offered an important advantage: It permitted the investigators to study multiple "exposures," such as hypertension, smoking, obesity, cholesterol levels, and other factors, as well as the complex interactions among the exposures, by using multivariable techniques. Thus, although a cohort study that begins with an exposed and an unexposed group focuses often on only one specific exposure, a cohort study that begins with a defined population can explore the roles of many exposures to the study outcome measure(s).

EXAMPLE 2: INCIDENCE OF BREAST CANCER AND PROGESTERONE DEFICIENCY

It has long been recognized that breast cancer is more common in women who are older at the time of their first pregnancy. A difficult question is raised by this observation: Is the relationship between late age at first pregnancy and increased risk of breast cancer related to the finding that early first pregnancy protects against breast cancer (and therefore such protection is missing in women who have a later pregnancy or no pregnancy), or are both a delayed first pregnancy and an increased risk of breast cancer the result of some third factor, such as an underlying hormonal abnormality?

It is difficult to tease apart these two interpretations. However, in 1978, Linda Cowan and coworkers[2] carried out a study designed to determine which of these two explanations was likely to be the correct one (Fig. 8.8). The researchers identified a population of women who

TABLE 8.3 **Derivation of the Framingham Study Population**			
	No. of Men	No. of Women	Total
Random sample	3,074	3,433	6,507
Respondents	2,024	2,445	4,469
Volunteers	312	428	740
Respondents free of CHD	1,975	2,418	4,393
Volunteers free of CHD	307	427	734
Total free of CHD: The Framingham Study Group	2,282	2,845	5,127

CHD, Coronary heart disease.
From Dawber TR, Kannel WB, Lyell LP. An approach to longitudinal studies in a community: the Framingham Study. *Ann NY Acad Sci.* 1993;107:539–556.

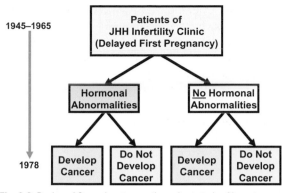

Fig. 8.8 Design of Cowan's retrospective cohort study of breast cancer. *JHH,* Johns Hopkins Hospital. (Data from Cowan LD, Gordis L, Tonascia JA, Jones GS. Breast cancer incidence in women with progesterone deficiency. *Am J Epidemiol.* 1981;114:209–217.)

were patients at the Johns Hopkins Hospital Infertility Clinic in Baltimore, Maryland, from 1945 to 1965. Because they were patients at this clinic, the subjects, by definition, all had a late age at first pregnancy. In the course of their diagnostic evaluations, detailed hormonal profiles were developed for each woman. The researchers were therefore able to separate the women with an underlying hormonal abnormality, including progesterone deficiency (exposed), from those without such a hormonal abnormality (unexposed) who had another cause of infertility, such as a problem with tubal patency or a husband's low sperm count. Both groups of women were then followed for subsequent development of breast cancer.

How could the results of this study design clarify the relationship between late age at first pregnancy and increased risk of breast cancer? If the explanation for the association of late age at first pregnancy and increased risk of breast cancer is that an early first pregnancy protects against breast cancer, we would not expect any difference in the incidence of breast cancer between the women who have a hormonal abnormality and those who do not (and none of the women would have had an early first pregnancy). However, if the explanation for the increased risk of breast cancer is that the underlying hormonal abnormality predisposes these women to breast cancer, we would expect to find a higher incidence of breast cancer in women with the hormonal abnormality than in those without this abnormality.

The study found that, when the development of breast cancer was considered for the entire group, the incidence was 1.8 times greater in women with hormonal abnormalities than in women without such abnormalities, but the finding was not statistically significant. However, when the occurrence of breast cancer was divided into categories of premenopausal and postmenopausal incidence, women with hormonal abnormalities had a 5.4 times greater risk of premenopausal occurrence of breast cancer (they developed breast cancer earlier); no difference was seen for postmenopausal occurrence of breast cancer. It is not clear whether this lack of a difference in the incidence of postmenopausal breast cancer represents the true absence of a difference or whether it can be attributed to the small number of women in this population who had reached menopause at the time the study was conducted.

What type of study design is this? Clearly, it is a cohort design because it compares exposed and unexposed persons. Furthermore, because the study was carried out in 1978 and the investigator used a roster of patients who had been seen at the Infertility Clinic from 1945 to 1965, it is a retrospective cohort design.

Cohort Studies for Investigating Childhood Health and Disease

A particularly appealing use of the cohort design is for long-term cohort studies of childhood health and disease. In recent years, there has been increasing recognition that experiences and exposures during fetal life may have long-lasting effects, even into adult life. Infections during pregnancy, as well as exposures to environmental toxins, hormonal abnormalities, or the use of drugs (either medications taken during pregnancy or substances abused during pregnancy), may have potentially damaging effects on the fetus and child, and these agents might have possible effects that last even into adult life. David Barker and his colleagues concluded from their studies that adult chronic disease is biologically programmed in intrauterine life or early infancy.[3] The importance of including a life course approach to the epidemiologic study of chronic disease throughout life has been emphasized.

In this chapter, we have discussed two types of cohort studies; both have applicability to the study of childhood health. In the first type of cohort study, we start with exposed and unexposed groups. For example, follow-up studies of fetuses exposed to radiation from atomic bombs in Hiroshima and Nagasaki during World War II have provided much information about cancer and other health problems resulting from intrauterine exposure to radiation.[4] The exposure dose was calibrated for the survivors on the basis of how far the pregnant women was from the point of the bomb drop and the nature of the barriers between that person and the point of the bomb drop. It was then possible to relate the risk of adverse outcome to the radiation dose that each person received. Another example is the cohort of pregnancies during the Dutch Famine in World War II.[5] Because the Dutch kept excellent records, it was possible to identify cohorts who were exposed to the severe famine at different times in gestation and to compare them with one another and with an unexposed group.

As discussed earlier in this chapter, in the second type of cohort study, we identify a group before any of its members become exposed or before the exposure has been identified. For example, infants born during a single week in 1946 in Great Britain were followed into childhood and later into adult life. The Collaborative Perinatal Study, begun in the United States in the 1950s, was a multicenter cohort study that followed more than 58,000 children from birth to age 7 years.[6]

Although the potential knowledge to be gained by such studies is very attractive, several challenging questions arise when such large cohort studies of children are envisioned and when such long-term follow-up is planned. Among the questions are the following:

1. At what point should the individuals in the cohort first be identified? When a cohort is initiated at birth and then followed (Fig. 8.9), data on prenatal exposures can be obtained only retrospectively by interview and from relevant records. Therefore some cohort studies have begun in the prenatal period, when the pregnancy is first identified. However, even when this is done, preconceptual and periconceptual data that may be needed to answer certain questions may only be obtained retrospectively. Therefore a cohort initiated prior to the time of conception (Fig. 8.10) is desirable for answering many questions because it permits concurrent gathering of

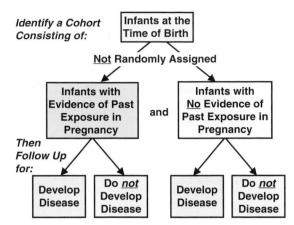

Fig. 8.9 Design of a cohort study to investigate the effects of exposures during pregnancy on disease throughout life: study beginning at birth.

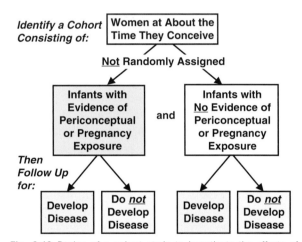

Fig. 8.10 Design of a cohort study to investigate the effects of exposures during pregnancy on disease throughout life: study beginning at about the time of conception.

data about exposures at the time of or preceding conception and then in the prenatal and perinatal periods. However, this is generally a logistically difficult and very expensive challenge.

2. Should the cohort be drawn from one center or from a few centers, or should it be a national sample drawn in an attempt to make the cohort representative of a national population? Will the findings of studies based on the cohort be broadly generalizable only if the cohort is drawn from a national sample? The National Children's Study (NCS) was a planned long-term study of 100,000 children and their parents in the United States which was designed to investigate environmental

influences on child health and development. The pilot study was initiated in 2009, and only 5,000 children were recruited by 2013 from 40 centers across the United States. Based on the recommendations of an expert panel, the National Institutes of Health (NIH) director closed the NCS in 2014. In 2016 the NIH launched a 7-year study called the Environmental Influences on Child Health Outcomes (ECHO) enrolling existing child (and parent in some cases) cohorts which will then continue to be followed using harmonized data collection. The resulting "synthetic cohort" (or a cohort of cohorts) should prove far more efficient than the planned NCS proposed cohort.

3. For how long should a cohort be followed? Eaton urged that a cohort should be established at the time of conception and followed into adult life or until death.[7] This approach would help to test Barker's hypothesis regarding the early origins of many chronic diseases. Recalling that federal funding is generally limited to 5 years, this is an impediment to long-term follow-up.

Which hypotheses and how many hypotheses should be tested in the cohort that will be established? A major problem associated with long-term follow-up of large cohorts is that, by the time the cohort has been established and followed for a number of years, the hypotheses that originally led to the establishment of the cohort may no longer be of sufficient interest or relevance because scientific and health knowledge has changed over time. Furthermore, as new knowledge leads to new hypotheses and to questions that were not originally anticipated when the study was initiated, data on the variables needed to test such new hypotheses and to answer such new questions may not be available in the data originally collected. An example from HIV/AIDS research illustrates these issues. In the early 1980s, when clusters of men were identified who had rare malignancies associated with compromised immune function, later to be defined as HIV/AIDS, the NIH launched the Multicenter AIDS Cohort Study in 1983 and enrolled the first participants in four US cities in 1984.[8] The goal was to identify risk factors for this viral disease and to elucidate the natural history of the disease. With the advent of highly active antiretroviral therapy in 1996, virtually all of the study participants who were already infected were then placed on treatment, and their immune systems were reconstituted. How then could the natural history of a treated infection remain relevant? Was there any use in continuing to follow this cohort? Indeed, a vast number of new, relevant questions unfolded, chief among them has become what is the impact of long-term antiretroviral therapy treatments upon natural aging and the incidence of chronic diseases (cancer, cardiovascular disease, and diabetes, among others)?[9] Furthermore, new genetic tests have been discovered over the past 15 years that provide new insights into why some participants do better than others on treatment.[10] It must be emphasized that cohort studies whose participants are examined periodically, such as the Atherosclerosis Risk in Communities (ARIC) study,[11] allow evaluation of new hypotheses based on information that is collected in follow-up examinations.

Potential Biases in Cohort Studies

A number of potential biases must be either avoided or taken into account in conducting cohort studies. Discussions of biases in relation to case-control studies were presented earlier; bias in relation to causal inference will be presented later. The definitions used for many types of biases often overlap, and in the interest of clarity, two major categories are commonly used: *selection bias* and *information bias*.

SELECTION BIASES

Nonparticipation and nonresponse can introduce major biases that can complicate the interpretation of the study findings. If participants refuse to join a cohort, might their characteristics differ sufficiently from those who consent to enroll, and might these differences lead to misguided inferences regarding exposures to outcomes? For example, if those who refuse to join a study are more likely to smoke than those who consent to participate, would our estimate of the effect of smoking on the disease outcome be biased? If smokers who refuse participation are more likely to develop the disease than those who participate, the impact would be to diminish the association toward the null. Similarly, loss to follow-up can be a serious problem: If people with the disease are selectively lost to follow-up, and those lost to follow-up differ from those not lost to follow-up, the incidence rates calculated in the exposed and unexposed groups will clearly be difficult to interpret.

INFORMATION BIASES

1. If the quality and extent of information obtained is different for exposed persons than for the unexposed persons, a significant bias can be introduced. This is particularly likely to occur in historical cohort studies, in which information is obtained from past records. As we will discuss next in connection with randomized trials, in any cohort study, it is essential that the quality of the information obtained be comparable in both exposed and unexposed individuals.

2. If the person who decides whether the disease has developed in each subject also knows whether that subject was exposed, and if that person is aware of the hypothesis being tested, that person's judgment as to whether the disease developed may be biased by that knowledge. This problem can be addressed by "masking" the person who is making the disease assessment and also by determining whether this person was, in fact, aware of each subject's exposure status.

3. As in any study, if the epidemiologists and statisticians who are analyzing the data have strong preconceptions, they may unintentionally introduce their biases into their data analyses and into their interpretation of the study findings.

When Is a Cohort Study Warranted?

Fig. 8.11A to C reviews the basic steps in a cohort study, beginning with identifying an exposed group and an unexposed group (see Fig. 8.11A). We then ascertain the rate of development of disease (incidence) in both the exposed and the unexposed groups (see Fig. 8.11B). If the exposure is associated with disease, we would expect to find a greater incidence rate of disease in the exposed group than in the unexposed group, as shown schematically in Fig. 8.11C.

Clearly, to carry out a cohort study, we must have some idea of which exposures are suspected a priori as possible causes of a disease and are therefore worth investigating. Consequently, a cohort study is indicated when good evidence suggests an association of a disease with a certain exposure or exposures (evidence obtained from either clinical observations or case-control or other types of studies). Often, we collect biologic specimens at study baseline (enrollment), allowing testing of these

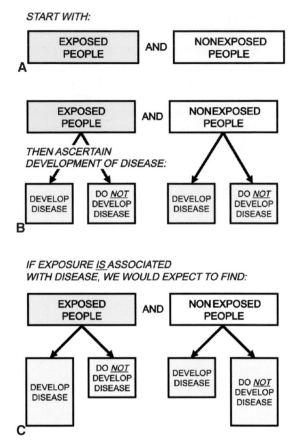

Fig. 8.11 Design of a cohort study. (A) Starting with exposed and unexposed groups. (B) Measuring the development of disease in both groups. (C) Expected findings if the exposure is associated with disease.

samples in the future, often when new test methods are developed and/or new hypotheses are generated. As an example, George Comstock collected serum specimens at the time of a community assessment in the 1960s in Washington County, Maryland. Decades later, these specimens were tested for "clues" to the development of cancer. Results from the Campaign Against Cancer and Heart Disease (CLUE II) cohort study that Dr. Comstock founded showed that high serum cholesterol increases the risk of high-grade prostate cancer and subsequently supports the hypothesis that cholesterol lowering is a potential mechanism by which statins, a cholesterol-lowering medications, could have anticancer effects.[12]

Because cohort studies often involve follow-up of populations over a long period, the cohort approach is particularly attractive when we can minimize attrition (losses to follow-up) of the study population. Consequently, such studies are generally easier to conduct when the interval between the exposure and the development of disease is short. An example of an association in which the interval between exposure and outcome is short is the relationship between rubella infection during pregnancy and the development of congenital malformations in the offspring.

Case-Control Studies Based Within a Defined Cohort

In recent years, considerable attention has focused on whether it is possible to take advantage of the benefits of both case-control and cohort study designs by combining some elements of both into a single study. The resulting combined study is in effect a hybrid design in which a case-control study is initiated within a cohort study. The general design is shown schematically in Fig. 8.12.

In this type of study, a population is identified and followed over time. At the time the population is identified, baseline data are obtained from records or interviews, from blood or urine tests, and in other ways. The population is then followed for a period of years. For most of the diseases that are studied, a small percentage of study participants manifest the disease, whereas most do not. As seen in Fig. 8.12, a case-control study is then carried out using as cases persons in whom the disease developed and using as

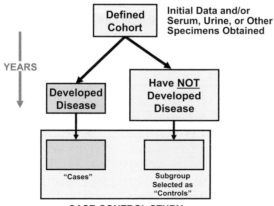

Fig. 8.12 Design of a case-control study initiated within a cohort.

controls a sample of those in whom the disease did not develop.

Such cohort-based case-control studies can be divided into two types, largely on the basis of the approach used for selecting the controls. These two types of studies are called *nested case-control studies* and *case-cohort studies*.

NESTED CASE-CONTROL STUDIES

In *nested case-control studies* the controls are a sample of individuals who are at risk for the disease *at the time each case of the disease develops*. This is shown schematically in Fig. 8.13A to I.

Fig. 8.13A shows the starting point as a defined cohort of individuals. Some of them develop the disease in question, but most do not. In this hypothetical example, the cohort is observed over a 5-year period. During this time, five cases develop—one case after 1 year, one after 2 years, two after 4 years, and one after 5 years.

Let us follow the sequence of steps over time. Fig. 8.13B to I shows the time sequence in which the cases develop after the start of observations. At the time each case or cases develop, the same number of controls is selected. The solid arrows on the left side of the figure denote the appearance of cases of the disease, and the dotted arrows on the right side denote the selection of controls who are disease free but who are at risk of developing the disease in question at the time the case develops the disease. Fig. 8.13B shows case #1 developing after 1 year, and Fig. 8.13C shows control #1 being selected at that time. Fig. 8.13D shows case #2 developing after 2 years, and Fig. 8.13E shows control #2 being selected at that time. Fig. 8.13F shows cases #3 and #4 developing after 4 years, and Fig. 8.13G shows controls #3 and #4 being selected at that time. Finally, Fig. 8.13H shows the final case (#5) developing after 5 years, and Fig. 8.13I shows control #5 being selected at this point.

Fig. 8.13I is also a summary of the design and the final study populations used in the nested case-control study. At the end of 5 years, five cases have appeared, and at the times the cases appeared a total of five controls were selected for study. In this way, the cases and controls are, in effect, matched on calendar time and length of follow-up. Because a control is selected each time a case develops, a control who is selected

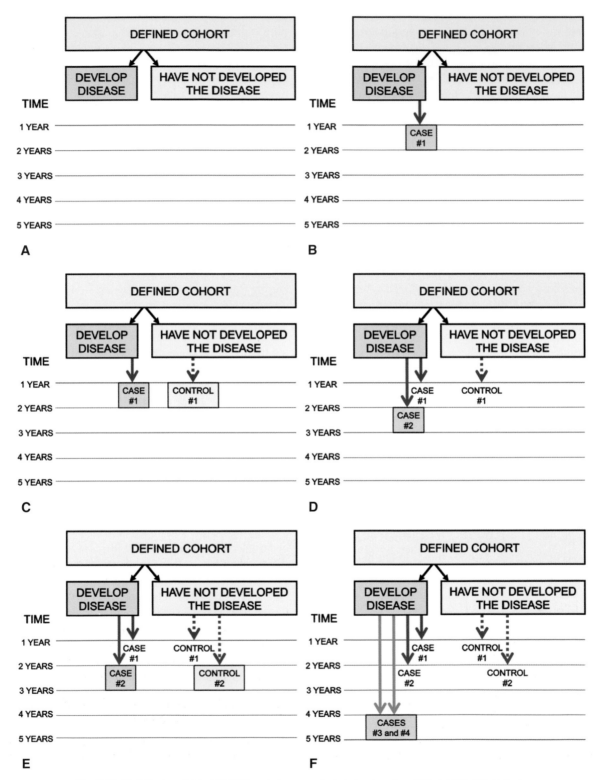

Fig. 8.13 (A–I) Design of a hypothetical nested case-control study: steps in selecting cases and controls.

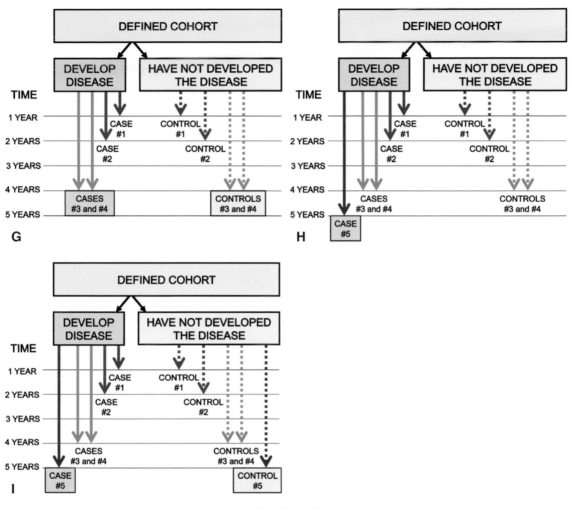

Fig. 8.13 cont'd

early in the study could later develop the disease and become a case in the same study.

CASE-COHORT STUDIES

The second type of cohort-based case-control study is the *case-cohort design* seen in Fig. 8.14. In the hypothetical case-cohort study seen here, cases develop at the same times that were seen in the nested case-control design just discussed, but the controls are randomly chosen from the defined cohort with which the study began. This subset of the full cohort is called the subcohort. An advantage of this design is that because controls are not individually matched to each case, it

is possible to study different diseases (different sets of cases) in the same case-cohort study using the same cohort for controls. In this design, in contrast to the nested case-control design, cases and controls are not matched on calendar time and length of follow-up; instead, exposure is characterized for the subcohort. This difference in study design needs to be taken into account in analyzing the study results.

ADVANTAGES OF EMBEDDING A CASE-CONTROL STUDY IN A DEFINED COHORT

What are the advantages of conducting a case-control study in a defined cohort? First, because interviews

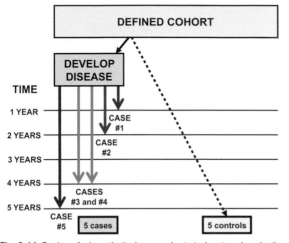

Fig. 8.14 Design of a hypothetical case-cohort study: steps in selecting cases and controls.

are completed or certain blood or urine specimens are obtained at the beginning of the study (at baseline), the data are obtained before any disease has developed. Consequently, the problem of possible recall bias discussed earlier in this chapter is eliminated. Second, if abnormalities in biologic characteristics such as laboratory values are found, because the specimens were obtained years before the development of clinical disease, it is more likely that these findings represent risk factors or other premorbid characteristics than a manifestation of early, subclinical disease. When such abnormalities are found in the traditional case-control study, we do not know whether they preceded the disease or were a result of the disease, particularly when the disease has a long subclinical (asymptomatic) phase, such as prostate cancer and chronic lymphocytic leukemia. Third, such a study is often more economical to conduct. One might ask, why perform a case-control study within a defined cohort? Why not perform a regular prospective cohort study? The answer is that in a cohort study of, say, 10,000 people, laboratory analyses of all the specimens obtained would have to be carried out, often at great cost, to define *exposed and unexposed* groups. However, in a case-control study within the same cohort, the specimens obtained initially are frozen or otherwise stored. Only after the disease has developed in some subjects is a case-control study begun and the specimens from the relatively small number of people who are included in the case-control

study are thawed and tested. Laboratory tests would not need to be performed on all 10,000 people in the original cohort. Thus the laboratory burden and costs are dramatically reduced.

Finally, in both nested case-control and case-cohort designs, cases and controls are derived from the same original cohort, so there is likely to be greater comparability between the cases and the controls than one might ordinarily find in a traditional case-control study. For all of these reasons, the cohort-based case-control study is an extremely valuable type of study design.

Conclusion

Several considerations can make the cohort design impractical. Often, strong evidence does not exist to justify mounting a large and expensive study for in-depth investigation of the role of a specific risk factor in the etiology of a disease. Even when such evidence is available, a cohort of exposed and unexposed persons often cannot be identified easily. In general, we do not have access to appropriate past records or other sources of data that enable us to conduct a retrospective cohort study; as a result, a long study is required because of the need for extended follow-up of the population after exposure. Furthermore, many of the diseases that are of interest today occur at very low rates. Consequently, very large cohorts must be enrolled in a study to ensure that enough cases develop by the end of the study period to permit valid analyses and conclusions.

In view of these considerations, an approach other than a cohort design is often needed—one that will surmount many of these difficulties. As we previously presented, such study designs—the case-control study and cross-sectional study designs—are being increasingly used. Later, we discuss the use of these study designs in estimating increased risk associated with an exposure.

REFERENCES

1. Kannel WB. CHD risk factors: a Framingham Study update. *Hosp Pract.* 1990;25:93–104.
2. Cowan LD, Gordis L, Tonascia JA, et al. Breast cancer incidence in women with progesterone deficiency. *Am J Epidemiol.* 1981;114:209–217.
3. Barker DJP, ed. *Fetal and Infant Origins of Adult Disease.* London: BMJ Books; 1992.
4. Yoshimoto Y, Kato H, Schull WJ. Cancer risk among in utero exposed survivors: a review of 45 years of study of Hiroshima

and Nagasaki atomic bomb survivors. *J Radiat Res (Tokyo)*. 1991;32(suppl):231–238. Also available as RERF Technical Report 4–88, and in *Lancet*. 1988;2:665–669.
5. Susser E, Hoek HW, Brown A. Neurodevelopmental disorders after prenatal famine: the story of the Dutch Famine Study. *Am J Epidemiol*. 1998;147:213–216.
6. Broman S. The collaborative perinatal project: an overview. In: Mednick SA, Harway M, Pinello KM, eds. *Handbook of Longitudinal Research*. Vol I. New York: Praeger; 1984.
7. Eaton WW. The logic for a conception-to-death cohort study. *Ann Epidemiol*. 2002;12:445–451.
8. Kaslow R, Ostrow DG, Detels R, et al; for the Multicenter AIDS Cohort Study. The Multicenter AIDS Cohort Study: rationale, organization, and selected characteristics of the participants. *Am J Epidemiol*. 1987;126:310–318.
9. Brown TT, Cole SR, Li X, et al. Antiretroviral therapy and the prevalence and incidence of diabetes mellitus in the Multicenter AIDS Cohort Study. *Arch Intern Med*. 2005;165:1179–1184.
10. Winkler C, Modi W, Smith MW, et al. Genetic restriction of AIDS pathogenesis by an SDF-1 chemokine gene variant. *Science*. 1998;279:389–393.
11. ARIC investigators. The Atherosclerosis Risk in Communities (ARIC) Study: design and objectives. *Am J Epidemiol*. 1989;129:687–702.
12. Mondul AM, Clipp SL, Helzlsouer KJ, et al. Association between plasma total cholesterol concentration and incident prostate cancer in the CLUE II cohort. *Cancer Causes Control*. 2010;21(1):61–68.

REVIEW QUESTIONS FOR CHAPTER 8

1 *In cohort studies of the role of a suspected factor in the etiology of a disease, it is essential that:*
 a. There be equal numbers of persons in both study groups
 b. At the beginning of the study, those with the disease and those without the disease have equal risks of having the factor
 c. The study group with the factor and the study group without the factor be representative of the general population
 d. The exposed and unexposed groups under study be as similar as possible with regard to possible confounding factors
 e. Both *b* and *c*

2 *Which of the following is not an advantage of a prospective cohort study?*
 a. It usually costs less than a case-control study
 b. Precise measurement of exposure is possible
 c. Incidence rates can be calculated
 d. Recall bias is minimized compared with a case-control study
 e. Many disease outcomes can be studied simultaneously

3 *Retrospective cohort studies are characterized by all of the following except:*
 a. The study groups are exposed and unexposed
 b. Incidence rates may be computed
 c. The required sample size is smaller than that needed for a prospective cohort study
 d. The required sample size is similar to that needed for a prospective cohort study
 e. They are useful for rare exposures

4 *A major problem resulting from the lack of randomization in a cohort study is:*
 a. The possibility that a factor that led to the exposure, rather than the exposure itself, might have caused the disease
 b. The possibility that a greater proportion of people in the study may have been exposed
 c. The possibility that a smaller proportion of people in the study may have been exposed
 d. That, without randomization, the study may take longer to carry out
 e. Planned crossover is more likely

5 *In a cohort study, the advantage of starting by selecting a defined population for study before any of its members become exposed, rather than starting by selecting exposed and unexposed individuals, is that:*
 a. The study can be completed more rapidly
 b. A number of outcomes can be studied simultaneously
 c. A number of exposures can be studied simultaneously
 d. The study will cost less to carry out
 e. *a* and *d*

6 *In 2010, investigators were interested in studying early-adult obesity as a risk factor for cancer mortality. The investigators obtained physician health reports on students who attended the University of Glasgow between 1948 and 1968. These reports included records of the students' heights and weights at the time they attended the university. The students were then followed through 2010. Mortality information was obtained using death certificates. This study can best be described as a:*

a. Nested case-control

b. Cross-sectional

c. Prospective cohort

d. Retrospective cohort

e. Population-based case-control

7 *From 1983 to 1988, blood samples were obtained from 3,450 HIV-negative men in the Multicenter AIDS Cohort Study (MACS) and stored in a national repository. In 2010 a researcher was interested in examining the association between levels of inflammation and HIV infection. Of the 3,450 men, 660 men were identified as HIV-infected cases. The researcher investigated the association between C-reactive protein (CRP) and HIV infection among these 660 cases and 660 controls, matched to the cases by age and ethnicity, who did not become infected with HIV. The researcher used the stored blood samples to measure the serum level of CRP, a marker of systemic inflammation. The study initiated in 2010 is an example of a:*

a. Nested case-cohort study

b. Nested case-control study

c. Retrospective cohort study

d. Cross-sectional study

e. Randomized clinical trial

Chapter 9

Comparing Cohort and Case-Control Studies

At this point in our discussion, we will review some of the material that has been covered to this point in Section II. Because the presentation proceeds in a stepwise manner, it is important to understand what has been discussed thus far.

First, let's compare the designs of cohort and case-control studies, as seen in Fig. 9.1. The important point that distinguishes between these two types of study designs is that, in a cohort study, exposed and unexposed persons are compared and, in a case-control study, persons with the disease (cases) and without the disease (controls) are compared (Fig. 9.2A). In cohort studies, we compare the incidence of disease in exposed and in unexposed individuals, and in case-control studies, we compare the proportions who have the exposure of interest in people with the disease and in people without the disease (see Fig. 9.2B).

Table 9.1 presents a detailed comparison of prospective cohort, retrospective (historical) cohort, and case-control study designs. If the reader has followed the discussion in Section II to this point, the entries in the table should be easy to understand.

When we begin a cohort study with exposed and unexposed groups, we can study only the specific exposure that distinguishes one group from the other. However, as shown in Fig. 9.3, we can study multiple outcomes or diseases in relation to the exposure of interest. Most cohort studies start with exposed and unexposed individuals. Less common is the situation where we start with a defined population in which the study population is selected on the basis of a factor not related to exposure, such as place of residence, and some members of the cohort become exposed and others are not exposed over time (Fig. 9.4). In a cohort study that starts with a defined population, it is possible to study multiple exposures. Thus, for example, in the Framingham Study, it was possible to study many exposures, including weight, blood pressure, cholesterol level, smoking, and physical activity among the participating individuals residing in Framingham, Massachusetts.

In cohort studies, incidence in both exposed and unexposed groups *can* be calculated, and we can therefore directly calculate the relative risk. Prospective cohort studies minimize the potential for recall and other bias in assessing the exposure and have greater validity of the exposure assessments. However, in retrospective cohort studies, which require data from the past, these problems may be significant. Cohort studies are desirable when the exposure of interest is rare. In a case-control design, we are unlikely to identify a sufficient number of exposed persons when we are dealing with a rare exposure. In prospective cohort studies in particular, we are likely to have better data on the temporal relationship between exposure and outcome (i.e., did the exposure precede the outcome?) Among the disadvantages of cohort studies is that they usually require large populations, and, in general, prospective cohort studies are especially expensive to carry out because follow-up of a large population over time is required. A greater potential bias for assessing the outcome is present in cohort studies than in case-control studies. Finally, cohort studies often become impractical when the disease under study is rare.

As seen in Table 9.1, case-control studies have a number of advantages. They are relatively inexpensive and require a relatively small number of subjects for study. They are desirable when the disease occurrence is rare, because if a cohort study were performed in such a circumstance, a tremendous number of people would have to be followed to generate enough people with the disease for study. As seen in Fig. 9.5, in a case-control study, because we begin with cases and controls, we are able to study more than one possible etiologic factor and to explore interactions among the factors.

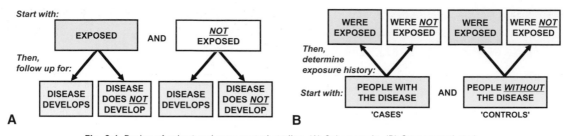

Fig. 9.1 Design of cohort and case-control studies. (A) Cohort study. (B) Case-control study.

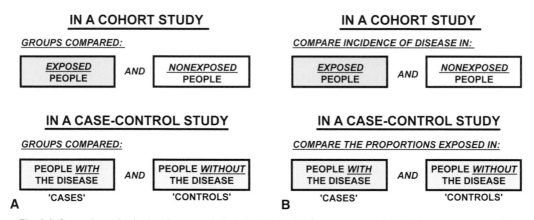

Fig. 9.2 Comparison of cohort and case-control study designs. (A) Groups compared. (B) Outcome measurements.

Because case-control studies often require data about past events or exposures, they are often encumbered by the difficulties encountered in using such data (including a potential for recall bias). Furthermore, as has been discussed in some detail, selection of an appropriate control group is one of the most difficult methodologic problems encountered in epidemiology. In addition, in most case-control studies, we cannot calculate disease incidence in either the total population or the exposed and unexposed groups without some supplemental information.

The nested case-control design combines elements of both cohort and case-control studies and offers a number of advantages. The possibility of recall bias is eliminated because the data on exposure are obtained before the disease develops. Exposure data are more likely to represent the pre-illness state because they are obtained years before clinical illness is diagnosed. Finally, the costs are lower than with a cohort study because laboratory tests need to be done only on specimens from subjects who are later chosen as cases

or controls; that is, we need to selectively do laboratory tests only on a subset of the overall cohort, thereby yielding considerable cost savings.

In addition to the cohort and case-control study designs, we have discussed the cross-sectional study design, in which data on both exposure and disease outcomes are collected simultaneously from each subject. The data from a cross-sectional study can be analyzed by comparing the prevalence of disease in exposed individuals with that in unexposed individuals or by comparing the prevalence of exposure in persons with the disease with that of persons without the disease. Although cross-sectional data are often obtained from representative surveys and can be very useful, they usually do not permit the investigator to determine the temporal relationship between exposure and the development of disease. As a result, their value for deriving causal inferences is somewhat limited. However, they can provide important directions for further research using cohort, case-control, and nested case-control designs.

TABLE 9.1	**Comparisons of Cohort and Case-Control Studies**		
	COHORT STUDIES		
	Prospective	**Retrospective**	**Case-Control Studies**
A. Study group	Exposed persons: $(a + b)$	Exposed persons: $(a + b)$	Persons with the disease (cases): $(a + c)$
B. Comparison group	Nonexposed persons: $(c + d)$	Nonexposed persons: $(c + d)$	Persons without disease (controls): $(b + d)$
C. Outcome measurements	Incidence in the exposed $\left(\dfrac{a}{a+b}\right)$ and Incidence in the nonexposed $\left(\dfrac{c}{c+d}\right)$	Incidence in the exposed $\left(\dfrac{a}{a+b}\right)$ and Incidence in the nonexposed $\left(\dfrac{c}{c+d}\right)$	Proportion of cases exposed $\left(\dfrac{a}{a+c}\right)$ and Proportion of controls exposed $\left(\dfrac{b}{b+d}\right)$
D. Measures of risk	Absolute risk Relative risk Odds ratio Attributable risk	Absolute risk Relative risk Odds ratio Attributable risk	— — Odds ratio Attributable risk[a]
E. Temporal relationship between exposure and disease	Easy to establish	Sometimes hard to establish	Sometimes hard to establish
F. Multiple associations	Possible to study associations of an exposure with several diseases[b]	Possible to study associations of an exposure with several diseases[b]	Possible to study associations of a disease with several exposures or factors
G. Time required for the study	Generally long because of need to follow the subjects	May be short	Relatively short
H. Cost of study	Expensive	Generally less expensive than a prospective study	Relatively inexpensive
I. Population size needed	Relatively large	Relatively large	Relatively small
J. Potential bias	Assessment of outcome	Susceptible to bias both in assessment of exposure and assessment of outcome	Assessment of exposure
K. Best when	Exposure is rare Disease is frequent among exposed	Exposure is rare Disease is frequent among exposed	Disease is rare Exposure is frequent among persons with disease
L. Problems	Selection of nonexposed comparison group often difficult Changes over time in criteria and methods	Selection of nonexposed comparison group often difficult Changes over time in criteria and methods	Selection of appropriate controls often difficult Incomplete information on exposure

[a]Additional information must be available.
[b]It is also possible to study multiple exposures when the study population is selected on the basis of a factor unrelated to the exposure.

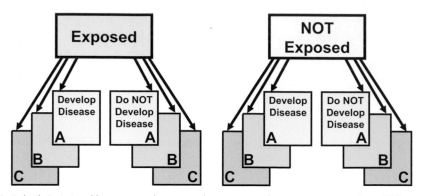

Fig. 9.3 In a cohort study that starts with an exposed group and a nonexposed group, we can study multiple outcomes but only one exposure.

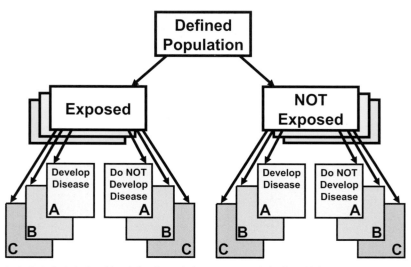

Fig. 9.4 In a cohort study that starts with a defined population, we can study both multiple exposures and multiple outcomes.

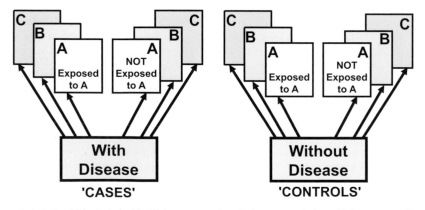

Fig. 9.5 In a case-control study which starts by identifying cases and controls, we can study multiple exposures but only one outcome.

Chapter 10

Assessing Preventive and Therapeutic Measures: Randomized Trials

All who drink of this treatment recover in a short time,
Except those whom it does not help, who all die,
It is obvious, therefore, that it fails only in incurable cases.

— Galen[1] (129–c. 199 CE)

Learning Objectives

- To describe the important elements of randomized trials.
- To define the purpose of randomization and of masking.
- To introduce design issues related to randomized trials, including stratified randomization, planned and unplanned crossovers, and factorial design.
- To illustrate the problems posed by noncompliance in randomized trials.

Some ways of quantifying the natural history of disease and of expressing disease prognosis were discussed in Chapter 6. Our objective, both in clinical practice and in public health, is to modify the natural history of a disease so as to prevent or delay death or disability and to improve the health of the patient or the population. The challenge is to select the best available preventive or therapeutic measures to achieve this goal. To do so, we need to carry out studies that determine the value of these measures. The randomized trial is considered the ideal design for evaluating both the efficacy and the side effects of new forms of intervention.

The notion of using a rigorous methodology to assess the efficacy of new drugs, or of any new modalities of care, is not recent. In 1883, Sir Francis Galton, the British anthropologist, explorer, and eugenicist, who had a strong interest in human intelligence, wrote as follows:

It is asserted by some, that men possess the faculty of obtaining results over which they have little or no direct personal control, by means of devout and earnest prayer, while others doubt the truth of this assertion. The question regards a matter of fact, that has to be determined by observation and not by authority; and it is one that appears to be a very suitable topic for statistical inquiry. … Are prayers answered, or are they not? … [D]o sick persons who pray, or are prayed for, recover on the average more rapidly than others?[2]

As with many pioneering ideas in science and medicine, many years were to pass before this suggestion was actually implemented. In 1965 Joyce and Welldon reported the results of a double-blind randomized trial of the efficacy of prayer.[3] The findings of this study did not indicate that patients who were prayed for derived any special benefits from that prayer. However, a more recent study by Byrd[4] evaluated the effectiveness of intercessory prayer in a coronary care unit population using a randomized double-blind protocol. The findings from this study suggested that prayer had a beneficial therapeutic effect. *Which is correct?*

In this chapter and the one following, we discuss study designs that can be used for evaluating approaches to treatment and prevention and focus on the use of the randomized trial. Although the term *randomized clinical trial* is often used together with its acronym, RCT, the randomized trial design also has major applicability to studies outside the clinical setting, such as community-based trials. For this reason, we use the term *randomized trial*. To facilitate our discussion, reference is generally made to treatments and drugs; the reader should bear in mind that the principles described apply equally to evaluations of preventive (such as screening programs for the early detection of disease) and other measures (e.g., behavioral interventions). Trials are essentially experiments which are under the control of the investigator. Compare this with observational studies reviewed in Chapter 7, where the investigator watches what unfolds but does not interfere or control.

Suggestions of many of the elements that are important to randomized trials can be seen in many anecdotal descriptions of early trials. In a review of the history of clinical trials, Bull described an unintentional trial conducted by Ambroise Paré (1510–1590), a leading figure in surgery during the Renaissance.[5] Paré lived at a time when the standard treatment for war wounds was the application of boiling oil. In 1537 Paré was responsible for the treatment of the wounded after the capture of the castle of Villaine. The wounded were so numerous that, he says:

At length my oil lacked and I was constrained to apply in its place a digestive made of yolks of eggs, oil of roses and turpentine. That night I could not sleep at my ease, fearing that by lack of cauterization I would find the wounded upon which I had not used the said oil, dead from the poison. I raised myself early to visit them, when beyond my hope I found those to whom I had applied the digestive medicament feeling but little pain, their wounds neither swollen nor inflamed, and having slept through the night. The others to whom I had applied the boiling oil were feverish with much pain and swelling about their wounds. Then I determined never again to burn thus so cruelly the poor wounded.

Although this was not a randomized trial, it was a form of unplanned trial, which has been carried out many times when a therapy thought to be the best available has been in short supply and has not been available for all of the patients who needed it.

A planned trial was described by the Scottish surgeon James Lind in 1747.[6] Lind became interested in scurvy, which killed thousands of British seamen each year. He was intrigued by the story of a sailor who had developed scurvy and had been put ashore on an isolated island, where he subsisted on a diet of grasses and then recovered from the scurvy. Lind conducted an experiment, which he described as follows:

I took 12 patients in the scurvy on board the Salisbury at sea. The cases were as similar as I could have them … they lay together in one place and had one diet common to them all. Two of these were ordered a quart of cider per day. … Two others took 25 gutts of elixir vitriol. … Two others took two spoonfuls of vinegar. … Two were put under a course of sea water. … Two others had two oranges and one lemon given them each day. … Two others took the bigness of nutmeg. The most sudden and visible good effects were perceived from the use of oranges and lemons, one of those who had taken them being at the end of 6 days fit for duty. … The other … was appointed nurse to the rest of the sick.

Interestingly, the idea of a dietary cause of scurvy proved unacceptable in Lind's day. Only 47 years later did the British Admiralty allow the experiment to be repeated—this time on an entire fleet of ships. The results were so dramatic that, in 1795, the Admiralty made lemon juice a required part of the standard diet of British seamen and later changed this to lime juice. Scurvy essentially disappeared from British sailors, who, even today, are referred to as "limeys."

Randomized trials can be used for many purposes. They can be used for evaluating new drugs and other treatments of disease, including tests of new health and medical care technology. Trials can also be used to assess new programs for screening and early detection, to compare different approaches to prevention, or new ways of organizing and delivering health services.

The basic design of a randomized trial is shown in Fig. 10.1.

We begin with a defined population in which participants are randomized to receive either a new

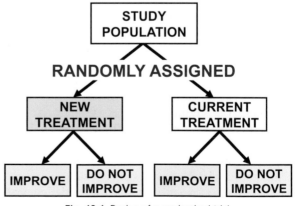

Fig. 10.1 Design of a randomized trial.

treatment or the current treatment, and we then follow the subjects in each group to see how many are improved in the new treatment group compared with how many are improved in the current treatment group (often referred to as "usual care" or "standard of care"). If the new treatment is associated with a better outcome, we would expect to find better outcomes in more of the new treatment group than the current treatment group.

We may choose to compare two groups receiving different therapies, or we may compare more than two groups. Although at times a new treatment may be compared with no treatment, often a decision is made not to use an untreated group. For example, if we wanted to evaluate a newly developed therapy for acquired immunodeficiency syndrome (AIDS), would we be willing to have a group of AIDS patients in our study who were untreated? The answer is clearly no; we would compare the newly developed therapy with a currently recommended regimen, which would clearly be better than no therapy at all.

Let us now turn to some of the issues that must be considered in the design of randomized trials. Chief among them is specification of the study "arms," or treatments. These must be clearly stated with criteria for their measurement, as well as the duration of the treatments and how long the study will last. First, let's start with who is eligible to be studied.

Selection of Subjects

The criteria for determining who will or will not be included in the study must be spelled out with great precision and *in writing before the study is begun.* An excellent test of the adequacy of these written criteria is to ask: If we have spelled out our criteria in writing and someone not involved in the study walks in off the street and applies our criteria to the same population, will that person select the same subjects whom we would have selected? There should be no element of subjective decision-making on the part of the investigator in deciding who is included or not included in the study. Any study procedure must in principle be replicable by others, just as is the case with laboratory experiments. Clearly, this is easier said than done because in randomized trials we are often dealing with relatively large populations. The principle is nevertheless

important, and the selection criteria must therefore be precisely stated.

Allocating Subjects to Treatment Groups Without Randomization

Before discussing the process of randomization, let us ask whether there might be some alternatives to randomization that could be used.

STUDIES WITHOUT COMPARISON

The first possible alternative is the *case study* or *case series* (as was presented in Chapter 7). In this type of study, no comparison is made with an untreated group or with a group that is receiving some other treatment. The following story was told by Dr. Earl Peacock when he was chairman of the Department of Surgery at the University of Arizona:

One day when I was a junior medical student, a very important Boston surgeon visited the school and delivered a great treatise on a large number of patients who had undergone successful operations for vascular reconstruction. At the end of the lecture, a young student at the back of the room timidly asked, "Do you have any controls?" Well, the great surgeon drew himself up to his full height, hit the desk, and said, "Do you mean did I not operate on half of the patients?" The hall grew very quiet then. The voice at the back of the room very hesitantly replied, "Yes, that's what I had in mind." Then the visitor's fist really came down as he thundered, "Of course not. That would have doomed half of them to their death." God, it was quiet then, and one could scarcely hear the small voice ask, "Which half?"[7]

The issue of comparison is important because we want to be able to derive a causal inference regarding the relationship of a treatment and subsequent outcome. The problem of inferring a causal relationship from a sequence of events without any comparison is demonstrated in a story cited by Ederer.[8]

During World War II, rescue workers, digging in the ruins of an apartment house blown up in the London blitz, found an old man lying naked in a bathtub, fully conscious. He said to his rescuers, "You know, that was the most amazing experience I ever had. When I pulled the plug and the water started down the drain, the whole house blew up."

The problem exemplified by this story is: If we administer a drug and the patient improves, can we attribute the improvement to the administration of that drug? Professor Hugo Muensch of Harvard University articulated his Second Law: "Results can always be improved by omitting controls."[9]

STUDIES WITH COMPARISON

If we therefore recognize the need for our study to include some type of comparison, what are the possible designs?

Historical Controls

We could use a comparison group from the past, called *historical controls*. We have a therapy today that we believe will be quite effective, and we would like to test it in a group of patients; we know that we need a comparison group. So, for comparison, we will go back to the records of patients with the same disease who were treated before the new therapy became available. This type of design seems inherently simple and attractive.

What are the problems in using historical controls? First, if today we decide to carry out the study just described, we may set up a very meticulous system for data collection from the patients currently being treated. But, of course, we cannot do that for the patients who were treated in the past, for whom we must abstract data from medical records which are likely useful for managing individual care but are fraught with error and omissions when used for research purposes. Consequently, if at the end of the study we find a difference in outcome between patients treated in the early period (historical controls) and patients treated in the later (current) period, we will not know whether there was a true difference in outcome or whether the observed difference was due only to a difference in the quality of the data collection. The data obtained from the study groups must be comparable in kind and quality; in studies using historical controls, this is often not the case.

The second problem is that if we observe a difference in outcome between the early group and the later group, we will not be sure that the difference is due to the therapy because many things other than the therapy

change over calendar time (e.g., ancillary supportive therapy, living conditions, nutrition, and lifestyles). This is often referred to as "secular changes." Hence, if we observe a difference and if we have ruled out differences in data quality as the reason for the observed difference, we will not know whether the difference is a result of the drug we are studying or of other changes that take place in many other factors that may be associated with the outcome over calendar time.

However, at times, this type of design may be useful. For example, when a disease is uniformly fatal and a new drug becomes available, a decline in case-fatality that parallels use of the drug would strongly support the conclusion that the new drug is having an effect. Examples include the discovery of insulin to treat diabetes, of penicillin to treat serious infections, and of tyrosine kinase inhibitors (TKIs) such as imatinib (Gleevec) to treat chronic myelocity leukemia. Nevertheless, the possibility that the decline could have resulted from other changes in the environment would still have to be ruled out.

Simultaneous Nonrandomized Controls

Because of the importance of the problems posed by historical controls and the difficulties of dealing with changes over calendar time, an alternative approach is to use simultaneous controls that are not selected in a randomized manner. The problem with selecting simultaneous controls in a nonrandomized manner is illustrated by the following story:

A sea captain was given samples of anti-nausea pills to test during a voyage. The need for controls was carefully explained to him. Upon return of the ship, the captain reported the results enthusiastically. "Practically every one of the controls was ill, and not one of the subjects had any trouble. Really wonderful stuff." A skeptic asked how he had chosen the controls and the subjects. "Oh, I gave the stuff to my seamen and used the passengers as controls."[10]

There are a number of possible approaches for selecting controls in such a nonrandomized fashion. One is to assign patients by the day of the month on which the patient is admitted to the hospital: for example, if admission is on an odd-numbered day of the month the patient is in group A, and if admission is on an even-numbered day of the month the patient is in group B. In a trial of anticoagulant therapy after World War II, in which this day-of-the-month method was used, it was discovered that more patients than expected were admitted on odd-numbered days. The investigators reported that "as physicians observed the benefits of anticoagulant therapy, they speeded up, where feasible, the hospitalization of those patients … who would routinely have been hospitalized on an even day in order to bring as many as possible under the odd-day deadline."[11]

The problem here is that the assignment system was predictable: it was possible for the physicians to know what the assignment of the next patient would be. The goal of randomization is to eliminate the possibility that the investigator will know what the assignment of the next patient will be, because such knowledge introduces the possibility of bias on the part of the investigator regarding the treatment group to which each participant will be assigned.

Many years ago a study was carried out of the effects of bacillus Calmette-Guérin (BCG) vaccination against tuberculosis in children from families with tuberculosis in New York City.[12] The physicians were told to divide the group of eligible children into a group to be immunized and a comparison or control group who were not immunized. As seen in Table 10.1, tuberculosis mortality was almost five times higher in the controls than in the vaccinated children. However, as the investigators wrote:

Subsequent experience has shown that by this method of selection, the tendency was to inoculate the children of the more intelligent and cooperative parents and to keep the children of the noncooperative parents as controls. This was probably of considerable error since the cooperative parent will not only keep more careful precautions, but will usually bring the child more regularly to the clinic for instruction as to child care and feeding.[12]

Recognizing that the vaccinations were selectively performed in children from families that were more likely to be conscious of health and related issues, the investigators realized that it was possible that the mortality rate from tuberculosis was lower in the vaccinated group not because of the vaccination itself but because these children were selected from more health-conscious families that had a lower risk of mortality from tuberculosis, with or without vaccination. To address this problem, a change was made in the study design: alternate children were vaccinated and the remainder served as controls. This does not constitute randomization, but it was a marked improvement over the initial design. As seen in Table 10.2, there was now no difference between the groups.

Allocating Subjects Using Randomization

In view of the problems discussed, randomization is the best approach in the design of a trial. Randomization means, in effect, tossing a coin to decide the assignment of a patient to a study group. The critical element of randomization is the unpredictability of the next assignment. Fig. 10.2 shows a comic strip cited by Ederer to demonstrate the problem of predictability of the next assignment.[13]

How is randomization accomplished? Although random allocation is currently usually done through computer programs, on occasion manual randomization is used either as a backup to computer-generation assignment or when access to a computer is limited. In this hypothetical example of manual assignment we use a selection from a table of random numbers

TABLE 10.1 **Results of a Trial of Bacillus Calmette-Guérin Vaccination: I**		TUBERCULOSIS DEATHS	
	No. of Children	Number	%
Vaccinated	445	3	0.67
Controls	545	18	3.30

Data from Levine MI, Sackett MF. Results of BCG immunization in New York City. *Am Rev Tuberculosis.* 1946;53:517–532.

TABLE 10.2 **Results of a Trial of Bacillus Calmette-Guérin Vaccination: II**		TUBERCULOSIS DEATHS	
	No. of Children	Number	%
Vaccinated	556	8	1.44
Controls	528	8	1.52

Data from Levine MI, Sackett MF. Results of BCG immunization in New York City. *Am Rev Tuberculosis.* 1946;53:517–532.

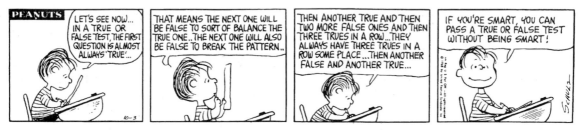

Fig. 10.2 How to predict the next patient's treatment assignment in a randomized study. (PEANUTS © UFS. Reprinted by permission.)

TABLE 10.3	**Table of Random Numbers**			
	00–04	**05–09**	**10–14**	**15–19**
00	56348	01458	36236	07253
01	09372	27651	30103	37004
02	44782	54023	61355	71692
03	04383	90952	57204	57810
04	98190	89997	98839	76129
05	16263	35632	88105	59090
06	62032	90741	13468	02647
07	48457	78538	22759	12188
08	36782	06157	73084	48094
09	63302	55103	19703	74741

BOX 10.1 EXAMPLES OF USING A RANDOM NUMBERS TABLE FOR ALLOCATING PATIENTS TO TREATMENT GROUPS IN A RANDOMIZED TRIAL

If we plan to compare two groups:
- We decide that even digits designate treatment A, odd digits designate treatment B, *or*
- We decide that digits 0–4 designate treatment A, digits 5–9 designate treatment B

If we plan to compare three groups:
- We decide that digits 1–3 designate treatment A, digits 4–6 designate treatment B, digits 7–9 designate treatment C, and digit 0 would be ignored

(Table 10.3). (Such random number tables are available in an appendix in most statistics textbooks or can be generated on computers.)

First, how do we look at Table 10.3? Note that the table is divided into 10 rows and 4 numbered columns (row numbers appear on the far left columns). The columns are numbered along the top, 00–04, 05–09, and so on. This means that the number in Column 00 is 5, the number in Column 01 is 6, the number in Column 03 is 3, etc. Similarly, the rows are numbered along the left, 00, 01, 02, and so on. Thus it is possible to refer to any digit in the table by giving its column and row numbers. This is important if the quality of the randomization process is to be checked by an outsider. How do we use this table? Let us say that we are conducting a study in which there will be two groups: therapy A and therapy B. In this example, we will consider every odd number an assignment to A and every even number an assignment to B. We close our eyes and put a finger anywhere on the table, and write down the column and row number that was our starting point. We also write down the direction we will

move in the table from that starting point (horizontally to the right, horizontally to the left, up, or down). Let us assume that we point to the "5" at the intersection of column 07 and row 07 and move horizontally to the right. The first patient, then, is designated by an odd number, 5, and will receive therapy A. The second patient is also designated by an odd number, 3, and will receive therapy A. The third is designated by an even number, 8, and will receive therapy B, and so on. Note that the next patient assignment is not predictable; it is *not* a strict alternation, which would be predictable and hence subject to investigator bias, knowingly or unknowingly.

There are many ways of using a table of random numbers for allocating patients to treatment groups in a randomized trial (Box 10.1). Although many approaches are valid, the important point is to spell out *in writing* whatever approach is selected for use, before randomization is actually begun.

Having decided conceptually how to use the random numbers for allocating patients, how do we make a practical decision as to which patients get which therapy? Let us assume, for example, that a decision has been made that odd digits will designate assignment to treatment A and even digits will designate treatment B. The treatment assignment that is designated by the random number is written on a card, and this card is placed inside an opaque envelope. Each envelope is labeled on the outside: Patient 1, Patient 2, Patient 3, and so on, to match the sequence in which the patients are enrolled in the study. For example, if the first random number is 2, a card for therapy B would be placed in the first envelope; if the next random number is 7, a card for therapy A in the second one, and so on, as determined by the random numbers.

The envelopes are then sealed. When the first patient is enrolled, envelope 1 is opened and the assignment is read; this process is repeated for each of the remaining patients in the study.

However, this process is not foolproof. The following anecdote illustrates the need for careful quality control of any randomized study:

In a randomized study comparing radical and simple mastectomy for breast cancer, one of the surgeons participating was convinced that radical mastectomy was the treatment of choice and could not reconcile himself to performing simple mastectomy on any of his patients who were included in the study. When randomization was carried out for his patients and an envelope was opened that indicated simple mastectomy for the next assignment, he would set the envelope aside and keep opening envelopes until he reached one with an assignment to radical mastectomy.

What is reflected here is the conflict experienced by many clinicians who enroll their own patients in randomized trials. On the one hand, the clinician has the obligation to do the best he or she can for the patient; on the other hand, when a clinician participates in a clinical trial, he or she is, in effect, asked to step aside from the usual decision-making role and essentially to "flip a coin" to decide which therapy the patient will receive. Thus there is often an underlying conflict between the clinician's role and the role of the physician participating in a clinical trial, and as a result, unintentional biases may occur.

This is such a common problem, particularly in large, multicentered trials, that randomization is not carried out by each participating clinical field center; rather, it is done by an impartial separate coordinating and statistical center. When a new patient is registered at a clinical center, the coordinating center is called or an assignment is downloaded by the coordinating center. A randomized assignment is then made for that patient by the coordinating center, and the assignment is noted in both the clinical and centralized locations.

What do we hope to accomplish by randomization? If we randomize properly, we achieve nonpredictability of the next assignment; we do not have to worry that any subjective biases of the investigators, either overt or covert, may be introduced into the process of selecting patients for one treatment group or the other. In addition, if the study is large enough and there are enough participants, we hope that randomization will increase the likelihood that the groups will be comparable to each other in regard to characteristics about which we may be concerned, such as sex, age, race, and severity of disease—all factors that may affect prognosis. Randomization is not a guarantee of comparability because chance may play a role in the process of random treatment assignment. However, if the treatment groups that are being randomized are large enough and the randomization procedure is free of bias, they will tend to be similar.

Fig. 10.3 presents a hypothetical example of the effect of lack of comparability on a comparison of mortality rates of the groups being studied. Let us assume a study population of 2,000 subjects with myocardial infarctions, of whom half receive an intervention and the other half do not. Let us further assume that of the 2,000 patients, 700 have an arrhythmia and 1,300 do not. Case-fatality in patients with the arrhythmia is 50%, and in patients without the arrhythmia it is 10%.

Let us look at the nonrandomized study on the left side of Fig. 10.3. Because there is no randomization, the intervention groups may not be comparable in the proportion of patients who have the arrhythmia. Perhaps 200 in the intervention group may have the arrhythmia (with a case-fatality of 50%) and 500 in the no-intervention group may have the arrhythmia (with its 50% case-fatality). The resulting case-fatality will be 18% in the intervention group and 30% in the no-intervention group. We might be tempted to

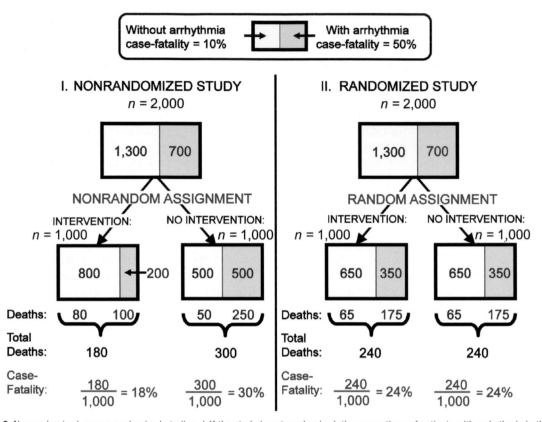

Fig. 10.3 Nonrandomized versus randomized studies. *I,* If the study is not randomized, the proportions of patients with arrhythmia in the two intervention groups may differ. In this example, individuals with arrhythmia are less likely to receive the intervention than individuals without arrhythmia. *II,* If the study is randomized, the proportions of patients with arrhythmia in the two intervention groups are more likely to be similar.

conclude that the intervention is more effective than not intervening.

However, let us now look at the randomized study on the right side of Fig. 10.3. As seen here, the groups are comparable, as is likely to occur when we randomize, so that 350 of the 1,000 patients in the intervention group and 350 of the 1,000 patients in the no-intervention group have the arrhythmia. When the case-fatality is calculated for this example, it is 24% in both groups. Thus the difference observed between intervention and no intervention when the groups were not comparable in terms of the arrhythmia was entirely due to the noncomparability and not to any effects of the intervention itself. (Please note that although Fig. 10.3 shows 1,000 participants in both the intervention and no-intervention group, randomization does *not*

guarantee an equal number of participants in each group; however, with large numbers, on average the two groups will generally be comparable.)

One might ask, if we are so concerned about the comparability of the groups, why not just match the groups on the specific variables about which we are concerned, rather than randomizing? The answer is that we can match only on variables that we know about and that we can measure. Thus we cannot match on many variables that may affect prognosis, such as an individual's genetic constitution, elements of an individual's immune status, or other variables of which we may not even be aware. In addition, if we match on a particular characteristic, we cannot analyze its association with the outcome because the two groups will already be identical. Randomization increases the likelihood that the groups will be comparable not only in terms of variables that we recognize and can measure, but also in terms of variables that we may not recognize, may not be able to test now, and may not be able to measure with today's technologies. However, at the end of the day, randomization cannot always guarantee comparability of the groups being studied. We can analyze whether there are important differences between the two groups that may be associated with the trial outcome.

What Is the Main Purpose of Randomization?

The main purpose of randomization is to prevent any potential biases on the part of the investigators from influencing the assignment of participants to different treatment groups. When participants are randomly assigned to different treatment groups, all decisions on treatment assignment are removed from the control of the investigators. Thus the use of randomization is crucial to protect the study from any biases that might be introduced consciously or subconsciously by the investigator into the assignment process.

As mentioned previously, although randomization often increases the comparability of the different treatment groups, randomization does not guarantee comparability. Another benefit of randomization is that to whatever extent it contributes to comparability, this contribution applies both to variables we can measure and to variables that we cannot measure and may not even be aware of, even though they may be important in interpreting the findings of the trial.

Stratified Randomization

Sometimes we may be particularly concerned about comparability of the groups in terms of one or a few important characteristics that we strongly think may influence prognosis or response to therapy in the groups being studied, but as we have just said, randomization does not ensure comparability. An option that can be used is *stratified randomization,* an assignment method that can be very helpful in increasing the likelihood of comparability of the study groups. In this section, we will show how this method is used to assign participants to different study groups.

For example, let us say that we are particularly concerned about age as a prognostic variable: prognosis is much worse in older patients than among the younger.

Therefore we are concerned that the two treatment groups be comparable in terms of age. Although one of the benefits of randomization is that it may increase the likelihood of such comparability, it does not guarantee it. It is still possible that after we randomize, we may, by chance, find that most of the older patients are in one group and most of the younger patients are in the other. Our results would then be impossible to interpret because the higher-risk patients would be clustered in one group and the lower-risk patients in the other. Any difference in outcome between intervention groups may then be attributable to this difference in the age distributions of the two groups rather than to the effects of the intervention.

In *stratified randomization,* we first stratify (stratum = layer) our study population by each variable that we consider important and then randomize participants to treatment groups within each stratum.

Let us consider the example shown in Fig. 10.4. We are studying 1,000 patients and are concerned that sex and age are important determinants of prognosis. If we randomize, we do not know what the composition of the groups may be in terms of sex and age; therefore we decide to use stratified randomization.

We first stratify the 1,000 patients by sex into 600 males and 400 females. We then separately stratify the males by age and the females by age. We now have four groups (strata): younger males, older males, younger females, and older females. We now randomize *within each group (stratum),* and the result is a new treatment group and a current treatment group for each of the four groups. As in randomization without stratification, we end up with two intervention groups, but having initially stratified the groups, we increase the likelihood that the two groups will be comparable in terms of sex and age. (As in Fig. 10.3, Fig. 10.4 shows that randomization results in an equal number of participants in each treatment group, although this result is *not* guaranteed by randomization.)

Data Collection on Subjects

As mentioned earlier, it is essential that the data collected for each of the study groups be of the same quality. We do not want any differences in results between the groups to be due to differences in the quality or completeness of the data that were collected in the

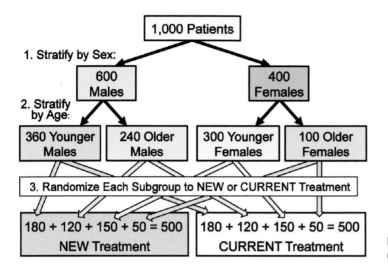

Fig. 10.4 Example of stratified randomization. See discussion in text.

study groups. Let us consider some of the variables about which data need to be obtained on the subjects.

TREATMENT (ASSIGNED AND RECEIVED)

What data are needed? First, we must know to which treatment group the patient was assigned. In addition, we must know which therapy the patient *actually* received. It is important to know, for example, if the patient was assigned to receive treatment A but did not comply. A patient may agree to be randomized but may later change his or her mind and refuse to comply. Conversely, it is also clearly important to know whether a patient who was not assigned to receive treatment A may have taken treatment A on his or her own, often without the investigators knowing.

OUTCOME

The need for comparable measurements in all study groups is particularly true for measurements of outcome. Such measurements include both improvement (the desired effect) and any side effects that may appear. There is therefore a need for explicitly stated criteria for all outcomes to be measured in a study. Once the criteria are explicitly stated, we must be certain that they are measured comparably in all study groups. In particular, the potential pitfall of outcomes being measured more carefully in those receiving a new drug than in those receiving currently available therapy must

be avoided. Blinding (masking), discussed later, can prevent much of this problem, but because blinding is not always possible, attention must be given to ensuring comparability of measurements and of data quality in all of the study groups.

All-Cause Mortality Outcome ("Public Health Outcome")

On occasion a medication or a preventive strategy for mortality that is effective with regard to the main outcome of interest does not increase event-free survival. For example, in the 13-year follow-up of the European Randomized Study of Screening for Prostate Cancer, there was a reduction of approximately 27% in prostate cancer mortality.[14] However, overall mortality (also known as "public health outcome") was similar in the two study groups, thus suggesting that effectiveness of screening with regard to all-cause mortality was null.

PROGNOSTIC PROFILE AT ENTRY

If we know the risk factors for a bad outcome, we want to verify that randomization has provided reasonable similarity between the two groups in terms of these risk factors. For example, if age is a significant risk factor, we would want to know that randomization has resulted in groups that are comparable for age. Data for prognostic factors should be obtained at the time of subject entry into the study, and then the two (or more) groups can be compared on these factors at baseline (i.e., before the treatment is provided). Another strategy to evaluate comparability is to examine an outcome totally unrelated to the treatment that is being evaluated. For example, if the randomized trial's objective is to evaluate a new medication for migraines, it is expected that mortality from cancer would be similar in the two groups.

MASKING (BLINDING)

Masking involves several components: First, we would like the subjects not to know which group they are assigned to. This is of particular importance when the outcome is a subjective measure, such as self-reported severity of headache or low back pain. If the patient knows that he or she is receiving a new therapy, enthusiasm and certain psychological factors on the part of the patient may operate to elicit a positive response even if the therapy itself had no positive biologic or clinical effect.

How can subjects be masked? One way is by using a *placebo*, an inert substance that looks, tastes, and smells like the active agent. However, use of a placebo does not automatically guarantee that the patients are masked (blinded). Some participants may try to determine whether they are taking the placebo or active drug. For example, in a randomized trial of vitamin C for the common cold, patients were blinded by use of a placebo and were then asked whether they knew or suspected which drug they were taking.

As seen in Table 10.4, of the 52 people who were receiving vitamin C and were willing to make a guess, 40 stated they had been receiving vitamin C. Of the 50 who were receiving placebo, 39 said they were receiving placebo. How did they know? They had bitten into the capsule and could tell by the bitter taste. Does it make any difference that they knew? The data suggest that the rate of colds was higher in subjects who received vitamin C but thought they were receiving placebo than in subjects who received placebo but thought they were receiving vitamin C. Thus we must be very concerned about lack of masking or blinding of the subjects and its potential effects on the results of the study, particularly when we are dealing with subjective end points.

Use of a placebo is also important for studying the rates of side effects and reactions. The Physicians' Health

TABLE 10.4 Randomized Trial of Vitamin C and Placebo for the Common Cold: Results of a Questionnaire Study to Determine Whether Subjects Suspected Which Agent They Had Been Given

	SUSPECTED DRUG		
Actual Drug	**Vitamin C**	**Placebo**	**Total**
Vitamin C	40	12	52
Placebo	11	39	50
Total	51	51	102

$P < .001$.

From Karlowski TR, Chalmers TC, Frenkel LD, et al. Ascorbic acid for the common cold. A prophylactic and therapeutic trial. *JAMA.* 1975;231:1038. Copyright 1975, American Medical Association.

TABLE 10.5 Physicians' Health Study: Side Effects According to Treatment Group

Side Effect	Aspirin Group (%)	Placebo Group (%)	*P*
GI symptoms (except ulcer)	34.8	34.2	.48
Upper GI tract ulcers	1.5	1.3	.08
Bleeding problems	27.0	20.4	<.00001

GI, Gastrointestinal.

Data from Steering Committee of the Physicians' Health Study Research Group. Final report on the aspirin component of the Ongoing Physicians' Health Study. *N Engl J Med.* 1989;321:129–135. Copyright 1989, Massachusetts Medical Society. All rights reserved.

Study was a randomized trial of the use of aspirin to prevent myocardial infarctions. Table 10.5 shows the side effects that were reported in groups receiving aspirin and those receiving placebo in this study.

Note the high rates of reported reactions in people receiving placebo. Thus it is not sufficient to say that 34% of the people receiving aspirin had gastrointestinal symptoms; what we really want to know is the extent to which the risk of side effects is increased in people taking aspirin compared with those not taking aspirin (i.e., those taking placebo). Thus the placebo plays a major role in identifying both the real benefits of an agent and its side effects. Sometimes it is possible to use a medication in both the new therapy and in the placebo groups to prevent the occurrence of the most obvious side effects of the therapy. In the aspirin example, a proton pump inhibitor, which is a class of medication that is used to prevent gastrointestinal symptoms from excess acid, could be given to both randomized groups, thus masking the participants with regard to the group to which they were allocated. In addition to blinding the subjects, we also want to mask (or blind) the observers or data collectors in regard to which group a patient is in. The masking of both participants and study personnel is called "double blinding." Some years ago, a study was being conducted to evaluate coronary care units in the treatment of myocardial infarction. It was planned in the following manner:

Patients who met strict criteria for categories of myocardial infarction [were to] be randomly assigned either to the group that was admitted immediately to the coronary care unit or to the group that was returned to their homes for domiciliary care. When the preliminary data were presented, it was apparent in the early phases of the experiment that the group of patients labeled as having been admitted to the coronary care unit did somewhat better than the patients sent home. An enthusiast for coronary care units was uncompromising in his insistence that the experiment was unethical and should be terminated and that the data showed that all such patients should be admitted to the coronary care unit. The statistician then revealed the headings of the data columns had been interchanged and that really the home care group seemed to have a slight advantage. The enthusiast then changed his mind and could not be persuaded to declare coronary care units unethical.[15]

The message of this example is that each of us comes to whatever study we are conducting with a certain number of subconscious or conscious biases and preconceptions. The methods discussed in this chapter and Chapter 11 are designed to shield the study from the biases of the investigators.

We will now turn to two other aspects of the design of randomized trials: crossover and factorial designs.

Crossover

Another important issue in clinical trials is *crossover.* Crossover may be of two types: planned or unplanned.

A *planned crossover* is shown in Fig. 10.5. In this example, a new treatment is being compared with current treatment. Subjects are randomized to new treatment or current treatment (see Fig. 10.5A). After being observed for a certain period of time on one therapy and after any changes are measured (see Fig. 10.5B), the patients are switched to the other therapy (see Fig. 10.5C). Both groups are then again observed for a certain period of time (see Fig. 10.5D). Changes in group 1 patients while they are on the new treatment can be compared with changes in these patients while they are on the current treatment (see Fig. 10.5E). Changes in group 2 patients while they are on the new treatment can also be compared with changes in these patients while they are on the current treatment (see Fig. 10.5F). Thus each patient can serve as his or her own control, holding constant the variation between individuals in many characteristics that could potentially affect a comparison of the effectiveness of two agents.

This type of design is very attractive and useful provided that certain cautions are taken into account. First is that of *carryover:* For example, if a subject is changed from therapy A to therapy B and observed under each therapy, the observations under therapy B will be valid only if there is no residual carryover from therapy A. There must be enough of a "washout period" to be sure none of therapy A, or its effects, remains before starting therapy B. Second, the order in which the therapies are given may elicit psychological responses. Patients may react differently to the first therapy given in a study as a result of the enthusiasm that is often accorded a new study; this enthusiasm may diminish over time. We therefore want to be sure that any differences observed are indeed due to the agents being evaluated, and not to any effect of the order in which they were administered. Finally, the planned crossover design is clearly not possible if the new therapy is surgical or if the new therapy cures the disease.

A more important consideration is that of an *unplanned crossover.* Fig. 10.6A shows the design of a randomized trial of coronary bypass surgery, comparing it with medical care for coronary heart disease.

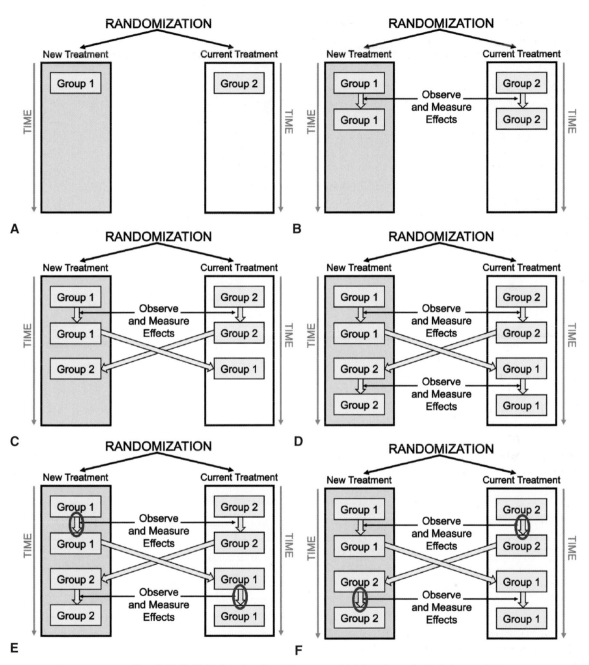

Fig. 10.5 (A–F) Design of a **planned crossover** trial. See discussion in text.

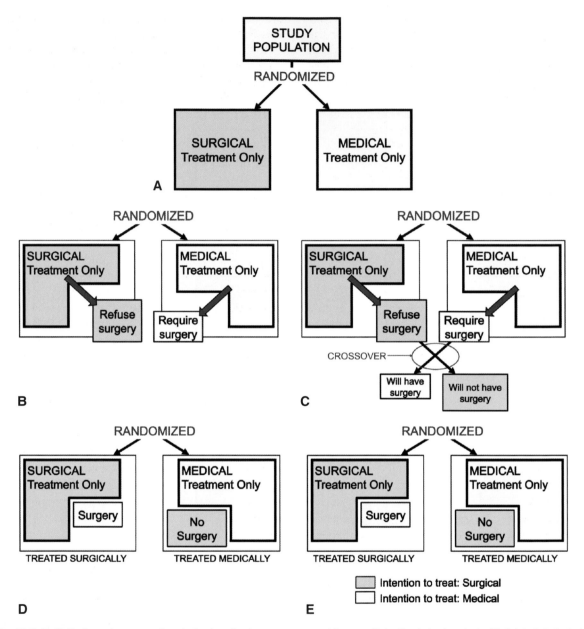

Fig. 10.6 (A–E) **Unplanned crossover** in a study of cardiac bypass surgery and the use of intention to treat analysis. (A) Original study design. (B–D) Unplanned crossovers. (E) Use of intention to treat analysis.

Randomization is carried out after informed consent has been obtained. Although the initial design is straightforward, in reality, unplanned crossovers may occur. Some subjects randomized to bypass surgery may begin to have second thoughts and decide not to

have the surgery (see Fig. 10.6B). They are therefore crossovers into the medical care group (see Fig. 10.6C). In addition, the condition of some subjects assigned to medical care may begin to deteriorate and urgent bypass surgery may be required (see Fig. 10.6B)—these subjects are crossovers from the medical to the surgical care group (see Fig. 10.6C). The patients seen on the left in Fig. 10.6D are now treated surgically, and those on the right in this figure are treated medically. Those treated surgically include some who were randomized to surgery (shown in pink) and some who crossed over to surgery (shown in yellow). Those treated medically include some who were randomized to medical treatment (shown in yellow) and some who crossed over to medical treatment (shown in pink).

Unplanned crossovers pose a serious challenge in analyzing the data. If we analyze according to the original assignment (called an *intention to treat analysis*), we will include in the surgical group some patients who received only medical care, and we will include in the medical group some patients who had surgery. In other words, we would compare the patients according to the treatment to which they were originally randomized, regardless of what treatment actually occurred. Fig. 10.6E shows an intention to treat analysis in which we compare the group in pink (randomized to surgical treatment) with the group in yellow (randomized to medical treatment). If, however, we analyze according to the treatment that the patients actually receive (*as treated analysis*), we will have broken, and therefore lost the benefits of, the randomization.

No perfect solution is available for this dilemma. Current practice is to perform the primary analysis by intention to treat—according to the original randomized assignment. We would hope that the results of other comparisons would be consistent with this primary approach. The bottom line is that because there are no perfect solutions, the number of unplanned crossovers must be kept to a minimum. Obviously, if we analyze according to the original randomization and there have been many crossovers, the interpretation of the study results will be questionable. If the number of crossovers becomes large, the problem of interpreting the study results may become insurmountable.

Factorial Design

An attractive alternative option in the study designs discussed in these chapters is the *factorial design*. Assuming that two drugs are to be tested, the anticipated outcomes for the two drugs are different, and their modes of action are independent, one can economically use the same study population for testing both drugs. This factorial type of design is shown in Fig. 10.7.

If the effects of the two treatments are indeed completely independent, we could evaluate the effects of treatment A by comparing the results in cells $a + c$ to the results in cells $b + d$ (Fig. 10.8A). Similarly, the results for treatment B could be evaluated by comparing the effects in cells $a + b$ to those in cells $c + d$ (see Fig. 10.8B). In the event that it is decided to terminate the study of treatment A, this design permits continuing the study to determine the effects of treatment B.

An example of a factorial design is seen in the Physicians' Health Study.[16] More than 22,000 physicians were randomized using a 2×2 factorial design that tested aspirin for primary prevention of cardiovascular disease and beta carotene for primary prevention of cancer. Each physician received one of four possible interventions: both aspirin and beta carotene, neither aspirin nor beta carotene, aspirin and beta carotene placebo, or beta carotene and aspirin placebo. The resulting four groups are shown in Figs. 10.9 and 10.10. The aspirin part of the study (Fig. 10.11A) was terminated early, on the advice of the external data monitoring board, because a statistically significant 44% decrease in the risk of first myocardial infarction was observed in the group taking aspirin. The randomized beta carotene component (see Fig. 10.11B) continued until the originally scheduled date of completion. After 12 years of beta carotene supplementation, no benefit or harm was observed in terms of the incidence of cancer or heart disease or death from all causes. Subsequent reports have shown greater risk of cancer with beta carotene in smokers.[17]

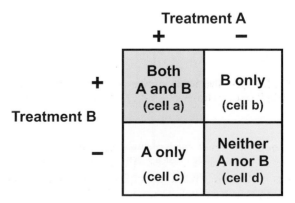

Fig. 10.7 Factorial design for studying the effects of two treatments.

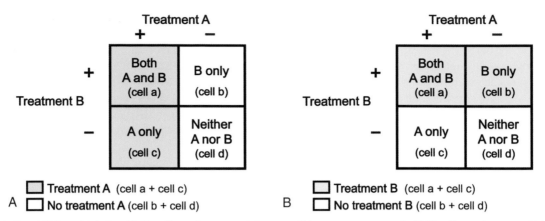

Fig. 10.8 (A and B) Factorial design. (A) The effects of treatment A *(orange cells)* versus no treatment A. (B) The effects of treatment B *(purple cells)* versus no treatment B.

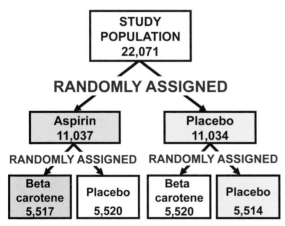

Fig. 10.9 Factorial design used in a study of aspirin and beta carotene.

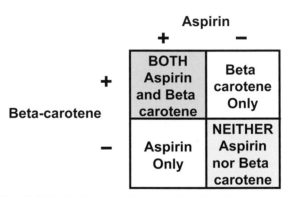

Fig. 10.10 Factorial design of the study of aspirin and beta carotene in 2 × 2 table format.

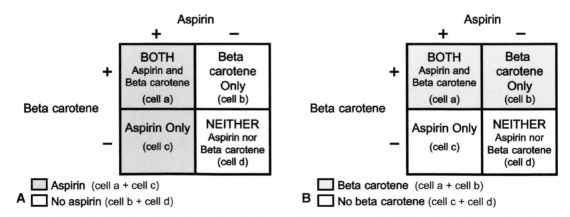

Fig. 10.11 (A and B) Factorial design. (A) The effects of aspirin *(orange cells)* versus no aspirin. (B) The effects of beta carotene *(purple cells)* versus no beta carotene.

Noncompliance

Patients may agree to be randomized, but following randomization they may not comply with the assigned treatment. Noncompliance may be overt or covert: On the one hand, people may overtly articulate their refusal to comply or may stop participating in the study. These noncompliers are also called *dropouts* from the study. On the other hand, people may just stop taking the agent assigned without admitting this to the investigator or the study staff. Whenever possible, checks on potential noncompliance are built into the study. These may include, for example, urine tests for the agent being tested or for one of its metabolites.

Another problem in randomized trials has been called *drop-ins*. Patients in one group may inadvertently take the agent assigned to the other group. For example, in a trial of the effect of aspirin for prevention of myocardial infarction, patients were randomized to aspirin or to no aspirin. However, a problem arose in that, because of the large number of over-the-counter preparations that contain aspirin, many of the control patients might well be taking aspirin without knowing it. Two steps were taken to address this problem: (1) controls were provided with lists of aspirin-containing over-the-counter preparations that they should avoid, and (2) urine tests for salicylates were carried out both in the aspirin group and in the controls.

The net effect of noncompliance on the study results will be to reduce any observed differences (i.e., driving the difference toward the null) because the treatment group will include some who did not receive the therapy, and the no-treatment group may include some who received the treatment. Thus the groups will be less different in terms of therapy than they would have been had there been no noncompliance, so that even if there is a difference in the effects of the treatments, it will appear much smaller.

One approach that was used in the Veterans Administration Study of the Treatment of Hypertension was to carry out a pilot study in which compliers and noncompliers were identified. When the actual full study was later carried out, the study population was limited to those who had been compliers during the pilot study (sometimes referred to as a "run-in period"). The problem with this approach is that when we want to generalize from the results of such a study, we can only do so to other populations of compliers, which may be different from the population in any free-living community, which would consist of both compliers and noncompliers.

Table 10.6 shows data from the Coronary Drug Project reported by Canner and coworkers.[18] This study was a comparison of clofibrate and placebo for lowering cholesterol. The table presents the mortality in the two groups.

No large difference in 5-year mortality was seen between the two groups. The investigators speculated that perhaps this was the result of the patients not having taken their medication. Table 10.7 shows the results of separating the clofibrate subjects into good compliers and poor compliers. Here we see the 5-year mortality was 24.6% in the poor-complier group

TABLE 10.6 Coronary Drug Project: 5-Year Mortality in Patients Given Clofibrate or Placebo

	No. of Patients	Mortality (%)
Clofibrate	1,065	18.2
Placebo	2,695	19.4

Modified from Canner PL, Forman SA, Prud'homme GJ, for the Coronary Drug Project Research Group. Influence of adherence to treatment and response to cholesterol on mortality in the coronary drug project. *N Engl J Med.* 1980;303:1038–1041.

TABLE 10.7 Coronary Drug Project: 5-Year Mortality in Patients Given Clofibrate or Placebo According to Level of Compliance

	No. of Patients	Mortality (%)
Clofibrate		
Poor complier (<80%)	357	24.6
Good complier (≥80%)	708	15.0
Placebo	2,695	19.4

Modified from Canner PL, Forman SA, Prud'homme GJ, for the Coronary Drug Project Research Group. Influence of adherence to treatment and response to cholesterol on mortality in the coronary drug project. *N Engl J Med.* 1980;303:1038–1041.

TABLE 10.8 Coronary Drug Project: 5-Year Mortality in Patients Given Clofibrate or Placebo According to Level of Compliance

	CLOFIBRATE		PLACEBO	
Compliance	No. of Patients	Mortality (%)	No. of Patients	Mortality (%)
Poor (<80%)	357	24.6	882	28.2
Good (≥80%)	708	15.0	1,813	15.1
Total Group	1,065	18.2	2,695	19.4

Modified from Canner PL, Forman SA, Prud'homme GJ, for the Coronary Drug Project Research Group. Influence of adherence to treatment and response of cholesterol on mortality in the coronary drug project. *N Engl J Med.* 1980;303:1038–1041.

compared with 15% in the good-complier group. We might thus be tempted to conclude that compliance was indeed the factor that produced the results seen in Table 10.6: no significant difference between the clofibrate and placebo groups.

Table 10.8 separates both groups, clofibrate and placebo, into compliers and noncompliers. Even in the placebo group, 5-year mortality in the poor compliers was higher than in the good compliers: 28% compared with 15%. One way to maximize compliance is to administer a single pill that includes a combination of two medications needed to achieve a therapeutic target. This is commonly called fixed-dose combinations (FDCs). A systematic review and meta-analysis found that the use of FDCs of antihypertensive medications is associated with a significant improvement in medication compliance or persistence, despite nonsignificant, yet beneficial trends in blood pressure and adverse effects.[19]

What can we learn from these tables? People who do not comply or who do not participate in studies differ from those who do comply and who do participate. Therefore, in conducting a study to evaluate a therapy or other intervention, we cannot offer the agent to a population and compare the effects in those who take the agent to the effects in those who refuse or do not, because the two groups are basically different in terms of many demographic, social, psychological, and cultural variables that may have important roles in determining outcome. These are all forms of *selection bias* that were discussed previously when we talked about observational study designs. Randomization, or some other approach that reduces selection bias, is essential in a valid clinical trial.

Conclusion

The randomized trial is generally considered the gold standard of study designs. When hierarchies of study design are created to assess the strength of the available evidence supporting clinical and public health policy, randomized trials are virtually always at the top of the list when study designs are ranked in order of descending quality. However, a recently developed observational study approach—Mendelian randomization—the discussion of which is not within the scope of this textbook, mimics random allocation if its rather stringent assumptions can be met.[20]

This chapter has discussed many of the components of the randomized trial that are designed to shield the study from any preconceptions and biases of the investigator and of others involved in conducting the study, as well as from other biases that might inadvertently be introduced. In Chapter 11 we will address some other issues relating to the design of randomized trials and will consider several interesting examples and applications of the randomized trial design. Later in this book, we will discuss the use of randomized trials and other study designs for evaluating health services and for studying the effectiveness of screening.

REFERENCES

1. Cited in Silverman WA. *Where's the Evidence? Debates in Modern Medicine.* New York: Oxford University Press; 1998.
2. Galton F. *Inquiries Into Human Faculty and Its Development.* London: Macmillan; 1883.
3. Joyce CRB, Welldon RMC. The efficacy of prayer: a double blind clinical trial. *J Chronic Dis.* 1965;18:367.
4. Byrd RC. Positive therapeutic effects of intercessory prayer in a coronary care unit population. *South Med J.* 1988;81:826.

5. Bull JP. The historical development of clinical therapeutic trials. *J Chronic Dis*. 1959;10:218.

6. Lind J. *A Treatise of the Scurvy*. Edinburgh: Sands, Murray & Cochran; 1753.

7. Peacock E. Cited in Tufte ER: *Data Analysis for Politics and Policy*. Englewood Cliffs, NJ: Prentice-Hall; 1974.

8. Ederer F. Why do we need controls? Why do we need to randomize? *Am J Ophthalmol*. 1975;79:758.

9. Bearman JE, Loewenson RB, Gullen WH. *Muensch's Postulates, Laws and Corollaries*. Biometrics Note No. 4. Bethesda, MD, Office of Biometry and Epidemiology, National Eye Institute, April 1974.

10. Wilson EB. Cited in Ederer F: Why do we need controls? Why do we need to randomize? *Am J Ophthalmol*. 1975;79:761.

11. Wright IS, Marple CD, Beck DF. Cited in Ederer F: Why do we need controls? Why do we need to randomize? *Am J Ophthalmol*. 1975;79:761.

12. Levine MI, Sackett MF. Results of BCG immunization in New York City. *Am Rev Tuber*. 1946;53:517–532.

13. Ederer F. Practical problems in collaborative clinical trials. *Am J Epidemiol*. 1975;102:111–118.

14. Schröder FH, Hugosson J, Roobol MJ, et al. Screening and prostate-cancer mortality in a randomized European study. *N Engl J Med*. 2009;360:1320–1328.

15. Cochrane AL. Cited in Ballintine EJ: Objective measurements and the double masked procedure. *Am J Ophthalmol*. 1975;79:764.

16. Hennekens CH, Buring JE, Manson JE. Lack of effect of long-term supplementation with beta carotene on the incidence of malignant neoplasms and cardiovascular disease. *N Engl J Med*. 1996;334:1145–1149.

17. Goralczyk R. Beta-carotene and lung cancer in smokers: review of hypotheses and status of research. *Nutr Cancer*. 2009;61(6):767–774.

18. Canner PL, Forman SA, Prud'homme GJ. Influence of adherence to treatment and response of cholesterol on mortality in the coronary drug project. *N Engl J Med*. 1980;303:1038–1041.

19. Gupta AK, Arshad S, Poulter NR. Compliance, safety, and effectiveness of fixed-dose combinations of antihypertensive agents: a meta-analysis. *Hypertension*. 2010;55(2):399–407.

20. Smith GD, Ebrhaim S. 'Mendelian randomization': Can genetic epidemiology contribute to understanding environmental determinants of disease? *Int J Epidemiol*. 2003;32(1):1–22.

Review Questions for Chapters 10 and 11 are at the end of Chapter 11.

Randomized Trials: Some Further Issues

Learning Objectives

- To define key concepts of epidemiologic study design in the context of randomized trials: sample size, type I error, type II error, power, generalizability (external validity), and internal validity.
- To calculate and interpret efficacy in a randomized trial.
- To describe the design and results of five historically important randomized trials.
- To define the four major phases of randomized trials that are used by the US Food and Drug Administration for evaluating new drugs in the United States.
- To introduce several ethical considerations as they relate to randomized trials.
- To discuss the rationale for requiring the registration of new randomized trials in advance of their launch.

Sample Size

At a scientific meeting some years ago, an investigator presented the results of a study he had conducted to evaluate a new drug in sheep. "After taking the drug," he reported, "one third of the sheep were markedly improved, one third of the sheep showed no change, and the other one ran away."

This story introduces one of the most frequent questions asked by physicians conducting trials of new agents, or for that matter by anyone conducting evaluative studies: "How many subjects do we have to study?" The time to answer this question is *before* the study is done. All too often studies are conducted, large amounts of money and other resources are invested, and only after the study has been completed do the investigators find that from the beginning they had too few subjects to obtain meaningful results.

The question of how many subjects are needed for study is not based on mystique. This section presents the logic of how to approach the question of sample size. Let's begin this discussion of sample size with Fig. 11.1.

We have two jars of beads, each containing 100 beads, some white and some blue. The jars are opaque ("masked"), so (despite their appearance in the figure) we cannot see the colors of the beads in the jars just by looking at the jars. We want to know whether the distribution of the beads by color differs in jars A and B. In other words, is there a larger (or smaller) proportion of blue beads in jar A than in jar B?

To answer this question, let's take a sample of 10 beads from jar A in one hand and a sample of 10 beads from jar B in the other. On the basis of the color distribution of the 10 beads in each hand, we will try to reach a conclusion about the color distribution of all 100 beads in each of the jars.

Let's assume that (as shown in Fig. 11.2) in one hand we have 9 blue beads and 1 white bead from jar A, and in the other hand we have 2 blue beads and 8 white beads from jar B. Can we conclude that 90% of the beads in jar A are blue and that 10% are white? Clearly we cannot. It is possible, for example, that of the 100 beads in jar A, 90 are white and 10 are blue, but *by chance* our 10-bead sample includes 9 blue and 1 white. This is possible but highly unlikely. Similarly, in regard to jar B we cannot conclude that 20% of the beads are blue and 80% are white. It is conceivable that 90 of the 100 beads are blue and 10 are white, but that *by chance* the 10-bead sample includes 2 blue beads and 8 white beads. This is conceivable but, again, highly unlikely.

On the basis of the distributions of the 10-bead samples in each hand, could we say that the distributions of the 100 beads in the two jars are different? Given the samples in each hand, could it be, for example, that the distribution of beads in each jar is 50 blue and 50 white? Again, it is possible, but it is not likely. We cannot exclude this possibility on the basis of our samples. We are looking at

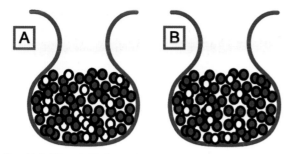

Fig. 11.1 (A) and (B) Two opaque jars, each holding 100 beads, some blue and some white.

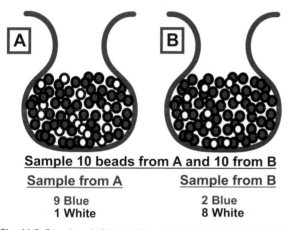

Sample 10 beads from A and 10 from B

Sample from A	Sample from B
9 Blue	2 Blue
1 White	8 White

Fig. 11.2 Samples of 10 beads from jar A and 10 beads from jar B.

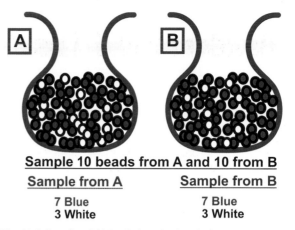

Sample 10 beads from A and 10 from B

Sample from A	Sample from B
7 Blue	7 Blue
3 White	3 White

Fig. 11.3 Samples of 10 beads from jar A and 10 beads from jar B.

BOX 11.1 FOUR POSSIBLE CONCLUSIONS WHEN TESTING WHETHER OR NOT THE TREATMENTS DIFFER

- **When, in reality, the treatments do <u>not</u> differ:**
  1. We may correctly conclude that they do <u>not</u> differ,
     or
  2. In error, we may conclude that they do differ.

- **When, in reality, the treatments <u>do</u> differ:**
  3. In error, we may conclude that they do not differ,
     or
  4. We may correctly conclude that they <u>do</u> differ.

samples and trying to draw a conclusion regarding a whole population—the jars from which we have drawn the samples.

Let's consider a second example, shown in Fig. 11.3. Again, we draw two samples. This time, the 10-bead sample from jar A consists of 7 blue beads and 3 white beads, and the 10-bead sample from jar B also consists of 7 blue beads and 3 white beads. Could the color distribution of the beads in the two jars be the same? Clearly, it could. Could we have drawn these two samples of 7 blue beads and 3 white beads from both jars if the distribution is actually 90 white beads and 10 blue beads in jar A and 90 blue beads and 10 white beads in jar B? Yes, possibly, but unlikely.

When we carry out a study we are only looking at the sample of subjects in our study, such as a sample of patients with a certain illness who are being treated with treatment A or with treatment B. From the study

results, we want to draw a conclusion that goes beyond the study population—is treatment A more effective than treatment B in the total universe of all patients with this disease who might be treated with treatment A or treatment B? The same issue that arose with the 10-bead samples arises when we want to derive a conclusion regarding all patients from the sample of patients included in our study. Rarely, if ever, is a study conducted in all patients with a disease or in all patients who might be treated with the drugs in question.

Given this background, let's now consider a trial in which groups receiving one of two therapies, therapy A and therapy B, are being compared. (Keep in mind the sampling of beads just discussed.) Before beginning our study, we can list the four possible study outcomes (Box 11.1):

1. It is possible that in reality there is no difference in efficacy between therapy A and therapy B. In

other words, therapy A is no better and no worse than therapy B. When we do our study, we correctly conclude on the basis of our samples that the two groups do not differ.

2. It is possible that in reality there is no difference in efficacy between therapy A and therapy B, but in our study we found a difference between the groups and therefore concluded, on the basis of our samples, that there is a difference between the therapies. This conclusion, based on our samples, is in error.

3. It is possible that in reality there is a difference in efficacy between therapy A and therapy B, but when we examine the groups in our study we find no difference between them. We therefore conclude, on the basis of our samples, that there is no difference between therapy A and therapy B. This conclusion is in error.

4. It is possible that in reality there is a difference in efficacy between therapy A and therapy B, and when we examine the groups in our study, we find that they differ. On the basis of these samples, we correctly conclude that therapy A differs from therapy B.

These four possibilities constitute all of the possible outcomes after we complete our study. Let's look at these four possibilities as presented in a 2 × 2 table (Fig. 11.4): Two columns represent reality—either therapy A differs from therapy B, or therapy A does not differ from therapy B. The two rows represent our decision: We conclude either that they differ or that

they do not differ. In this figure, the four possibilities that were just listed are represented as four cells in a 2 × 2 table. If there is no difference, and on the basis of the samples included in our study we conclude there is no difference, this is a correct decision (*cell a*). If there is a difference, and on the basis of our study we conclude that there is a difference (*cell d*), this too is a correct decision. In the best of all worlds, all of the possibilities would fall into one of these two cells. Unfortunately, this is rarely, if ever, the case. There are times when there is no difference between the therapies, but on the basis of the samples of subjects included in our study, we erroneously conclude that they differ (*cell c*). This is called a *type I error*. It is also possible that there really is a difference between the therapies, but on the basis of the samples included in our study we erroneously conclude that there is no difference (*cell b*); this is called a *type II error*. (In this situation, the therapies differ, but we fail to detect the difference in our study samples.)

The *probability* that we will make a type I error is designated α, and the *probability* that we will make a type II error is designated β (as shown in Fig. 11.5).

α is the so-called *P* value, which is seen in many published papers and has been sanctified by many years of use. When you see "*P* < .05," the reference is to α. What does *P* < .05 mean? It tells us that we have concluded that therapy A differs from therapy B on the basis of the sample of subjects included in our study, which we found to differ. The probability that such a difference could have arisen by chance alone,

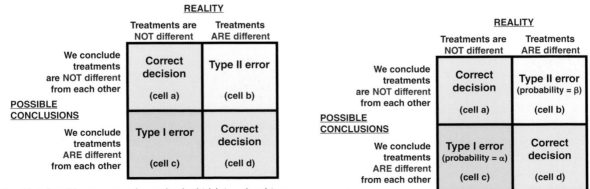

Fig. 11.4 Possible outcomes of a randomized trial: type I and type II errors.

Fig. 11.5 Possible outcomes of a randomized trial: α and β.

and that this difference between our groups does not reflect any true difference between therapies A and B, is only 0.05 (or 1 in 20).

Let's now direct our attention to the right half of this 2 × 2 table, which shows the two possibilities when there is a true difference between therapies A and B, as shown in Fig. 11.6. If, as seen here, the reality is that there is a difference between the therapies, there are only two possibilities: (1) We might conclude, in error, that the therapies do not differ (type II error). The probability of making a type II error is designated β. Or (2) we might conclude, correctly, that the therapies differ. Because the total of all probabilities must equal 1 and the probability of a type II error = β, the probability that we will correctly decide on the basis of our study that the therapies differ if there is a difference will equal 1 − β. This probability, 1 − β, is called the *power* of the study. It tells us how good our study is at correctly identifying a difference between the therapies if in reality they are different. How likely is our study not to miss a difference if one exists?

The full 2 × 2 table in Fig. 11.7 includes all of the terms that have been discussed. Table 11.1 provides multiple definitions of these terms that are commonly used in the epidemiologic literature.

How do these concepts help us to arrive at an estimate of the sample size that we need? If we ask the question "How many people do we have to study in a clinical trial?," we must be able to specify a number of items as listed in Box 11.2.

First, we must specify the expected difference in response rate. Let's say that the existing therapy cures 40% of patients, and we are going to test a new therapy. We must be able to say whether we expect the new

REALITY

	Treatments are NOT different	Treatments ARE different
POSSIBLE CONCLUSIONS We conclude treatments are NOT different from each other	Correct decision	Type II error (probability = β)
We conclude treatments ARE different from each other	Type I error (probability = α)	Correct decision (probability = 1 - β) (power)

Fig. 11.7 Possible outcomes of a randomized trial: summary.

TABLE 11.1	**Summary of Terms**
Term	**Definitions**
α	= Probability of making a type I error
	= Probability of concluding the treatments differ when in reality they do not differ
β	= Probability of making a type II error
	= Probability of concluding that the treatments do not differ when in reality they do differ
Power	= 1 − Probability of making a type II error
	= 1 − β
	= Probability of correctly concluding that the treatments differ
	= Probability of detecting a difference between the treatments if the treatments do in fact differ

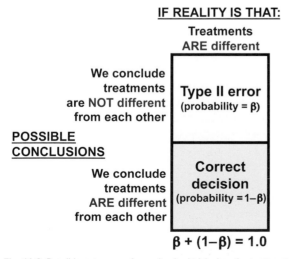

IF REALITY IS THAT:

Treatments ARE different

POSSIBLE CONCLUSIONS We conclude treatments are NOT different from each other	Type II error (probability = β)
We conclude treatments ARE different from each other	Correct decision (probability = 1−β)

$$\beta + (1-\beta) = 1.0$$

Fig. 11.6 Possible outcomes of a randomized trial when the treatments differ.

BOX 11.2 WHAT MUST BE SPECIFIED TO ESTIMATE THE SAMPLE SIZE NEEDED IN A RANDOMIZED TRIAL?

1. The difference in response rates to be detected
2. An estimate of the response rate in one of the groups
3. Level of statistical significance (α)
4. The value of the power desired (1 − β)
5. Whether the test should be one-sided or two-sided

therapy to cure 50%, 60%, or some other proportion of treated patients. That is, will the new therapy be 10% better than the current therapy and cure 50% of people, 20% better than current therapy and cure 60%, or some other difference? What is the size of the difference between current therapy and new therapy that we want to be able to detect with our study? Does the size of the difference make clinical sense?

How do we generally arrive at such an estimate of how much better the new therapy will be? What if we do not have information on which to base an estimate of the improvement in effectiveness that might be anticipated? Perhaps we are studying a new therapy for which we have no prior experience. One approach is to search for data in human populations for similar diseases and therapies. We can also search for relevant data from animal studies. At times, we simply have no way of producing such an estimate. In this situation, we can make a guess (say, 30% improvement) but *bracket* the estimate—that is, calculate the sample size needed based on a 40% improvement in response rate and also calculate the sample size needed based on a 20% improvement in response rate. This is sometimes referred to as a "sensitivity analysis."

Second, we must have an estimate of the clinical outcome (rate of cure, rate of improvement) in one of the groups. In the example just used, we said the current cure rate is 40%. This is the estimate of the response rate for the current treatment group based on current clinical experience.

Third, we must specify the level of α with which we will be satisfied. The choice is up to the investigator; there is nothing sacred about any specific value, but values of 0.05 or 0.01 are commonly used in research.

Fourth, we must specify the power of the study. Again, no specific value is sacred, but powers of 80% or 90% are commonly used. We do not want to miss a difference if one exists!

Finally, we must specify whether the test should be one-sided or two-sided. What does this mean? Our present cure rate is 40%, and we are trying a new therapy that we believe will have a higher cure rate— perhaps 50% or 60%. We want to detect a difference that is in the direction of improvement with the new therapy—an increase in cure rate. So we might say we will only test for a difference in that direction (improvement) because that is the direction in which we are interested—that is, a one-sided test.

The problem is that in the history of medicine and of public health we have at times been surprised to find that new therapies that we thought would be beneficial have actually been harmful or may lead to significant side effects. If such a possibility exists, we would want to find a difference in cure rate *in either direction* from the current rate in our study—that is, we would use a two-sided test, testing not only for a difference that is better than the current cure rate, but also allowing for one that is worse than the current rate. Clinicians and other investigators often prefer to use a one-sided test in their studies because such tests require smaller sample sizes than two-sided tests. Because the number of patients available for study is often limited, a one-sided test is attractive. At times investigators may make a practical decision to use a one-sided test, even if there is no conceptual justification for this decision.

Opinions differ on this subject. Some believe that if the investigator is only interested in one direction— improvement—a one-sided test is justified. Others believe that as long as the difference could go in either direction, a two-sided test is required. In a situation in which a particular disease is currently 100% fatal, any difference with a new therapy could only be in the direction of improvement, then a one-sided test would be appropriate.

Let's now turn to the application of these five factors to estimate the needed sample size from a sample size table. Tables 11.2 and 11.3 are selections from sample size tables published by Gehan in 1979.[1] (Similar tables are available as appendices in standard statistics textbooks.) Both tables give the number of patients needed *in each group* to detect various differences in cure rates with an α of 0.05 and a power $(1 - \beta)$ of 0.80. Table 11.2 is intended to be used for a two-sided test and Table 11.3 for a one-sided test.

Let's say that we are conducting a clinical trial of two therapies: one that is currently in use (the "standard of care") and one that is new. The current therapy has a cure rate of 40%, and we believe that the new therapy may have a cure rate of 60%—that is, we wish to detect an improvement in cure rate of 20%. How many subjects do we have to study? Let's say we will use an α of 0.05, a power of 80%, and a two-sided test. We therefore

TABLE 11.2 Number of Patients Needed in Each Group to Detect Various Differences in Cure Rates; α = 0.05; Power (1 − β) = 0.80 (Two-Sided Test)

Lower of the Two Cure Rates	DIFFERENCES IN CURE RATES BETWEEN THE TWO TREATMENT GROUPS													
	0.05	0.10	0.15	0.20	0.25	0.30	0.35	0.40	0.45	0.50	0.55	0.60	0.65	0.70
0.05	420	130	69	44	36	31	23	20	17	14	13	11	10	8
0.10	680	195	96	59	41	35	29	23	19	17	13	12	11	8
0.15	910	250	120	71	48	39	31	25	20	17	15	12	11	9
0.20	1,090	290	135	80	53	42	33	26	22	18	16	12	11	9
0.25	1,250	330	150	88	57	44	35	28	22	18	16	12	11	—
0.30	1,380	360	160	93	60	44	36	29	22	18	15	12	—	—
0.35	1,470	370	170	96	61	44	36	28	22	17	13	—	—	—
0.40	1,530	390	175	97	61	44	35	26	20	17	—	—	—	—
0.45	1,560	390	175	96	60	42	33	25	19	—	—	—	—	—
0.50	1,560	390	170	93	57	40	31	23	—	—	—	—	—	—

Modified from Gehan E. Clinical trials in cancer research. *Environ Health Perspect.* 1979;32:31.

TABLE 11.3 Number of Patients Needed in Each Group to Detect Various Differences in Cure Rates; α = 0.05; Power (1 − β) = 0.80 (One-Sided Test)

Lower of the Two Cure Rates	DIFFERENCES IN CURE RATES BETWEEN THE TWO TREATMENT GROUPS													
	0.05	0.10	0.15	0.20	0.25	0.30	0.35	0.40	0.45	0.50	0.55	0.60	0.65	0.70
0.05	330	105	55	40	33	24	20	17	13	12	10	9	9	8
0.10	540	155	76	47	37	30	23	19	16	13	11	11	9	8
0.15	710	200	94	56	43	32	26	22	17	15	11	10	9	8
0.20	860	230	110	63	42	36	27	23	17	15	12	10	9	8
0.25	980	260	120	69	45	37	31	23	17	15	12	10	9	—
0.30	1,080	280	130	73	47	37	31	23	17	15	11	10	—	—
0.35	1,160	300	135	75	48	37	31	23	17	15	11	—	—	—
0.40	1,210	310	135	76	48	37	30	23	17	13	—	—	—	—
0.45	1,230	310	135	75	47	36	26	22	16	—	—	—	—	—
0.50	1,230	310	135	73	45	36	26	19	—	—	—	—	—	—

Modified from Gehan E. Clinical trials in cancer research. *Environ Health Perspect.* 1979;32:31.

will use Table 11.2. The first column of this table is designated the lower of the two cure rates. As the current cure rate is 40%, and we expect a cure rate of 60% with our new therapy, the lower of the two cure rates is 40%, and we move to that row of the table. We expect the new therapy to have a cure rate of 60%, so the difference in cure rates will be 20%. We therefore move down the 20% column (the difference in cure rates) to the point at which it intersects the row of 40% (the lower of the cure rates), where we find the value 97. We need 97 subjects *in each of our study groups.*

Another approach is to use the table in a reverse direction. For example, let's consider a clinic for people who have a certain rare disease. Each year the clinic treats 30 patients with the disease and wishes to test a new therapy. Given this maximum number of 30 patients, we could ask, "What size difference in cure rates could we hope to detect?" We may find a difference of a certain size that may be acceptable, or we may find that the number of subjects available for study is simply too small. If the number of patients is too small, we have several options: We can decide not to do the study, and such a decision should be made early on, before most of the effort has been invested. Or we could decide to extend the study in time to accumulate more subjects. Finally, we could decide to collaborate with investigators at other institutions to increase the total number of subjects available for the study. In a study that uses only a single site, any biases in selecting participants may be difficult to identify, but in a multicenter study, the presence of any such bias at one of the centers would be more readily detectable.

This section has demonstrated the use of a sample size table. Formulas and computer programs are also available for calculating sample size. Sample sizes can be calculated not only for randomized trials but also for cohort and case-control studies, as discussed earlier.

Recruitment and Retention of Study Participants

A major challenge in the conduct of randomized trials is to recruit a sufficient number of eligible and willing volunteers. Failure to recruit a sufficient number of volunteers can leave a well-designed trial without enough participants to yield statistically valid results. Potential participants must also be willing to be randomized for the trial. Trials may be significantly delayed by this problem of limited recruitment, and costs of completing such trials may be increased since it may take longer to do the overall study. However, given the pressures to recruit a sufficient number of participants, a high level of vigilance is needed to be sure that no coercion, either overt or covert, has been used by study investigators, consciously or subconsciously, to convince possible participants to enroll in a study. Within the limits of a randomized trial, participants must be fully informed of the risks and what arrangements have been made for their compensation if untoward effects should occur. Appropriate arrangements must also be made to cover participants' expenses, such as transportation, accommodations if needed, and the participants' time, particularly if participation is associated with loss of income. However, payment of cash incentives to prospective volunteers will often risk subtle or overt coercion; biases and distortion of the study results may occur, particularly if large incentives are paid.

At times, enrollment as a participant in a study has been marketed to potential volunteers on the basis that only through participation will a participant have a chance of being treated with the newest available treatments. However, the justification for conducting a randomized trial is that we do not know which therapy is better. It is therefore critical that the persons

conducting the trial avoid being overly zealous in promising the participants benefits that have not yet been conclusively demonstrated to be associated with the therapy being tested. Institutional Review Boards oversee all of the ethical issues involved in research studies, and no research participants can be recruited until the research protocol is approved.

A related problem is that of retaining volunteers for the full duration of the study. Losses to follow-up and other forms of noncompliance can make this issue a major concern. Participants may lose interest in the study over time, or find participation too inconvenient, particularly over the long term (such as years of follow-up). Investigators must develop an appreciation of why participants often drop out of studies and develop appropriate measures to prevent losses to follow-up.

Ways of Expressing the Results of Randomized Trials

The results of randomized trials can be expressed in a number of ways. The risks of death or of developing a disease or complication in each group can be calculated, and the *reduction in risk* (efficacy) can then be calculated. *Efficacy* of an agent being tested, such as a vaccine, can be expressed in terms of the rates of developing disease in the vaccine and placebo groups:

$$\text{Efficacy} = \frac{\left(\begin{array}{c}\text{Rate in those who}\\\text{received the placebo}\end{array}\right) - \left(\begin{array}{c}\text{Rate in those who}\\\text{received the vaccine}\end{array}\right)}{\text{Rate in those who received the placebo}}$$

This formula tells us the extent of the reduction in disease by use of the vaccine. Risks are often calculated per *person-years* of observation.

Efficacy, or how well a treatment works under "ideal" conditions (such as that in a clinical trial), may be differentiated from effectiveness, or how well a treatment works in "real-life" situations. Although randomized trials most often evaluate efficacy of a treatment, the two terms (efficacious and effective) are often (wrongly) used interchangeably. Efficacy and effectiveness will be discussed later.

Another approach to reporting results from randomized trials is to calculate the *ratio of the risks* in the two treatment groups (the relative risk), which will be discussed later. In addition, often we compare the *survival curves* for each of the groups, as we previously illustrated, to determine whether they differ significantly.

A major objective of randomized trials is to have an impact on the way clinical medicine and public health are practiced. But at times practitioners may find it difficult to place the findings of such trials in a perspective that seems relevant to their practices. Another approach, therefore, for expressing the results of randomized trials is to estimate the *number of patients who would need to be treated* (NNT) to prevent one adverse outcome such as one death. This can be calculated by:

$$NNT = \dfrac{1}{\left(\begin{array}{c}\text{Rate in}\\\text{untreated group}\end{array}\right) - \left(\begin{array}{c}\text{Rate in}\\\text{treated group}\end{array}\right)}$$

Thus if, for example, the mortality rate in the untreated group is 17% and mortality in the treated group is 12%, we would need to treat:

$$\frac{1}{17\% - 12\%} = \frac{1}{0.05} = 20$$

people to prevent one death. Estimates of NNT are usually rounded up to the next highest whole number. This approach can be used in studies of various interventions, including both treatment and prevention.

For example, as mentioned in Chapter 10, in the European Randomized Study of Screening for Prostate Cancer, there was a reduction of about 27% in prostate cancer mortality.[2] Thus if in 100 screened individuals 27 prostate cancer deaths were avoided, screening would have to be conducted in $(100 \div 27 = 1 \div 0.27) \approx 4$ individuals in order to prevent one prostate cancer death. The same approach can also be used to look at the risk of side effects by calculating the *number needed to harm* (NNH) to cause one additional person to be harmed. These estimates are subject to considerable error and are generally presented with 95% confidence intervals so that they can be properly interpreted. In addition, they have other limitations: they do not take into account quality of life and are of limited value to patients. These estimates can nevertheless help practitioners to estimate the size of the effect they might expect to observe by using the new treatment or preventive measure in their practices.

Interpreting the Results of Randomized Trials

GENERALIZABILITY OF RESULTS BEYOND THE STUDY POPULATION

Whenever we carry out a trial, the ultimate objective is to generalize the results beyond the study population itself. Let's consider an example. Suppose we want to evaluate a new drug for lupus erythematosus (a connective tissue disease) using a randomized trial. The diagrams in Fig. 11.8 represent a randomized trial in which a defined population is identified from a total population, and a subset of that defined population is the study population. For example, the *total population* might be all patients with lupus erythematosus, the *defined population* might be all patients with lupus erythematosus in our community, and the *study population* could be patients with the disease who receive their medical care from one of several clinics in our community.

If we carry out a study in patients recruited from several clinics in our community and find a new therapy to be better than a therapy that is currently used (the standard of care), we would like to be able to say that the new therapy is better for the disease regardless of where the patients are treated, and not just for patients in those clinics. Our ability to apply the results obtained in our study population to a broader population is called the *generalizability*, or *external validity*, of the study. We want to be able to *generalize* from the study findings to all patients with the disease in our community. To do so, we must know to what extent the patients we have studied are representative of the defined population—that is, of all patients with the disease in question in our community (see Fig. 11.8A). We must characterize those who did not participate in the study and identify characteristics of study patients that might differ from those in patients who did not participate in the study. Such differences may preclude our generalizing the results of the study to other patients who were not included in the study. We may also wish to generalize our results, not just to all patients with the disease in our community, but to all patients with the disease, regardless of where they live—that is, to

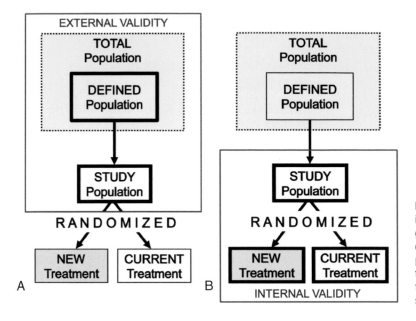

Fig. 11.8 (A) External validity (generalizability) in a randomized trial. Findings of the study are generalizable from the study population to the defined population and, presumably, to the total population. (B) Internal validity in a randomized trial. The study was done properly, and the findings of the study are therefore valid in the study population.

the total population of patients with the disease. Rarely, however, is the total population for a randomized trial known (let alone enumerated). Although it is hoped that the defined population is representative of the total population, this assumption is rarely, if ever, verified.

External validity should be distinguished from *internal validity* (see Fig. 11.8B). A randomized trial is *internally valid* if the randomization has been properly done and the study is free of other biases and is without any of the major methodologic problems that have been discussed. Essentially it should be ideally concluded that the observed differences in the outcomes in the two groups being compared are attributed to the hypothesized exposure under study, aside from sampling errors. Randomized trials are considered the gold standard of study designs because randomization, if correctly conducted, prevents biases on the part of the study investigators from influencing the treatment assignment for each patient. If our study is sufficiently large, randomization will also most likely lead to comparability between treatment groups on factors that may be important for the outcome, such as age, sex, race, and so on, as well as for factors we have not measured or may not even be aware of as important. The issues of internal validity and of external validity (generalizability) are basic concerns in the conduct of

any randomized trial and in observational study designs, discussed in prior chapters. Because randomized trials usually study volunteers, their external validity tends to be lower than that of observational studies. The opposite is true for internal validity, given that comparability between groups is much more likely in clinical trials.

WHAT CAN THE RESULTS OF A RANDOMIZED TRIAL TELL A TREATING PHYSICIAN ABOUT AN INDIVIDUAL PATIENT?

Let's consider a simple hypothetical scenario. A physician is about to prescribe a treatment for one of her patients. The physician is familiar with a recently published high-quality randomized trial that compared Therapy A to Therapy B for the condition with which her patient presents (Fig. 11.9A). As seen in the diagram, in the trial, a much greater proportion of patients who received Therapy A had a good result (blue portions of the bars) than the proportion of patients who had a good result who received Therapy B. The trial results were therefore reported as showing that Therapy A is superior to Therapy B for this condition.

The physician is well aware of the results reported for the randomized trial. However, before prescribing therapy for her patient on the basis of reported trial

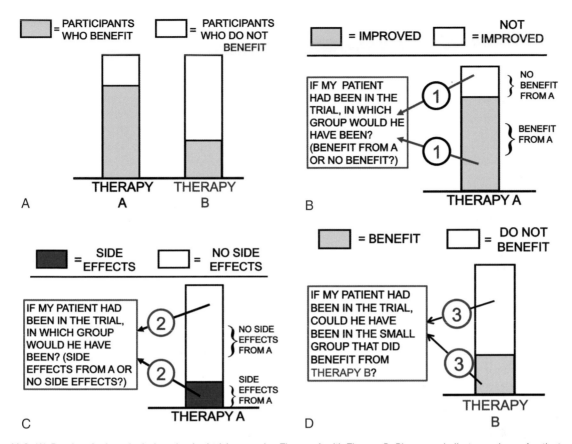

Fig. 11.9 (A) Results of a hypothetical randomized trial comparing Therapy A with Therapy B. Blue areas indicate numbers of patients who benefited from each therapy, and white areas indicate those who did not respond to each therapy. (B) Physician's first question. (C) Physician's second question. (D) Physician's third question. (See explanation in text below.)

results, the physician has a few questions she would like to have answered which could provide her with valuable guidance for selecting the better therapy *for this patient*. Only three of her questions will be listed here as examples:

1. "If my patient had participated in the randomized trial and had been in the group that was randomized to receive Therapy A (see Fig. 11.9B), would he have been among those who improved (shown in blue) or would he have been among those who did not respond to Therapy A (the top white part of the bar)?"

2. "If my patient had been a participant in the randomized trial and had been in the group that received Therapy A (see Fig. 11.9C), would he

have been among those who developed side effects (shown in red) or would he have been among those who did not show any side effects from Therapy A (the top white part of the bar)?"

3. "If my patient had been a participant in the randomized trial and had been in the group receiving Therapy B (see Fig. 11.9D), would he have been in the group who improved after receiving Therapy B (shown in blue) or would he have been among those who did not respond to Therapy B (the top white part of the bar)?"

Unfortunately, most randomized trials do not provide the information the physician would need to characterize an individual patient sufficiently to predict what responses her patient might have to the therapies available. She is generally not given enough information to tell her whether it would be reasonable for her to generalize from the randomized trial results to a specific patient before selecting and initiating treatment. If she does generalize to her patient, from which subgroup of participants in the trial should she generalize?

Another limiting factor in many randomized trials is that even if we assume that dropouts from the trial were kept to a minimum and that the participants had all agreed to be randomized, the question remains: Can we assume that in the "real" nonrandomized world, a given patient would respond in the same way that a randomized patient might respond in a trial? What do we know about the personalities and preferences of participants in randomized trials that would indicate to us if a specific patient to be treated has similar characteristics including the same values, personality, and concerns? Is a person who agrees to be randomized similar to a general population from which a specific patient may have come for treatment? As David Mant pointed out, participants in randomized trials are usually not representative of the general population.[3] Participants in trials are generally healthier, younger, and better educated than people coming in for treatment. A final question to address is whether we have lost our concern about individuals when we reduce everyone in a study to being part of a study group, often only examining the results for the group as a whole but losing sight of individual differences and preferences.

COMPARATIVE EFFECTIVENESS RESEARCH

Some randomized trials are designed to compare a new therapy to a placebo. Other randomized trials focus on comparing a new treatment with an older accepted treatment in order to determine whether the new treatment is superior to the established treatment. Two examples of trials used for evaluating widely accepted interventions are discussed later in this chapter. In recent years, interest has also developed in what has been termed comparative effectiveness research (CER), in which two or more existing interventions are compared in order "to determine which intervention would work best in a given population or for a given patient."[4] In this type of approach, results from other types of study designs, which are discussed in prior chapters, may be used together with the findings of randomized trials to try to answer these questions.

Another issue relates to the costs of interventions. For example, many treatments of human immuno-deficiency virus (HIV) infections are very expensive, and such treatments may be affordable in high-income countries but may not be affordable in many low- and middle-income countries. As newer and less expensive (generic) medications are developed, studies are often conducted to determine whether the newer, less expensive alternatives are as effective as the more expensive interventions whose effectiveness has already been documented. Such studies are often referred to as *equivalence studies* and are designed to determine whether the less expensive interventions are as effective as the more expensive treatments. The term *non-inferiority studies* has also been used for such evaluations. These studies should be distinguished from *superiority studies,* in which newly developed agents are evaluated to determine whether they are more effective (superior) than currently available interventions.

Four Phases in Testing New Drugs in the United States

As new drugs are developed, the US Food and Drug Administration follows a standard sequence of four phases for testing and evaluating these new agents:

Phase I trials: These trials are clinical pharmacologic studies—small studies of 20 to 80 patients that look at safety issues with the new drug or other treatment. Toxic and pharmacologic effects are examined, including safety, safe ranges of human dosage, and the side effects observed with the new treatment. If the drug passes these studies, it then undergoes *phase II* studies.

Phase II trials: Phase II studies consist of clinical investigations of 100 to 300 patients in order to evaluate the efficacy of the new drug or treatment and to further assess its relative safety. If the drug passes phase II studies, it is then tested in *phase III* trials.

Phase III trials: These studies are large-scale randomized controlled trials for efficacy and relative safety. These studies often include 1,000 to 3,000 or more participants. Recruiting such large numbers of participants may be very difficult and often necessitates recruiting from more than one study center. When recruitment difficulties are anticipated from the beginning, the study may be designed in its planning stage as a multicenter trial. If the drug passes phase III testing, it can be approved and licensed for marketing.

Phase IV studies: It has been increasingly recognized that certain adverse effects of drugs, such as carcinogenesis (cancer) and teratogenesis (congenital malformations), may not become manifest for many years. It is also possible that such adverse effects of new drugs may be so infrequent that they may not be detectable even in relatively large randomized clinical trials, but may become evident only when the drug is in use by large populations after marketing has begun. For this reason, *phase IV* studies, which are also called *postmarketing surveillance*, are important for monitoring new agents as they come into general use by the public. Phase IV studies are not randomized studies and are not really trials at all, unlike phase I, II, and III trials. Since phase IV studies ascertain side effects of a new treatment after the drug has been marketed, participants are not randomized. For the findings from such postmarketing surveillance to be valid, a very high-quality system for reporting of adverse effects is essential. While the focus of phase IV studies is often on the numbers of side effects reported and the number of people who received the new agent and developed side effects, phase IV studies are often very valuable in providing additional evidence on benefits and to help optimize the use of the new agent.

The rigorous sequence described above has protected the American public against many hazardous agents. In recent years, however, pressure to speed up the processing of new agents for treating HIV and acquired immunodeficiency syndrome (AIDS) has led to a reexamination of this approval process. It seems likely that whatever modifications are ultimately made in the approval process will not remain limited to drugs used against AIDS but will in fact have extensive ramifications for the general process of approving new drugs. The changes made in the future will therefore have major implications for the health of the public both in the United States and throughout the world.

Five Major Randomized Trials in the United States

THE HYPERTENSION DETECTION AND FOLLOW-UP PROGRAM

Whether or not to aggressively control blood pressure in hypertensive individuals is a continuous clinical challenge. In the 1960s, a Veterans Administration study demonstrated that treating people who experience quite elevated blood pressure can significantly reduce their mortality, laying the groundwork for blood pressure control in the United States.[5] The question of whether antihypertensive therapy benefits people with only modestly elevated blood pressure (diastolic blood pressure of 90 to 104 mm Hg) was left unanswered. Although we might be able to reduce blood pressure in such persons, side effects of antihypertensive agents are a concern. Unless some health benefit to the patients can be demonstrated, use of these antihypertensive agents would not be justified in people whose blood pressure is only minimally elevated.

The multicenter Hypertension Detection and Follow-up Program (HDFP) study was thus designed to investigate the benefits of treating mild to moderate hypertension. In this study, of 22,994 subjects who were eligible because they had elevated diastolic blood pressure, 10,940 were randomized either to the stepped care or to the referred care group (Fig. 11.10).

Stepped care meant treatment according to a precisely defined protocol, under which treatment was changed when a specified decrease in blood pressure had not occurred during a certain period. The comparison group posed a problem: from the standpoint of study design, a group receiving *no care* for hypertension might have been desirable. However, the investigators believed it was ethically unjustifiable to withhold antihypertensive care from known hypertensive subjects. Thus the subjects in the comparison group were referred back to their own physicians (usual care [UC]), and this group was therefore called the *referred care group*. Mortality in both groups over a 5-year period was then investigated.[6]

Fig. 11.11 shows that at every interval following entry into the study, the patients in the stepped care group had lower mortality than did those in the referred care group. In Fig. 11.11 we see that the same pattern held in those with only mild increases in blood pressure.

The results are shown in greater detail in Table 11.4, in which the data are presented according to diastolic blood pressure at entry into the study prior to antihypertensive treatment. The right-hand column shows the percentage reduction in mortality for the

stepped care group: the greatest reduction occurred in those subjects with a minimal increase in diastolic pressure.

This study has had considerable impact in encouraging physicians to treat even mild to moderate elevations in blood pressure. It has been criticized, however, because of the absence of an untreated group for comparison. Not only were these patients referred back to their own physicians, but there was no monitoring of the care that was provided to them by their physicians. Therefore some problems remain in interpreting these data. Even today, people differ on whether there was indeed a legitimate ethical objection to including an untreated placebo group in this study or whether

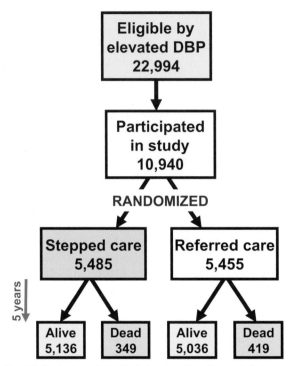

Fig. 11.10 Design of the Hypertension Detection and Follow-up Program. *DBP*, Diastolic blood pressure.

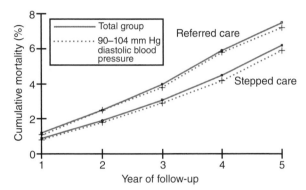

Fig. 11.11 Cumulative all-cause mortality by blood pressure status and type of care received in the Hypertension Detection and Follow-up Program. (Modified from Hypertension Detection and Follow-up Program Cooperative Group: Five-year findings of the Hypertension Detection and Follow-up Program: I. Reduction in mortality of persons with high blood pressure, including mild hypertension. *JAMA.* 1979;242:2562–2571.)

TABLE 11.4   **Mortality From All Causes During the Hypertension Detection and Follow-Up Program**

Diastolic Blood Pressure at Entry (mm Hg)	Stepped Care	Referred Care	5-YEAR DEATH RATE		Mortality Reduction in SC Group (%)
			SC	RC	
90–104	3,903	3,922	5.9	7.4	20.3
105–114	1,048	1,004	6.7	7.7	13.0
≥115	534	529	9.0	9.7	7.2
Total	5,485	5,455	6.4	7.7	16.9

RC, Referred care; *SC,* stepped care.

From Hypertension Detection and Follow-up Program Cooperative Group. Five-year findings of the Hypertension Detection and Follow-up Program: I. Reduction in mortality of persons with high blood pressure, including mild hypertension. *JAMA.* 1979;242:2562–2571.

there was an ethical problem in designing an expensive study that was difficult to mount and left so much uncertainty and difficulty in interpretation.

THE MULTIPLE RISK FACTOR INTERVENTION TRIAL

A serious problem in large-scale trials that require the investment of tremendous resources, financial and otherwise, and take years to complete is that their interpretation is often clouded by a problem in design or methodology that may not have been appreciated at an early stage of the study. The Multiple Risk Factor Intervention Trial (MRFIT) was a randomized study designed to determine whether mortality from myocardial infarction could be reduced by changes in lifestyle and other measures. In this study, one group received special intervention (SI), consisting of stepped care for hypertension and intensive education and counseling about lifestyle changes. The comparison group received its UC in the community. Over an average follow-up period of 7 years, levels of coronary heart disease (CHD) risk factors declined more in SI men than in UC men (Fig. 11.12).

However, by the end of the study, no statistically significant differences were evident between the groups in either CHD mortality or all-cause mortality (Fig. 11.13). What may have led to this?

Serious problems complicated the interpretation of these results. First, the study was conducted at a time when mortality from coronary disease was declining in the United States. In addition, it was not clear whether the lack of difference found in this study was because lifestyle changes made no difference or because the control group, on its own, had made the same lifestyle changes as those made by many other people in the United States during this period. Widespread dietary changes, increases in exercise, and smoking cessation occurred in much of the population, so the control group may have been "contaminated" with some of the behavior changes that had been encouraged in the study group in a formal and structured manner.

This study also shows the problem of using intermediate measures as end points of efficacy in randomized trials. Because any effect on mortality may take years to manifest, it is tempting to use measures that might be affected sooner by the intervention ("proxy indicators"). However, as seen here, although the intervention succeeded in reducing smoking, cholesterol levels, and

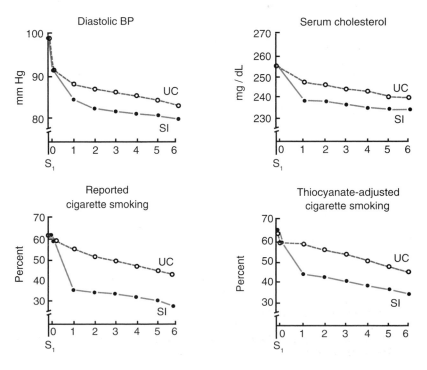

Fig. 11.12 Mean risk factor levels by year of follow-up for Multiple Risk Factor Intervention Trial Research Group participants. *BP*, Blood pressure; S_1, first screening visit; *SI*, special intervention; *UC*, usual care. (From Multiple Risk Factor Intervention Trial Research Group. Multiple Risk Factor Intervention Trial: risk factor changes and mortality results. *JAMA*. 1982;248:1465–1477.)

diastolic blood pressure, one could not conclude on the basis of these changes that the intervention was effective, because the objective of the study was to determine whether the intervention could reduce CHD mortality, which it did not.

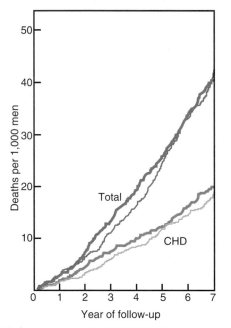

Fig. 11.13 Cumulative coronary heart disease *(CHD)* and total mortality rates for Multiple Risk Factor Intervention Trial Research Group participants. The heavy line indicates men receiving usual care; the thin line indicates men receiving special intervention. (From Multiple Risk Factor Intervention Trial Research Group. Multiple Risk Factor Intervention Trial: risk factor changes and mortality results. *JAMA.* 1982;248:1465–1477.)

Because of these problems, which often occur in very large and expensive studies, some have advocated that the same financial investment in a number of smaller studies by different investigators in different populations might be a wiser choice: If the results were consistent, they might be more credible due to generalizability, despite the problems of smaller sample size (affecting statistical power) that would occur in the individual studies.

STUDY OF BREAST CANCER PREVENTION USING TAMOXIFEN

The observation that women treated with tamoxifen for breast cancer had a lower incidence of cancer in the other (contralateral) breast suggested that tamoxifen might have value in preventing breast cancer. To test this hypothesis, a randomized trial was initiated in 1992. By September 1997, 13,388 women 35 years of age or older had been enrolled in the trial and had been randomly assigned to receive either placebo or 20 mg per day of tamoxifen for 5 years. In March 1998, an independent, data-monitoring committee decided that the evidence of a reduction in breast cancer risk was sufficiently strong to warrant stopping the study before its planned end date. As seen in Fig. 11.14, cumulative rates of both invasive and noninvasive breast cancer were markedly reduced in women receiving tamoxifen. At the same time, as seen in Fig. 11.15, rates of invasive endometrial cancer were increased in the tamoxifen group. When the decision is being made

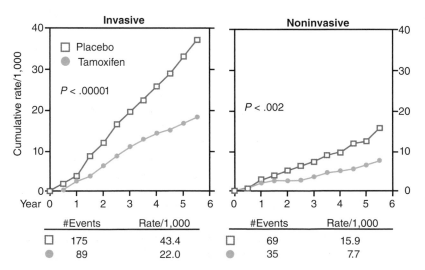

Fig. 11.14 Cumulative rates of invasive and noninvasive breast cancer occurring in participants receiving placebo or tamoxifen. (From Fisher B, Costantino JP, Wickerham DL, et al. Tamoxifen for prevention of breast cancer: report of the National Surgical Adjuvant Breast and Bowel Project P-1 Study. *J Natl Cancer Inst.* 1998;90:1371–1388.)

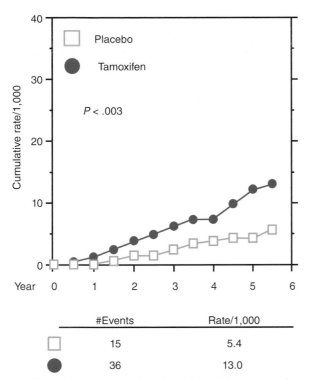

Fig. 11.15 Cumulative rates of invasive endometrial cancer occurring in participants receiving placebo or tamoxifen. (From Fisher B, Costantino JP, Wickerham DL, et al. Tamoxifen for prevention of breast cancer: report of the National Surgical Adjuvant Breast and Bowel Project P-1 Study. *J Natl Cancer Inst.* 1998;90:1371–1388.)

whether to use tamoxifen for breast cancer prevention, the potential benefits of tamoxifen must be weighed against the increased incidence of unanticipated side effects—in this case endometrial cancer. The picture is further complicated by the fact that at the time the results of this trial were published, two smaller studies in Europe did not find a similar reduction as reported in the US study. Thus the issue here is one of benefit versus harm; in addition, the question arises why other studies have not demonstrated the same marked effect on breast cancer incidence and how the results of those studies should be taken into account in developing public policy in this area.

Randomized Trials for Evaluating Widely Accepted Interventions

Randomized controlled trials can be used for two major purposes: (1) to evaluate new forms of intervention before they are approved and recommended for general use and (2) to evaluate interventions that are highly controversial or that have been widely used or recommended without ever having been adequately evaluated. In assessing the impact that randomized controlled trials have on medical practice, the latter use demonstrates the challenge of changing approaches used in existing medical practice that may not have been well evaluated. Two examples of such use are presented in this section.

A TRIAL OF ARTHROSCOPIC KNEE SURGERY FOR OSTEOARTHRITIS

About 6% of adults older than 30 years of age and 12% of adults older than 65 years of age have significant knee pain due to osteoarthritis. In the United States, a frequently performed operation for patients with knee pain and evidence of osteoarthritis has been arthroscopic surgery with lavage (washing out) or débridement (cleaning out) of the knee joint using an arthroscope. It has been estimated that the procedure is performed on more than 225,000 middle-aged and older adults each year, at an annual cost of more than $1 billion.

In a number of randomized controlled trials in which patients receiving débridement or lavage of the knee were compared with controls receiving no treatment, those who were treated reported more improvement in knee pain than those who were untreated. Other studies, however, in which only saline was injected into the knee, also reported improvement of knee symptoms. Thus it became clear that the perceived benefits might be related more to patient expectations (like a placebo effect) than to actual effectiveness, because the subjective improvements reported by patients were more likely when patients were not masked as to whether they received or did not receive surgical treatment. In order to resolve the question of whether arthroscopic lavage or débridement reduces symptoms of knee pain in patients with osteoarthritis, a randomized controlled trial was needed in which the controls would have a sham treatment. In July 2002, a beautifully conducted randomized trial of this procedure, using sham arthroscopy for the controls, was reported by Moseley and colleagues.[7]

The design of this study is shown in Fig. 11.16. One hundred eighty veterans were randomized to a group receiving arthroscopic débridement (59), a group receiving arthroscopic lavage (61), or a placebo group receiving a sham (placebo) intervention (60). The sham intervention consisted of a skin incision and simulated débridement without insertion of an arthroscope. Outcomes that were measured included level of knee pain, as determined by self-reports, and physical function, as determined by both self-reports and direct observation. These outcomes were assessed over a 2-year period. Raters who assessed pain and functional levels in the participants as well as the participants themselves were blinded to the treatment group assignment of each patient.

The results are shown in Figs. 11.17 and 11.18. At no point did either arthroscopic intervention group have greater pain relief than the placebo group (see Fig. 11.17). Moreover, at no point did either intervention group have significantly greater improvement in physical function than the placebo (sham intervention) group (see Fig. 11.18).

The principal investigator of the study, Dr. Nelda Wray, of the Houston Veterans Affairs Medical Center, where the trial was performed, summarized the results by saying, "Our study shows that the surgery is no better than the placebo—the procedure itself is useless." One month after publication of this study, the Department of Veterans Affairs issued an advisory to its physicians, stating that the procedure should not be performed pending additional review. The advisory statement said that knee pain was not a sufficient indicator for the surgery unless there was also evidence of "anatomic or mechanical abnormalities," which presumably could be improved by such a procedure.

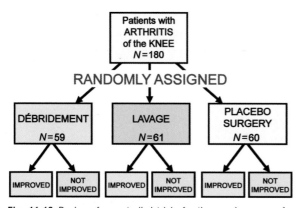

Fig. 11.16 Design of a controlled trial of arthroscopic surgery for osteoarthritis of the knee. (Based on Moseley JB, O'Malley K, Petersen NJ, et al. A controlled trial of arthroscopic surgery for osteoarthritis of the knee. *N Engl J Med.* 2002;347:81–88.)

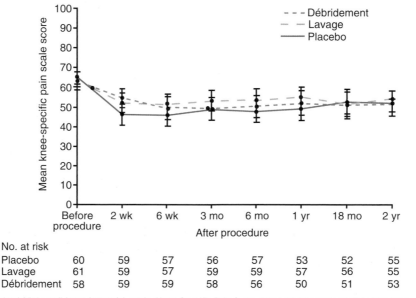

Fig. 11.17 Mean values (and 95% confidence intervals) on the Knee-Specific Pain Scale. Assessments were made before the procedure and 2 weeks, 6 weeks, 3 months, 6 months, 12 months, 18 months, and 24 months after the procedure. Higher scores indicate more severe pain. (From Moseley JB, O'Malley K, Petersen NJ, et al. A controlled trial of arthroscopic surgery for osteoarthritis of the knee. *N Engl J Med.* 2002;347(2):81–88.)

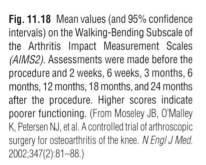

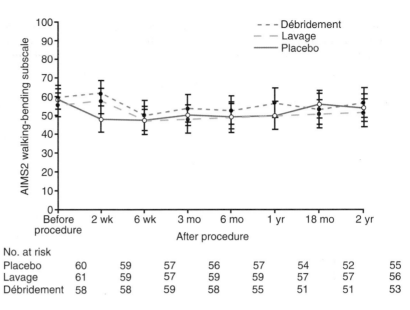

Fig. 11.18 Mean values (and 95% confidence intervals) on the Walking-Bending Subscale of the Arthritis Impact Measurement Scales *(AIMS2)*. Assessments were made before the procedure and 2 weeks, 6 weeks, 3 months, 6 months, 12 months, 18 months, and 24 months after the procedure. Higher scores indicate poorer functioning. (From Moseley JB, O'Malley K, Petersen NJ, et al. A controlled trial of arthroscopic surgery for osteoarthritis of the knee. *N Engl J Med.* 2002;347(2):81–88.)

No. at risk

Placebo	60	59	57	56	57	54	52	55
Lavage	61	59	57	59	59	57	57	56
Débridement	58	58	59	58	55	51	51	53

EFFECT OF GROUP PSYCHOSOCIAL SUPPORT ON SURVIVAL OF PATIENTS WITH METASTATIC BREAST CANCER

In 1989, a study was reported in which women with metastatic breast cancer were randomly assigned to supportive-expressive group therapy (a behavioral intervention) or to a control group. Supportive-expressive therapy is a standardized treatment for patients with life-threatening illness that encourages a group of participants, led by a therapist, to express their feelings and concerns about their illness and its impact. This study showed a survival benefit, although a survival analysis had not been originally planned in the study. Other trials of other psychosocial interventions have shown no survival benefit.

To clarify this issue, Goodwin and colleagues[8] conducted a multicenter randomized trial in which 235 women with metastatic breast cancer were randomized either to a group that received supportive-expressive therapy or to a control group that did not receive this intervention (Fig. 11.19). Of the 235 women, 158 were assigned to the intervention group and 77 to the control group.

Over the period of the study, survival was not prolonged in patients who received supportive-expressive therapy (Fig. 11.20). However, mood

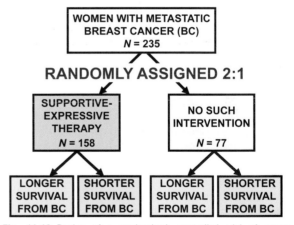

Fig. 11.19 Design of a randomized, controlled trial of group psychosocial support on survival in patients with metastatic breast cancer. (Data from Goodwin PJ, Leszcz M, Ennis M, et al. The effect of group psychosocial support on survival in metastatic breast cancer. *N Engl J Med.* 2001;345(24):1719–1726.)

and pain perception were improved, particularly in women who were the most distressed at study entry. Although the findings in the literature are still mixed regarding survival and additional studies are being conducted, the results of this study suggest that there is no survival benefit from this intervention. Therefore the wishes of women who choose to cope with their

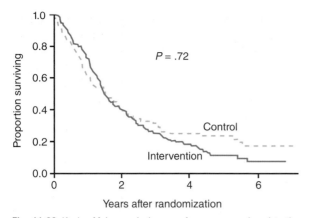

Fig. 11.20 Kaplan-Meier survival curves for women assigned to the intervention group and the control group. There was no significant difference in survival between the two groups. (From Goodwin PJ, Leszcz M, Ennis M, et al. The effect of group psychosocial support on survival in metastatic breast cancer. *N Engl J Med.* 2001;345(24):1719–1726.)

illness in different ways, including not sharing their feelings in a group, should be respected. Furthermore, it should not be suggested to women who prefer not to participate in such group therapy at this difficult time in their lives that their refusal may be hastening their own deaths.

Registration of Clinical Trials

It has long been recognized that not all results of clinical trials are published. This can pose a serious problem when the results from all published clinical trials are reviewed. For example, if clinical trials of a new drug are reviewed but only those that show beneficial results have been published and those showing negative results (for some reason) have not been published, an erroneous conclusion that *all* studies of the new drug have shown a clear benefit might be drawn from the published studies. This type of common problem is called *publication bias* or *non-publication bias*. For example, Liebeskind and colleagues[9] identified 178 controlled clinical trials of acute ischemic stroke reported in English over a 45-year period from 1955 to 1999 through a systematic search of several large databases. These trials enrolled a total of 73,949 subjects and evaluated 75 agents or other types of intervention. They found the issue of publication bias to be an important factor in reviewing the literature on trials of acute ischemic strokes. Trials in which the tested agent was shown to be harmful were substantially more likely *not* to be published than trials in which results indicated the tested agent was neutral or beneficial.

Several factors account for the problem of publication bias. Journals are eager to publish results from studies showing dramatic effects, rather than results from studies showing no benefit from a new drug, device, or other medical intervention. Both researchers and journals appear less interested in studies showing either that a new treatment is inferior to current treatment or that the findings are not clear one way or the other (null findings). An even more important issue is contributing to this problem: Companies that develop new drugs and fund studies of these drugs frequently want to keep the results unpublished when they show no benefits, or show serious side effects, or when the drug studied is shown to be less effective than currently available agents. The companies are clearly concerned that the results of such studies could adversely affect sales of the product and significantly impact the large potential profits they anticipate from the new agent. The net result, however, is concealment of the data, giving a picture of the agent—including its effectiveness and safety—that is not complete, so that regulators, physicians, and the public are prevented from making an evidence-based decision (i.e., a decision based on the total information generated through clinical trials).

The extent of the risk to public health from selective reporting of clinical trials and the frequency with which this selective reporting occurs led the International Committee of Medical Journal Editors to adopt a policy, which became effective in 2005, that *all* clinical trials of medical interventions must be registered in a public trials registry before any participants are enrolled in the study.[10] Medical interventions include drugs, surgical procedures, devices, behavioral treatments, and processes of health care. Registration in a registry accessible to the public at no charge is required before any clinical trial will be considered for publication by the major journals that have agreed to this policy. The federal repository for clinical trials is found at ClinicalTrials.gov on the internet. As of 2017, all NIH-funded clinical trials are expected to register and submit study results to ClinicalTrials.gov, according to the "*NIH Policy on Dissemination of NIH-Funded Clinical Trial Information*" (NOT-OD-16-149).[11]

Ethical Considerations

Many ethical issues arise in the context of clinical trials. One frequently raised question is whether randomization itself is ethical. How can we knowingly withhold a drug from patients, particularly those with serious and life-threatening diseases? Randomization is ethical only when we do not know whether drug A is better than drug B. We may have some indication that one treatment is better than the other (and often this is the rationale for conducting a trial in the first place), but we are not certain. Often, however, it is not clear at what point we "know" that drug A is better than drug B. The question may be better stated as, "When do we have adequate evidence to support the conclusion that drug A is better than drug B?" One question that has received considerable attention in recent years is whether it is ethical to use a placebo.[12] Implicit in this question is the issue of whether it is ethical to withhold a treatment that has been shown to be effective.[13]

The question can also be posed in the reverse: "Is it ethical not to randomize?" When we are considering drugs, preventive measures, or systems of health care delivery that apply to large numbers of people, both in the United States and in other countries, the mandate may be to carry out a randomized trial to resolve questions of benefit and harm, and not to continue to subject people to unnecessary toxic effects and raise false hopes, often at tremendous expense. Hence the question about the ethics of randomization should be asked in both directions: randomizing and not randomizing.

Another important question is whether truly informed consent can be obtained in studies. Many protocols for multicentered clinical trials require that patients be entered into the study immediately after diagnosis. The patient may be incapable of giving consent at that time, and the family may be so shocked by the diagnosis that has just been received and by its implications that they have great difficulty in dealing with the notion of randomization and agreement to be randomized. For example, much of the progress of recent decades in the treatment of childhood leukemia has been a result of the rigorous multicentered protocols that have required enrollment of the child immediately after the diagnosis of leukemia has been made. Clearly, at such a time the parents are so distressed that one may question whether they are capable of giving truly informed consent. Nevertheless, only through such rigorous trials has the progress been made that has saved the lives of so many children with acute leukemia.

Finally, under what circumstances should a trial be stopped earlier than originally planned? This is also a difficult issue and may arise because either harmful effects or beneficial effects of the agent become apparent early, before the full sample has been enrolled, or before subjects have been studied for the full follow-up period. In many studies, an outside data and safety monitoring board reviews the data as they are received, and the board makes that decision, as seen, for example, in the Physicians' Health Study discussed in Chapter 10, in which two medications were simultaneously tested in a factorial design: aspirin was tested for primary prevention of cardiovascular disease and beta carotene for primary prevention of cancer. The external data monitoring board decided that the findings for aspirin were sufficiently clear that the aspirin part of the study should be terminated but that the beta carotene portion of the study should be continued.

Conclusion

The randomized trial is the gold standard for evaluating the efficacy of therapeutic, preventive, and other measures in both clinical medicine and public health. This chapter and Chapter 10 have provided an overview of approaches to study design in randomized trials and the measures used to minimize or avoid selection and other types of bias. From a societal viewpoint, generalizability and ethical concerns are major considerations, and these issues have been discussed.

Epilogue

We conclude this discussion of randomized trials by citing an article by Caroline and Schwartz, which was published in the journal *Chest* in 1975. The article was titled "Chicken Soup Rebound and Relapse of Pneumonia: Report of a Case."[14]

The authors introduced their topic by saying:

Chicken soup has long been recognized to possess unusual therapeutic potency against a wide variety of viral and bacterial agents. Indeed, as early as the 12th century, the theologian, philosopher and physician, Moses Maimonides wrote, "Chicken soup ... is recommended as an excellent food as well as medication." Previous anecdotal reports regarding the therapeutic efficacy of this agent, however, have failed to provide details regarding the appropriate length of therapy. What follows is a case report in which abrupt withdrawal of chicken soup led to a severe relapse of pneumonia.[14]

The authors then present a case report of a 47-year-old physician who was treated with chicken soup for pneumonia. Chicken soup administration was terminated prematurely, and the patient suffered a relapse. Chicken soup being unavailable, the relapse was treated with intravenous penicillin.

The authors' discussion is of particular interest. It reads in part:

The therapeutic efficacy of chicken soup was first discovered several thousand years ago when an epidemic highly fatal to young Egyptian males seemed not to affect an ethnic minority residing in the same area. Contemporary epidemiologic inquiry revealed that the diet of the group not afflicted by the epidemic contained large amounts of a preparation made by boiling chicken with various vegetables and herbs. It is notable in this regard that the dietary injunctions given to Moses on Mount Sinai, while restricting consumption of no less than 19 types of fowl, exempted chicken from the prohibition. Some scholars believe that the recipe for chicken soup was transmitted to Moses on the same occasion, but was relegated to the oral tradition when the scriptures were canonized. … While chicken soup is now widely employed against a variety of organic and functional disorders, its manufacture remains largely in the hands of private individuals and standardization has proved nearly impossible. Preliminary investigation into the pharmacology of chicken soup (Bohbymycetin) has shown that it is readily absorbed after oral administration. … Parenteral administration is not recommended.[14]

This report stimulated several letters to the editor. In one, Dr. Laurence F. Greene, Professor of Urology at the Mayo Clinic, wrote:

You may be interested to know that we have successfully treated male impotence with another chicken-derived compound, sodium cytarabine hexamethylacetyl lututria tetrazolamine (Schmaltz [Upjohn]). This compound,

when applied in ointment form to the penis, not only cures impotence, but also increases libido and prevents premature ejaculation. … Preliminary studies indicate that its effects are dose related inasmuch as intercourse continues for 5 minutes when 5% ointment is applied, 15 minutes when 15% ointment is applied, and so forth.

We have received a grant in the sum of $650,000 from the National Scientific Foundation to carry out a prospective randomized, controlled double-blind study. Unfortunately, we are unable to obtain a suitable number of subjects inasmuch as each volunteer refuses to participate unless we assure him that he will be a subject rather than a control.[15]

REFERENCES

1. Gehan E. Clinical trials in cancer research. *Environ Health Perspect.* 1979;32:31.
2. Schröder FH, Hugosson J, Roobol MJ, et al. Screening and prostate-cancer mortality in a randomized European study. *N Engl J Med.* 2009;360:1320–1328.
3. Mant D. Can randomized trials inform clinical decisions about individual patients? *Lancet.* 1999;353:743–746.
4. Institute of Medicine. *Initial National Priorities for Comparative Effectiveness Research.* Washington, DC: National Academy Press; 2009. http://www.nap.edu/catalog.php?record_id=12648. Accessed October 5, 2017.
5. Veterans Administration Cooperative Study Group on Hypertensive Agents. Effects of treatment on morbidity in hypertension: results in patients with diastolic blood pressure averaging 115 through 129 mm Hg. *JAMA.* 1967;213:1028–1034.
6. Hypertension Detection and Follow-up Program Cooperative Group. Five year findings of the Hypertension Detection and Follow-up Program: I. Reduction of mortality of persons with high blood pressure, including mild hypertension. *JAMA.* 1979; 242:2562.
7. Moseley JB, O'Malley K, Petersen NJ, et al. A controlled trial of arthroscopic surgery for osteoarthritis of the knee. *N Engl J Med.* 2002;347:81–88.
8. Goodwin PJ, Leszcz M, Ennis M, et al. The effect of group psychosocial support on survival in metastatic breast cancer. *N Engl J Med.* 2001;345:1719–1726.
9. Liebeskind DS, Kidwell CS, Sayre JW, et al. Evidence of publication bias in reporting acute stroke clinical trials. *Neurology.* 2006;67:973–979.
10. DeAngelis CD, Drazen JM, Frizelle FA. Clinical trial registration: a statement from the International Committee of Medical Journal Editors. *JAMA.* 2004;292:1363–1364.
11. National Institutes of Health. *NIH policy on the dissemination of NIH-funded clinical trial information.* https://grants.nih.gov/grants/guide/notice-files/NOT-OD-16-149.html. Accessed October 5, 2017.
12. Emanuel EJ, Miller FG. The ethics of placebo-controlled trials: a middle ground. *N Engl J Med.* 2001;345:915–919.
13. Huston P, Peterson R. Withholding proven treatment in clinical research. *N Engl J Med.* 2001;345:912–914.
14. Caroline NL, Schwartz H. Chicken soup rebound and relapse of pneumonia: report of a case. *Chest.* 1975;67:215–216.
15. Greene LF. The chicken soup controversy [letter]. *Chest.* 1975;68:605.

REVIEW QUESTIONS FOR CHAPTERS 10 AND 11

1 *The major purpose of random assignment in a clinical trial is to:*

a. Help ensure that study subjects are representative of the general population

b. Facilitate double blinding (masking)

c. Facilitate the measurement of outcome variables

d. Ensure that the study groups have comparable baseline characteristics

e. Reduce selection bias in the allocation of treatment

2 *An advertisement in a medical journal stated that "2,000 subjects with sore throats were treated with our new medicine. Within 4 days, 94% were asymptomatic." The advertisement claims that the medicine was effective. Based on the evidence given above, the claim:*

a. Is correct

b. May be incorrect because the conclusion is not based on a rate

c. May be incorrect because of failure to recognize a long-term cohort phenomenon

d. May be incorrect because no test of statistical significance was used

e. May be incorrect because no control or comparison group was involved

3 *The purpose of a* double blind *or double masked study is to:*

a. Achieve comparability of treated and untreated subjects

b. Reduce the effects of sampling variation

c. Avoid observer and subject bias

d. Avoid observer bias and sampling variation

e. Avoid subject bias and sampling variation

4 *In many studies examining the association between estrogens and endometrial cancer of the uterus, a one-sided significance test was used. The underlying assumption justifying a one-sided rather than a two-sided test is:*

a. The distribution of the proportion exposed followed a "normal" pattern

b. The expectation before doing the study was that estrogens cause endometrial cancer of the uterus

c. The pattern of association could be expressed by a straight-line function

d. Type II error was the most important potential error to avoid

e. Only one control group was being used

5 *In a randomized trial, a planned crossover design:*

a. Eliminates the problem of a possible order effect

b. Must take into account the problem of possible residual effects of the first therapy

c. Requires stratified randomization

d. Eliminates the need for monitoring compliance and noncompliance

e. Enhances the generalizability of the results of the study

6 *A randomized trial comparing the efficacy of two drugs showed a difference between the two (with a P value $< .05$). Assume that in reality, however, the two drugs do not differ. This is therefore an example of the following:*

a. Type I error (α error)

b. Type II error (β error)

c. $1 - \alpha$

d. $1 - \beta$

e. None of the above

7 *All of the following are potential benefits of a randomized clinical trial, except:*

a. The likelihood that the study groups will be comparable is increased

b. Self-selection for a particular treatment is eliminated

c. The external validity of the study is increased

d. Assignment of the next subject cannot be predicted

e. The therapy that a subject receives is not influenced by either conscious or subconscious bias of the investigator

Number of Patients Needed in an Experimental and a Control Group for a Given Probability of Obtaining a Significant Result (Two-Sided Test)

Lower of the Two Cure Rates	DIFFERENCES IN THE CURE RATES BETWEEN THE TWO TREATMENT GROUPS					
	0.05	0.10	0.15	0.20	0.25	0.30
0.05	420	130	69	44	36	31
0.10	680	195	96	59	41	35
0.15	910	250	120	71	48	39
0.20	1,090	290	135	80	53	42
0.25	1,250	330	150	88	57	44
0.30	1,380	360	160	93	60	44
0.35	1,470	370	170	96	61	44
0.40	1,530	390	175	97	61	44

$\alpha = 0.05$; power $(1 - \beta) = 0.80$.
Data from Gehan E. Clinical trials in cancer research. *Environ Health Perspect.* 1979;32:31.

Question 8 is based on the above table.

8 *A drug company maintains that a new drug G for a certain disease has a 50% cure rate as compared with drug H, which has only a 25% cure rate. You are asked to design a clinical trial comparing drugs G and H. Using the preceding table, estimate the number of patients needed in each therapy group to detect such a difference with $\alpha = 0.05$, two-sided, and $\beta = 0.20$.*

The number of patients needed in each therapy group is _____.

Use your knowledge on study design to answer question 9.

9 *Choose the best study design from the list below for each of the following research questions. Each study design can only be used once.*

a. Ecologic study
b. Cross-sectional study
c. Case-control study
d. Prospective cohort
e. Randomized trial

9a. _____ An investigator wishes to determine if the prevalence of syphilis is higher among men than women.

9b. _____ A researcher believes that a rare disease may be associated with use of a common lawn fertilizer.

9c. _____ Health officials in Baltimore City believe that a smoking cessation program in combination with nicotine patches will be more effective than a cessation program alone.

9d. _____ Investigators want to determine the risk of potential health outcomes from heavy drinking among young adults.

9e. _____ A researcher believes that the county-level rate of hospitalization for cardiovascular disease will increase with increasing levels of outdoor air pollution.

Questions 10 and 11 involve the following randomized controlled trial, which explores the effects of a drug in reducing recurrent strokes:

Given the increasing burden of cardiovascular disease, a researcher designs a randomized controlled trial targeting patients who have experienced a stroke within the past 30 days. The trial is testing whether Drug A reduces the likelihood of stroke recurrence compared with the current standard of care (superiority trial). In the trial, 300 stroke patients are randomized into two groups where Group 1 receives Drug A and Group 2 receives standard of care. The investigator compared the cumulative incidence of a recurrent stroke between both groups. Some patients randomized to standard of care obtain Drug A through other means. Meanwhile, some participants randomized to Drug A ended up not taking it. The results from the randomized controlled trial are below:

	GROUP 1		GROUP 2	
	RANDOMIZED TO DRUG A		RANDOMIZED TO STANDARD OF CARE	
	Took Drug A	Standard of Care	Took Drug A	Standard of Care
Had a recurrent stroke	10	20	5	40
Did not have a recurrent stroke	80	40	15	90

10 *With an intention-to-treat analysis, calculate the cumulative incidence ratio for recurrent stroke using standard of care as the reference. Answers should be rounded to two decimal places.*

Cumulative Incidence Ratio = _____

11 *With a per-protocol analysis, calculate the cumulative incidence ratio for recurrent stroke using standard of care as the reference. Answers should be rounded to two decimal places.*

Cumulative Incidence Ratio = _____

Chapter 12

Estimating Risk: Is There an Association?

Learning Objectives

- To explore the concept of absolute risk.
- To introduce and compare relative risk and odds ratio as measures of association between an exposure and a disease.
- To calculate and interpret a relative risk in a cohort study.
- To calculate and interpret an odds ratio in a cohort study and in a case-control study and to describe when the odds ratio is a good estimate of the relative risk.
- To calculate and interpret an odds ratio in a matched-pairs case-control study.

In the previous chapters, we discussed the basic study designs that are commonly used in epidemiologic investigations. These are shown diagrammatically in Figs. 12.1 through 12.3.

Recall that the fundamental difference between a randomized trial and a cohort study is that, in a cohort study, subjects are not randomly assigned to be exposed or to remain unexposed, because randomization to exposure to possibly toxic or carcinogenic agents clearly would not be acceptable. Otherwise, cohort studies and randomized trials are essentially equivalent. Consequently, cohort studies are used in many studies of etiology because this study design enables us to capitalize on populations that have had a documented specified exposure and to compare them with populations that have not had that exposure. Case-control studies are also used to address questions of etiology, although often at a more exploratory phase. Regardless of which design is used, the objective is to determine whether there is an excess risk (incidence) or perhaps a reduced risk of (or protected from) a certain disease in association with a specified exposure

or characteristic. As stated earlier, incidence is a measure of risk of disease. Risk can be defined as the probability of an event (such as developing a disease) occurring.

Before describing these comparative approaches, we will discuss the concept of absolute risk.

Absolute Risk

The incidence of a disease in a population is termed the *absolute risk*. Absolute risk can indicate the magnitude of the risk in a group of people with a certain exposure, but because it does not take into consideration the risk of disease in unexposed individuals, it does not indicate whether the exposure is associated with an increased risk of the disease. Comparison is fundamental to epidemiology. Nevertheless, absolute risk may have important implications in both clinical medicine and public health policy. For example, a woman who contracts rubella in the first trimester of pregnancy and asks her physician, "What is the risk that my child will be malformed?" is given a certain number as an answer. On the basis of this information, she may decide to abort her pregnancy or to continue her pregnancy. She is not explicitly given comparative data, but an implicit comparison is generally being made: The woman is wondering not only what her risk is, but she also is wondering how that risk compares with what it would have been had she not contracted rubella (this is call the *counterfactual* in causal inference terms, to be discussed later in this book). So, although absolute risk does not stipulate any explicit comparison, an implicit comparison is often made whenever we look at the incidence of a disease. However, to address the question of association, we must use approaches that involve explicit comparisons.

How Do We Determine Whether a Certain Disease Is Associated With a Certain Exposure?

To determine whether an association exists between a specified exposure and a particular disease, we must determine, often using data obtained in cross-section, case-control, or cohort studies, whether there is an excess risk of the disease in persons who have been exposed to a certain agent. Let us consider the results of an investigation of a foodborne disease outbreak. The suspect foods were identified, and for each food, the attack rate (or incidence rate) of the disease was calculated for those who ate the food (exposed) and for those who did not eat the food (unexposed), as shown in Table 12.1.

How can we determine whether an excess risk is associated with each of the food items? One approach, shown in column C of Table 12.2, is to calculate the *ratio* of the attack rate (those we suspect

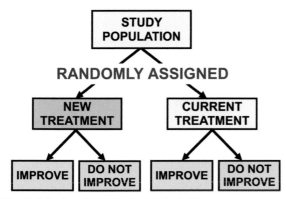

Fig. 12.1 Design of a randomized clinical trial.

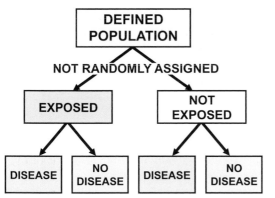

Fig. 12.2 Design of a cohort study.

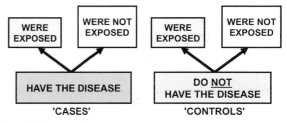

Fig. 12.3 Design of a case-control study.

TABLE 12.1 **Foodborne Disease Outbreak: I. Percent of People Sick Among Those Who Ate and Those Who Did Not Eat Specific Foods**		
Food	Ate (% Sick)	Did Not Eat (% Sick)
Egg salad	83	30
Macaroni	76	67
Cottage cheese	71	69
Tuna salad	78	50
Ice cream	78	64
Other	72	50

TABLE 12.2 **Foodborne Disease Outbreak: II. Ways of Calculating Excess Risk**				
Food	(A) Ate (% Sick)	(B) Did not eat (% Sick)	(C) (A)/(B)	(D) (A) − (B) (%)
Egg salad	83	30	2.77	53
Macaroni	76	67	1.13	9
Cottage cheese	71	69	1.03	2
Tuna salad	78	50	1.56	28
Ice cream	78	64	1.21	14
Other	72	50	1.44	22

were ill) in those who ate each food to the attack rate in those who did not eat the food. An alternate approach for identifying any excess risk in exposed individuals is shown in column D. We can subtract the risk in those who did not eat the food from the risk in those who did eat the food. The *difference* represents the excess absolute risk in those who were exposed.

Thus, as seen in this foodborne outbreak, to determine whether a certain exposure is associated with a certain disease, we must determine whether there is an excess risk of disease in exposed populations by comparing the risk of disease (in this case food poisoning) in exposed populations to the risk of disease in unexposed populations. We have just seen that such an excess risk can be calculated in the two following ways:

1. The *ratio* of the risks (or of the incidence rates):

$$\frac{\text{Disease risk in exposed}}{\text{Disease risk in unexposed}}$$

2. The *difference* in the risks (or in the incidence rates):

$$\left(\begin{array}{c}\text{Disease risk}\\\text{in exposed}\end{array}\right) - \left(\begin{array}{c}\text{Disease risk}\\\text{in unexposed}\end{array}\right)$$

Does the method that we choose to calculate excess risk make any difference? Let us consider a hypothetical example of two communities, A and B, seen in Table 12.3.

In community A, the incidence of a disease in exposed persons is 40% and the incidence in unexposed persons is 10%. Is there an excess risk associated with exposure? As in the food poisoning example, we can

calculate the ratio of the rates or the difference between the rates. The *ratio* of the incidence rates is 4.0. If we calculate the *difference* in incidence rates, it is 30%. In community B, the incidence in exposed persons is 90% and the incidence in unexposed persons is 60%. If we calculate the *ratio* of the incidence of exposed to unexposed persons in population B, it is 90/60, or 1.5. If we calculate the *difference* in the incidence in exposed and unexposed persons in community B it is, again, 30%.

What do these two measures tell us? Is there a difference in what we learn from the ratio of the incidence rates compared with the difference in the incidence rates? This question is the theme of this chapter and Chapter 13.

Relative Risk

CONCEPT OF RELATIVE RISK

Both case-control and cohort studies are designed to determine whether there is an association between exposure to a factor and development of a disease. If an association exists, how strong is it? If we carry out a cohort study, we can put the question another way: "What is the ratio of the risk of disease in exposed individuals to the risk of disease in unexposed individuals?" This ratio is called the *relative risk* (RR):

$$\text{Relative risk} = \frac{\text{Risk in exposed}}{\text{Risk in unexposed}}$$

The relative risk can also be defined as the probability of an event (developing a disease) occurring in exposed people compared with the probability of the event in unexposed people, or as the ratio of these two probabilities.

INTERPRETING THE RELATIVE RISK

How do we interpret the value of a relative risk?

1. If the relative risk is equal to 1, the numerator equals the denominator, and the risk in exposed persons equals the risk in unexposed persons. Therefore no evidence exists for any increased risk in exposed individuals or for any association of the disease with the exposure in question.
2. If the relative risk is greater than 1, the numerator is greater than the denominator, and the risk in

TABLE 12.3 Example Comparing Two Ways of Calculating Excess Risk

	POPULATION	
	A	B
Incidence (%)		
In exposed	40	90
In unexposed	10	60
Difference in incidence rates (%)	30	30
Ratio of incidence rates	4.0	1.5

exposed persons is greater than the risk in unexposed persons. This is evidence of a positive association, which may be causal (as discussed in a later chapter).

3. If the relative risk is less than 1, the numerator is less than the denominator, and the risk in exposed persons is less than the risk in unexposed persons. This is evidence of a negative association, which may be indicative of a protective effect. Such a finding can be observed in people who are given an effective vaccine ("exposed" to the vaccine).

These three possibilities are summarized in Table 12.4.

CALCULATING THE RELATIVE RISK IN COHORT STUDIES

In a *cohort* study the relative risk can be calculated *directly*. Recall the design of a cohort study, seen here in Table 12.5.

In this table, we see that the incidence in exposed individuals is

$$\frac{a}{a+b}$$

and the incidence in unexposed individuals is

$$\frac{c}{c+d}$$

We calculate the relative risk as follows:

$$\text{Relative risk} = \frac{\text{Incidence in exposed}}{\text{Incidence in unexposed}} = \frac{\left(\dfrac{a}{a+b}\right)}{\left(\dfrac{c}{c+d}\right)}$$

Table 12.6 shows a hypothetical cohort study of 3,000 smokers and 5,000 nonsmokers to investigate the relation of smoking to the development of coronary heart disease (CHD) over a 1-year period.

TABLE 12.4 Interpreting Relative Risk (RR) of a Disease	
If RR = 1	Risk in exposed equal to risk in unexposed (no association)
If RR > 1	Risk in exposed greater than risk in unexposed (positive association; possibly causal)
If RR < 1	Risk in exposed less than risk in unexposed (negative association; possibly protective)

TABLE 12.5 Risk Calculations in a Cohort Study

		THEN FOLLOW TO SEE WHETHER			
		Disease Develops	Disease Does Not Develop	Totals	Incidence Rates of Disease
First, Select	Exposed	a	b	$a + b$	$\dfrac{a}{a+b}$
	Not exposed	c	d	$c + d$	$\dfrac{c}{c+d}$

$\dfrac{a}{a+b}$ = Incidence in exposed $\dfrac{c}{c+d}$ = Incidence in nonexposed

TABLE 12.6 Smoking and Coronary Heart Disease (CHD): A Hypothetical Cohort Study of 3,000 Cigarette Smokers and 5,000 Nonsmokers

	CHD Develops	CHD Does Not Develop	Totals	Incidence per 1,000 per Year
Smoke cigarettes	84	2,916	3,000	28.0
Do not smoke cigarettes	87	4,913	5,000	17.4

In this example:

$$\text{Incidence among the exposed} = \frac{84}{3,000}$$

$$= 28.0 \text{ per } 1,000$$

and

$$\text{Incidence among the unexposed} = \frac{87}{5,000}$$

$$= 17.4 \text{ per } 1,000$$

Consequently,

$$\text{Relative risk} = \frac{\text{Incidence in exposed}}{\text{Incidence in unexposed}}$$

$$= \frac{28.0}{17.4} = 1.61$$

A similar expression of risks is seen in an historical example in Table 12.7, which shows data from the first 12 years of the Framingham Study relating risk of coronary disease to age, sex, and cholesterol level.

First, direct your attention to the upper part of the table, which shows incidence rates per 1,000 population in Framingham by age, sex, and serum cholesterol level.

In men the association of risk to cholesterol level seems dose related; risk increases for both age groups with increases in cholesterol level. The relationship is not as consistent in women.

In the lower half of the table, the values have been converted to relative risks. The authors have taken the incidence rate of 38.2 in younger men with low cholesterol levels and assigned it a risk of 1.0; these subjects are considered "unexposed." All other risks in the table are expressed in relation to this risk of 1.0. For example, the incidence of 157.5 in younger men with a cholesterol level greater than 250 mg/dL is compared with the 38.2 incidence rate; by dividing 157.5 by 38.2 we obtain a relative risk of 4.1. Using these relative risks, it is easier to compare the risks and to identify any trends. Although the lowest risk in men has been chosen as the standard and set at 1.0, the authors could have chosen to set any of the values in the table at 1.0 and to make all others relative to it. Thus, when describing the relative risk, the numerator and denominator categories should be specified (e.g., in Table 12.7 the risk of younger men with cholesterol levels ≥250 mg/dL is approximately four times higher than that of younger men whose cholesterol levels are <190 mg/dL). One reason for choosing a low value as the standard is that most of the other values will be greater than 1.0; for most people, the table is easier

TABLE 12.7   Relationship Between Serum Cholesterol Levels and Risk of Coronary Heart Disease by Age and Sex: Framingham Study During First 12 Years

Serum Cholesterol (mg/dL)	MEN		WOMEN	
	30–49 Years	50–62 Years	30–49 Years	50–62 Years
	Incidence Rates (per 1,000)			
<190	38.2	105.7	11.1	155.2
190–219	44.1	187.5	9.1	88.9
220–249	95.0	201.1	24.3	96.3
250+	157.5	267.8	50.4	121.5
	Relative Risks[a]			
<190	1.0	2.8	0.3	4.1
190–219	1.2	4.9	0.2	2.3
220–249	2.5	5.3	0.6	2.5
250+	4.1	7.0	1.3	3.2

[a]Incidence for each subgroup is compared with that of males 30 to 49 years of age, with serum cholesterol levels less than 190 mg/dL (risk = 1.0).

From Truett J, Cornfield J, Kannel W. A multivariate analysis of the risk of coronary heart disease in Framingham. *J Chronic Dis*. 1967;20:511–524.

to read when fewer values are completely to the right of the decimal.

Fig. 12.4 shows data based on merging 2,282 middle-aged men followed for 10 years in the Framingham Study and 1,838 middle-aged men followed for 8 years in Albany, New York. The data relate smoking, cholesterol level, and blood pressure to risk of myocardial infarction and death from CHD. Recall that at this point in history, these associations were not yet known, although currently we all agree that they are now established risk factors for heart disease. The authors have assigned a value of 1 to the lowest of the risks in each of the two parts of the figure, and the other risks are calculated relative to this value. On the left is shown the risk in nonsmokers with low cholesterol levels (which has been set at 1) and the risk in nonsmokers with high cholesterol levels; risks for smokers with low and high cholesterol levels are each calculated relative to risks for nonsmokers with low cholesterol levels. Note that the risk is higher with high cholesterol levels, and that this holds both in smokers and in nonsmokers (although the risk is higher in smokers even when cholesterol levels are low). Thus both smoking and elevated cholesterol levels contribute to the risk of myocardial infarction and death from CHD. A comparable analysis with blood pressure and smoking is shown on the right side of the figure.

Odds Ratio (Relative Odds)

We have seen that, to calculate a relative risk, we must have values for the incidence of the disease in the exposed and the incidence in the unexposed, as can be obtained from a cohort study. However, in a *case-control* study, we do not know the incidence in the exposed population or the incidence in the unexposed population because we start with diseased people (cases) and nondiseased people (controls). Hence in a case-control study we *cannot* calculate the relative risk directly. In this section we will see how another measure of association, the *odds ratio* (OR), can be obtained from either a cohort or a case-control study and can be used instead of the relative risk. We will also see that even though we cannot calculate a relative risk from a case-control study, under many conditions we can obtain a very good *estimate* of the relative risk from a case-control study using the odds ratio.

DEFINING THE ODDS RATIO IN COHORT AND IN CASE-CONTROL STUDIES

In previous chapters we discussed the *proportion* of the exposed population in whom disease develops and the *proportion* of the unexposed population in whom disease develops in a cohort study. Similarly, in case-control studies, we have discussed the *proportion* of the cases who were exposed and the *proportion* of the controls who were exposed (Table 12.8).

An alternate approach is to use the concept of *odds*. When betting at the racetrack, you typically consider the odds of each horse winning—the so-called handicapping system. Suppose we are betting on a horse named Epi Beauty, which has a 60% probability of winning the race (*P*). Epi Beauty therefore has a 40% probability of losing (1 − *P*). If these are the probabilities, what

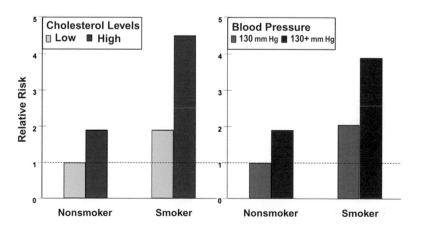

Fig. 12.4 Relative risk for myocardial infarction and death from coronary heart disease in men aged 30 to 62 years by serum cholesterol *(left)* and blood pressure levels *(right)* in relation to cigarette smoking. High cholesterol levels are defined as 220 mg/dL or greater. (Data from Doyle JT, Dawber TR, Kannel WB, et al. The relationship of cigarette smoking to coronary heart disease. *JAMA.* 1964;190:886.)

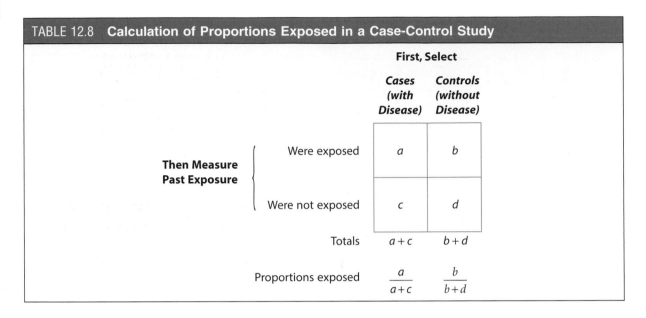

TABLE 12.8 **Calculation of Proportions Exposed in a Case-Control Study**

		First, Select	
		Cases (with Disease)	*Controls (without Disease)*
Then Measure Past Exposure	Were exposed	*a*	*b*
	Were not exposed	*c*	*d*
	Totals	*a + c*	*b + d*
	Proportions exposed	$\dfrac{a}{a+c}$	$\dfrac{b}{b+d}$

are the *odds* that the horse will win the race? To answer this, we must keep in mind that *the odds of an event can be defined as the ratio of the number of ways the event can occur to the number of ways the event cannot occur.* Consequently, the odds of Epi Beauty winning, as defined previously, are as follows:

$$Odds = \frac{\text{Probability that Epi Beauty will win the race}}{\text{Probability that Epi Beauty will lose the race}}$$

Recall that, if *P* is the probability that Epi Beauty will win the race, $1 - P$ equals the probability that Epi Beauty will lose the race. Consequently, the odds of Epi Beauty winning are:

$$Odds = \frac{P}{1-P} \quad \text{or} \quad \frac{60\%}{40\%} = 1.5:1 = 1.5$$

It is important to keep in mind the distinction between *probability* and *odds*. In the previous example:

$$\text{Probability of winning} = 60\%$$

and

$$\text{Odds of winning} = \frac{60\%}{40\%} = 1.5$$

Odds Ratio in Cohort Studies

Let us examine how the concept of odds can be applied to both cohort and case-control studies. Let us first consider the cohort study design shown in Fig. 12.5A. Our first question is, "What is the *probability (P)* that the disease will develop in an exposed person?" The answer to this is the incidence of the disease in the top row (exposed persons), which equals $\dfrac{a}{a+b}$. Next let us ask, "What are the *odds* that the disease will develop in an exposed person?" Again, looking only at the top row in Fig. 12.5A, we see that there are $(a + b)$ exposed persons; the odds that the disease will develop in them are $a : b$, or $\dfrac{a}{b}$. (Recall $\dfrac{P}{1-P}$ from the Epi Beauty example.) Similarly, looking only at the bottom row of this table, there are $(c + d)$ unexposed persons; the probability that the disease will develop in unexposed persons is $\dfrac{c}{c+d}$ and the odds of the disease developing in these unexposed persons are $c : d$, or $\dfrac{c}{d}$.

Just as the ratio of the incidence in the exposed to the incidence in the unexposed can be used to measure an association of exposure and disease, we can also look at the ratio of the odds that the disease will develop

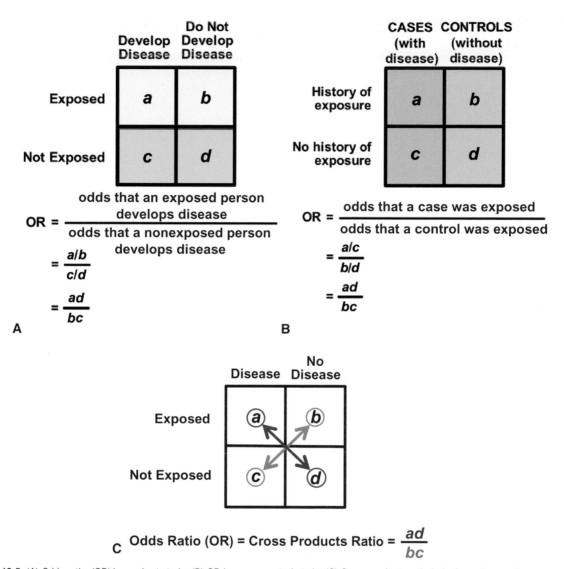

Fig. 12.5 (A) Odds ratio *(OR)* in a cohort study. (B) OR in a case-control study. (C) Cross-products ratio in both a cohort and a case-control study.

in an exposed person to the odds that it will develop in an unexposed person. Either measure of association is valid in a cohort study.

In a cohort study, to answer the question of whether there is an association between the exposure and the disease, we can either use the relative risk discussed in the previous section or we can use the odds ratio (also called the *relative odds*). In a *cohort study* the odds ratio

is defined as the *ratio of the odds of developing disease in exposed persons to the odds of developing disease in unexposed persons*, and it can be calculated as follows:

$$\frac{\left(\dfrac{a}{b}\right)}{\left(\dfrac{c}{d}\right)} = \frac{ad}{bc}$$

Odds Ratio in a Case-Control Study

As just discussed, in a *case-control study*, we cannot calculate the relative risk directly to determine whether there is an association between the exposure and the disease. This is because, having started with cases and controls rather than with exposed and unexposed persons, we do not have information about the incidence of disease in exposed versus unexposed persons. However, although we can use the odds ratio as a measure of the association between exposure and disease in a case-control study, we ask somewhat different questions: "What are the odds that a case was exposed?" Looking at the left-hand column in Fig. 12.5B, we see that the *odds* of a case having been exposed are $a : c$, or $\frac{a}{c}$. Next, we ask, "What are the odds that a control was exposed?" Looking at the right-hand column, we see that the *odds* of a control having been exposed are $b : d$, or $\frac{b}{d}$.

We can then calculate the odds ratio, which, in a case-control study, is defined as the ratio of the odds that the cases were exposed to the odds that the controls were exposed. This is calculated as follows:

$$\frac{\left(\dfrac{a}{c}\right)}{\left(\dfrac{b}{d}\right)} = \frac{ad}{bc}$$

Thus, interestingly, $\frac{ad}{bc}$ represents the odds ratio (or relative odds) in *both* cohort (see Fig. 12.5A) and case-control (see Fig. 12.5B) studies. In both types of studies the odds ratio is an excellent measure of whether a certain exposure is associated with a specific disease. The *odds ratio* is also known as the *cross-products ratio*, because it can be obtained by multiplying both diagonal cells in a 2 × 2 table and then dividing $\frac{ad}{bc}$, as seen in Fig. 12.5C. Note that, when calculating the odds ratio as a cross-products ratio, the format of the table must be exactly as shown in Table 12.5 (i.e., cases on the left hand side column and exposed individuals in the upper row). Failure to do so will result in an incorrectly calculated odds ratio.

Note also that, in both cohort and case-control studies, the odds ratio can be calculated as the cross-products ratio, which means that the odds ratio of exposure from a case-control study equals the odds ratio of disease. For example, in a case-control study of Alzheimer disease, a condition that is fairly common in the elderly, Tolppanen et al.,[1] using a 5-year lag time, found that cases had an odds of past brain injury 1.23 times higher than that in controls. When reporting these results, it would be correct but not too useful to say that the odds of past brain injury (exposure) in cases was 2.4 times greater than that in controls. However, because epidemiology is always concerned with identifying predictors of disease and as the odds ratio of exposure is the same as the odds ratio of disease, a more useful description of this result would be that the odds of developing Alzheimer disease in individuals with a brain injury (exposure) was 1.23 times higher than in those without an episode of brain injury. In other words, even in case-control studies, the interpretation of the odds ratio is always prospective. (Note that, because Alzheimer disease is common in the elderly, the odds ratio in this example is generally not considered to be a good estimate of the relative risk and thus the odds ratio must be described in terms of odds, not of risks. See also the section below, titled "When Is the Odds Ratio a Good Estimate of the Relative Risk?")

The odds ratio or the cross-products ratio can be viewed as the ratio of the product of the two cells that support the hypothesis of an association (cells *a* and *d*—diseased people who were exposed and nondiseased people who were not exposed), to the product of the two cells that negate the hypothesis of an association (cells *b* and *c*—nondiseased people who were exposed and diseased people who were not exposed).

Interpreting the Odds Ratio

We interpret the odds ratio just as we have interpreted the relative risk. If the exposure is not related to the disease, the odds ratio will equal 1. If the exposure is positively related to the disease, the odds ratio will be greater than 1. If the exposure is negatively related to the disease (i.e., it is protective), the odds ratio will be less than 1.

WHEN IS THE ODDS RATIO A GOOD ESTIMATE OF THE RELATIVE RISK?

In a case-control study, only the odds ratio can be calculated as a measure of association, whereas in a cohort study, either the relative risk or the odds ratio is a valid measure of association. However, many people are more comfortable using the relative risk, and this is the more frequently used measure of association reported in the literature when cohort studies are published. Even when the odds ratio is used, people are often interested in knowing how well it approximates the relative risk. Even prestigious clinical journals have been known to publish reports of case-control studies and to label a column of results as *relative risks*. Having read the discussion in this chapter, you should now be aghast to see such a presentation because you now know that relative risks cannot be calculated directly from a case-control study! Clearly, what is meant is an *estimate* of relative risks based on the odds ratios that are obtained in the case-control studies.

When is the odds ratio (relative odds) obtained in a case-control study a good approximation of the relative risk in the population? When the following three conditions are met:

1. When the *cases* studied are representative, with regard to history of exposure, of all people with the disease in the population from which the cases were drawn.
2. When the *controls* studied are representative, with regard to history of exposure, of all people without the disease in the population from which the cases were drawn.
3. When the disease being studied does not occur frequently.

This third condition—also known as the "rarity assumption"—has a statistical, rather than a public health, meaning. For example, a disease with an incidence of 4% in the exposed individuals and 2% in the unexposed cannot be said to be infrequent from the population viewpoint. However, from the viewpoint of the rarity assumption, the disease is rare and thus the relative risk (2.0) and the odds ratio (2.04) are virtually the same.

The third condition (that the disease occurrence is not frequent) can be intuitively explained as follows:

Recall that there are $(a + b)$ exposed persons. Because most diseases with which we are dealing occur infrequently, very few persons in an exposed population will actually develop the disease; consequently, a is very small compared with b, and one can approximate $(a + b)$ as b, or $(a + b) \cong b$. Similarly, very few unexposed

persons $(c + d)$ develop the disease, and we can approximate $(c + d)$ as d, or $(c + d) \cong d$. Therefore we may calculate a relative risk as follows:

$$\frac{\left(\dfrac{a}{a+b}\right)}{\left(\dfrac{c}{c+d}\right)} \cong \frac{\left(\dfrac{a}{b}\right)}{\left(\dfrac{c}{d}\right)}$$

From performing this calculation, we obtain $\dfrac{ad}{bc}$, which is the odds ratio. For the committed reader, a neater and more sophisticated derivation is provided in the appendix to this chapter.

Figs. 12.6 and 12.7 show two examples of cohort studies that demonstrate how the odds ratio provides a good approximation of the relative risk when the occurrence of a disease is infrequent but not when it is frequent. In Fig. 12.6 the occurrence of disease is infrequent and we see that the relative risk is 2. If we now calculate an odds (cross-products) ratio, we find it to be 2.02, which is a very close approximation.

Now, let us examine Fig. 12.7, in which the occurrence of disease is more frequent. Although the relative risk is again 2.0, the odds ratio is 3.0, which is considerably different from the relative risk.

We therefore see that the odds ratio is in itself a valid measure of association without considering relative

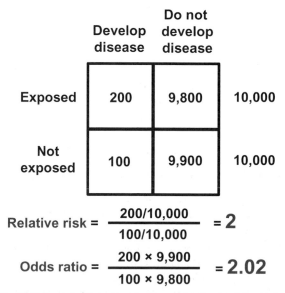

Fig. 12.6 Example: The odds ratio is a good estimate of the relative risk when a disease is infrequent.

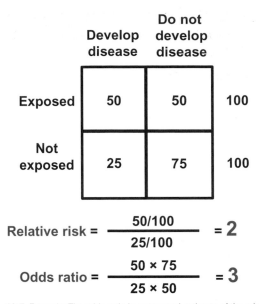

$$\text{Relative risk} = \frac{50/100}{25/100} = 2$$

$$\text{Odds ratio} = \frac{50 \times 75}{25 \times 50} = 3$$

Fig. 12.7 Example: The odds ratio is *not* a good estimate of the relative risk when a disease is *not* infrequent.

CASES	CONTROLS
E	N
E	E
N	N
E	N
N	E
N	N
E	N
E	E
E	N
N	N

E = Exposed
N = Not Exposed

Fig. 12.8 A case-control study of 10 cases and 10 unmatched controls.

risk. However, if you choose to use the relative risk as the index of association, when the disease occurrence is infrequent, the odds ratio is a very good approximation of the relative risk.

Remember:

- The relative odds (odds ratio) is a useful measure of association, in and of itself, in both case-control and cohort studies.
- In a cohort study the relative risk can be calculated directly.
- In a case-control study the relative risk cannot be calculated directly, so that the relative odds or odds ratio (cross-products ratio) is used as an estimate of the relative risk when the risk of the disease is low.

The case-control study conducted by Arvonen et al.[2] is an example of the odds ratio as a good estimate of the relative risk. These authors found an odds ratio of 2.4 for the association of cow's milk allergy in infancy (exposure) with the development of juvenile idiopathic arthritis. Because the incidence of this disease is very low (approximately 13.9 per 100,000),[3] an accurate interpretation of the odds ratio would be that the *risk* of the disease in the exposed individuals is more than two times higher than that in the unexposed.

EXAMPLES OF CALCULATING ODDS RATIOS IN CASE-CONTROL STUDIES

In this section, we will calculate odds ratios in two case-control studies (one in which the controls were *not* matched to the cases, and the other in which they *were* matched). For purposes of these examples, let us assume the following: our research budget is incredibly small, so we have carried out a case-control study of only 10 cases and 10 controls. This disease may have just been recognized and there are very few identified cases to date; however, the disease itself is very lethal! N indicates an unexposed individual, and E indicates an *exposed* individual.

Calculating the Odds Ratio in an Unmatched Case-Control Study

Let us assume that this case-control study is done without any matching of controls to cases and that we obtain the results seen in Fig. 12.8. Thus 6 of the 10 cases were exposed and 3 of the 10 controls were exposed. If we arrange these data in a 2 × 2 table, we obtain the following:

The odds ratio in this *unmatched* study equals the ratio of the cross-products:

$$\text{Odds ratio} = \frac{ad}{bc}$$

$$\text{Odds ratio} = \frac{6 \times 7}{4 \times 3} = \frac{42}{12} = 3.5$$

TABLE 12.9	**Example of Calculating an Odds Ratio from a Case-Control Study**

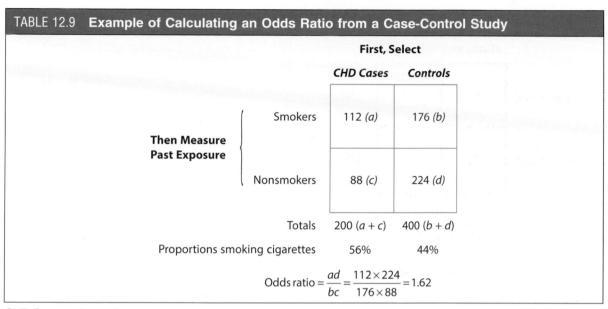

First, Select

		CHD Cases	*Controls*
Then Measure Past Exposure	Smokers	112 *(a)*	176 *(b)*
	Nonsmokers	88 *(c)*	224 *(d)*
	Totals	200 *(a + c)*	400 *(b + d)*
	Proportions smoking cigarettes	56%	44%

$$\text{Odds ratio} = \frac{ad}{bc} = \frac{112 \times 224}{176 \times 88} = 1.62$$

CHD, Coronary heart disease.

Table 12.9 shows data from an unmatched case-control study of smoking and CHD. The letters *a, b, c,* and *d* have been inserted to identify the cells of the 2 × 2 table that are used for the calculation. The odds ratio, as calculated from these data, is as follows:

$$\text{Odds ratio} = \frac{ad}{bc} = \frac{112 \times 224}{176 \times 88} = 1.62$$

Calculating the Odds Ratio in a Matched-Pairs Case-Control Study

As discussed previously, in selecting the study population in case-control studies, controls are often selected by matching each one to a case according to variables that are known to be related to disease risk, such as sex, age, or race (using individual matching or matched pairs). The results are then analyzed in terms of case-control pairs rather than for individual subjects.

What types of case-control combinations are possible in regard to exposure history? Clearly, if exposure is dichotomous (a person is either exposed or not exposed), only the following four types of case-control pairs are possible:

Concordant pairs
1. Pairs in which *both* the case and the control were exposed
2. Pairs in which *neither* the case nor the control was exposed

Discordant pairs
3. Pairs in which the case was exposed but the control was not
4. Pairs in which the control was exposed but the case was not

Note that the case-control pairs that had the same exposure experience are termed *concordant pairs* and those with different exposure experience are termed *discordant pairs.* These possibilities are shown schematically in a 2 × 2 table. Note that unlike other 2 × 2 tables that we have examined previously, the figure in each cell represents pairs of subjects (i.e., *case-control pairs*), *not* individual subjects. Thus the table contains *a* pairs—in which both the case and the control were exposed; *b* pairs—in which the case was exposed and the control was not; *c* pairs—in which the case was not exposed and the control was exposed; and *d* pairs—in which neither the case nor the control was exposed.

Calculation of the odds ratio in such a matched-pair study is based on the *discordant pairs* only (*b* and *c*). The concordant pairs (*a* and *d*, in which cases and controls were either both exposed or both not exposed) are ignored because they do not contribute to our knowledge of how cases and controls differ in regard to past history of exposure.

The odds ratio for matched pairs is therefore the ratio of the discordant pairs (i.e., the ratio of the number of pairs in which the case was exposed and the control was not, to the number of pairs in which the control was exposed and the case was not). The odds ratio for the preceding 2 × 2 table is as follows:

$$\text{Matched pairs odds ratio} = \frac{b}{c}$$

Again, the matched-pairs odds ratio can be viewed as the ratio of the number of pairs that support the hypothesis of an association (pairs in which the case was exposed and the control was not) to the number of pairs that negate the hypothesis of an association (pairs in which the control was exposed and the case was not).

Let us now look at an example of an odds ratio calculation in a matched-pairs case-control study (Fig. 12.9). Let us return to our low-budget study, which included only 10 cases and 10 controls: now our study is designed so that each control has been individually matched to a case, resulting in 10 case-control *pairs*

(the horizontal arrows indicate the matching of pairs). If we use these findings to construct a 2 × 2 table for *pairs*, we obtain the following:

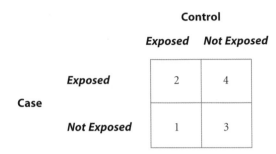

Note that there are two pairs in which *both* the case and the control were exposed and three pairs in which *neither* the case *nor* the control was exposed. These concordant pairs are ignored in the analysis of matched pairs.

There are four pairs in which the case was exposed and the control was not and one pair in which the control was exposed and the case was not.

Hence the odds ratio for matched pairs is as follows:

$$\text{Matched pairs odds ratio} = \frac{b}{c} = \frac{4}{1} = 4$$

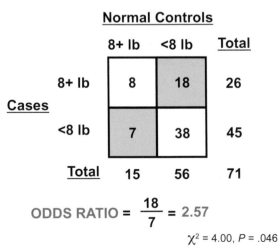

$$\text{ODDS RATIO} = \frac{18}{7} = 2.57$$

$$\chi^2 = 4.00, P = .046$$

Fig. 12.10 Birth weight of index child: matched-pairs comparison of cases and normal controls (≥8 lb vs. <8 lb). (Data from Gold E, Gordis L, Tonascia J, et al. Risk factors for brain tumors in children. *Am J Epidemiol.* 1979;109:309–319.)

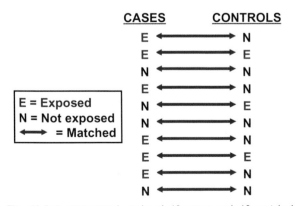

Fig. 12.9 A case-control study of 10 cases and 10 matched controls.

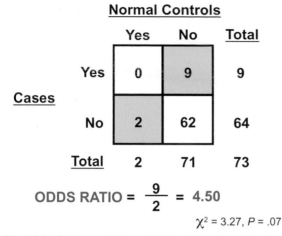

Normal Controls

		Yes	No	Total
Cases	Yes	0	9	9
	No	2	62	64
	Total	2	71	73

$$\text{ODDS RATIO} = \frac{9}{2} = 4.50$$

$\chi^2 = 3.27, P = .07$

Fig. 12.11 Exposure of index child to sick pets: matched-pairs comparison of cases and normal controls. (Data from Gold E, Gordis L, Tonascia J, et al. Risk factors for brain tumors in children. *Am J Epidemiol.* 1979;109:309–319.)

Figs. 12.10 and 12.11 present data selected from the case-control study of brain tumors in children that was discussed in a previous chapter. Data are shown for two variables. Fig. 12.10 presents a matched-pairs analysis for birth weight. A number of studies have suggested that children with higher birth weights are at increased risk for certain childhood cancers. In this analysis, *exposure* is defined as birth weight greater than 8 lb. The result is an odds ratio of 2.57.

In Fig. 12.11 a matched-pairs analysis is presented for exposure to sick pets. Many years ago, the Tri-State Leukemia Study found that more cases of leukemia than controls had family pets. Interest in oncogenic viruses stimulated an interest in exposure to sick pets as a possible source of such agents. Gold and coworkers explored this question in their case-control study,[4] and the results are shown in Fig. 12.11. Although the odds ratio was 4.5, the number of discordant pairs was very small.

Although the above-mentioned examples are a bit historical, the way the calculation of both RR and OR is done is the same in more contemporary research articles. However, the current presentation of the results focuses more on adjustment to potential confounding variables.

Conclusion

This chapter has introduced the concepts of absolute risk, relative risk, and odds ratio. In Chapter 13 we turn to another important aspect of risk: the attributable risk. We will then review the study designs and indices of risk that have been discussed before addressing the use of these concepts in deriving causal inferences.

REFERENCES

1. Tolppanen AM, TAipale H, Hartikainen S. Head or brain injuries and Alzheimer's disease: a nested case-control regiser study. *Alzheimers Dement.* 2017;13:1371–1379.
2. Arvonen M, Virta LJ, Pokka T, et al. Cow's milk allergy in infancy and later development of juvenile idiopathic arthritis: a register-based case-control study. *Am J Epidemiol.* 2017;186: 237–244.
3. Towner SR, Michet CJ Jr, O'Fallon WM, et al. The epidemiology of juvenile arthritis in Rochester, Minnesota 1960-1979. *Arthritis Rheum.* 1983;26:1208–1213.
4. Gold E, Gordis L, Tonascia J, et al. Risk factors for brain tumors in children. *Am J Epidemiol.* 1979;109:309–319.

REVIEW QUESTIONS FOR CHAPTER 12

1 *Of 2,872 persons who had received radiation treatment in childhood because of an enlarged thymus, cancer of the thyroid developed in 24 and a benign thyroid tumor developed in 52. A comparison group consisted of 5,055 children who had received no such treatment (brothers and sisters of the children who had received radiation treatment). During the follow-up period, none of the comparison group developed thyroid cancer, but benign thyroid tumors developed in six. Calculate the relative risk for benign thyroid tumors:* _____

Questions 2 and 3 are based on the information given in the following table.

In a small pilot study, 12 women with uterine cancer and 12 with no apparent disease were contacted and asked whether they had ever used estrogen. Each woman with cancer was matched by age, race, weight, and parity to a woman without disease. The results are shown below:

Pair No.	Women With Uterine Cancer	Women Without Uterine Cancer
1	Estrogen user	Estrogen nonuser
2	Estrogen nonuser	Estrogen nonuser
3	Estrogen user	Estrogen user
4	Estrogen user	Estrogen user
5	Estrogen user	Estrogen nonuser
6	Estrogen nonuser	Estrogen nonuser
7	Estrogen user	Estrogen nonuser
8	Estrogen user	Estrogen nonuser
9	Estrogen nonuser	Estrogen user
10	Estrogen nonuser	Estrogen user
11	Estrogen user	Estrogen nonuser
12	Estrogen user	Estrogen nonuser

2 *What is the* estimated *relative risk of cancer when analyzing this study as a matched-pairs study?*

a. 0.25

b. 0.33

c. 1.00

d. 3.00

e. 4.20

3 *Unmatch the pairs. What is the* estimated *relative risk of cancer when analyzing this study as an* unmatched *study design?*

a. 0.70

b. 1.43

c. 2.80

d. 3.00

e. 4.00

4 *In a study of a disease in which all cases that developed were ascertained, if the relative risk for the association between a factor and the disease is equal to or less than 1.0, then:*

a. There is no association between the factor and the disease

b. The factor protects against development of the disease

c. Either matching or randomization has been unsuccessful

d. The comparison group used was unsuitable, and a valid comparison is not possible

e. There is either no association or a negative association between the factor and the disease

Questions 5 through 7 are based on the following information.

Talbot and colleagues carried out a study of sudden unexpected death in women. Data on smoking history are shown in the following table.

Smoking History for Cases of Atherosclerotic Heart Disease Sudden Death and Controls (Current Smoker, 1+ Pack/Day) [Matched Pairs], Allegheny County, 1980				
		Controls		
	Cases	**Smoking 1+ Pack/ Day**	**Smoking <1 Pack/ Day**	**Totals**
Smoking 1+ pack/day		2	36	38
Smoking <1 pack/day		8	34	42
Totals		10	70	80

Modified from Talbott E, Kuller LH, Perper J, Murphy PA. Sudden unexpected death in women: biologic and psychosocial origins. *Am J Epidemiol.* 1981;114:671–682.

5 Calculate the matched-pairs odds ratio for these data. _____

6 Using data from the table, unmatch the pairs and calculate an unmatched odds ratio. _____

7 What are the odds that the controls smoke 1+ pack/day? _____

Questions 8 and 9 are based on the information given in the following table.

Rates of Atherosclerotic Heart Disease (ASHD) per 10,000 Population, by Age and Sex, Framingham, Massachusetts				
	MEN		**WOMEN**	
Age at Beginning of Study (year)	ASHD Rates at Initial Exam	Yearly Follow-up Exams (Mean Annual Incidence)	ASHD Rates at Initial Exam	Yearly Follow-up Exams (Mean Annual Incidence)
29–34	76.7	19.4	0.0	0.0
35–44	90.7	40.0	17.2	2.1
45–54	167.6	106.5	111.1	29.4
55–62	505.4	209.1	211.1	117.8

8 The relative risk for developing ASHD subsequent to entering this study in men as compared with women is:
a. Approximately equal in all age groups
b. Highest in the oldest age group
c. Lowest in the youngest and oldest age groups, and highest at ages 35 to 44 and 45 to 54 years
d. Highest in the youngest and oldest age groups, and lowest at ages 35 to 44 and 45 to 54 years
e. Lowest in the oldest age group

9 *The most likely explanation for the differences in rates of ASHD between the* initial *examination and the yearly* follow-up *examinations in men is:*

a. The prevalence and incidence of ASHD increase with age in men

b. Case-fatality of ASHD is higher at younger ages in men

c. A classic cohort effect explains these results

d. The case-fatality in ASHD is highest in the first 24 hours following a heart attack

e. The initial examination measures the prevalence of ASHD, whereas the subsequent examinations primarily measure the incidence of ASHD

Question 10 is based on the following information.

A matched case-control study is conducted to explore the relationship of C-reactive protein (CRP) and progression to AIDS in South Africa. Each case is matched to one control; they are selected from separate HIV-care clinics from the United States. The cases and controls are matched by age and sex, which are known confounders of the relationship between CRP and progression to AIDS. The exposure was a high CRP value, defined as ≥2 mg/L. The following distribution of exposure was observed among 145 case-control pairs.

		CONTROL	
		+	−
Case	+	25	31
	−	16	73

10 *Calculate the odds ratio (OR) for the case-control study*

OR = _____

Questions 11 and 12 involve a case-control study exploring the relationship between use of aspirin and odds of prostate cancer in a study with 375 cases and 407 controls.

Aspirin Use	Case	Control
Never	198	174
Ever	177	233

11 *What is the odds ratio for prostate cancer comparing never versus ever aspirin? (*Ever use *is the reference category).*

_____

12 *Provide a one-sentence interpretation of the odds ratio you obtained in Question 11:*

13 *Which of the following generally cannot be estimated in a case-control study?*

a. Relative risk

b. Incidence rate

c. Prevalence of exposure in the source population

d. Odds ratio of disease

e. Odds ratio of exposure

Appendix to Chapter 12

Derivation of the relationship of the odds ratio and the relative risk can be demonstrated by the following algebra. Recall that:

$$\text{Relative risk (RR)} = \frac{\left(\dfrac{a}{a+b}\right)}{\left(\dfrac{c}{c+d}\right)}$$

$$\text{The odds ratio (OR)} = \frac{ad}{bc}$$

The relationship of the relative risk to the odds ratio can therefore be expressed as the ratio of the RR to the OR:

(1) FORMULA 1:

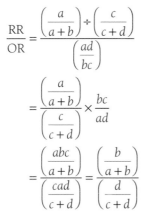

$$\frac{\text{RR}}{\text{OR}} = \frac{\left(\dfrac{a}{a+b}\right) \div \left(\dfrac{c}{c+d}\right)}{\left(\dfrac{ad}{bc}\right)}$$

$$= \frac{\left(\dfrac{a}{a+b}\right)}{\left(\dfrac{c}{c+d}\right)} \times \frac{bc}{ad}$$

$$= \frac{\left(\dfrac{abc}{a+b}\right)}{\left(\dfrac{cad}{c+d}\right)} = \frac{\left(\dfrac{b}{a+b}\right)}{\left(\dfrac{d}{c+d}\right)}$$

Since

$$\frac{b}{a+b} = \frac{a+b-a}{a+b} = \frac{a+b}{a+b} - \frac{a}{a+b} = 1 - \frac{a}{a+b}$$

and

$$\frac{d}{c+d} = \frac{c+d-c}{c+d} = \frac{c+d}{c+d} - \frac{c}{c+d} = 1 - \frac{c}{c+d}$$

the relationship of the relative risk to the odds ratio can therefore be reduced to the following equation:

(2) FORMULA 2:

$$\frac{\text{RR}}{\text{OR}} = \frac{1 - \left(\dfrac{a}{a+b}\right)}{1 - \left(\dfrac{c}{c+d}\right)}$$

If we then multiply Formula 2 by the OR:

(3) FORMULA 3:

$$\text{RR} = \frac{1 - \left(\dfrac{a}{a+b}\right)}{1 - \left(\dfrac{c}{c+d}\right)} \times \text{OR}$$

If a disease is rare, both $\dfrac{a}{a+b}$ and $\dfrac{c}{c+d}$ will be very small, so that the terms in parentheses in Formula 3 will be approximately 1, and the odds ratio will then approximate the relative risk.

It also is of interest to examine this relationship in a different form. Recall the definition of *odds* (i.e., the ratio of the number of ways the event can occur to the number of ways the event cannot occur):

$$O = \frac{P}{1-P}$$

where O is the *odds* that the disease will develop and P is the *risk* that the disease will develop. Note that, as P becomes smaller, the denominator $1 - P$ approaches 1, with the result that:

$$\frac{P}{1-P} \cong \frac{P}{1} = P$$

(i.e., the *odds* become a good approximation of the *risk*). Thus, if the risk is low (the disease is rare), the *odds* that the disease will develop are a good approximation of the *risk* that it will develop.

Now, consider an exposed group and an unexposed group. If the risk of a disease is very low, the *ratio* of the *odds* in the exposed group to the *odds* in the unexposed group closely approximates the *ratio* of the *risk* in the exposed group to the *risk* in the unexposed group *(the relative risk)*.

That is, when *P* is very small:

$$\frac{O_{exp}}{O_{nonexp}} \cong \frac{P_{exp}}{P_{nonexp}}$$

where:

O_{exp} is the odds of the disease developing in the exposed population,

O_{nonexp} is the odds of the disease developing in the unexposed population,

P_{exp} is the probability (or risk) of the disease developing in the exposed population, and

P_{nonexp} is the probability (or risk) of the disease developing in the unexposed population.

This ratio of odds is the *odds ratio* (relative odds).

Chapter 13

More on Risk: Estimating the Potential for Prevention

Learning Objectives

- To calculate and interpret the attributable risk for the exposed group.
- To calculate and interpret the population attributable risk.
- To describe how attributable risk is used to estimate the potential for prevention.

Attributable Risk

Our discussion in Chapter 12 addressed the relative risk and the odds ratio, which is often used as a surrogate for the relative risk in a case-control study. The *relative risk* is an important measure of the *strength of the association*, which is a major consideration in deriving causal inferences. In this chapter, we turn to a different question: *How much of the disease that occurs can be attributed to a certain exposure?* This is answered by another measure of risk, the *attributable risk*, which is defined as the amount or proportion of disease incidence (or disease risk) that can be attributed to a specific exposure. For example, how much of the coronary heart disease (CHD) risk experienced by smokers can be attributed to smoking? How much can be attributed to host genetics? Whereas the relative risk is important in establishing etiologic relationships, the attributable risk is in many ways more important in clinical practice and in public health, because it addresses a different question: *How much of the risk (incidence) of disease can we hope to prevent if we are able to eliminate exposure to the agent in question?*

We can calculate the attributable risk for exposed persons (e.g., the attributable risk of CHD in smokers) or the attributable risk for the total population, which includes both exposed and unexposed persons (e.g., the attributable risk of CHD in a total population, which consists of both smokers and nonsmokers). These calculations and their uses and interpretations are discussed in this chapter.

ATTRIBUTABLE RISK FOR THE EXPOSED GROUP

Fig. 13.1 offers a schematic introduction to this concept. Consider two groups: one exposed and the other not exposed. In Fig. 13.1A, the total risk of the disease in the exposed group is indicated by the full height of the bar on the left, and the total risk of disease in the unexposed group is indicated by the full height of the bar on the right. As seen here, the total risk of the disease is higher in the exposed group than in the unexposed group. We can ask the following question: In the exposed persons, how much of the total risk of disease is actually due to exposure (e.g., in a group of smokers, how much of the risk of CHD is due to smoking)?

How can this question be answered? Let's start by addressing the unexposed persons, designated by the bar on the right. Although they are not exposed, they have some risk of disease (albeit at a lower level than that of the exposed persons). That is, the risk of the disease is not zero even in unexposed persons. For instance, in this example of smoking and CHD, nonsmokers may have some risks of CHD, possibly due to obesity, blood pressure, cholesterol levels, and other factors. This risk is termed *background risk*. Every person shares the background risk regardless of whether or not he or she has had the specific exposure in question (in this case, tobacco smoking; see Fig. 13.1B). Thus both unexposed and exposed persons have this background risk. Therefore the total risk of the disease in exposed individuals is the sum of the background risk that any person has and the additional risk due to the exposure in question. If we want to know how much of the total risk in exposed persons is due to the exposure, we should subtract the background risk from

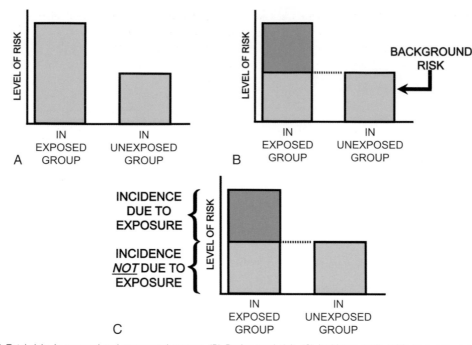

Fig. 13.1 (A) Total risks in exposed and unexposed groups. (B) Background risk. (C) Incidence attributable to exposure and incidence not attributable to exposure.

the total risk (see Fig. 13.1C). Because the risk in the unexposed group is equal to the background risk, we can calculate the risk in the exposed group that is a result of the specific exposure by subtracting the risk in the unexposed group (the background risk) from the total risk in the exposed group.

Thus the incidence of a disease that is attributable to the exposure in the exposed group can be calculated as follows:

Formula 13.1

$$\left(\begin{array}{c}\text{Incidence in}\\\text{exposed group}\end{array}\right) - \left(\begin{array}{c}\text{Incidence in}\\\text{unexposed group}\end{array}\right)$$

We could instead ask, "What proportion of the risk in exposed persons is due to the exposure?" We could then express the attributable risk as the proportion of the total incidence in the exposed group that is attributable to the exposure by simply dividing Formula 13.1 by the incidence in the exposed group, as follows:

Formula 13.2

$$\frac{\left(\begin{array}{c}\text{Incidence in}\\\text{exposed group}\end{array}\right) - \left(\begin{array}{c}\text{Incidence in}\\\text{unexposed group}\end{array}\right)}{\text{Incidence in exposed group}}$$

The attributable risk expresses the most that we can hope to accomplish in reducing the risk of the disease if we completely eliminate the exposure. For example, if all smokers were induced to stop smoking, how much of a reduction could we anticipate in CHD rates? From a practical programmatic standpoint, the attributable risk may be more relevant than the relative risk. The relative risk is a measure of the strength of the association, but the attributable risk indicates the potential for prevention if the exposure could be eliminated.

The practicing clinician is mainly interested in the attributable risk in the exposed group: For example, when a physician advises a patient to stop smoking, he or she is in effect telling the patient that stopping smoking will reduce the risk of CHD. Implicit in this advice is the physician's estimate that the patient's risk will be reduced by a certain proportion if he or she stops smoking; the risk reduction is motivating the physician to give that advice. Although the physician often does not have a specific value in mind for the attributable risk, he or she is in effect relying on an attributable risk for an exposed group (smokers) to which the patient belongs. The physician is implicitly addressing the question: In a population of smokers, how much of the CHD that they experience is due to smoking, and consequently, how much of the CHD could be prevented if they did not smoke? Thus attributable risk tells us the potential for prevention.

If all the incidence of a disease were the result of a single factor, the attributable risk for that disease would be 100%. However, this is rarely if ever the case. Both the concept and the calculation of attributable risk imply that not all of the disease incidence is due to a single specific exposure, as the disease even develops in some unexposed individuals. Fig. 13.2 recapitulates this concept.

ATTRIBUTABLE RISK FOR THE TOTAL POPULATION—POPULATION ATTRIBUTABLE RISK

Let's turn to a somewhat different question relating to attributable risk. Assume that we know how to eliminate smoking. We tell the mayor that we have a highly effective way to eliminate smoking in the community, and we want her to provide the funds to support such a program. The mayor responds that she is delighted to hear the news, but asks, "What will the impact of your smoking cessation program be on coronary heart disease incidence rates in our city?" This question differs from that which was just discussed. For if we talk about CHD rates in the entire population of a city, and not just in exposed individuals, we are talking about a population that is composed of both smokers and nonsmokers. The mayor is not asking what impact we will have on smokers in this city, but rather what impact will we have on the entire population of the city, which includes both smokers and nonsmokers.

Let's consider this question further. In addition to the assumption that we have an evidence-based successful smoking cessation program, let's also assume that everyone in the city smokes. (Heaven forbid!) We now want to calculate the attributable risk. Clearly, because everyone in the city smokes, the attributable risk for the entire population of the city would equal the attributable risk for the exposed population. If everybody smokes, the attributable risk for the exposed group tells us what we can hope to accomplish with a smoking cessation program in the total population.

Now let's assume that an ideal situation exists and that nobody in the city smokes. What will be the potential for preventing CHD through the use of a completely effective smoking cessation program that we wish to apply to the population of the city? The answer is zero; because there are no exposed people in the city, a program that aims at eliminating the exposure does not make sense and would therefore have no effect on the risk of CHD. Therefore the spectrum of potential effect runs from a maximum (if everybody smokes) to zero (if nobody smokes). Of course, in reality, the answer is generally somewhere in between, because some members of the population smoke and some do not. The latter group (all nonsmokers) clearly will not benefit from a smoking cessation program, regardless of how effective it is.

To this point, we have discussed the concept and calculation of attributable risk for *an exposed group*. For example, in a population of smokers, how much of the CHD that they experience is due to smoking,

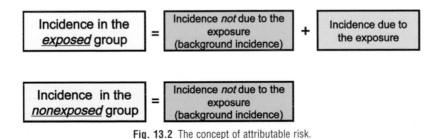

Fig. 13.2 The concept of attributable risk.

and consequently, how much of the CHD could be prevented if they did not smoke? However, to answer the mayor's question as to what effect the smoking cessation program will have on the city's population as a whole, we need to calculate the *attributable risk for the total population:* What proportion of the disease incidence in a *total population* (including both exposed and unexposed people) can be attributed to a specific exposure? What would be the total impact of a prevention program on the community? If we want to calculate the attributable risk in the total population, the calculation is similar to that for exposed people, but we begin with the *incidence in the total population* and again subtract the background risk, or the incidence in the unexposed population. The incidence in the total population that is due to the exposure[a] can be calculated as shown in Formula 13.3:

Formula 13.3

$$\left(\begin{array}{c}\text{Incidence in}\\\text{total population}\end{array}\right)-\left(\begin{array}{c}\text{Incidence in}\\\text{unexposed group}\\\text{(background risk)}\end{array}\right)$$

Again, if we prefer to express this as the proportion of the incidence in the total population that is attributable to the exposure, Formula 13.3 can be divided by the incidence in the total population:

Formula 13.4

$$\frac{\left(\begin{array}{c}\text{Incidence in}\\\text{total population}\end{array}\right)-\left(\begin{array}{c}\text{Incidence in}\\\text{unexposed group}\end{array}\right)}{\text{Incidence in total population}}$$

The attributable risk for the total population (population attributable risk [PAR]) is a valuable concept for the public health worker. The question addressed is: What proportion of CHD in the total population can be attributed to smoking? This question could be reworded as follows: If smoking were eliminated, what proportion of the incidence of CHD in the total population (which consists of both smokers and nonsmokers) would be prevented? The answer is: the attributable

risk in the total population, also called the PAR—or the PAR (as discussed earlier).[b]

From a public health standpoint, this is often both the critical issue and the question that is raised by policy makers and by those responsible for funding prevention programs. They may want to know what the proposed program is going to do for the community as a whole. How is it going to change the burden on the health care system or the burden of suffering in the entire community, not just in exposed individuals? For example, if all smokers in the community stopped smoking, what would be the impact of this change on the incidence of CHD in the total population of the community (which includes both smokers and nonsmokers)?

AN EXAMPLE OF AN ATTRIBUTABLE RISK CALCULATION FOR THE EXPOSED GROUP

This section presents a step-by-step calculation of the attributable risk in both an exposed group and in a total population. We will use the hypothetical example previously presented of a cohort study of smoking and CHD. The data are again shown in Table 13.1.

The incidence of CHD in the exposed group (smokers) that is attributable to the exposure is calculated using Formula 13.1:

Formula 13.1

$$\left(\begin{array}{c}\text{Incidence in}\\\text{exposed group}\end{array}\right)-\left(\begin{array}{c}\text{Incidence in}\\\text{unexposed group}\end{array}\right)$$
$$=\frac{28.0-17.4}{1,000}=\frac{10.6}{1,000}$$

What does this mean? It means that 10.6 of the 28/1,000 incident cases in smokers are attributable to the fact that these people smoke. Stated another way,

---

[a]The incidence in the population that is due to the exposure can also be calculated as follows: Attributable risk for the exposed group × Proportion of the population exposed.

[b]Another way to calculate the attributable risk for the total population is to use Levin's formula, which is given in the appendix to this chapter. Levin's formula allows the estimation of the PAR using case-control data by replacing the relative risk with the odds ratio (if the disease is relatively rare). It requires, however, an estimate of the prevalence of the exposure in the reference population. Note that Levin's formula only applies to PARs based on unadjusted relative risks.

TABLE 13.1 Smoking and Coronary Heart Disease (CHD): A Hypothetical Cohort Study of 3,000 Cigarette Smokers and 5,000 Nonsmokers

	CHD Develops	CHD Does Not Develop	Total	Incidence Per 1,000 Per Year
Smoke cigarettes	84	2,916	3,000	28.0
Do not smoke cigarettes	87	4,913	5,000	17.4

$$\text{Incidence among smokers} = \frac{84}{3,000} = 28.0 \text{ per } 1.000$$

$$\text{Incidence among nonsmokers} = \frac{87}{5,000} = 17.4 \text{ per } 1,000$$

---

if we had an effective smoking cessation campaign, we could hope to prevent 10.6 of the $\frac{28}{1,000}$ incident cases of CHD that smokers experience.

If we prefer, we can express this as a proportion. The proportion of the total incidence in the exposed group that is attributable to the exposure can be calculated by dividing Formula 13.1 by the incidence in the exposed group (Formula 13.2):

Formula 13.2

$$\frac{\left(\begin{array}{c}\text{Incidence in}\\ \text{exposed group}\end{array}\right) - \left(\begin{array}{c}\text{Incidence in}\\ \text{unexposed group}\end{array}\right)}{\text{Incidence in exposed group}}$$

$$= \frac{28.0 - 17.4}{28.0} = \frac{10.6}{28.0} = 0.379 = 37.9\%$$

Thus 37.9% of the incidence from CHD among smokers may be attributable to smoking and could presumably be prevented by eliminating smoking.

AN EXAMPLE OF AN ATTRIBUTABLE RISK CALCULATION IN THE TOTAL POPULATION (POPULATION ATTRIBUTABLE RISK)

Using the same example, let's calculate the PAR—that is, the attributable risk for the total population. The question we are asking is: What can we hope to accomplish with our smoking cessation program *in the total population* (i.e., the entire community, which consists of both smokers and nonsmokers)?

Remember that in the total population, the incidence that is due to smoking (the exposure) can be calculated by subtracting the background risk (i.e., the incidence

in the nonsmokers, or unexposed) from the incidence in the total population:

Formula 13.3

$$\left(\begin{array}{c}\text{Incidence in}\\ \text{total population}\end{array}\right) - \left(\begin{array}{c}\text{Incidence in}\\ \text{unexposed group}\end{array}\right)$$

To calculate Formula 13.3, we must know either the incidence of the disease (CHD) in the total population (which we often do not know) or all of the following three values, from which we can then calculate the incidence in the total population:
1. The incidence among smokers
2. The incidence among nonsmokers
3. The proportion of the total population that smokes

In this example, we know that the incidence among the smokers is 28.0 per 1,000 and the incidence among the nonsmokers is 17.4 per 1,000. However, we do not know the incidence in the total population. Let's assume that, from some other source of information, we know that the proportion of smokers in the population is 44% (and therefore the proportion of nonsmokers is 56%). The incidence in the total population can then be calculated as follows:

$$\left(\begin{array}{c}\text{Incidence}\\ \text{in smokers}\end{array}\right)\left(\begin{array}{c}\text{% Smokers}\\ \text{in population}\end{array}\right)$$
$$+ \left(\begin{array}{c}\text{Incidence in}\\ \text{nonsmokers}\end{array}\right)\left(\begin{array}{c}\text{% Nonsmokers}\\ \text{in population}\end{array}\right)$$

(We are simply weighting the calculation of the incidence in the total population, taking into account the proportion of the population that smokes and the proportion of the population that does not smoke.)

So, in this example, the incidence in the total population can be calculated as follows:

$$\left(\frac{28.0}{1,000}\right)(0.44) + \left(\frac{17.4}{1,000}\right)(0.56) = \frac{22.1}{1,000}$$

We now have the values needed for using Formula 13.3 to calculate the attributable risk in the total population:

Formula 13.3

$$\left(\begin{array}{c}\text{Incidence in}\\\text{total population}\end{array}\right) - \left(\begin{array}{c}\text{Incidence in}\\\text{unexposed group}\end{array}\right)$$

$$= \frac{22.1}{1,000} - \frac{17.4}{1,000} = \frac{4.7}{1,000}$$

What does this tell us? How much of the total risk of CHD in this population (which consists of both smokers and nonsmokers) is attributable to smoking? If we had an effective prevention program (smoking cessation) in this population, how much of a reduction in CHD incidence could we anticipate, at best, in the total population (of both smokers and nonsmokers)?

If we prefer to calculate the proportion of the incidence in the total population that is attributable to the exposure, we can do so by dividing Formula 13.3 by the incidence in the total population, as in Formula 13.4:

Formula 13.4

$$\frac{\left(\begin{array}{c}\text{Incidence in}\\\text{total population}\end{array}\right) - \left(\begin{array}{c}\text{Incidence in}\\\text{unexposed group}\end{array}\right)}{\text{Incidence in total population}}$$

$$= \frac{22.1 - 17.4}{22.1} = 21.3\%$$

Thus 21.3% of the incidence of CHD in the total population can be attributed to smoking, and if an effective prevention program eliminated smoking, the best that we could hope to achieve would be a reduction of 21.3% in the incidence of CHD in the total population (which includes both smokers and nonsmokers).

Attributable risk is a critical concept in virtually any area of public health and in clinical practice, in particular in relation to questions regarding the potential of preventive measures. For example, Lim and colleagues[1] estimated the actual causes of death worldwide in 2010. These estimates used published data and applied attributable risk calculations as well as other approaches. Their estimates are shown in Fig. 13.3. The authors reported that dietary risk factors and physical inactivity accounted for 30% of all deaths.

It is also of interest that in the legal arena, in which toxic tort litigation has become increasingly common, the concept of attributable risk for the exposed individuals has taken on great importance. One of the legal criteria used in finding a company responsible for an environmental injury, for example, is whether it is "more likely than not" that the company caused the injury. It has been suggested that an attributable risk of greater than 50% might represent a quantitative determination of the legal definition of "more likely than not."

Comparison of Relative Risk and Attributable Risk

In earlier chapters, we discussed several measures of risk and of excess risk. The relative risk and the odds ratio are important as measures of the strength of the association, which is a critical consideration in deriving a causal inference. The attributable risk is a measure of how much of the disease risk is attributable to a certain exposure. Consequently, the attributable risk is useful in answering the question of how much disease can be prevented if we have an effective means of eliminating the exposure in question. Thus the relative risk is valuable in etiologic studies of disease, whereas the attributable risk has major applications in clinical practice and public health.

Table 13.2 shows a classic example from a study by Doll and Peto[2] that relates mortality from lung cancer and CHD in smokers and nonsmokers, and provides an illuminating comparison of relative risk and attributable risk in the same set of data.

Let's first examine the data for lung cancer. (Note that in this example, we are using mortality as a surrogate for risk.) We see that the lung cancer mortality

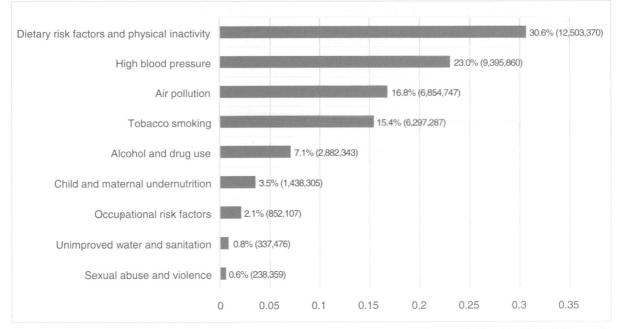

Fig. 13.3 Deaths attributable to selected risk factors or risk factor clusters in 2010, worldwide. (Data modified from Lim SS, Vos T, Flaxman AD, et al. A comparative risk assessment of burden of disease and injury attributable to 67 risk factors and risk factor clusters in 21 regions, 1990–2010: a systematic analysis for the Global Burden of Disease Study 2010. *Lancet.* 2012;380:2224–2260.)

TABLE 13.2 Lung Cancer and Coronary Heart Disease Mortality in Male British Physicians: Smokers vs. Nonsmokers

	AGE-ADJUSTED DEATH RATES PER 100,000		Relative Risk	Attributable Risk (Deaths per 100,000)	% Attributable Risk
	Smokers	Nonsmokers			
Lung cancer	140	10	14.0	130	92.9
Coronary heart disease	669	413	1.6	256	38.3

From Doll R, Peto R. Mortality in relation to smoking: twenty years' observation on male British doctors. *Br Med J.* 1976;2:1525–1536.

risk is 140 for smokers and 10 for nonsmokers. We can calculate the relative risk as $\frac{140}{10} = 14$.

Now let's look at the data for CHD. The CHD mortality rate is 669 in smokers and 413 in nonsmokers. The relative risk can be calculated as $\frac{669}{413} = 1.6$. Thus the relative risk is much higher for smoking and lung cancer than it is for smoking and CHD.

Now let's turn to the attributable risks in smokers. How much of the total risk in smokers can we attribute

to smoking? To calculate the attributable risk, we subtract the background risk—the risk in the unexposed group (nonsmokers)—from the risk in the exposed group (smokers). With the data for lung cancer used, 140 − 10 = 130.

To calculate the attributable risk for CHD and smoking, we subtract the risk in the unexposed group (nonsmokers) from the risk in the exposed group (smokers), 669 − 413 = 256. That is, of the total 669 deaths per 100,000 in smokers, 256 can be attributed to smoking.

If we prefer to express the attributable risk for lung cancer and smoking as a proportion (i.e., the proportion of the lung cancer risk in smokers that can be attributed to smoking), we divide the attributable risk by the risk in smokers:

$$\frac{(140-10)}{140} = 92.9\%$$

If we prefer to express the attributable risk of CHD and smoking as a proportion (the proportion of the CHD risk in smokers that can be attributed to smoking), we divide the attributable risk by the risk in smokers:

$$\frac{(669-413)}{669} = 38.3\%$$

What does this table tell us? First, we see a tremendous difference in the relative risks for lung cancer and for CHD in relation to smoking: 14.0 for lung cancer compared with 1.6 for CHD (i.e., much stronger association exists for smoking and lung cancer than for smoking and CHD). However, the attributable risk is almost twice as high (256) for CHD as it is for lung cancer (130). If we choose to express the attributable risk as a proportion, we find that 92.9% of lung cancer deaths in smokers can be attributed to smoking (and are potentially preventable by eliminating smoking), compared with only 38.3% of deaths from CHD in smokers that can be attributed to smoking.

Thus the relative risk is much higher for lung cancer than for CHD, and the attributable risk expressed as a proportion is also much higher for lung cancer. However, if an effective smoking cessation program were available today and smoking was eliminated, would the preventive impact be greater on mortality from lung cancer or from CHD? If we examine the table, we see that if smoking were eliminated, 256 deaths per 100,000 from CHD would be prevented in contrast to only 130 from lung cancer, despite the fact that the relative risk is higher for lung cancer and despite the fact that the proportion of deaths attributable to smoking is greater for lung cancer. Why is this so? This is a result of the fact that the mortality level in smokers is much higher for CHD than for lung cancer (669 compared to 140) and that the attributable risk in those exposed to smoking (the difference between total risk in smokers and background risk) is much greater for CHD than for lung cancer.

It is important to emphasize that, as the attributable risk implies that a certain proportion of the risk can be prevented, it should be estimated only when there is reasonable certainty that the association of the risk factor with the disease is causal.[3] In addition, for risk factors with a cumulative exposure, it is more appropriate to define attributable risk as the proportion of the risk (either in the exposed or in the population) that can be attributed to a given exposure than as the proportion that can be eliminated by cessation of exposure. For example, according to the US Surgeon General's Report from 2010, the lung cancer risk in former smokers 15 years after quitting is one-half that in current smokers, which means that it is still considerably higher than the risk in never-smokers.

Conclusion

In this chapter, we have introduced the concept of attributable risk and described how it is calculated and interpreted. Attributable risk is summarized in the four calculations shown in Table 13.3.

The concepts of relative risk and attributable risk are essential for understanding causation and the potential for prevention. Several measures of risk have now been discussed: (1) absolute risk, (2) relative risk, (3) odds ratios, and (4) attributable risk. In Chapter 14, we will

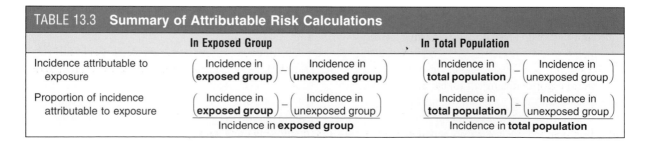

TABLE 13.3	**Summary of Attributable Risk Calculations**		
	In Exposed Group	**In Total Population**	
Incidence attributable to exposure	$\left(\begin{array}{c}\text{Incidence in}\\ \textbf{exposed group}\end{array}\right) - \left(\begin{array}{c}\text{Incidence in}\\ \textbf{unexposed group}\end{array}\right)$	$\left(\begin{array}{c}\text{Incidence in}\\ \textbf{total population}\end{array}\right) - \left(\begin{array}{c}\text{Incidence in}\\ \text{unexposed group}\end{array}\right)$	
Proportion of incidence attributable to exposure	$\dfrac{\left(\begin{array}{c}\text{Incidence in}\\ \textbf{exposed group}\end{array}\right) - \left(\begin{array}{c}\text{Incidence in}\\ \text{unexposed group}\end{array}\right)}{\text{Incidence in } \textbf{exposed group}}$	$\dfrac{\left(\begin{array}{c}\text{Incidence in}\\ \textbf{total population}\end{array}\right) - \left(\begin{array}{c}\text{Incidence in}\\ \text{unexposed group}\end{array}\right)}{\text{Incidence in } \textbf{total population}}$	

briefly review study designs and concepts of risk before proceeding to a discussion of how we use estimates of excess risk to derive causal inferences.

REFERENCES

1. Lim SS, Vos T, Flaxman AD, et al. A comparative risk assessment of burden of disease and injury attributable to 67 risk factors and risk factor clusters in 21 regions, 1990-2010: a systematic analysis for the Global Burden of Disease Study 2010. *Lancet.* 2012;380:2224–2260.
2. Doll R, Peto R. Mortality in relation to smoking: twenty years' observations on male British doctors. *Br Med J.* 1976;2:1525–1536.
3. Rothman K, Greenland S. *Modern Epidemiology.* 3rd ed. Philadelphia: Wolters Kluwer Health/Lipincott; 2008.
4. Levin ML. The occurrence of lung cancer in man. *Acta Unio Int Contra Cancrum.* 1953;9:531.
5. Leviton A. Definitions of attributable risk. *Am J Epidemiol.* 1973;98:231.

REVIEW QUESTIONS FOR CHAPTER 13

1 *Several studies have found that approximately 85% of cases of lung cancer are due to cigarette smoking. This measure is an example of:*

a. An incidence rate

b. An attributable risk

c. A relative risk

d. A prevalence risk

e. A proportionate mortality ratio

Questions 2 and 3 refer to the following information:

The results of a 10-year cohort study of smoking and coronary heart disease (CHD) are shown below:

	OUTCOME AFTER 10 YEARS	
At Beginning of Study	**CHD Developed**	**CHD Did Not Develop**
2,000 Healthy smokers	65	1,935
4,000 Healthy nonsmokers	20	3,980

2 *The incidence of CHD in smokers that can be attributed to smoking is:* _____

3 *The proportion of the total incidence of CHD in smokers that is attributable to smoking is:* _____

Questions 4 and 5 are based on the following information:

In a cohort study of smoking and lung cancer, the incidence of lung cancer among smokers was found to be 9/1,000 and the incidence among nonsmokers was 1/1,000. From another source we know that 45% of the total population were smokers.

4 *The incidence of lung cancer attributable to smoking in the total population is:* _____

5 *The proportion of the risk in the total population that is attributable to smoking is:* _____

Appendix to Chapter 13: Levin's Formula for the Attributable Risk for the Total Population

Another way to calculate this proportion for the total population is to use Levin's formula[4]:

$$\frac{p(r-1)}{p(r-1)+1}$$

where p is the proportion of the population with the characteristic or exposure and r is the relative risk (or odds ratio).

Leviton[5] has shown that Levin's formula[4] and the following formula are algebraically identical:

$$\frac{\left(\begin{array}{c}\text{Incidence in}\\\text{total population}\end{array}\right)-\left(\begin{array}{c}\text{Incidence in}\\\text{unexposed group}\end{array}\right)}{\text{Incidence in total population}}$$

Chapter 14

From Association to Causation: Deriving Inferences From Epidemiologic Studies

Not everything that can be counted counts, and not everything that counts can be counted.

—William Bruce Cameron, 1963[1]

Learning Objectives

- To describe a frequent sequence of study designs used to address questions of etiology in human populations.
- To differentiate between real and spurious associations in observational studies.
- To define the concepts of "necessary" and "sufficient" in the context of causal relationships.
- To present guidelines for judging whether an association is causal based on the guidelines set forth by the US Surgeon General and to discuss the application of these guidelines to broader questions of causal inference.
- To describe how the guidelines for causation originally proposed by the US Surgeon General have been modified and used by the US Public Health Service and the US Preventive Services Task Force.

In previous chapters, we discussed a variety of designs of epidemiologic studies that are used to determine whether an association exists between an exposure and a disease outcome (Fig. 14.1A). We then addressed different types of risk measurement that are used to quantitatively express an excess in risk. If we determine that an exposure is associated with a disease, the next question is whether the observed association reflects a causal relationship (see Fig. 14.1B).

Although Figs. 14.1A and B refer to an environmental exposure, they could just as well have specified a genetic characteristic or some other risk characteristic or a specific combination of environmental and genetic factors. As we shall see in the chapter on genetics and environmental factors, studies of disease etiology generally address the contributions of both genetic and environmental factors and their interactions.

This chapter discusses the derivation of causal inferences in epidemiology. Let us begin by asking, "What approaches are available for studying the etiology of disease?"

Approaches for Studying Disease Etiology

If we are interested in whether a certain substance is carcinogenic in human beings, a first step in the study of the substance's effect might be to expose animals to the carcinogen in a controlled laboratory environment. Although such animal studies afford us the opportunity to control the exposure dose and other environmental conditions and genetic factors precisely and to keep loss to follow-up to a minimum, at the conclusion of the study we are left with the problem of having to extrapolate data across species (i.e., from animal to human populations). Certain diseases seen in humans have neither occurred nor been produced in animals. It is also difficult to extrapolate animal doses to human doses, and species differ in their responses. Thus, although such toxicologic studies can be useful, they still leave a gnawing uncertainty as to whether the animal findings can be generalized to human beings.

We can also use *in vitro* systems, such as cell culture or organ culture. However, because these are artificial systems, we are again left with the difficulty of extrapolating from artificial systems to intact, whole human organisms.

In view of these limitations, if we want to be able to draw a conclusion as to whether a substance causes disease in human beings, we need to make *observations in human populations*. Because we cannot ethically or

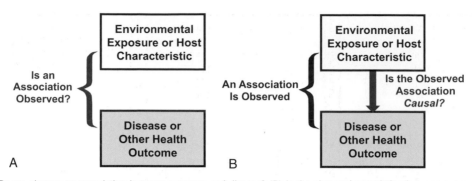

Fig. 14.1 (A) Do we observe an association between exposure and disease? (B) Is the observed association between exposure and disease causal?

practically randomize human beings to exposure to a suspected carcinogen, we are dependent on nonrandomized observations, such as those that come from case-control and cohort studies.

APPROACHES TO ETIOLOGY IN HUMAN POPULATIONS

Epidemiology often capitalizes on what have been called "unplanned" or "natural" experiments. (Some think that this phrase is a contradiction in terms, in that the word "experiment" implies a planned exposure.) What we mean by *unplanned* or *natural* experiments is that we take advantage of groups of people who have been exposed for nonstudy purposes, such as occupational cohorts in specific industries or persons exposed to toxic chemicals. Examples include people affected by the poison gas leak disaster at a pesticide manufacturing plant in Bhopal, India, in 1984 and residents of Hiroshima and Nagasaki, Japan, who were exposed to radiation from the atomic bombs dropped on both cities by US forces in 1945. Each of these exposed groups can be compared with an unexposed group (e.g., residents of Chennai, India or Tokyo, Japan) to determine whether there is an increased risk of a certain adverse effect in persons who have been exposed.

In conducting human studies, the sequence shown in Fig. 14.2 is frequently followed. The initial step may consist of *clinical observations* at the bedside. For example, when the surgeon Alton Ochsner observed that virtually every patient on whom he operated for lung cancer gave a history of cigarette smoking, he was among the first to suggest a possible causal relationship.[2] A second step is to try to identify *routinely available*

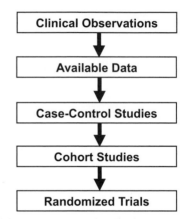

Fig. 14.2 A frequent sequence of studies in human populations.

data, the analysis of which might shed light on the question. We can then carry out *new studies* such as the cohort and case-control studies, as discussed in prior chapters, which are specifically designed to determine whether there is an association between an exposure and a disease, and whether a causal relationship exists.

The usual first step in carrying out new studies to explore a relationship is often a *case-control study*. For example, if Ochsner had wanted to further explore his suggestion that cigarette smoking may be associated with lung cancer, he would have compared the smoking histories of a group of his patients with lung cancer with those of a group of patients without lung cancer—a case-control study.

If a case-control study yields evidence that a certain exposure is suspect, we might next do a *cohort study*

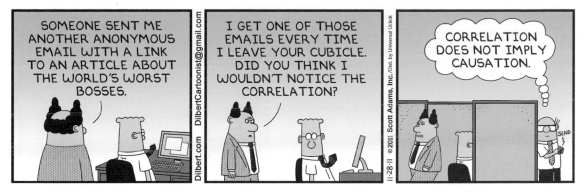

Fig. 14.3 Another example of association or causation. (DILBERT © 2011 Scott Adams. Used by permission of ANDREWS MCMEEL SYNDICATION. All rights reserved.)

(e.g., comparing smokers and nonsmokers and determining the rate of lung cancer in each group or comparing workers exposed to an industrial toxin with workers without such an exposure). Although, in theory, a randomized trial might be the next step, as discussed earlier, randomized trials are almost never used to study the effects of putative toxins or carcinogens and are generally used only for studying potentially *beneficial* agents.

Conceptually, a two-step process is followed in carrying out studies and evaluating evidence. However, in practice, this process often becomes interactive and deviates from a fixed sequence:

1. We determine whether there is an association or correlation between an exposure or characteristic and the risk of a disease (Fig. 14.3). To do so, we use:
    a. Studies of group characteristics: ecologic studies (discussed in Chapter 7)
    b. Studies of individual characteristics: cohort, case-control, and other types of studies
2. If an association is demonstrated, we determine whether the observed association is likely to be a causal one.

Types of Associations

REAL OR SPURIOUS ASSOCIATIONS

Let us turn next to the types of associations that we might observe in a cohort or case-control study. If we observe an association, we start by asking the question, "Is it a true (real) association or a false (spurious) one?"

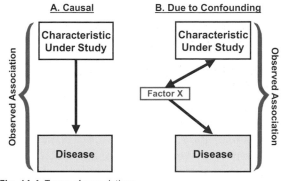

Fig. 14.4 Types of associations.

For example, if we designed a study to select controls in such a way that they tended to be unexposed, we might observe an association of exposure with disease (i.e., more frequent exposure in cases than in controls). This would not be a true association but only a result of the study design. Recall that this issue was raised in Chapter 7 regarding a study of coffee consumption and cancer of the pancreas. The possibility was suggested that the controls selected for the study had a lower rate of coffee consumption than was found in the general population.

INTERPRETING REAL ASSOCIATIONS

If the observed association is real, is it causal? Fig. 14.4 shows two possibilities. Fig. 14.4A shows a causal association: we observe an association of exposure and disease, as indicated by the bracket, and the exposure induces development of the disease, as indicated by the arrow. Fig. 14.4B shows the same observed association of exposure and disease, but they are associated only because they are both linked to a third factor, which is called a confounding variable and designated here as *factor X*. This association is a result of confounding and is noncausal. Confounding is discussed in greater detail in Chapter 15.

In Chapter 7 we discussed this issue in relation to McMahon's study of coffee and cancer of the pancreas. McMahon observed an association of coffee consumption with risk of pancreatic cancer. Cigarette smoking was known to be associated with pancreatic cancer, and coffee drinking and cigarette smoking are closely associated (few smokers at the time of that report did not drink coffee) (Fig. 14.5). Therefore, was the observed association of coffee drinking and cancer of the pancreas likely to be a causal relationship, or could the association be due to the fact that coffee and cigarette smoking are associated and that cigarette smoking is a known risk factor for cancer of the pancreas?

The same issue is exemplified by the observed association of increased serum cholesterol level and risk of coronary heart disease (CHD) (Fig. 14.6). Is physical inactivity a causal factor for increased risk of colon cancer, or is the observed association due to confounding? That is, are we observing an association of physical inactivity and colon cancer because both are associated with a factor X (such as a smoking), which might cause people to have both physical inactivity and an increased risk of colon cancer?

Is this distinction really important? What difference does it make? The answer is that it makes a tremendous difference from both clinical and public health standpoints. If the relationship is causal, we will succeed in reducing the risk of colon cancer if we promote physical activity, both for the individual but also at the population level. However, if the relationship is due to confounding, then the increased risk of colon cancer is caused by factor X. Therefore increasing physical activity will have no effect on the risk of colon cancer. Thus it is extremely important for us to be able to distinguish between an association due to a causal relationship and an association due to confounding (which is noncausal).

Let us look at another example. For many years it has been known that cigarette smoking by pregnant women is associated with low birth weight in their infants. As seen in Fig. 14.7 the effect is not just the

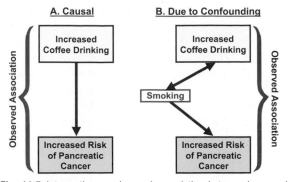

Fig. 14.5 Interpreting an observed association between increased coffee drinking and increased risk of pancreatic cancer.

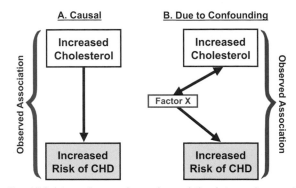

Fig. 14.6 Interpreting an observed association between increased cholesterol level and increased risk of coronary heart disease *(CHD)*.

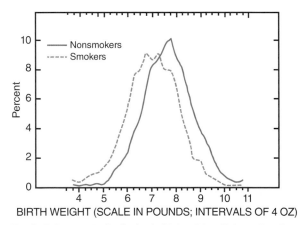

Fig. 14.7 Percentage distribution by birth weight of infants of mothers who did not smoke during pregnancy and of those mothers who smoked 1 pack of cigarettes or more per day. (From US Department of Health, Education, and Welfare. *The Health Consequences of Smoking.* Washington, DC: Public Health Service; 1973:105.)

result of the birth of a few low-birth-weight babies in this group of women. Rather, the entire weight distribution curve is shifted to the left in the babies born to smokers. The reduction in birth weight is also not a result of shorter pregnancies. The babies of smokers are smaller than those of nonsmokers at each gestational age (Fig. 14.8). A dose-response relationship is also seen (Fig. 14.9). The more a woman smokes, the greater her risk of having a low-birth-weight baby. For many years the interpretation of this association was the subject of great controversy. Many believed the association reflected a causal relation. Others, including a leading statistician, Jacob Yerushalmy, believed the association was due to confounding and was not causal. He wrote as follows:

A comparison of smokers and nonsmokers shows that the two differ markedly along many environmental, behavioral and biologic variables. For example, smokers are less likely to use contraceptives and to plan the pregnancy. Smokers are more likely to drink coffee, beer and whiskey and the nonsmoker, tea, milk and wine. The smoker is more likely than the nonsmoker to indulge in these habits to excess. In general, the nonsmokers are revealed to be more moderate than the smokers who are shown to be more extreme and carefree in their mode of life. Some biologic differences are also noted between them: Thus smokers have a higher twinning rate only in whites and their age for menarche is lower than for nonsmokers.[3]

In view of these many differences between smokers and nonsmokers, Yerushalmy believed that it was not the *smoking* that caused the low birth weight but rather that the low weight was attributable to *other characteristics of the smokers*. It is interesting to examine a study that Yerushalmy carried out to support his position at the time (Fig. 14.10).[3]

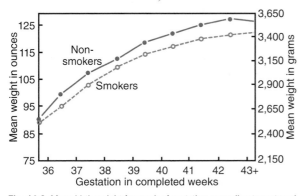

Fig. 14.8 Mean birth weight for week of gestation according to maternal smoking habit. (From US Department of Health, Education, and Welfare. *The Health Consequences of Smoking.* Washington, DC: Public Health Service; 1973:104.)

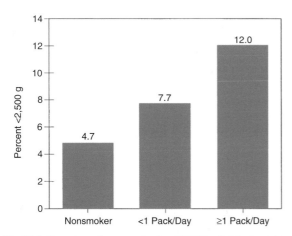

Fig. 14.9 Percentage of pregnancies (*n* = 50,267) with infant weighing less than 2,500 g, by maternal cigarette smoking category. (Redrawn from Ontario Department of Health. *Second Report of the Perinatal Mortality Study in Ten University Teaching Hospitals.* Vol. I. Toronto, Ontario: Department of Health, Ontario Perinatal Mortality Study Committee; 1967:275.)

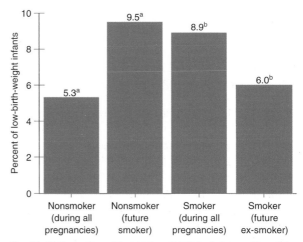

Fig. 14.10 Percentage of low-birth-weight infants by smoking status of their mothers ([a]*P* < .01; [b]*P* < .02). (Redrawn from Yerushalmy J. Infants with low birth weight born before their mothers started to smoke cigarettes. *Am J Obstet Gynecol.* 1972;112:277–284.)

Yerushalmy examined the results of one pregnancy (the study pregnancy) in a population of women who had had several pregnancies. The rate of low-birth-weight babies in the study pregnancy was 5.3% for women who were nonsmokers in *all* of their pregnancies. However, if they were smokers in all of their pregnancies, the rate of low birth weight in the study pregnancy was almost 9%. When he examined pregnancies of women who were nonsmokers during the study pregnancy, but who later became smokers, he found that their rate of low-birth-weight babies was approximately equal to that of women who smoked in all pregnancies. When he examined pregnancies of women who were smokers in the study pregnancy but who subsequently stopped smoking, he found that their rate of low birth weight in the study pregnancy was similar to that of women who were nonsmokers in all of their pregnancies.

On the basis of these data, Yerushalmy came to the conclusion that it was not the smoking but rather some characteristic of the smoker that caused the low birth weight. Today, however, it is virtually universally accepted that smoking is a cause of low birth weight. The causal nature of this relation has also been demonstrated in randomized trials that have reduced the frequency of low birth weight by initiating programs for smoking cessation in pregnant women. Although this issue has now largely been resolved, it is illuminating to review both the controversy and the study because they exemplify the reasoning that is necessary in trying to distinguish causal from noncausal interpretations of observed associations.

Types of Causal Relationships

A causal pathway can be either *direct* or *indirect* (Fig. 14.11). In *direct* causation a factor directly causes a disease without any intermediate step. In *indirect* causation a factor causes a disease but only through an intermediate step or steps. In human biology, intermediate steps are virtually always present in any causal process.

If a relationship is causal, four types of causal relationships are possible: (1) necessary and sufficient; (2) necessary but not sufficient; (3) sufficient but not necessary; and (4) neither sufficient nor necessary.

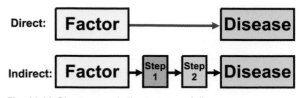

Fig. 14.11 Direct versus indirect causes of disease.

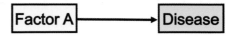

Fig. 14.12 Types of causal relationships: I. Factor A is both necessary and sufficient.

NECESSARY AND SUFFICIENT

In the first type of causal relationship a factor is both necessary and sufficient for producing the disease. Without that factor, the disease never develops (the factor is necessary), and in the presence of that factor, the disease always develops (the factor is sufficient) (Fig. 14.12). This situation rarely if ever occurs. For example, in most infectious diseases, a number of people are exposed, some of whom will manifest the disease and others who will not. Members of households of a person with tuberculosis do not uniformly acquire the disease from the index case. If the exposure dose is assumed to be the same, there are likely differences in immune status, genetic susceptibility, or other characteristics that determine who develops the disease and who does not. A one-to-one relationship of exposure to disease, which is a consequence of a necessary and sufficient relationship, rarely if ever occurs.

NECESSARY BUT NOT SUFFICIENT

In another model, each factor is necessary but not in itself sufficient to cause the disease (Fig. 14.13). Thus multiple factors are required, often in a specific temporal sequence. For example, carcinogenesis is considered to be a multistage process involving both initiation and promotion. For cancer to result, a promoter must act after an initiator has acted. Action of an initiator or a promoter alone will not produce a cancer.

Again, in tuberculosis, the tubercle bacillus is clearly a necessary factor, even though its presence may not

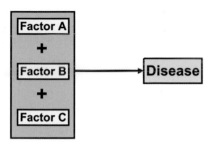

Fig. 14.13 Types of causal relationships: II. Each factor is necessary, but not sufficient.

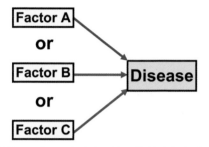

Fig. 14.14 Types of causal relationships: III. Each factor is sufficient, but not necessary.

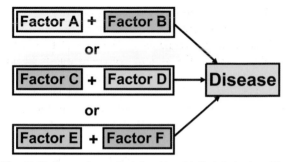

Fig. 14.15 Types of causal relationships: IV. Each factor is neither sufficient nor necessary.

be sufficient to produce the disease in every infected individual. Another example is the relationship of *Helicobacter pylori* to noncardia gastric adenocarcinoma.[4] Although this bacterium is widely regarded as a necessary cause of this cancer, most individuals who are infected with *H. pylori* do not develop this cancer, a phenomenon that explains why *H. pylori* infection prevalence is very high in many populations, yet gastric adenocarcinoma remains relatively rare in these same populations. Thus, in addition to *H. pylori*, individuals have to be exposed to other risk factors (e.g., smoking and intake of foods containing nitrates) to develop gastric cancer. (The relationship of *H. pylori* to gastric ulcers is discussed later in this chapter.)

SUFFICIENT BUT NOT NECESSARY

In this model the factor alone can produce the disease but so can other factors that are acting alone (Fig. 14.14). Thus either radiation exposure or benzene exposure can each produce leukemia without the presence of the other. However, even in this situation, cancer does not develop in everyone who has experienced radiation or benzene exposure, so although both factors are not

needed, other cofactors probably are. Thus the criterion of *sufficient* is rarely met by a single factor.

NEITHER SUFFICIENT NOR NECESSARY

In the fourth model a factor by itself is neither sufficient nor necessary to produce disease (Fig. 14.15). This is a more complex model, which probably most accurately represents the causal relationships that operate in most chronic diseases. An example is that of the often non-overlapping nature of risk factor clusters for the development of CHD; for instance, individuals may develop CHD if they are exposed to smoking, diabetes, and low high-density lipoprotein (HDL) or to a combination of hypercholesterolemia, hypertension, and physical inactivity. Each of these CHD risk factors is neither sufficient nor necessary. Interestingly, recognizing that many, if not most, individual risk factors are neither sufficient nor necessary, Rothman has proposed a model consistent with Fig. 14.15, in which a "sufficient cause" is formed by a *constellation* of risk factors, termed by him "component causes." In Rothman's conceptualization, a pie chart formed by a number of "component causes" represents the "sufficient cause." Thus Rothman's "sufficient cause" is actually a cluster of "component causes."[5] Hypothetical (yet not illogical) examples of Rothman-defined two "sufficient causes" for athero-sclerotic disease are seen in Fig. 14.16.

Evidence for a Causal Relationship

Many years ago, when the major disease problems faced by humans were primarily infectious in origin, the question arose as to what evidence would be necessary to prove that an organism causes a disease. In 1840

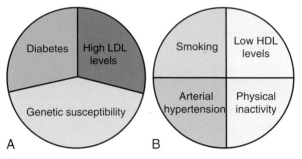

Fig. 14.16 (A–B) Hypothetical examples of of sufficient causes of atherosclerotic disease. *HDL*, High-density lipoprotein; *LDL*, low-density lipoprotein.

Henle proposed postulates for causation that were expanded by Koch in the 1880s.[6] The postulates for causation were as follows:

1. The organism is *always* found with the disease.
2. The organism is *not* found with any other disease.
3. The organism, when isolated from one who has the disease and cultured through several generations, produces the disease (in experimental animals).

Koch added that "[E]ven when an infectious disease cannot be transmitted to animals, the 'regular' and 'exclusive' presence of the organism [postulates 1 and 2] proves a causal relationship."[6]

These postulates, although not perfect, proved very useful for infectious diseases. However, as apparently noninfectious diseases assumed increasing importance toward the middle of the 20th century, the issue arose as to what would represent strong evidence of causation in diseases that were generally not of infectious origin. In such diseases there was no organism that could be isolated, cultured, and grown in animals. Specifically, as attention was directed to a possible relationship between smoking and lung cancer, the US Surgeon General appointed an expert committee to review the evidence. The committee developed a set of guidelines,[7] which have been revised over the years. The next few pages present a modified list of these guidelines (Box 14.1) with some brief comments.

Guidelines for Judging Whether an Observed Association Is Causal

1. Temporal Relationship. It is clear that if a factor is believed to be the cause of a disease, exposure to the

BOX 14.1 GUIDELINES FOR JUDGING WHETHER AN OBSERVED ASSOCIATION IS CAUSAL

1. Temporal relationship
2. Strength of the association
3. Dose-response relationship
4. Replication of the findings
5. Biologic plausibility
6. Consideration of alternate explanations
7. Cessation of exposure
8. Consistency with other knowledge
9. Specificity of the association

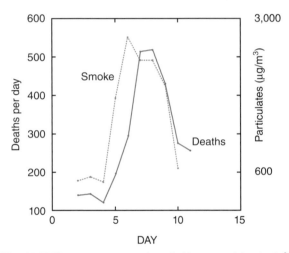

Fig. 14.17 The mean concentration of airborne particles (μg/m³) from the four inner monitoring stations in London and the count of daily deaths in the London Administrative County during the beginning of December 1952. (From Schwartz J. Air pollution and daily mortality: a review and meta analysis. *Environ Res.* 1994;64:36–52.)

factor must occur before the disease develops. Fig. 14.17 shows the number of deaths per day and the mean concentration of airborne particles in London in early December 1952.[8] The pattern of a rise in particle concentration followed by a rise in mortality and a subsequent decline in particle concentration followed by a decline in mortality strongly supported the increase in mortality being due to the increase in air pollution. This example demonstrates the use of ecologic data for exploring a temporal relationship. Further investigation revealed that the increased mortality consisted almost entirely of respiratory and cardiovascular deaths and was highest in the elderly.

It is often easier to establish a temporal relationship in a prospective cohort study than in a case-control study or a retrospective (nonconcurrent) cohort study. In the latter two types of studies, exposure information may need to be located or re-created from past records and the timing may therefore be imprecise.

The temporal relationship of exposure and disease is important not only for clarifying the *order* in which the two occur but also in regard to the *length of the interval* between exposure and disease. For example, asbestos has been clearly linked to increased risk of lung cancer, but the latent period between the exposure and the appearance of lung cancer is at least 15 to 20 years. Therefore, if, for example, lung cancer develops after only 3 years since the asbestos exposure, it is probably safe to conclude that the lung cancer was not a result of this exposure.

2. Strength of the Association. The strength of the association is measured by the relative risk (or odds ratio). The stronger the association, the more likely it is that the relation is causal. For example, the relative risk for the relationship of high blood pressure (exposure) to stroke (outcome) is very high. In a population-based study conducted in Sweden, the relative risk was found to be greater than 5.0 in individuals with severe hypertension.[9] There is little or no doubt that high blood pressure levels cause stroke.

3. Dose-Response Relationship. As the dose of exposure increases, the risk of disease also increases. Fig. 14.18 shows an example of the dose-response relationship for cigarette smoking and lung cancer. Another example is given by the Swedish study mentioned above, in which, using normal blood pressure levels as the reference category, the adjusted relative risk for stroke increased in a graded fashion from 2.84 in individuals with prehypertension to 3.90 in those with moderately severe hypertension to 5.43 in those with levels consistent with severe hypertension. If a dose-response relationship is present, it is strong evidence for a causal relationship. However, the absence of a dose-response relationship does not necessarily rule out a causal relationship. In some cases in which a *threshold* may exist, no disease may develop up to a certain level of exposure (a threshold); above this level, disease may develop.

4. Replication of the Findings. If the relationship is causal, we would expect to find it consistently in

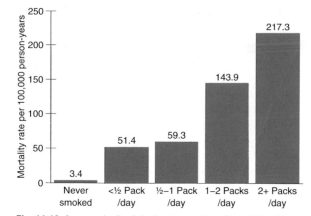

Fig. 14.18 Age-standardized death rates due to well-established cases of bronchogenic carcinoma (exclusive of adenocarcinoma) by current amount of smoking. (Modified from Hammond EC, Horn D. Smoking and death rates: report on 44 months of follow-up of 187,783 men: II. Death rates by cause. *JAMA.* 1958;166:1294–1508. Copyright 1958, American Medical Association.)

different studies and in different populations. Replication of findings is particularly important in epidemiology. If an association is observed, we would also expect it to be seen consistently within subgroups of the population and in different populations, unless there is a clear reason to expect different results.

5. Biologic Plausibility. Biologic plausibility refers to coherence with the current body of biologic knowledge. Examples may be cited to demonstrate that epidemiologic observations have sometimes preceded biologic knowledge. Thus, as discussed in an earlier chapter, Gregg's observations on rubella and congenital cataracts preceded any knowledge of teratogenic viruses. Similarly, the implication of high oxygen concentration in the causation of retrolental fibroplasia, a form of blindness that occurs in premature infants, preceded any biologic knowledge supporting such a relationship. Nevertheless, we seek consistency of the epidemiologic findings with existing biologic knowledge, and when this is not the case, interpreting the meaning of the observed association may be difficult. We may then be more demanding in our requirements about the size and significance of any differences observed and in having the study replicated by other investigators in other populations.

6. Consideration of Alternate Explanations. We have discussed the problem in interpreting an observed association in regard to whether a relationship is causal or is the result of confounding. In judging whether a reported association is causal, the extent to which the investigators have taken other possible explanations into account and the extent to which they have ruled out such explanations are important considerations.

7. Cessation of Exposure. If a factor is a cause of a disease, we would expect the risk of the disease to decline when exposure to the factor is reduced or eliminated. Fig. 14.19 shows such historical data for cigarette smoking and lung cancer. Another example

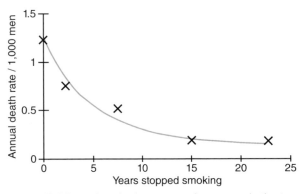

Fig. 14.19 Effects of terminating exposure: lung cancer death rates, standardized for age and amount smoked, among men continuing to smoke cigarettes and men who gave up smoking for different periods. The corresponding rate for nonsmokers was 0.07 per 1,000. (Modified from Doll R, Hill AB. Mortality in relation to smoking: ten years' observations of British doctors. *BMJ.* 1964;1:1399–1410.)

was the rapid decrease of CHD, diabetes, and stroke rates following a dramatic decrease in energy intake and thus obesity due to the economic Cuban economic crisis of 1989–2000.[10]

Eosinophilia-myalgia syndrome (EMS) reached epidemic proportions in 1989. Characterized by severe muscle pain and a high blood eosinophil count, the syndrome was found to be associated with manufactured preparations of L-tryptophan. In November 1989 a nationwide recall by the US Food and Drug Administration of over-the-counter preparations of L-tryptophan was followed by dramatic reductions in numbers of cases of EMS reported each month (Fig. 14.20). This is another example of a reduction in incidence being related to cessation of exposure, which adds to the strength of the causal inference regarding the exposure.

When cessation data are available, they provide helpful supporting evidence for a causal association. However, in certain cases the pathogenic process may have been irreversibly initiated and the disease occurrence may have been determined by the time the exposure is removed. Emphysema is not reversed with cessation of smoking, but its progression is reduced.

8. Consistency With Other Knowledge. If a relationship is causal, we would expect the findings to be consistent with other data. For example, Fig. 14.21 shows data regarding lung cancer rates in men and women and cigarette smoking in men and women.

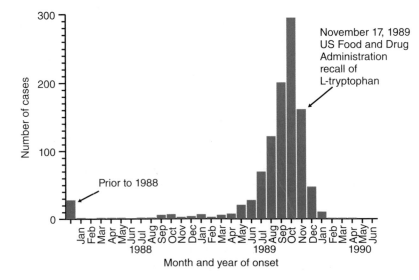

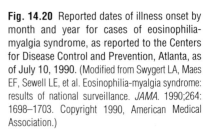

Fig. 14.20 Reported dates of illness onset by month and year for cases of eosinophilia-myalgia syndrome, as reported to the Centers for Disease Control and Prevention, Atlanta, as of July 10, 1990. (Modified from Swygert LA, Maes EF, Sewell LE, et al. Eosinophilia-myalgia syndrome: results of national surveillance. *JAMA.* 1990;264: 1698–1703. Copyright 1990, American Medical Association.)

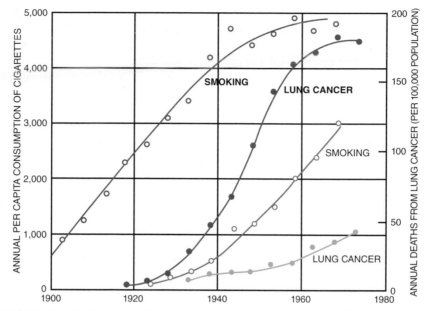

Fig. 14.21 Parallel trends between cigarette consumption and lung cancer in men *(two curves on left)* and in women *(two curves on right)* in England and Wales. (From Cairns J. The cancer problem. *Sci Am.* 1975;233:64–72, 77–78.)

We see a consistent direction in the curves, with the increase in lung cancer rates following the increase in cigarette sales for both men and women. These data are consistent with what we would expect if the relationship between smoking and lung cancer is established as a causal one. Although the absence of such consistency would not completely rule out this hypothesis, if we observed rising lung cancer rates after a period of declining cigarette sales, for example, we would need to explain how this observation could be consistent with a causal hypothesis.

9. Specificity of the Association. An association is specific when a certain exposure is associated with only one disease; this is the weakest of all the guidelines and should probably be deleted from the list. Cigarette manufacturers have pointed out that the diseases attributed to cigarette smoking do not meet the requirements of this guideline because cigarette smoking has been linked to lung cancer, pancreatic cancer, bladder cancer, heart disease, emphysema, and other conditions.

The possibility of such multiple effects from a single factor is not, in fact, surprising: regardless of the tissue that comprises them, all cells have common

characteristics, including DNA, RNA, and various subcellular structures, so a single agent could have effects in multiple tissues. Furthermore, cigarettes are not a single factor but constitute a mixture of a large number of compounds; consequently, a large number of effects might be anticipated.

When specificity of an association is found, it provides additional support for a causal inference. However, as with a dose-response relationship, absence of specificity in no way negates a causal relationship.

Any conclusion that an observed association is causal is greatly strengthened when different types of evidence from multiple sources support such reasoning. Thus it is not so much a count of the number of guidelines present that is relevant to causal inference but rather an *assessment of the total pattern of evidence observed* that may be consistent with one or more of the guidelines. Sir Austin Bradford Hill eloquently expressed this sentiment in an essay written in 1965:

Here then are nine different viewpoints [guidelines] from all of which we should study association before we cry causation. What I do not believe—and this has been suggested—that we can usefully lay down some hard-and-fast rules of evidence that must be obeyed before we can accept cause and effect. None of my nine viewpoints can bring indisputable evidence for or against the cause-and-effect hypothesis and none can be required as a sine qua non. What they can do, with greater or less strength, is to help us to make up our minds on the fundamental question—is there any other way of explaining the set of facts before us, is there any other answer equally, or more, likely than cause and effect?[11]

Deriving Causal Inferences: Two Examples

PEPTIC ULCERS AND GASTRIC CANCER IN RELATION TO INFECTION WITH *HELICOBACTER PYLORI*

Although the preceding guidelines do not permit a quantitative estimation of whether an association is causal, they can nevertheless be very helpful, as seen in the following examples.

Until the 1980s the major causes of peptic ulcer disease were considered to be stress and lifestyle factors, including smoking. Peptic ulcer disease had long been attributed to the effects of gastric acid. Susceptibility to gastric acid had been linked to cigarette smoking, alcohol consumption, and use of nonsteroidal antiinflammatory agents. Therapy was primarily directed at inhibiting acid secretion and protecting mucosal surfaces from acid. Although these therapies helped healing, relapses were common.

In 1984 Australian physicians Drs. Barry J. Marshall and J. Robin Warren reported that they had observed small curved bacteria colonizing the lower part of the stomach in patients with gastritis and peptic ulcers.[12] After several attempts, Marshall succeeded in cultivating a hitherto unknown bacterial species (later named *H. pylori*) from several of these biopsies (Fig. 14.22). Together they found that the organism was present in almost all patients with gastric inflammation or peptic ulcer. Many of these patients had biopsies performed which showed evidence of inflammation present in the gastric mucosa close to where the bacteria were seen. Based on these results, they proposed that *H. pylori* is involved in the etiology of these diseases. It was subsequently shown that the ulcer was often not cured until *H. pylori* had been eliminated.

It is now firmly established that *H. pylori* causes more than 90% of duodenal ulcers and up to 80%

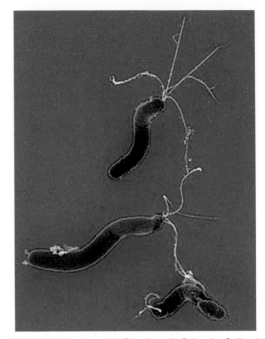

Fig. 14.22 *Helicobacter pylori.* (Encyclopædia Britannica Online. http://www.britannica.com/EBchecked/topic/450889/peptic-ulcer?overlay=true&assemblyId=94921. Accessed November 2017.)

of gastric ulcers. The link between *H. pylori* infection and subsequent gastritis and peptic ulcer disease has been established through studies of human volunteers, antibiotic treatment studies, and epidemiologic studies. Thus many of the study designs discussed in previous chapters and many of the guidelines for causal inferences discussed earlier in this chapter were involved in elucidating the role of *H. pylori* in peptic ulcer and gastritis. In 2005 the Nobel Prize for Physiology or Medicine was shared by Drs. Marshall and Warren "for their discovery of the bacterium *H. pylori* and its role in gastritis and peptic ulcer disease."

Box 14.2 categorizes this evidence according to several of the guidelines for causation just discussed. Thus, as seen here, the guidelines can be extremely helpful in characterizing the evidence supporting a causal relationship.

Increasing evidence now also supports the association of *H. pylori* infection and the development of gastric cancer. Uemura and coworkers[13] prospectively studied 1,526 Japanese patients who had duodenal or gastric

BOX 14.2 ASSESSMENT OF THE EVIDENCE SUGGESTING *HELICOBACTER PYLORI* AS A CAUSATIVE AGENT OF DUODENAL ULCERS

1. Temporal relationship
   - *Helicobacter pylori* is clearly linked to chronic gastritis. Approximately 11% of chronic gastritis patients will go on to have duodenal ulcers over a 10-year period.
   - In one study of 454 patients who underwent endoscopy 10 years earlier, 34 of 321 patients who had been positive for *H. pylori* (11%) had duodenal ulcer compared with 1 of 133 *H. pylori*–negative patients (0.8%).
2. Strength of the association
   - *H. pylori* is found in at least 90% of patients with duodenal ulcer. In at least one population reported to lack duodenal ulcers, a northern Australian aboriginal tribe that is isolated from other people, it has never been found.
3. Dose-response relationship
   - Density of *H. pylori* per square millimeter of gastric mucosa is higher in patients with duodenal ulcer than in patients without duodenal ulcer. Also see item 2 above.
4. Replication of the findings
   - Many of the observations regarding *H. pylori* have been replicated repeatedly.
5. Biologic plausibility
   - Although originally it was difficult to envision a bacterium that infects the stomach antrum causing ulcers in the duodenum, it is now recognized that *H. pylori* has binding sites on antral cells and can follow these cells into the duodenum.
   - *H. pylori* also induces mediators of inflammation.
   - *H. pylori*–infected mucosa is weakened and is susceptible to the damaging effects of acid.
6. Consideration of alternate explanations
   - Data suggest that smoking can increase the risk of duodenal ulcer in *H. pylori*–infected patients but is not a risk factor in patients in whom *H. pylori* has been eradicated.
7. Cessation of exposure
   - Eradication of *H. pylori* heals duodenal ulcers at the same rate as histamine receptor antagonists.
   - Long-term ulcer recurrence rates were zero after *H. pylori* was eradicated using triple-antimicrobial therapy, compared with a 60%–80% relapse rate often found in patients with duodenal ulcers treated with histamine receptor antagonists.
8. Consistency with other knowledge
   - Prevalence of *H. pylori* infection is the same in men as in women. The incidence of duodenal ulcer, which in earlier years was believed to be higher in men than in women, has been equal in recent years.
   - The prevalence of ulcer disease is believed to have peaked in the latter part of the 19th century, and the prevalence of *H. pylori* may have been much higher at that time because of poor living conditions. This reasoning is also based on current observations that the prevalence of *H. pylori* is much higher in developing countries.
9. Specificity of the association
   - Prevalence of *H. pylori* in patients with duodenal ulcers is 90%–100%. However, it is found in some patients with gastric ulcer and even in asymptomatic individuals.

Data from Megraud F, Lamouliatte H. Helicobacter pylori *and duodenal ulcer: evidence suggesting causation.* Dig Dis Sci. *1992;37:769–772; and DeCross AJ, Marshall BJ. The role of* Helicobacter pylori *in acid-peptic disease.* Am J Med Sci. *1993;306:381–392.*

ulcers, gastric hyperplasia, or nonulcer hyperplasia. Of this group, 1,246 had *H. pylori* infection and 280 did not. The mean follow-up period was 7.8 years. Gastric cancers developed in 36 (2.9%) of the infected patients but in none of the uninfected patients. Individuals who carry antibodies to *H. pylori* may have a 2 to 3 times higher risk of stomach cancer than those who do not (Fig. 14.23). The risk of stomach cancer also appears to be related to the type of strain of *H. pylori* which is infecting a person. Evidence is accumulating to support the idea that therapy against *H. pylori* may prevent gastric cancer. In the future, gastric cancer may come to be viewed as a largely preventable cancer of infectious origin.

AGE OF ONSET OF ALCOHOL USE AND LIFETIME ALCOHOL ABUSE

In 1997 Grant and Dawson[14] reported data on the relationship of age at first use of alcohol and prevalence of lifetime alcohol dependence and abuse. They analyzed data from 27,616 current and former drinkers who were interviewed as part of the 1992 National Longitudinal Alcohol Epidemiologic Survey. The rates of lifetime *dependence* decreased from more than 40%

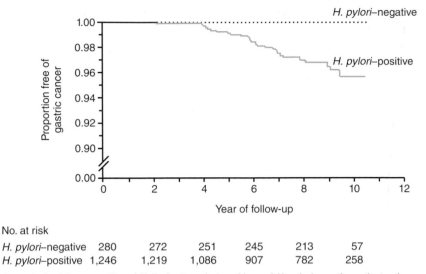

No. at risk

H. pylori–negative	280	272	251	245	213	57
H. pylori–positive	1,246	1,219	1,086	907	782	258

Fig. 14.23 Kaplan-Meier analysis of the proportion of *Helicobacter pylori*–positive and *H. pylori*–negative patients who remained free of gastric cancer. During follow-up, gastric cancer developed in 36 of the 1,246 *H. pylori*–infected patients (2.9%) but in none of the 280 uninfected patients (*P* < .001). (From Uemura N, Okamoto S, Yamomoto S, et al. *Helicobacter pylori* infection and the development of gastric cancer. *N Engl J Med.* 2001; 345:784–789.)

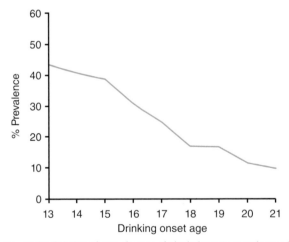

Fig. 14.24 Relation of age of onset of alcohol use to prevalence of lifetime alcohol abuse. (Modified from Grant BF, Dawson DA. Age at onset of alcohol use and its association with DSM-IV alcohol abuse and dependence: results from the National Longitudinal Alcohol Epidemiologic Survey. *J Subst Abuse.* 1997;9:103–110.)

among individuals who began drinking at age 14 years or younger to approximately 10% among those who started drinking at age 20 years or older (Fig. 14.24). The configuration of the curve in Fig. 14.24 suggests a dose-response relationship as has been observed for

longer duration of smoking associated with increased risk of lung cancer. However, the data may also point to a period of particularly high susceptibility, namely, that the period of preadolescence and early adolescence is a period of increased risk for developing a disorder of alcohol use. Therefore preventive interventions should be targeted to this group in the hope of delaying drinking onset. However, adopting such an approach assumes that the relationship between early onset of drinking and subsequent lifetime abuse is a causal one, so that delaying age at onset of drinking would reduce the risk of lifetime alcohol dependence. Another possible explanation is that those who are destined for lifetime alcohol dependence tend to begin drinking earlier but that the earlier age at drinking onset is not necessarily a cause of the later dependence. Further research is therefore needed to explain the intriguing association that has been observed. We shall return to this example in Chapter 16.

Modifications of the Guidelines for Causal Inferences

In 1986 the US Public Health Service brought together a group of 19 experts to examine the scientific basis of the content of prenatal care and to answer the question: Which measures implemented during prenatal care have actually been demonstrated to be associated with improved outcome? The panel's report was issued in 1989 and served as the basis of a comprehensive report.[15] As the panel began its deliberations, it became clear that questions of causation were at the heart of the panel's task and that guidelines were needed for assessing the relationship of prenatal measures to health outcomes. A subcommittee reviewed the current guidelines (just enumerated in the preceding text) and defined a process for using evidence that includes (1) categorization of the evidence by the quality of its sources and (2) evaluation of the evidence of a causal relationship using standardized guidelines.[16] These recommendations are excerpted in Box 14.3. Although these modified guidelines clearly use the original components, they establish reasonable priorities in weighting them. They thus define an approach for looking at causation that

may have applicability far beyond questions of the effectiveness of prenatal measures.

A similar approach, ranking studies by the quality of the study and its evidence, is used by the US Preventive Services Task Force, which is responsible for developing clinical practice guidelines for prevention and screening (Table 14.1).[17] The Task Force is an independent committee of experts supported by the US government. Members include experts in primary care, prevention, evidence-based medicine, and research methods. Various clinical areas and experience in preventive medicine, public health, and health policy are also represented.

For each topic the Task Force considers, it defines the questions that need to be addressed and identifies and retrieves the relevant evidence. The quality of each individual study is assessed, after which the strength of the totality of available evidence is judged. Estimates are made of the balance of benefits and harms. This

TABLE 14.1	US Preventive Services Task Force Levels of Certainty[a] Regarding Net Benefit
High	The available evidence usually includes consistent results from well-designed, well-conducted studies in representative primary care populations. These studies assess the effects of the preventive service on health outcomes. This conclusion is therefore unlikely to be strongly affected by the results of future studies.
Moderate	The available evidence is sufficient to determine the effects of the preventive service on health outcomes, but confidence in the estimate is constrained by such factors as: • The number, size, or quality of individual studies. • Inconsistency of findings across individual studies. • Limited generalizability of findings to routine primary care practice. • Lack of coherence in the chain of evidence. As more information becomes available, the magnitude or direction of the observed effect could change, and this change may be large enough to alter the conclusion.
Low	The available evidence is insufficient to assess effects on health outcomes. Evidence is insufficient because of: • The limited number or size of studies. • Important flaws in study design or methods. • Inconsistency of findings across individual studies. • Gaps in the chain of evidence. • Findings not generalizable to routine primary care practice. • A lack of information on important health outcomes. More information may allow an estimation of effects on health outcomes.

[a]The US Preventive Services Task Force (USPSTF) defines certainty as "likelihood that the USPSTF assessment of the net benefit of a preventive service is correct." The net benefit is defined as benefit minus harm of the preventive service as implemented in a general, primary care population. The USPSTF assigns a certainty level based on the nature of the overall evidence available to assess the net benefit of a preventive service.
Modified from US Preventive Services Task Force Procedure Manual. December 2015. https://www.uspreventiveservicestaskforce.org/Home/GetFile/6/7/procedure-manual_2015/pdf. Accessed October 25, 2017.

BOX 14.3 PROCESS FOR USING THE EVIDENCE IN DEVELOPING RECOMMENDATIONS ON THE EFFECTIVENESS OF PRENATAL INTERVENTIONS

Stage I: Categorizing the Evidence by the Quality of Its Source. *(In each category, studies are listed in descending order of quality.)*

1. Trials (planned interventions with contemporaneous assignment of treatment and nontreatment)
   a. Randomized, double-blind, placebo-controlled with sufficient power appropriately analyzed.
   b. Randomized but blindness not achieved.
   c. Nonrandomized trials with good control of confounding, that are well conducted in other respects.
   d. Randomized but with deficiencies in execution or analysis (insufficient power, major losses to follow-up, suspect randomization, analysis with exclusions).
   e. Nonrandomized trials with deficiencies in execution or analysis.
2. Cohort or case-control studies
   a. Hypothesis specified before analysis, good data, confounders accounted for.
   b. As above but hypothesis not specified before analysis.
   c. Post hoc, with problem(s) in the data or the analysis.
3. Time-series studies
   a. Analyses that take confounding into account.
   b. Analyses that do not consider confounding.
4. Case-series studies: Series of case reports without any specific comparison group

Among other issues that must be considered in reviewing the evidence are the precision of definition of the outcome being measured, the degree to which the study methodology has been described, adequacy of the sample size, and the degree to which characteristics of the population studied and of the intervention being evaluated have been described.

A study can be well designed and carried out in an exemplary fashion (internal validity), but if the population studied is an unusual or highly selected one, the results may not be generalizable (external validity).

Stage II: Guidelines for Evaluating the Evidence of a Causal Relationship. *(In each category, studies are listed in descending priority order.)*

1. Major criteria
   a. Temporal relationship: An intervention can be considered evidence of a reduction in risk of disease or abnormality only if the intervention was applied before the time the disease or abnormality would have developed.
   b. Biologic plausibility: A biologically plausible mechanism should be able to explain why such a relationship would be expected to occur.
   c. Consistency: Single studies are rarely definitive. Study findings that are replicated in different populations and by different investigators carry more weight than those that are not. If the findings of studies are inconsistent, the inconsistency must be explained.
   d. Alternative explanations (confounding): The extent to which alternative explanations have been explored is an important criterion in judging causality.
2. Other considerations
   a. Dose-response relationship: If a factor is indeed the cause of a disease, usually (but not invariably) the greater the exposure to the factor, the greater the risk of the disease. Such a dose-response relationship may not always be seen because many important biologic relationships are dichotomous and reach a threshold level for observed effects.
   b. Strength of the association: The strength of the association is usually measured by the extent to which the relative risk or odds depart from unity, either greater than 1 (in the case of disease-causing exposures) or less than 1 (in the case of preventive interventions).
   c. Cessation effects: If an intervention has a beneficial effect, the benefit should cease when it is removed from a population (unless carryover effect is operant).

Modified from Gordis L, Kleinman JC, Klerman LV, et al. Criteria for evaluating evidence regarding the effectiveness of prenatal interventions. In: Merkatz IR, Thompson JE, eds. New Perspectives on Prenatal Care. New York: Elsevier; 1990:31–38.

balance is expressed as the net benefit (the difference between benefits and harms). The Task Force prepares recommendations for preventive interventions based on these considerations.

Fig. 14.25 shows a generic example of the analytic plan prepared by the Task Force as a framework for evaluating the evidence for a screening program. The straight arrows show possible pathways of benefit, and the blue curved arrows show possible adverse effects relating to different stages. The primary question (question 1 in the figure) is generally one of whether screening is effective in reducing the risk of an adverse outcome such as mortality and, if so, to what extent.

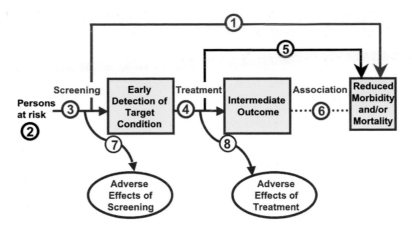

Fig. 14.25 Generic analytic framework for screening topics used by the US Preventive Services Task Force. Numbers refer to key questions in the figure. (1) Does screening for X reduce morbidity and/or mortality? (2) Can a group at high risk for X be identified on clinical grounds? (3) Are there accurate (i.e., sensitive and specific) screening tests available? (4) Are treatments available that make a difference in intermediate outcomes when the disease is caught early or detected by screening? (5) Are treatments available that make a difference in morbidity or mortality when the disease is caught early or detected by screening? (6) How strong is the association between the intermediate outcomes and patient outcomes? (7) What are the harms of the screening test? (8) What are the harms of the treatment? (Modified from US Preventive Services Task Force Procedure Manual. December 2015. https://www.uspreventiveservicestaskforce.org/Home/GetFile/6/7/procedure-manual_2015/pdf. Accessed October 25, 2017.)

Deliberations of the Task Force often deal with the different steps or linkages that comprise this overall pathway. The purple arrow in the figure (step 5) shows the relation of treatment to outcome. Red arrows in the figure, steps 3, 4, and 6, show individual components of question 1. These assessments generally depend on a review of relevant randomized trials to prepare a chain of supporting evidence on which to base an answer to question 1. The evidence for each linkage is summarized in the evidence review and then summarized across the different linkages to provide an overall assessment of the supporting evidence for the preventive service being evaluated.

The certainty of net benefit is graded on a three-point scale: high, moderate, or low (see Table 14.1). The recommendations of the Task Force are based on a combined consideration of the certainty and the magnitude of the net benefit as shown in the matrix in Fig. 14.26, in which a grading system of A, B, C, D, and *Insufficient* is used. The meaning of each grade is explained in Table 14.2.

The work of the Task Force has dealt with screening for many diseases and conditions. Some examples will illustrate the breadth of the Task Force's activities. It has reviewed the evidence for screening for different cancers,

Certainty of Net Benefit	Magnitude of Net Benefit			
	Substantial	Moderate	Small	Zero/Negative
High	A	B	C	D
Moderate	B	B	C	D
Low	Insufficient (I)			

Fig. 14.26 Grid used by the US Preventive Services Task Force for assessing the certainty of benefit and the magnitude of net benefit in determining the grade of its recommendations. (Modified from US Preventive Services Task Force Procedure Manual. December 2015. https://www.uspreventiveservicestaskforce.org/Home/GetFile/6/7/procedure-manual_2015/pdf. Accessed October 25, 2017.)

for cardiovascular diseases including hypertension, CHD, and abdominal aortic aneurysm, for infectious diseases, including gonorrhea, syphilis, chlamydia, and hepatitis B and C, and for mental conditions such as dementia, depression, and suicide risk, and screening for glaucoma and for type 2 diabetes. The Task Force has also reviewed the evidence for the effectiveness of counseling for many conditions such as counseling to prevent tobacco use and tobacco-related diseases, counseling to prevent alcohol misuse, counseling to promote a healthy diet, and counseling to promote physical activity. The above issues have been addressed

TABLE 14.2	What the US Preventive Services Task Force (USPSTF) Grades Mean and Suggestions for Practice	
Grade	**Grade Definitions**	**Suggestions for Practice**
A	The USPSTF recommends the service. There is high certainty that the net benefit is substantial.	Offer or provide this service.
B	The USPSTF recommends the service. There is high certainty that the net benefit is moderate or there is moderate certainty that the net benefit is moderate to substantial.	Offer or provide this service.
C	*Note: The following statement is undergoing revision.* Clinicians may provide this service to selected patients depending on individual circumstances. However, for most individuals without signs or symptoms there is likely to be only a small benefit from this service.	Offer or provide this service only if there are other considerations that support the offering or providing the service in an individual patient.
D	The USPSTF recommends against the service. There is moderate or high certainty that the service has no net benefit or that the harms outweigh the benefits.	Discourage the use of this service.
I	The USPSTF concludes that the current evidence is insufficient to assess the balance of benefits and harms of the service. Evidence is lacking, of poor quality, or conflicting, and the balance of benefits and harms cannot be determined.	Read the clinical considerations section of USPSTF Recommendation Statement. If offered, patients should understand the uncertainty about the balance of benefits and harms.

Modified from US Preventive Services Task Force Procedure Manual. December 2015. https://www.uspreventiveservicestaskforce.org/Home/GetFile/6/7/procedure-manual_2015/pdf. Accessed October 25, 2017.

in adults, but childhood conditions have also been reviewed by the Task Force, including prevention of dental caries in preschool children, screening for scoliosis in adolescents, newborn hearing screening, screening for visual impairment in children younger than 5 years of age, and screening for obesity in children and adolescents. These and many more evidence reviews and recommendations of the Task Force can be found on the website of the Agency for Health Care Research and Quality (https://www.ahrq.gov). The deliberations and recommendations of the Task Force provide a highly useful model of assessing the strength of the evidence and moving from causal inferences to policy recommendations.

Conclusion

Although causal guidelines discussed in this chapter are often referred to as *criteria*, this term does not seem entirely appropriate. While it may be a desirable goal to place causal inferences on a firm quantitative and structural foundation, at present we generally do not have all the information needed for doing so. The list presented in this chapter should therefore only

be considered as guidelines that can be of most value when coupled with reasoned judgment about the entire body of available evidence in making decisions about causation.

In the next chapter, we address several additional issues that need to be considered in deriving causal inferences from epidemiologic studies.

REFERENCES

1. Cameron WB. *Informal Sociology: A Casual Introduction to Sociological Thinking*. New York: Random House; 1963:13. (This quotation was also attributed to Albert Einstein some years later.)
2. Ochsner A, DeBakey M. Primary pulmonary malignancy. *Surg Gynecol Obstet*. 1939;68:435.
3. Yerushalmy J. Infants with low birth weight born before their mothers started to smoke cigarettes. *Am J Obstet Gynecol*. 1972;112:277–284.
4. de Martel C, Forman D, Plummer M. Gastric cancer: epidemiology and risk factors. *Gastroenterol Clin North Am*. 2013;42:219–240.
5. Rothman KJ. *Modern Epidemiology*. Boston/Toronto: Little Brown and Company; 1986:[Chapter 2].
6. Evans AS. *Causation and Disease: A Chronological Journey*. New York: Plenum; 1993:13–39.
7. US Department of Health, Education and Welfare. *Smoking and Health: Report of the Advisory Committee to the Surgeon General*. Washington, DC: Public Health Service; 1964.
8. Schwartz J. Air pollution and daily mortality: a review and meta analysis. *Environ Res*. 1994;64:36–52.

9. Li C, Engstrom G, Hedblad B, et al. Blood pressure control and risk of stroke. A population-based cohort study. *Stroke.* 2005;36:725–730.

10. Franco M, Ordunez P, Caballero B, et al. Impact of energy intake, physical activity, and population-wide weight loss on cardiovascular disease and diabetes mortality in Cuba, 1980-2005. *Am J Epidemiol.* 2007;166:1374–1380.

11. Hill AB. The environment and disease: association or causation? *Proc R Soc Med.* 1965;58:295–300.

12. Marshall BJ, Warren JR. Unidentified curved bacilli in the stomachs of patients with gastritis and peptic ulceration. *Lancet.* 1984;1:1311–1315.

13. Uemura N, Okamoto S, Yamamoto S, et al. *Helicobacter pylori* infection and the development of gastric cancer. *N Engl J Med.* 2001;345:784–789.

14. Grant BF, Dawson DA. Age at onset of alcohol use and its association with DSM-IV alcohol abuse and dependence: results from the National Longitudinal Alcohol Epidemiologic Survey. *J Subst Abuse.* 1997;9:103–110.

15. Merkatz IR, Thompson JE, eds. *New Perspectives on Prenatal Care.* New York: Elsevier; 1990.

16. Gordis L, Kleinman JC, Klerman LV, et al. Criteria for evaluating evidence regarding the effectiveness of prenatal interventions. In: Merkatz IR, Thompson JE, eds. *New Perspectives on Prenatal Care.* New York: Elsevier; 1990:31–38.

17. US Preventive Services Task Force. *Procedure Manual.* December 2015. https://www.uspreventiveservicestaskforce.org/Home/GetFile/6/7/procedure-manual_2015/pdf. Accessed October 25, 2017.

REVIEW QUESTIONS FOR CHAPTER 14

1 In a large case-control study of patients with pancreatic cancer, 17% of the patients were found to be diabetic at the time of diagnosis, compared with 4% of a well-matched control group (matched by age, sex, ethnic group, and several other characteristics) that was examined for diabetes at the same time as the cases were diagnosed. It was concluded that the diabetes played a causal role in the pancreatic cancer. This conclusion:

a. Is correct

b. May be incorrect because there is no control or comparison group

c. May be incorrect because of failure to establish the time sequence between onset of the diabetes and diagnosis of pancreatic cancer

d. May be incorrect because of less complete ascertainment of diabetes in the pancreatic cancer cases

e. May be incorrect because of more complete ascertainment of pancreatic cancer in nondiabetic persons

2 An investigator examined cases of fetal death in 27,000 pregnancies and classified mothers according to whether they had experienced sexual intercourse within 1 month before delivery. It was found that 11% of the mothers of fetuses that died and 2.5% of the mothers of fetuses that survived had had sexual intercourse during the period. It was concluded that intercourse during the month preceding delivery caused the fetal deaths. This conclusion:

a. May be incorrect because mothers who had intercourse during the month before childbirth may differ in other important characteristics from those who did not

b. May be incorrect because there is no comparison group

c. May be incorrect because prevalence rates are used where incidence rates are needed

d. May be incorrect because of failure to achieve a high level of statistical significance

e. Both *b* and *c*

3 All of the following are important criteria when making causal inferences except:

a. Consistency with existing knowledge

b. Dose-response relationship

c. Consistency of association in several studies

d. Strength of association

e. Predictive value

Questions 4 and 5 are based on the following information:

Factor A, B, or C can each individually cause a certain disease without the other two factors but only when followed by exposure to factor X. Exposure to factor X alone is not followed by the disease, but the disease never occurs in the absence of exposure to factor X.

4 *Factor X is:*
   a. A necessary and sufficient cause
   b. A necessary but not sufficient cause
   c. A sufficient but not necessary cause

   d. Neither necessary nor sufficient
   e. None of the above

5 *Factor A is:*
   a. A necessary and sufficient cause
   b. A necessary but not sufficient cause
   c. A sufficient but not necessary cause

   d. Neither necessary nor sufficient
   e. None of the above

Chapter 15

More on Causal Inference: Bias, Confounding, and Interaction

Learning Objectives

- To review some possible biases in epidemiologic studies, including selection bias and information bias.
- To define confounding and to discuss possible ways to deal with confounding in the design and/or analysis of an observational (nonrandomized) study.
- To define interaction and to present a framework for detecting whether (and to what extent) two factors interact to influence the risk of a disease.

In this chapter, we expand on the discussion of causation that was begun in Chapter 14. We now focus on three important issues in making causal inferences: (1) bias, (2) confounding, and (3) interaction. These three issues are important for any type of study design, although if a randomized study is done properly, bias and confounding will be kept to a minimum. Examples of each issue are described in the context of specific study designs, but it should be kept in mind that these issues can affect all types of study designs, and are not limited to the types of studies that have been selected as examples in this chapter.

Bias

Bias has been addressed in many of the previous chapters because it is a major consideration in any type of epidemiologic study design. Therefore only a few additional comments will be made here.

What do we mean by *bias?* Bias has been defined as "any systematic error in the design, conduct or analysis of a study that results in a mistaken estimate of an exposure's effect on the risk of disease."[1]

SELECTION BIAS

What types of bias do we encounter in epidemiologic studies? The first is *selection bias.* If the way in which cases and controls, or exposed and unexposed individuals, were selected is such that an apparent association is observed—even if, in reality, exposure and disease are not associated—the apparent association is the result of selection bias.

Selection bias may result from nonresponse of potential study participants. For example, if we are studying the possible relationship of an exposure and a disease outcome and the response rate of potential subjects is higher in people with the disease who were exposed than in people with the disease who were not exposed, an apparent association could be observed even if in reality there is no association. Alternatively, the association, even if real, may be inflated by having greater participation among people with the disease who were exposed. The opposite may also lead to bias (i.e., when those who are both diseased and exposed are less likely to participate in the study).

In general, people who refuse to participate in a study often differ from those who participate in regard to many demographic, socioeconomic, cultural, lifestyle, and health status factors.[2] One study that attempted to characterize nonresponders was reported by Ronmark et al. in 1999.[3] In the course of carrying out a prevalence study of asthma, chronic bronchitis, and respiratory symptoms, they studied the characteristics of nonresponders and the reasons for nonresponse. In this study, 9,132 people living in Sweden were invited to participate. Data were obtained by a mailed questionnaire, and the response rate was 85%. A sample of nonresponders was contacted by telephone and interviewed using the same questionnaire used in the main study. The authors found a significantly higher proportion of current smokers and manual laborers among the nonresponders than among the study participants. In addition, the prevalence rates of wheezing, chronic cough, sputum production, attacks of breathlessness, asthma, and use of asthma medications were significantly higher among the nonresponders than among the responders. Thus the study inferences were diminished by the loss of participation from the nonresponders, as the associations that were found in the respondents were skewed toward the null.

In most studies no information can be obtained from the nonresponders, and hence nonresponse may introduce a serious bias into the study that may be difficult (or perhaps impossible) to assess. It is therefore important to keep nonresponse to a minimum. For example, the UK Biobank recruited 500,000 men and women ages 40 to 69 over 5 years to evaluate risk factors for the major diseases of middle and old age.[4] While a very large number for a cohort study, only 5% of the adults approached agreed to participate in the study. The extent to which the recruited sample represents the target population may be of concern. However, since all UK citizens are included in the National Health Service, comparisons of the cohort to the target population can be estimated. In addition, any nonresponders should be characterized as much as possible by using whatever information is available to determine ways in which they differ from responders (estimated age, sex, geographic location, etc.) and to gauge the likely impact of their nonresponse on the results of the study.

In cohort studies, participant losses during follow-up may also result in selection bias. However, since there is baseline information on these losses at the time of enrollment, it is possible to compare those who are lost with those who are not lost to observation on a number of sociodemographic and other factors. In the United States and other countries, it is also possible to link information on nonrespondents to a national death registry, thus allowing a comparison of mortality rates of the outcome under study for respondents and nonrespondents. This type of linkage is particularly useful when the primary outcome of the study is mortality.[5–8] It is important to keep in mind the distinction between *selecting subjects for a study* and *selection bias*. Virtually every study conducted in human populations selects study subjects from a larger (target) population. The nature of this selection

potentially affects the *generalizability* or *external validity* of the study but does not necessarily affect the validity of the comparisons made within the study or the study's *internal validity*. On the other hand, when a systematic error is made in selecting one or more of the study groups that will be compared, *selection bias* may result. Such a bias can result in odds ratios (ORs) or relative risks (RRs) that may not be correct estimates and consequently lead to invalid inferences regarding the associations of exposure and disease. Selection bias can therefore arise as an error in selecting a study group or groups within the study, and can have a major impact on the internal validity of the study and the legitimacy of the inference regarding the association of exposure and outcome. Selecting the study population from a larger target population should not be confused with selection bias, which results from a systematic error in selecting subjects in one or more of the study groups, such as exposed or unexposed participants, or cases or controls.

An interesting "classic" example of selection bias was demonstrated in 1974 with the publication of data that appeared to suggest a relationship between use of reserpine (a commonly used antihypertensive agent) and the risk of breast cancer. Three articles supporting such an association were published in the same issue of the *Lancet* in September 1974.[9–11] The three papers reported three studies conducted in Boston, Great Britain, and Helsinki, respectively.

Let's consider one of these articles, which exemplifies the problem of selection bias. Heinonen et al.[11] reported a matched-pair case-control study carried out in surgical patients at a hospital in Helsinki. Women with breast cancer were compared with women without breast cancer in terms of use of reserpine. Women with newly diagnosed breast cancer were identified from a hospital discharge register and from records that logged operations at the hospital. They served as "cases," and each was pair-matched by age and year of her operation to a control who was a woman admitted for elective surgery for some benign condition. A total of 438 case-control pairs were available for analysis. As seen in Table 15.1, there were 45 pairs in which the case used reserpine and the control did not, and 23 pairs in which the control used reserpine and the case did not. The resulting matched pair odds ratio (OR) was 45/23, or 1.96.

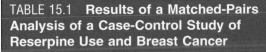

TABLE 15.1 **Results of a Matched-Pairs Analysis of a Case-Control Study of Reserpine Use and Breast Cancer**		
	Controls	
Breast Cancer Cases	*Used Reserpine*	*Did Not Use Reserpine*
Used Reserpine	8	45
Did Not Use Reserpine	23	362

$$\text{Matched-pairs odds ratio} = \frac{45}{23} = 1.96$$

Modified from Heinonen OP, Shapiro S, Tuominen L, Turunen MI. Reserpine use in relation to breast cancer. *Lancet.* 1974;2:675–677.

A problem was recognized, however, in the method used for selecting controls. In selecting the controls, the authors excluded women who had had the following surgeries: cholecystectomy, thyroidectomy for thyrotoxicosis, surgery for renal disease, and any cardiac operation, sympathectomy, or vascular graft. They were excluded because at the time the study was conducted, reserpine was one of the agents often used in treating these conditions. The authors were concerned that if patients with these conditions were included in this case-control study, the prevalence of reserpine use in the controls would be artificially high, so that even if reserpine use was increased in breast cancer cases, the increase might not be detected.

Unfortunately, in trying to address this concern, the authors created a different problem because these exclusions were not applied to the cases. By excluding patients with these conditions from the controls, they created a control group in which the prevalence of reserpine use was artificially lower because a large group of potential reserpine users was excluded. Thus, even if in reality reserpine use was not increased in women who developed breast cancer, this study could show a difference in reserpine use between the cases and the controls only because of the way the controls were selected.

This type of selection bias has been called *exclusion bias.*[12] It results when investigators apply different eligibility ("inclusion") criteria to the cases and to the controls, in regard to which clinical conditions in the past would permit eligibility in the study and which would serve as the basis for exclusion. Horwitz and Feinstein[12] tried to replicate the reserpine study in 257 women with breast cancer and 257 controls, calculating ORs in two ways: first, including all the women and, second, after excluding from the controls women with a history of cardiovascular disease. The OR including all women was 1.1, but when women with cardiovascular disease were excluded, the OR rose to 2.5. These findings support the suggestion that the apparent relation of reserpine use and breast cancer in the Helsinki study resulted from selection bias due to the different criteria for selecting controls in the study. The study that dealt with coffee drinking and pancreatic cancer[13] had a similar problem, as discussed in Chapter 7.

The application of the same eligibility criteria to the selection of cases and controls should ideally result in the phenomenon coined by Schlesselman as *compensating bias.*[1] A corollary of this notion is that when the bias in selecting cases and controls is of the same magnitude, compensating bias is achieved. A hypothetical example of compensating bias is a case-control study in which both cases and controls are identified through a screening program. Individuals who decide to undergo a screening examination do not know before the screening whether they will be cases or controls, and thus the self-selection for screening is independent of the screening result. In colon cancer, for example, individuals who choose to undergo a colonoscopy are more likely to have a family history of colon cancer and to have a history of colon polyps. However, as the self-selection process is the same for those who are subsequently found to have colon cancer and those who are not, compensating bias is achieved and, as a result, the OR is unbiased. In other words, these selection factors (family history and a history of colon polyps) are equally inflated (biased) in both cases and controls, and thus when calculating the OR, the "inflation (bias) factor" cancels out. If individuals with a family history of colon cancer are twice as likely to be included in the study, then:

$$\text{Odds Ratio} = \frac{\text{Odds of exposure in cases} \times 2.0}{\text{Odds of exposure in controls} \times 2.0}$$

$$= \frac{\text{Odds of exposure in cases}}{\text{Odds of exposure in controls}} \times 1.0$$

$$= \text{True Odds Ratio}$$

This phenomenon explains why the measure of association may be unbiased even if each exposure frequency is biased.

INFORMATION BIAS

Information bias can occur when the means for obtaining information about the subjects in the study are flawed so that some of the information gathered regarding exposures and/or disease outcomes is incorrect.

Given inaccuracies in methods of data acquisition, we may at times misclassify subjects and thereby introduce a misclassification bias. For example, in a case-control study, some people who have the disease (cases) may be unknowingly misclassified as controls, and some without the disease (controls) may be misclassified as cases. This may result, for example, from limited sensitivity and specificity of the diagnostic tests involved or from inadequacy of information derived from medical or other records. Another possibility is that we may misclassify a person's exposure status: we may believe the person was exposed when the person was not exposed, or we may believe that the person was not exposed when, in fact, exposure did occur. If exposure data are based on interviews, for example, subjects may either not be aware of their exposure or may erroneously think that it did not occur. It is also possible that research participants may hold back information if they think it might be potentially embarrassing. If ascertainment of exposure is based on old records, data may be lost, incomplete, or inaccurate.

Misclassification may occur in two forms: differential and nondifferential. In *differential misclassification*, the rate of misclassification differs in different study groups. For example, misclassification of exposure may occur such that unexposed cases are misclassified as being exposed more often than the unexposed controls are

misclassified as being exposed. This was seen in the hypothetical example of recall bias (maternal reports of infection during pregnancy and babies born with congenital malformations) presented in the discussion of case-control studies (see Chapter 7). Women who had a baby with a malformation tended to remember (or report) more mild infections that occurred during their pregnancies than mothers of infants without malformations. Controls were probably less likely to remember a mild infection during the pregnancy. Thus there was a tendency for differential misclassification in regard to prenatal infection, in that more unexposed cases were misclassified as exposed than unexposed controls. The result was an apparent association of malformations with infections, even though none existed. So, a differential misclassification bias can lead either to an apparent association even if one does not really exist or to an apparent lack of association when one does in fact exist.

In contrast, *nondifferential misclassification* results from the degree of inaccuracy that characterizes how information is obtained from any study group—either or both cases and controls or exposed and unexposed persons. Such misclassification is not related to exposure status or to case or control status; it is just a problem inherent in the *data collection methods*. The usual effect of nondifferential misclassification is that the relative risk (RR) or OR tends to be diluted, and it is shifted toward 1.0. In other words, we are less likely to detect an association, even if one really exists.

This can be seen intuitively. Let's say that in reality there is a strong association of an exposure and a disease—that is, people without the disease have much less exposure than do people with the disease. Unfortunately, by mistake, we have included some diseased persons in our control group (false negatives) and some nondiseased persons in our case group (false positives). We have, in other words, misclassified some of the subjects in regard to diagnosis. In this situation, our controls will not have such a low rate of exposure because some diseased people have been mistakenly included in this group, and our cases will not have such a high rate of exposure because some nondiseased people have been mistakenly included in the case group. As a result, a smaller difference in exposure will be found between our cases and our controls than actually exists between diseased and nondiseased people.

BOX 15.1 SOME TYPES AND SOURCES OF INFORMATION BIAS

> Bias in abstracting records
> Bias in interviewing
> Bias from surrogate interviews
> Surveillance bias
> Recall bias
> Reporting bias

Some of the types and sources of information bias in epidemiologic studies are shown in Box 15.1.

Bias may be introduced in the way that information is abstracted from medical, employment, or other records, or from the manner in which interviewers ask questions. Bias may also result from *surrogate interviews.* What does this mean? Suppose that we are carrying out a case-control study of pancreatic cancer. The case-fatality from this disease is very high, and the survival time is quite short (median treated survival is under 1 year). When we prepare to interview cases, we find that many of them have died and that many of those who have survived are too ill to be interviewed. We may then approach a family member to obtain information about the case's employment history, diet, and other exposures and characteristics. The person interviewed is most often a spouse or a child. Several problems arise in obtaining information from such surrogates. First, they may not have accurate information about the case's history. A spouse may not know accurately if at all the work-related exposures of the case. Children often know even less than do spouses. Second, there is evidence that when a wife reports on her husband's work and lifestyle after he dies, she tends to elevate his occupational level and lifestyle. She may ascribe to him a higher occupation category than that in which he was actually engaged. She may also convert him posthumously to a nondrinker or nonsmoker, or both.

If a population is monitored over a period of time, disease ascertainment may be better in the monitored population than in the general population, and may introduce a *surveillance bias,* which leads to an erroneous estimate of the RR or OR. For example, some years ago a great deal of interest centered on the possible relationship of oral contraceptive use with thrombophlebitis. It was suggested that physicians monitored patients who had been prescribed oral contraceptives much more closely than they monitored their other patients. As a result, they were more apt to identify cases of thrombophlebitis that developed in those patients who were taking oral contraceptives (and who were therefore being more closely monitored) than among other patients not prescribed oral contraceptives who were therefore not as well monitored. As a result, just through better ascertainment of thrombophlebitis in women receiving oral contraceptives, an apparent association of thrombophlebitis with oral contraceptive use may be observed, even if no true association exists.

In Chapter 7, we discussed *recall bias* in case-control studies. This bias operates to enhance recall in cases compared with controls. Thus a certain piece of information, such as a potentially relevant exposure, may be recalled by a case but forgotten by a control (as we saw in infection recall among women who had a baby with a congenital malformation). A related type of bias is *reporting bias,* in which a subject may be reluctant to report an exposure he is aware of because of attitudes, beliefs, and perceptions. This is commonly an issue in HIV/AIDS studies, where risk factors include sexual practices and substance use, which may be subject to significant reporting bias. Methodologic approaches to overcome this bias have been developed to avoid participants from trying to "look good." Audio Computer-Assisted Self-Interviewing (ACASI) was developed to allow study participants to answer sensitive questions to a computer rather than being verbally asked the questions by an interviewer, with some important results.[14,15] If such underreporting is more frequent either among the cases or among the controls, a bias may result. One example is presented below.

The term *wish bias* was coined by Wynder and coworkers[16] to denote the bias introduced by subjects who have developed a disease and who, in attempting to answer the question "Why me?," seek to show, often unintentionally, that the disease is not their fault. Thus they may deny certain exposures related to lifestyle (such as smoking or drinking); if they are contemplating litigation, they may overemphasize workplace-related exposures. Wish bias can be considered one type of reporting bias.

A point to remember is that *bias is a result of an error in the design or conduct of a study.* Efforts should therefore be made to reduce or eliminate bias or, at the very least, to recognize it and take it into account when interpreting the findings of a study. However, the data needed to document and assess the type and extent of bias may not always be available.

Let's consider an example. The relationship of induced abortion to risk of breast cancer has been a subject of considerable interest in recent years. Although in general no association has been reported for *spontaneous* abortion and risk of breast cancer, the data have been mixed in regard to the possible relationship of *induced* abortion and breast cancer. It was suggested that reporting bias might have played a role in those case-control studies that reported a positive association: healthy controls may have been more reluctant than women with breast cancer to report that they had had an induced abortion.

A study of induced abortion and risk of breast cancer provided an opportunity for the investigators to assess the extent and possible role of such reporting bias which is one type of information bias. Rookus and van Leeuwen[17] reported a case-control study in the Netherlands in which an overall estimated adjusted RR was 1.9 for induced abortion and breast cancer in parous women. (No association was found in nulliparous women.) They then compared the findings in two regions of the country—the southeastern region, which has a greater Roman Catholic, more conservative population, and the western region including Amsterdam, which has more liberal attitudes toward abortion. This difference in attitudes is reflected in the fact that the rates of induced abortions in the southeast have always been lower than in the west. As seen in Table 15.2, the authors found the association of induced abortion and breast cancer to be much stronger in the conservative southeast (estimated adjusted RR = 14.6) than in the more liberal west (estimated adjusted RR = 1.3), suggesting that the overall finding of an association of breast cancer and induced abortion in this study was largely attributable to underreporting of abortions by the controls in the southeast. Furthermore, since this study was part of a population-based case-control study of oral contraceptive use and breast cancer risk, it was possible to seek support for the possibility of such an underreporting bias as an explanation for regional differences. In the analysis of reported oral contraceptive use, when women's responses were compared with their physicians' prescriptions, controls

TABLE 15.2 Relative Risks[a] (RR) and 95% Confidence Intervals (CI) of the Development of Breast Cancer at Ages 20 to 45 Years in Relation to Previous Induced Abortions Reported by Parous Women in All Regions and in Western and Southeastern Regions of the Netherlands

	Unadjusted RR	Adjusted RR[b]	95% CI
All regions	1.8	1.9	1.1–3.2
Western region	1.2	1.3	0.7–2.6
Southeastern region	12.3	14.6	1.8–120

[a]Relative risks estimated using conditional logistic regression methods for matched pairs.
[b]Adjusted for spontaneous or induced abortion, age at first full-term pregnancy, number of full-term pregnancies, weeks of breast-feeding, family history of breast cancer, and use of injectable contraceptives.
Modified from Rookus MA, van Leeuwen FE. Induced abortion and risk for breast cancer: reporting (recall) bias in a Dutch case-control study. *J Natl Cancer Inst.* 1996;88:1759–1764.

in the southeastern region were found to have underreported the duration of their oral contraceptive use by more than 6 months more than controls in the western region.

Even location of the interview may influence the truthfulness of the information provided by the study subjects. D'Avanzo and her colleagues found different proportions of reported alcohol consumption when interviewing patients in the hospital and then again at home: when interviewed in the hospital, 62% claimed to be drinkers, but 72% reported they were drinkers upon subsequent home interviews.[18]

Confounding

A problem posed in many epidemiologic studies is that we observe a true association and are tempted to suggest a causal inference when, in fact, the relationship may not be causal. This brings us to the subject of *confounding*, one of the most important problems in observational epidemiologic studies.

What do we mean by *confounding?* In a study of whether exposure A is a cause of disease B, we say that a third factor, factor X, is a confounder *if the following are true*:

1. Factor X is a known risk factor for disease B.
2. Factor X is associated with exposure A, but is not a result of exposure A.

Recall the example we discussed in Chapter 7 of the relationship between coffee and cancer of the pancreas. Smoking was a confounder, because although we were interested in a possible relationship between coffee drinking (exposure A) and pancreatic cancer (disease B), the following are true of smoking (factor X):

1. Smoking is a known risk factor for pancreatic cancer.
2. Smoking is associated with coffee drinking, but is not a result of coffee drinking.

Thus if an association is observed between coffee drinking and cancer of the pancreas, it may be (1) that coffee actually causes cancer of the pancreas, or (2) that the observed association of coffee drinking and cancer of the pancreas may be a result of confounding by cigarette smoking (i.e., we observe the association of coffee drinking and pancreatic cancer because cigarette smoking is a risk factor for pancreatic cancer and cigarette smoking is associated with coffee drinking; Fig. 15.1).

When we observe an association, we ask whether it is causal (see Fig. 15.1A) or whether it is a result of confounding by a third factor that is both a risk factor for the disease and is associated with the putative exposure in question (see Fig. 15.1B).

Let's look at a hypothetical example: Table 15.3 shows data from an unmatched case-control study of an exposure and a disease, in which 100 cases and 100 controls were studied.

We calculate an unmatched OR of 1.95. The question arises: Is this association of the exposure with the disease a causal one, or could it have resulted from differences in the age distributions of the cases and controls? In other words, is the observed relationship confounded by age? The first question to ask in addressing this issue is whether age is related to being a case or a control. This question is answered by the analysis in Table 15.4.

We see that 80% of the controls are younger than 40 years of age, compared with only 50% of the cases. Thus older age is associated with being a case (having the disease), and younger age is associated with being a control (not having the disease).

The next question is whether age is related to exposure status.

Table 15.5 looks at the relationship of age to exposure for all 200 subjects studied, regardless of their

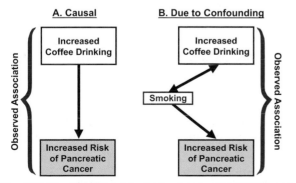

Fig. 15.1 The association between increased coffee drinking and increased risk of pancreatic cancer.

TABLE 15.3 **Hypothetical Example of Confounding in an Unmatched Case-Control Study: I. Numbers of Exposed and Nonexposed Cases and Controls**

Exposed	Cases	Controls
Yes	30	18
No	70	82
Total	100	100

$$\text{Odds ratio} = \frac{30 \times 82}{70 \times 18} = 1.95$$

TABLE 15.4 **Hypothetical Example of Confounding in an Unmatched Case-Control Study: II. Distribution of Cases and Controls by Age**

Age (yr)	Cases	Controls
<40	50	80
≥40	50	20
Total	100	100

TABLE 15.5 Hypothetical Example of Confounding in an Unmatched Case-Control Study: III. Relationship of Exposure to Age

Age (yr)	Total	Exposed	Not Exposed	% Exposed
<40	130	13	117	10
≥40	70	35	35	50

TABLE 15.6 Hypothetical Example of Confounding in an Unmatched Case-Control Study: IV. Calculations of Odds Ratios After Stratifying by Age

Age (yr)	Exposed	Cases	Controls	Odds Ratio
<40	Yes	5	8	$\dfrac{5 \times 72}{45 \times 8} = \dfrac{360}{360} = 1.0$
	No	45	72	
	Totals	**50**	**80**	
≥40	Yes	25	10	$\dfrac{25 \times 10}{25 \times 10} = \dfrac{250}{250} = 1.0$
	No	25	10	
	Totals	**50**	**20**	

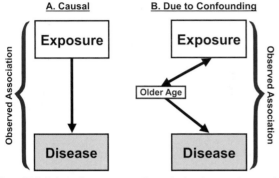

Fig. **15.2** Schematic representation of the issue of potential confounding.

BOX 15.2 APPROACHES TO HANDLING CONFOUNDING

In designing and carrying out the study:
1. Individual matching
2. Group matching

In the analysis of data:
1. Stratification
2. Adjustment

case-control status. We see that 130 people were younger than 40 years (the 50 + 80 in the top row of Table 15.4), and of these, 13 (10%) were exposed. Among the 70 subjects who were older than 40 years, 35 (50%) were exposed. Thus age is clearly related to exposure. So, at this point, we know that age is related to being a case (the cases were older than the controls); we also know that being exposed is related to older age.

As shown in Fig. 15.2, the question is: Is the association of exposure and disease causal (see Fig. 15.2A), or could we be seeing an association of exposure with disease only because there is an age difference between cases and controls, and older age is also related to being exposed (see Fig. 15.2B)? In other words, does exposure cause the disease, or is the observed association between the exposure and disease a result of confounding by a third factor (in this case, age)?

How can we clarify this issue? One approach is seen in Table 15.6. We can carry out a stratified analysis with subjects in two age groups: younger than 40 years and older than 40 years. Within each stratum a 2 × 2 table is created, and an OR is calculated for each. When we calculate the OR separately for the younger

and the older subjects, we find the OR to be 1.0 in each stratum. Thus the only reason we originally had an OR of 1.95 in Table 15.3 was because there was a difference in age distributions between the cases and the controls. Therefore in this example age is a confounder.

How can we address the problem of confounding? As seen in Box 15.2, the issue of confounding can be addressed either in designing and carrying out a study or in analysis of the data. In *designing and carrying out a case-control study*, we can match the cases to the controls, as discussed in Chapter 7 (by either group matching or individual matching), for the factor that we suspect could be a possible confounder. In this example, we could match by age to eliminate any age difference between the cases and the controls. If, after matching in this way, we then observe an association of exposure and disease, we would know that we could not attribute the observed association to age differences in cases and controls.

Alternatively, we can handle the problem of confounding in the *data analysis* in one of two ways: stratification or adjustment. Let's briefly discuss stratification, which was just demonstrated in the hypothetical example (see Table 15.6). Say we are interested in the relationship of smoking and lung cancer. We want to know whether the observed higher risks of lung cancer in smokers could be a result of confounding by air pollution and/or urbanization. Perhaps we are observing a relationship of smoking and lung cancer not because smoking causes lung cancer, but because air pollution causes lung cancer and smoking is more frequent in polluted areas (such as urban areas). Perhaps smoking is more common in cities than in rural areas.

How can we address this question? One approach would be to stratify the data by degree of urbanization—rural, town, or major city. We could then calculate the lung cancer rates in smokers and nonsmokers in each urbanization stratum (Table 15.7).

If the relationship of lung cancer to smoking is due to smoking, and not to the confounding effect of pollution and/or urbanization, then *in each stratum of urbanization* the incidence of lung cancer should be higher in smokers than in nonsmokers. It would

then be clear that the observed association of smoking and lung cancer could not be due to degree of urbanization.

We may prefer not just to dichotomize smoking groups into smokers and nonsmokers, but also to include in the analysis the number of cigarettes smoked per day (which of course is subject to some error, being estimated by study participants).

In Table 15.8, we have expanded cigarette smoking into categories of amount subjects said that they smoked per day. Again, we can calculate the incidence in each cell of the table. If the observed association of cigarette smoking and lung cancer is not due to confounding by urbanization or pollution or both, we would expect to see a dose-response pattern *in each stratum of urbanization.*

Fig. 15.3 shows actual age-adjusted lung cancer mortality rates per 100,000 person-years by urban-rural

TABLE 15.7 An Example of Stratification: Lung Cancer Rates by Smoking Status and Degree of Urbanization

Degree of Urbanization	CANCER RATES	
	Nonsmokers	Smokers
None		
Slight		
Town		
City		
Totals		

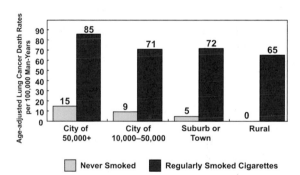

Fig. **15.3** Age-adjusted lung cancer death rates per 100,000 person-years by urban-rural classification and by smoking category. (Modified from Hammond EC, Horn D. Smoking and death rates: report on 44 months of follow-up of 187,783 men: II. death rates by cause. *JAMA.* 1958;166:1294–1308. Copyright 1958, American Medical Association.)

TABLE 15.8 An Example of Further Stratification: Lung Cancer Rates by Smoking Level and Degree of Urbanization

Degree of Urbanization	CANCER RATES			
	Nonsmokers	SMOKERS		
		<1 Pack/Day	1 Pack/Day	>1 Packs/Day
None				
Slight				
Town				
City				
Totals				

classification and smoking category in one of the classic epidemiologic reports on smoking and lung cancer mortality. For each degree of urbanization, lung cancer mortality rates in smokers are shown by the blue bars, and nonsmoker mortality rates are indicated by light green bars. We see that in every level (or stratum) of urbanization, lung cancer mortality is higher in smokers than in nonsmokers. Therefore the observed association of smoking and lung cancer cannot be attributed to level of urbanization. By examining each stratum separately, we are, in effect, holding urbanization constant, and we still find much higher lung cancer mortality in smokers than in nonsmokers.

At the same time, it is interesting to examine the data for nonsmokers (shown by the green bars). If we draw a line connecting the tops of these bars, we see that the higher the urbanization level, the higher the incidence of lung cancer in nonsmokers (Fig. 15.4). Thus there is a dose-response relationship of lung cancer and urbanization in nonsmokers. However, as we have seen, this relationship cannot explain the association of lung cancer with smoking, as the latter relationship holds within each level of urbanization.

Fig. 15.5 shows the relationship among smoking, drinking, and cancer of the esophagus. Four strata (levels) of the amount smoked are shown. Within each smoking stratum, the risk of esophageal cancer is plotted in relation to the amount of alcohol consumed.

What do we observe? The more a person reports smoking, the higher the levels of esophageal cancer. However, within each stratum of smoking, there is a dose-response relationship of esophageal cancer and the amount of alcohol consumed. Therefore we cannot attribute to smoking the effects of alcohol consumption on esophageal cancer. Both smoking and alcohol have separate effects on the risk of esophageal cancer.

It is important to note that in this presentation of data, we cannot compare smokers with nonsmokers or drinkers with nondrinkers because the authors have pooled the group that smokes 0 to 9 g of tobacco per day, and they have also pooled nondrinkers with minimal drinkers. Thus we have no rates for persons who are truly *unexposed* to alcohol or tobacco. It would have been preferable to have kept the data for unexposed persons separate so that RRs could have been calculated based on rates in unexposed persons. Mixing nondrinkers with light drinkers and nonsmokers with light smokers makes it difficult to properly analyze the data.

Two final points on confounding: First, when we identify a confounder, we generally consider it a problem and want to find ways to address the issue of confounding. However, sometimes finding a confounded relationship can also be enlightening. Even if an apparent association between exposure A (the factor in which we are primarily interested) and disease B is actually due to some third confounding factor X, so that

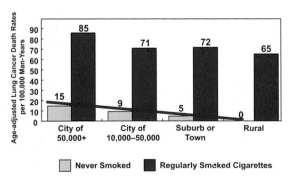

Fig. 15.4 Relationship of degree of urbanization to lung cancer death rates in nonsmokers. The *sloping line* connects the age-adjusted lung cancer death rates per 100,000 person-years by urban-rural classification in nonsmokers. (Modified from Hammond EC, Horn D. Smoking and death rates: report on 44 months of follow-up of 187,783 men: II. death rates by cause. *JAMA.* 1958;166:1294–1308. Copyright 1958, American Medical Association.)

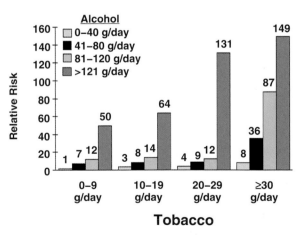

Fig. 15.5 Relative risk of developing cancer of the esophagus in relation to smoking and drinking habits. (Modified from Tuyns AJ, Pequignot G, Jensen OM. Esophageal cancer in Ille-et-Vilaine in relation to levels of alcohol and tobacco consumption: risks are multiplying. *Bull Cancer.* 1977;64:45–60.)

exposure A is not causally related to disease B, screening for exposure A can nevertheless be useful because it permits us to identify people who are at elevated risk for the disease and direct appropriate preventive and therapeutic interventions to them. Thus a confounded relationship may still be a helpful guide in screening populations even when we do not identify the specific etiologic agent involved.

Second, confounding is not an error in the study, but rather is a true phenomenon that is identified in a study and must be understood. Bias is a result of an error in the way that the study has been carried out, but confounding is a valid finding that describes the nature of the relationship among several factors and the risk of disease. However, *failure to take confounding into account in interpreting the results of a study* is indeed an error in the conduct of the study and can bias the conclusions of the study.

Interaction

To this point, our discussion has generally assumed the presence of a single exposure (risk factor) in the etiology of a disease. Although this approach is useful for discussion purposes, in real life, we rarely deal with single causes. In the previous examples of the relationship of lung cancer to smoking and urbanization and the relationship of esophageal cancer to drinking and smoking, we have already seen more than one factor involved in disease etiology. In this section, we ask the question: How do multiple factors interact in causing a disease?

What do we mean by *interaction*? MacMahon[19] defined interaction as follows: "When the incidence rate of disease in the presence of two or more risk factors differs from the incidence rate expected to result from their individual effects." The effect can be greater than what we would expect (positive interaction, synergism) or less than what we would expect (negative interaction, antagonism). The problem is to determine what we would *expect* to result from the individual effects of the exposures.

Fig. 15.6 shows an algorithm for exploring the possibility of interaction.

In examining our data, the first question is whether an association has been observed between an exposure and a disease. If so, is it due to confounding? If we

1. **Is there an association?**
2. **If so, is it due to confounding?**
3. **Is there an association equally strong in strata formed on the basis of a third variable?**

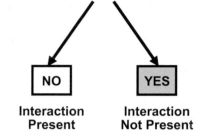

Fig. 15.6 Questions to ask regarding the nature of the relationship between exposure and outcome.

TABLE 15.9 Incidence Rates for Groups Exposed to Neither Risk Factor or to One or Two Risk Factors (Hypothetical Data)

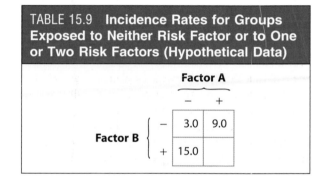

		Factor A −	Factor A +
Factor B	−	3.0	9.0
	+	15.0	

decide that it is *not* due to confounding—that is, the association is causal—then we ask whether the association is equally strong in each of the strata that are formed on the basis of some third variable. For example, is the association of smoking and lung cancer equally strong in strata formed on the basis of degree of urbanization? If the association is equally strong in all strata, there is no interaction. But if the association is of different strengths in different strata formed on the basis of age, for example (if the association is stronger in older people than in younger people), an interaction has been observed between age and exposure in producing the disease. If there was no interaction, we would expect the association to be of the same strength in each stratum.

Let's look more closely at interaction. Table 15.9 shows the incidence in persons exposed to either one of two risk factors (A or B), to both factors, or to neither factor, in a hypothetical example.

In persons with neither exposure, the incidence is 3.0. In persons exposed to factor A only and not to factor B, the incidence is 9.0. In persons exposed to factor B only and not to factor A, the incidence is 15.0. These are the individual effects of each factor considered separately.

What would we expect the incidence to be in persons who are exposed to both factors A and B (the lower right-hand cell in Table 15.9) if those people experienced the risk resulting from the independent contributions of both factors? The answer depends on the type of model that we propose. Let's assume that when there are two exposures, the effect of one exposure is *added* to the effect of the second exposure—that is, the model is *additive*. What, then, would we expect to see in the lower right-hand cell of the table? Let's use as an example the people who have neither exposure, whose risk in the absence of both exposures is 3.0. How does exposure to factor A affect their risk? It adds 6.0 to the 3.0 to produce a risk of 9.0. If factor A adds a risk of 6.0 to the risk that exists without factor A, it should have the same effect both in people exposed to factor B and in those not exposed to factor B. Because factor A adds 6.0 to the 3.0, it would also be expected to add 6.0 to the 15.0 rate of people exposed to factor B when they have exposure to A added as well. Thus we would expect the effects of exposures to both factors to yield an incidence of 21.0.

We can also view this as follows: If factor B adds 12.0 to the 3.0 incidence of people with neither exposure, we would expect it to add 12.0 to any group, including the group exposed only to factor A, whose incidence is 9.0. Therefore the effect of exposure to both A and B would be expected to equal 9.0 added to 12.0, or 21.0. (Remember that the 3.0 is a background risk that is present in the absence of both A and B. When we calculate the combined effect of factors A and B, we cannot just add 9.0 and 15.0—we must be sure that we do not count the background risk [3.0] twice.) The left-hand side of Table 15.10 shows the completed table from the partial data presented in Table 15.9.

Recall that when we discuss differences in risks, we are talking about *attributable risks*. This is shown on the right side of Table 15.10. If we examine persons who have neither exposure, they have a background risk, but the attributable risk—that is, the risk

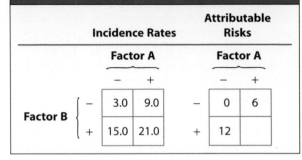

TABLE 15.10 Incidence Rates and Attributable Risks for Groups Exposed to Neither Risk Factor or to One or Two Risk Factors (Hypothetical Data in an Additive Model: I)

	Incidence Rates		Attributable Risks	
	Factor A		Factor A	
	−	+	−	+
Factor B −	3.0	9.0	0	6
Factor B +	15.0	21.0	12	

TABLE 15.11 Incidence Rates and Attributable Risks for Groups Exposed to Neither Risk Factor or to One or Two Risk Factors (Hypothetical Data in an Additive Model: II)

	Incidence Rates		Attributable Risks	
	Factor A		Factor A	
	−	+	−	+
Factor B −	3.0	9.0	0	6
Factor B +	15.0	21.0	12	18

attributable to exposure to factor A or B—is 0. As stated earlier, exposure only to factor A adds 6, and exposure only to factor B adds 12. What will the attributable risk be for both exposures? The answer is 18—that is, 18 more than the background risk. The additive model is summarized in Table 15.11.

What if an additive model does not describe correctly the effect of exposure to two independent factors? Perhaps a second exposure does not *add* to the effect of the first exposure but instead *multiplies* the effect of the first exposure. If having a certain exposure doubles a person's risk, we might expect it to double that risk regardless of whether that person had another exposure.

For example, if the effect of alcohol is to double a person's risk for a certain cancer, we might expect it to double that risk for both smokers and nonsmokers. The appropriate model for the effects of two independent factors might therefore be a *multiplicative* rather than an additive model.

Let's return to our original data on risk resulting from neither exposure, or from exposure to factor A or B. These data are shown again in Table 15.12.

We see that exposure to factor A triples the risk, compared with that seen when factor A is absent (9.0 compared with 3.0). What would we therefore expect to find in the lower right-hand cell of the table when both exposures are present? Since in the absence of factor B, factor A has tripled the risk of 3.0, we would also expect it to triple the risk of 15.0 observed when exposure to factor B is present. If so, the effect from exposure to both factors would be 45.0. Again, we can calculate this in a different fashion. Factor B multiplies the risk by 5 (15.0 compared with 3.0) when factor A is absent. We would therefore expect it to have the same effect when factor A is present. Because the risk when factor A is present is 9.0, we would expect the presence of factor B to yield a risk of 45.0 (9.0 × 5; Table 15.13).

The left-hand side of Table 15.13 shows the completed incidence rate table. Our discussion of a multiplicative model is of an *RR model*. This is shown on the right-hand side of the table. What value would we expect to find in the blank cell?

If we now assign the background risk (3.0) a value of 1, against which to compare the other values in the table, exposure to factor A triples the risk, yielding an RR of 3 for factor A in the absence of factor B. Factor

B multiplies the risk by 5, yielding an RR of 5 for exposure to factor B in the absence of factor A. When both factors A and B are operating, we would expect to see an RR of 15 (45.0/3.0) as seen on the left or 3 × 5 as seen on the right in Table 15.14.

We have considered two models thus far: additive and multiplicative. Several questions remain: What would we expect to see as a result of the independent effects of two risk factors? Do we expect an additive model or a multiplicative model?

The answers may not be obvious. If two factors are operating and the incidence is 21.0, the result is consistent with an additive model. If the incidence

TABLE 15.13 Incidence Rates and Relative Risks for Groups Exposed to Neither Risk Factor or to One or Two Risk Factors (Hypothetical Data in a Multiplicative Model: I)

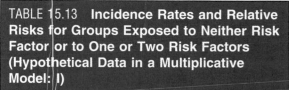

	Incidence Rates		Relative Risks	
	Factor A		Factor A	
	−	+	−	+
Factor B −	3.0	9.0	1	3
Factor B +	15.0	45.0	5	

TABLE 15.14 Incidence Rates and Relative Risks for Groups Exposed to Neither Risk Factor or to One or Two Risk Factors (Hypothetical Data in a Multiplicative Model: II)

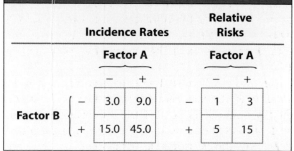

	Incidence Rates		Relative Risks	
	Factor A		Factor A	
	−	+	−	+
Factor B −	3.0	9.0	1	3
Factor B +	15.0	45.0	5	15

TABLE 15.12 Incidence Rates for Groups Exposed to Neither Risk Factor or to One or Two Risk Factors (Hypothetical Data)

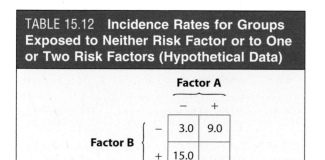

	Factor A	
	−	+
Factor B −	3.0	9.0
Factor B +	15.0	

is 45.0, the result is consistent with a multiplicative model. However, if the incidence resulting from two factors is 60.0, for example, even the value for a multiplicative model is clearly exceeded, and an interaction is present—that is, an effect greater than would be expected from the independent effects of the two separate factors.

However, if the incidence is 30.0, it is less than expected from a multiplicative model but still more than expected from an additive model. Then we would ask, "Is this more than we would expect from the independent effects of the two factors?" It is difficult to know the answer without more information about the biology of the disease, the mechanisms involved in the pathogenesis of the disease, and how such factors operate at cellular and molecular levels. Most experts accept any effect greater than additive as evidence of positive interaction, which is also called *synergism.* However, this opinion is often based on statistical considerations, whereas the validity of the model should ideally be based on biologic knowledge. The model may differ from one disease to another and from one exposure to another.

Let's consider a few examples. In a cohort study of smoking and lung cancer, Hammond and colleagues[20] studied the risk of lung cancer in 17,800 asbestos workers in the United States and in 73,763 men who were not exposed to asbestos in relation to their smoking habits. Table 15.15 shows the findings for deaths from lung cancer in relation to exposure. If the relationship between smoking and asbestos exposure were additive, we would expect the risk in those exposed to both smoking and asbestos (the lower right-hand cell) to

be 58.4 + 122.6 − 11.3, or 169.7 (recall that the 11.3 background risk is subtracted to avoid counting it twice). Clearly, the observed value of 601.6 is much greater than the expected additive value. In fact, the data in Table 15.15 closely approximate a multiplicative model and strongly suggest synergism between asbestos exposure and tobacco smoking.

A second example is seen in Table 15.16, which shows the RR of oral cancer by presence or absence of two exposures: smoking and alcohol consumption. The risk is set at 1.00 for persons with neither exposure. Is there evidence of an interaction? What would we expect the risk to be if the effect were multiplicative? We would expect 1.53 × 1.23, or 1.88. Clearly the observed effect of 5.71 is higher than a multiplicative effect and indicates the presence of interaction.

Let's look at more detailed data for these relationships using dose data for alcohol consumption and for smoking (Table 15.17).

Again, the risk in those who do not drink and do not smoke is set at 1.0. In those with the highest level of alcohol consumption and the highest level of smoking, the risk is 15.50. Is an interaction evident? The data appear to support this. The highest values in smokers who are nondrinkers and in drinkers who are nonsmokers are 2.43 and 2.33, respectively; the value of 15.5 clearly exceeds the resulting product of 5.66 that would be expected with a multiplicative effect.

However, a problem with these data should be mentioned. Note that each category of smoking or

TABLE 15.15 Deaths From Lung Cancer (Per 100,000) Among Individuals With and Without Exposure to Cigarette Smoking and Asbestos

Cigarette Smoking	ASBESTOS EXPOSURE	
	No	Yes
No	11.3	58.4
Yes	122.6	601.6

Modified from Hammond EC, Selikoff IJ, Seidman H. Asbestos exposure, cigarette smoking and death rates. *Ann NY Acad Sci.* 1979;330:473–490.

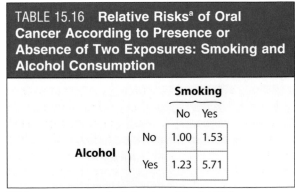

TABLE 15.16 Relative Risks[a] of Oral Cancer According to Presence or Absence of Two Exposures: Smoking and Alcohol Consumption

		Smoking	
		No	Yes
Alcohol	No	1.00	1.53
	Yes	1.23	5.71

[a]Risks are expressed relative to a risk of 1.00 for persons who neither smoked nor drank alcohol.

From Rothman K, Keller A. The effect of joint exposure to alcohol and tobacco on risk of cancer of the mouth and pharynx. *J Chronic Dis.* 1972;25:711–716.

TABLE 15.17 Risk Ratios[a] for Oral Cancer According to Level of Exposure to Alcohol and Smoking: I

Alcohol Consumption (oz/day)	CIGARETTE EQUIVALENTS PER DAY			
	0	<20	20–39	≥40
0	1.00	1.52	1.43	2.43
<0.4	0.40	1.67	3.18	3.25
0.4–1.5	1.60	4.36	4.46	8.21
>1.5	2.33	4.13	9.59	15.50

[a]Risks are expressed relative to a risk of 1.00 for persons who neither smoked nor drank.
From Rothman K, Keller A. The effect of joint exposure to alcohol and tobacco on risk of cancer of the mouth and pharynx. *J Chronic Dis.* 1972;25:711–716.

TABLE 15.18 Risk Ratios[a] for Oral Cancer According to Level of Exposure to Alcohol and Smoking: II

Alcohol Consumption (oz/day)	CIGARETTE EQUIVALENTS PER DAY			
	0	<20	20–39	≥40
None	1.00	1.52	1.43	2.43
<0.4	0.40	1.67	3.18	3.25
0.4–1.5	1.60	4.36	4.46	8.21
>1.5	2.33	4.13	9.59	15.50

[a]Risks are expressed relative to a risk of 1.00 for persons who neither smoked nor drank.
From Rothman K, Keller A. The effect of joint exposure to alcohol and tobacco on risk of cancer of the mouth and pharynx. *J Chronic Dis.* 1972;25:711–716.

TABLE 15.19 Relative Risks of Lung Cancer According to Smoking and Radiation Exposure in Two Populations

Radiation Level	URANIUM WORKERS (SMOKING LEVEL)		A-BOMB SURVIVORS (SMOKING LEVEL)	
	Low	High	Low	High
Low	1.0	7.7	1.0	9.7
High	18.2	146.8	6.2	14.2

From Blot WJ, Akiba S, Kato H. Ionizing radiation and lung cancer: a review including preliminary results from a case-control study among A-bomb survivors. In: Prentice RL, Thompson DJ, eds. *Atomic Bomb Survivor Data: Utilization and Analysis.* Philadelphia: Society for Industrial and Applied Mathematics; 1984:235–248.

drinking has upper and lower boundaries, except for the highest categories, which have no upper boundaries. Therefore the high risk of 15.50 could result from the presence of a few extreme outliers—either extraordinarily heavy smokers or extraordinarily heavy drinkers.

Is there a way to avoid this problem and still use the data shown here? We could ignore the right-hand column and the bottom row and look only at the resulting 3 × 3 table (Table 15.18). Now all of the categories have both upper and lower boundaries. If the model was multiplicative, we would expect to see 1.43 × 1.60, or 2.29, rather than the 4.46 actually observed. Thus we still see evidence of interaction, but much weaker evidence than we had seen in the full table, with its indefinite high-exposure categories. This

suggests that the problem of the lack of upper boundaries of categories was indeed a contributor to the high value of 15.50 seen in the 4 × 4 table.

As we have said, the decision as to whether an additive model or a multiplicative model is most relevant in a given situation should depend on the biology of the disease. Table 15.19 shows data regarding the risks of cancer from radiation and smoking in two different populations: uranium workers (left) and survivors of the 1945 atomic bombing of Japan (right). Low and high levels of smoking and low and high levels of radiation are shown for both groups in Table 15.19.

What kind of model is suggested by Table 15.19? Clearly a multiplicative relationship is suggested; 146.8 is close to the product of 7.7 × 18.2 (140.1). The columns on the right suggest an additive model; 14.2 is close to the sum of 9.7 + 6.2 − 1.0 (14.9). Therefore, although the data address radiation and smoking in two populations, in one setting, the exposures relate in an additive way, and in the other, they relate in a multiplicative way. It is not known whether this is a result of differences in radiation exposure in uranium mines compared with that from atomic bombs. Such a hypothesis is not unreasonable; we know that there was even a difference in the radiation emitted by the atomic bombs at Hiroshima and Nagasaki and that the dose-response curves for cancer were different in the two cities. Further, the location of survivors in each city may have varied. In any case, the fact that two exposures that are ostensibly the same (or, at least, similar) may have different interrelationships in different

TABLE 15.20 Risks[a] of Liver Cancer for Persons Exposed to Aflatoxin or Chronic Hepatitis B Infection: An Example of Interaction

	Aflatoxin-Negative	Aflatoxin-Positive
HBsAg negative	1.0	3.4
HBsAg positive	7.3	59.4

[a]Adjusted for cigarette smoking.

HBsAg, hepatitis B surface antigen.

Modified from Qian GS, Ross RK, Yu MC, et al. A follow-up study of urinary markers of aflatoxin exposure and liver cancer risk in Shanghai, People's Republic of China. *Cancer Epidemiol Biomarkers Prev.* 1994;3:3–10.

settings is an intriguing observation that requires further exploration.

Finally, a dramatic example of interaction is seen in the relationship of aflatoxin and chronic hepatitis B infection to the risk of liver cancer (Table 15.20). In this Chinese study, hepatitis B infection alone multiplied the risk of liver cancer by 7.3; aflatoxin exposure alone multiplied the risk by 3.4. However, when both exposures were present, the RR rose to 59.4, far in excess of what we might expect in both an additive and a multiplicative model.[a] Such an observation of synergy is of major clinical and public health interest, but also suggests important directions for further laboratory research into the etiology and pathogenesis of liver cancer.

The finding of an additive interaction or synergism may also have practical policy implications involving issues such as who is responsible for a disease and who should pay compensation to the victims. For example, earlier in this chapter we discussed the relationship of smoking and asbestos exposure in producing cancer, a relationship that clearly is strongly interactive or synergistic. Litigation against asbestos manufacturers dates back at least to the 1970s, and large awards were made by the cou rts. In 1998, at a time of increasing legal actions against the tobacco companies, a coalition of some of the victims of asbestos exposure joined forces with asbestos manufacturers to demand that Congress set aside a large amount of money from any national tobacco settlement bill to compensate people whose cancer was caused by the combined exposure to both asbestos and tobacco, a claim they justified by pointing to the synergistic relationship of these exposures. Those who objected to this demand claimed that those making the demand were in effect freeing the asbestos manufacturers from paying their obligation (shifting it to tobacco manufacturers) and were doing so only because they believed that it might be easier to obtain significantly higher compensation from tobacco companies than from asbestos manufacturers. In so doing, they were willing to forge an alliance with asbestos manufacturers who had previously been found responsible for their disease. The basis for this approach was the well-documented synergism of asbestos and tobacco smoking in causing cancer.

Conclusion

This chapter has reviewed the concepts of bias, confounding, and interaction in relation to the derivation of causal inferences. Biases reflect inadequacies in the design or conduct of a study, and clearly affect the validity of the findings. Biases therefore need to be assessed and, if possible, eliminated. Confounding and interaction, on the other hand, describe the reality of the interrelationships between certain exposures and a certain disease outcome. Confounding and interaction characterize virtually every situation in which etiology is addressed, because most causal questions involve the relationships of multiple exposures and multiple, possibly etiologic, factors. Such relationships are particularly important in investigating the roles of genetic and environmental factors in disease causation and in assigning responsibility for adverse health outcomes from environmental exposures. Assessing the relative contributions of genetic and environmental factors is discussed in the following chapter.

---

[a]A simple formula to calculate additive expected joint relative risk (RR) or odds ratio (OR) is [RR or OR for the isolated effect of factor A] + [RR or OR for the isolated effect of factor B] − 1.0. In the example, the additive expected joint RR is 7.3 + 3.4 − 1.0 = 9.7, which is much lower than the observed RR of 59.4, thus defining a strong additive interaction. (This approach is particularly useful in case-control studies, in which absolute differences in rates are not available.) The formula for the multiplicative expected joint RR or OR is based on multiplying the independent RRs or ORs; in the example, 7.3 × 3.4 = 24.8, which is also much lower than the observed RR of 59.4. Thus it can be concluded that there are both additive and multiplicative interactions.

REFERENCES

1. Schlesselman JJ. *Case-Control Studies: Design, Conduct, and Analysis.* New York: Oxford University Press; 1982.
2. Johson TJ. *Handbook of Health Survey Methods.* Hoboken, NJ: John Wiley & Sons; 2015.
3. Ronmark E, Lundqvist A, Lundback B, et al. Non-responders to a postal questionnaire on respiratory symptoms and diseases. *Eur J Epidemiol.* 1999;15:293–299.
4. Collins R. What make the UK Biobank special? *Lancet.* 2012;379:1173–1174.
5. Pinsky PF, Prorok PC, Yu K, et al. Extended mortality results for prostate cancer screening in the PLCO trial with median follow-up of 15 years. *Cancer.* 2017;123:592–599.
6. Loprinzi PD, Davis RE. Socioecological risk predictors of physical activity and associated mortality. *Am J Health Promot.* 2018;32:106–111.
7. Dobson AJ, Hockey R, Brown WJ, et al. Cohort profile update: Australian Longitudinal Study on Women's Health. *Int J Epidemiol.* 2015;44:1547a–1547f.
8. Koton S, Schneider AL, Rosamond WD, et al. Stroke incidence and mortality trends in US communities, 1987-2011. *JAMA.* 2014;312:259–268.
9. Boston Collaborative Drug Surveillance Program. Reserpine and breast cancer. *Lancet.* 1974;2:669–671.
10. Armstrong B, Stevens B, Doll R. Retrospective study of the association between use of Rauwolfia derivatives and breast cancer in English women. *Lancet.* 1974;2:672–675.
11. Heinonen OP, Shapiro S, Tuominen L, et al. Reserpine use in relation to breast cancer. *Lancet.* 1974;2:675–677.
12. Horwitz RI, Feinstein AR. Exclusion bias and the false relationship of reserpine and breast cancer. *Arch Intern Med.* 1985;145:1873–1875.
13. MacMahon B, Yens S, Trichopoulos D, et al. Coffee and cancer of the pancreas. *N Engl J Med.* 1981;304:630–633.
14. Metzger DS, Koblin B, Turner C, et al. Randomized controlled trial of audio computer-assisted self-interviewing: utility and acceptability in longitudinal studies. *Am J Epid.* 2000;152:99–107.
15. Macalino GE, Celentano DD, Latkin C, et al. Risk behaviors by audio computer-assisted self-interviews among HIV-seropositive and HIV-seronegative injection drug users. *AIDS Educ Prev.* 2002;14:367–378.
16. Wynder EL, Higgins IT, Harris RE. The wish bias. *J Clin Epidemiol.* 1991;43:619–621.
17. Rookus MA, van Leeuwen FE. Induced abortion and risk for breast cancer: reporting (recall) bias in a Dutch case-control study. *J Natl Cancer Inst.* 1996;88:1759–1764.
18. D'Avanzo B, LaVecchia C, Katsouyanni K, et al. Reliability of information on cigarette smoking and beverage consumption provided by hospital controls. *Epidemiology.* 1996;7:312–315.
19. MacMahon B. Concepts of multiple factors. In: Lee DH, Kotin P, eds. *Multiple Factors in the Causation of Environmentally Induced Disease.* New York: Academic Press; 1972.
20. Hammond EC, Selikoff IJ, Seidman H. Asbestos exposure, cigarette smoking and death rates. *Ann NY Acad Sci.* 1979;330:473–490.

REVIEW QUESTIONS FOR CHAPTER 15

1 *Which of the following is an approach to handling confounding?*
   a. Individual matching
   b. Stratification
   c. Group matching
   d. Adjustment
   e. All of the above

2 *Which of the following approaches can handle confounding at the design stage of the study?*
   a. Stratification
   b. Adjustment
   c. Restriction
   d. Regression

3 *It has been suggested that physicians may examine women who use oral contraceptives more often or more thoroughly than women who do not. If so, and if an association is observed between phlebitis and oral contraceptive use, the association may be due to:*
   a. Selection bias
   b. Interviewer bias
   c. Surveillance bias
   d. Nonresponse bias
   e. Recall bias

Questions 4 through 7 are based on the information given below:

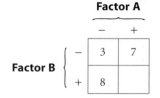

4 *Fill in the blank cell in the first table using the additive model of interaction:* _____

5 *Fill in the blank cell in the first table using the multiplicative model of interaction:* _____
Convert the numbers in the above table to attributable risks for the additive model (below, left) and relative risks for the multiplicative model (below, right).

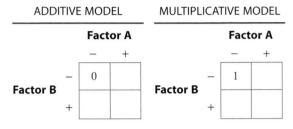

6 *Fill in the bottom right cell of the table at the bottom of the left column for the attributable risk of having both factors A and B (additive model):* _____

7 *Fill in the bottom right cell of the table at the bottom of the left column for the relative risk of having both factors A and B (multiplicative model):* _____

Question 8 is based on the information given below:
In a case-control study of the relationship of radiation exposure and thyroid cancer, 50 cases admitted for thyroid cancer and 100 "controls" admitted during the same period for treatment of hernias were studied. Only the cases were interviewed, and 20 of the cases were found to have been exposed to x-ray therapy in the past, based on the interviews and medical records. The controls were not interviewed, but a review of their hospital records when they were admitted for hernia surgery revealed that only two controls had been exposed to x-ray therapy in the past.

8 *Based on the description given above, what source of bias is least likely to be present in this study?*
   a. Recall bias
   b. Bias due to controls being nonrepresentative of the nondiseased population
   c. Bias due to use of different methods of ascertainment of exposure in the cases and controls
   d. Bias due to loss of subjects from the control group over time
   e. Selection bias for exposure to x-ray therapy in the past

9 *In 1990, a case-control study was conducted to investigate the positive association between artificial sweetener use and bladder cancer. Controls were selected from a hospital sample of patients diagnosed with obesity-related conditions. Obesity-related conditions have been positively associated with artificial sweetener use. How would the use of these patients as controls affect the estimate of the association between artificial sweetener use and bladder cancer?*
   a. The estimate of association would accurately reflect the true association regardless of the association between artificial sweetener use and obesity-related conditions
   b. The estimate of association would tend to underestimate the true association
   c. More information is needed on the strength of association between artificial sweetener use and obesity-related conditions before any judgment can be made
   d. The estimate of association would tend to overestimate the true association
   e. More information is needed on the strength of association between artificial sweetener use and bladder cancer before any judgment can be made

Chapter 16

Identifying the Roles of Genetic and Environmental Factors in Disease Causation

To produce another Wolfgang Amadeus Mozart, we would need not only Wolfgang's genome but his mother's uterus, his father's music lessons, his parents' friends and his own, the state of music in 18th century Austria, Haydn's patronage, and on and on, in ever-widening circles. Without Mozart's set of genes, the rest would not suffice; there was, after all, only one Wolfgang Amadeus Mozart. But we have no right to the converse assumption: that his genome, cultivated in another world at another time, would result in the same musical genius. If a particular strain of wheat yields different harvests under different conditions of climate, soil, and cultivation, how can we assume that so much more complex a genome as that of a human being would yield its desired crop of operas, symphonies, and chamber music under different circumstances of nurture?[1]

—Leon Eisenberg, MD, DSc, child psychiatrist, social psychiatrist, and medical educator (1922–2009)

Learning Objectives

- To examine how epidemiologic study designs can clarify the roles of genetic and environmental factors in risk of disease and their possible interactions.
- To show how genetic markers are used to map genes controlling risk of different diseases, including complex diseases.
- To test for interaction between genes and environmental risk factors.
- To discuss how innovative epidemiologic and molecular biology methods can help to define the etiologic roles of environmental and genetic risk factors, and potentially permit development of individualized treatments of disease.

In previous chapters, we discussed study designs for identifying causes of disease focusing primarily on the possible etiologic role of environmental factors. However, to prevent disease, we must also consider both the part played by host genetic factors and environmental factors. Human beings clearly differ from one another in physical characteristics, personality, and other factors. These phenotypes can be either qualitative or quantitative. A qualitative phenotype is a trait that can be categorized into two (or more) mutually exclusive groups (e.g. affected or unaffected; unaffected, mildly or severely affected). For example, a person can be classified dichotomously as either having hypertension or not. The underlying quantitative phenotype is a continuous measurement of the person's blood pressure. Genetic epidemiology aims to understand the contribution of host genetics to complex diseases and quantitative phenotypes, and to identify their relative importance. A glossary of genetic terms appears at the end of this chapter.

Traditional Genetics

Traditional medical genetics has focused primarily on single-gene traits that follow the transmission patterns outlined by Gregor Mendel, a 19th century Austrian monk. Mendelian diseases are typically rare in the population, and can be classified by their transmission as autosomal dominant, autosomal recessive, X-linked dominant, or X-linked recessive. Some Mendelian diseases, for example, cystic fibrosis (the most common autosomal recessive disease in populations of Northern European ancestry, with a birth prevalence of 1/2,500 livebirths among non-Hispanic whites in the United States) and sickle cell disease (the most common hemoglobinopathy among populations of West African ancestry with a birth prevalence of 1/360 live births among African Americans) are almost always due to mutations in a single gene (respectively *CFTR* on chromosome 7 and *beta globin* on chromosome 11). Although cystic fibrosis was a lethal disease of childhood for most of human history due to its severe nutritional and pulmonary effects, today patients do survive into adulthood with appropriate medical care. There are hundreds of different mutations identified in *CFTR*, but one three-base-pair deletion (Δ508) is by far the most common. Carrier screening followed by appropriate genetic counseling can reduce the burden of this disease in some populations,[1] while newborn screening aids in early identification and treatment of affected individuals early in life. Sickle cell disease is a debilitating disease with an elevated overall mortality rate, but is not uniformly lethal.[2] Universal newborn screening for sickle cell disease in the United States was first introduced in 1975,[3] and now allows early diagnosis, initiation of penicillin prophylaxis, and comprehensive care of affected children, which have significantly reduced childhood mortality from this disease.[4]

Although Mendelian diseases are not individually common enough to be considered a major public health burden across all populations, when all Mendelian diseases are considered together they do represent a major public health problem, especially for the pediatric health care system. Furthermore, newborn screening programs have been used for over 50 years to identify infants with inborn errors of metabolism (many of which reflect Mendelian diseases), and these programs are now functioning in most developed and many developing countries. Thus, while each of the 30 to 60 diseases commonly included in current newborn screening programs in the United States is quite rare, the sensitivity and specificity of screening tests are high enough, and the costs are low enough, to make this a valuable tool for public health.[5] For example, phenylketonuria is characterized by a genetically determined deficiency of phenylalanine hydroxylase, and a child homozygous for this mutation cannot metabolize the essential amino acid phenylalanine. The resulting excess phenylalanine levels lead to severe mental retardation. While we cannot prevent occurrence of this genotype, through newborn screening we can reduce or eliminate dietary phenylalanine for affected children and therefore prevent severe mental retardation. Thus, from standpoints of both clinical medicine and public health, newborn screening programs can identify those at risk at the earliest opportunity and maximize the effects of available intervention.

Complex Diseases

Most human diseases, however, are controlled by some combination of genetic *and* environmental factors acting together. The spectrum of genetic control over diseases varies from strictly genetic to strictly environmental, and some diseases fall in the middle range where both genes and environmental factors influence risk. These include some congenital malformations and cancers, where there is strong and compelling evidence for familial aggregation of risk (the hallmark of genetic control), but also recognized environmental risk factors (e.g., in utero exposure to viruses, exposures to carcinogens for cancers, etc.). Unlike the traditional single gene diseases, a complex disease likely reflects effects of one or more genes (that may interact with each other) and the environment, and there is often some degree of etiologic heterogeneity where multiple genes can lead to disease.

Clearly, disease does not necessarily develop in everyone exposed to any one environmental risk factor. Even if the relative risk of developing the disease is high given exposure to a specific factor, the notion of attributable risk conveys the message that not all occurrences of a disease are due only to the exposure in question. For example, the relationship between cigarette smoking and lung cancer has been clearly documented. However, lung cancer does not develop in everyone who smokes, and it can develop in nonsmokers. Either another environment factor is needed in addition to cigarette smoking, or individuals differ in their genetic susceptibility or both contribute to risk.

The interaction of genetic and environmental factors was succinctly described many years ago by Lancelot Hogben, who wrote:

Our genes cannot make bricks without straw. The individual differences which men and women display are partly due to the fact that they receive different genes from their parents and partly due to the fact that the same genes live in different houses.[6]

HOW EPIDEMIOLOGIC STUDY DESIGNS CAN CLARIFY THE ROLES OF GENETIC AND ENVIRONMENTAL FACTORS IN RISK TO DISEASE

In this chapter, we discuss how some common epidemiologic study designs can be extended to identify when genetic factors contribute to disease causation. Clearly, if genetic factors do influence risk of disease, relatives of cases (individuals with the disease) should be at a higher risk than relatives of controls (individuals without the disease). Therefore when doing a conventional case-control study it is quite possible to assess familial aggregation by simply asking about the disease status in relatives of both cases and controls. Reliable information can be garnered on first-degree relatives (parents, siblings, and children), and most individuals have some information on second-degree relatives (half-siblings, avuncular relatives, grandparents/grandchildren, etc.). However, beyond close family members it becomes more difficult to obtain reliable information through direct interview of only the index person (i.e., the case or control), and such information is likely subject to information and selection bias.

Such reported data on the prevalence of disease in relatives can be summarized as a simple binary variable (i.e., family history positive or negative) or stratified by type of relatives (i.e., number of affected male relatives). Either way, family history information is treated as a risk factor, and a risk ratio can be computed and tested for its statistical significance. If valid baseline information on risk in the population by age, gender, and birth cohort is available for the disease, this risk ratio can be viewed as a standardized incidence ratio for the entire family. Note, however, that families share more than genes. Common exposure to environmental factors (e.g., passive smoking, diet) may explain, at least partly, the level of familial aggregation.

TWIN STUDIES

Studies of twins have been of great value in identifying the relative contributions of genetic and environmental factors to the causation of human disease. There are two types of twins: monozygotic or MZ (identical) and dizygotic or DZ (fraternal). MZ twins arise from the same fertilized ovum and share 100% of their genetic material. However, DZ twins are genetically like other siblings and thus share, on the average, 50% of their genetic material.

If we look at the occurrence of a disease in MZ twins—who, in effect, have identical genetic material—what are the possible findings? Both twins (twin A and twin B) may have the disease, or both twins may not have the disease, that is, the pair may be *concordant* for the disease. It is also possible that twin A has the disease and twin B does not (or vice versa); that is, the twin pairs are *discordant* for the disease.

If MZ twins are concordant for a disease, what does that tell us about the role of genetic factors? Could the disease be genetic? Yes, because the twins have identical genetic material. Could it be environmental? Yes, because it is well recognized that parents often raise MZ twins similarly, and they obviously shared the same in utero exposures, so they are exposed to many of the same environmental factors. However, even if shared exposure to environmental factors were the same for MZ and DZ twins, type of placentation may influence twin concordance. MZ twins' placentas can be either monochorionic or dichorionic, whereas in DZ twins they are always dichorionic. Thus, in utero exposure to an environmental factor to the same degree in MZ and DZ twins may result in more concordance in the outcome for the former than for the latter, as placental blood vessel anastomoses in monochorionic placentas that characterize many MZ twins may lead to a greater sharing of the environmental exposure than that in dichorionic placentas. It is, for example, interesting that in MZ, but not in DZ twins whose mothers had been equally exposed to thalidomide during pregnancy, concordance for birth defects was almost universal.[7] Thus, observing concordance in MZ twins does not prove a disease is genetic or environmental in origin, but observing discordance in MZ twins does indicate some role for environmental risk factors. Because the discordant MZ twins share the same genetic material, the disease would have to be at least partly environmental in origin.

In DZ twins, both environmental and genetic factors are operating. If a disease is genetic, we would expect lower concordance in DZ twins than in MZ twins, because they share fewer alleles on average. One key assumption of twin studies is that both MZ and DZ twins share environmental factors to the same degree, which may be violated if MZ twins are treated more similarly than DZ twins by their parents and other family members. Other key assumptions are the absence of assortative mating and inbreeding among parents of twins.[8]

How do we calculate the rates of concordance and discordance in twins? Fig. 16.1 shows a cross-tabulation of twins 1 and 2. The numbers in each cell are the numbers of *twin pairs*: thus, there are *a* pairs (in which both twin 1 and 2 have the disease); *d* pairs (in which neither twin 1 nor 2 has the disease); *b* pairs (in which twin 1 does not have the disease but twin 2 does); and *c* pairs (in which twin 1 has the disease but twin 2 does not).

If we want to calculate the concordance rate in twins, most twins will fall into the *d* category; that is, neither will have the disease. We therefore usually look at the other three cells—those twin pairs in which at least one of the twins has the disease. We can calculate the concordance rate in twin pairs in which at least one twin has the disease as follows:

$$\text{Concordance rate} = \frac{a}{a+b+c}$$

We can also calculate the discordance rate in all twin pairs in which at least one twin has the disease as:

$$\text{Discordance rate} = \frac{b+c}{a+b+c}$$

Table 16.1 shows concordance data for leukemia in monozygotic and dizygotic twin pairs. We see the percentage of concordant pairs is notably high for congenital leukemia, which strongly suggests a major genetic component when the disease occurs near the time of birth. However, the number of twins is small (especially for DZ twins) with perinatal/congenital leukemia and there would be confounding between truly genetic causes and intra-uterine factors, which are shared by all twins.

How are concordance data used? Let us look at a few examples. Table 16.2 shows reported concordance rates for alcoholism in monozygotic and dizygotic twins reported by several studies.[9–12] Almost all the reported studies show higher concordance rates for monozygotic than for dizygotic twins; the findings from only one study of a relatively small number of twins were not consistent with the findings of the other studies. Thus, these data from the literature strongly suggest a genetic component in the etiology of alcoholism.

It should be pointed out that zygosity is often based on different information across twin studies, and when

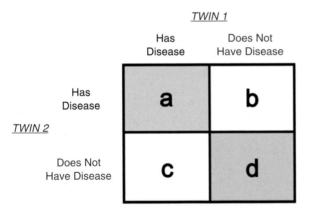

Fig. 16.1 Concordance in twins for a dichotomous variable, such as leukemia.

TABLE 16.1	Age Distribution in Published Clinical Reports of Childhood Leukemia in Twins, 1928–74				

	MONOZYGOTIC PAIRS		DIZYGOTIC PAIRS	
	Concordant	Discordant	Concordant	Discordant
Perinatal–congenital	14	1	1	1
Age 2–7 years	6	13	3	5
Age 7–12 years	1	8	–	1
Age 12 years and older	5	14	0	3
Total	**26**	**36**	**4**	**10**

From Keith L, Brown ER, Ames B, et al. Leukemia in twins: antenatal and postnatal factors. *Acta Genet Med Gemellol.* 1976;25:336–341.

TABLE 16.2   Concordance for Alcoholism in Monozygotic (MZ) and Dizygotic (DZ) Twin Pairs Identified Through an Alcoholic Member

| | | CONCORDANCE | | |
Author (Year)	No. of Twin Pairs	MZ (%)	DZ (%)	Ratio of MZ:DZ Concordance
Kaij (1960)	174	71	32	2.2
Hrubec et al. (1981)	15,924	26	13	2.0
Murray et al. (1983)	56	21	25	0.8
Pickens et al. (1991)	86 (M)	59	36	1.6
	44 (F)	25	5	5.0

Modified from Lumeng L, Crabb DW. Genetic aspects and risk factors in alcoholism and alcoholic liver disease. *Gastroenterology.* 1994;107:572–578.

examining data such as those shown in Tables 16.1 and 16.2, we must ask how twin pairs were labeled MZ or DZ? (Remember the caveat discussed earlier: If you are shown differences between groups or changes over time, the first question to ask is: Are they real? If you are convinced that a difference or change is real and not artefactual, then and only then should you proceed to interpret the findings.) The best way to classify zygosity is by comparing genetic markers between co-twins (which should consistently show 100% identity for MZ twins and 50% for DZ twins); however, DNA may not always be available. Questionnaire data collected from the twins or their parents are generally accurate enough if questions are included about how often one twin was mistaken for their co-twin by parents, teachers, or other family members, and how physically similar they appeared in childhood. This classification of zygosity is almost as accurate as tests using genetic markers.

So far, we have discussed concordance for a discrete variable, such as leukemia or schizophrenia, which is either present or absent. However, we are often interested in determining concordance for a continuous phenotype, such as blood pressure. In this case, we would plot the data for twin 1 against the data for twin 2 for all twin pairs and calculate the intra-class correlation coefficient (r), which measures the correlation of identical values, as seen in Fig. 16.2. The correlation coefficient ranges from −1 to +1. A correlation coefficient of +1 indicates a full positive correlation, 0 indicates no correlation, and −1 indicates a full inverse correlation. If we plot such data for MZ twin pairs and for DZ twin pairs, as shown in Fig. 16.3, we would expect to find a stronger correlation for MZ twins compared to DZ

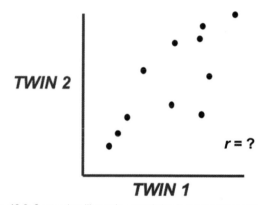

Fig. 16.2 Scatterplots illustrating correlation in twins for a continuous variable, such as systolic blood pressure. This is typically summarized as a correlation coefficient r^2.

twins if the quantitative phenotype is under genetic control. Using quantitative phenotypes within a classic twin design offers the opportunity to estimate a purely additive genetic component (due to transmitted alleles at unobserved genes), a residual component (reflecting random factors not shared between co-twins), and either a shared environmental component or a genetic component (that represents interaction between alleles at a single gene).[8] It is important to realize these latter two components are confounded with one another under the classic twin design where only data on the twins themselves are available. Extending the study to include other family members of the twins creates more contrasts thus allowing further modeling using more elaborate statistical tools.

Table 16.3 shows correlation coefficients for systolic blood pressure among relatives. The highest coefficient is seen in MZ twins; the values for DZ twins and ordinary

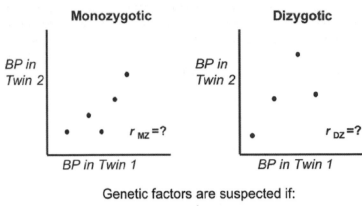

Fig. 16.3 Scatterplots illustrating correlation for continuous variables, such as blood pressure *(BP)*, in monozygotic and dizygotic twins to explore the etiologic role of genetic factors in controlling a continuous variable. Monozygotic twins should have a higher correlation than dizygotic twins.

TABLE 16.3	**Correlation Among Relatives for Systolic Blood Pressure**
Relatives Compared	**Correlation Coefficients**
Monozygotic twins	0.55
Dizygotic twins	0.25
Siblings	0.18
Parents and offspring	0.34
Spouses	0.07

Modified from Feinleib M, Garrison MS, Borhani N, et al. Studies of hypertension in twins. In: Paul O, ed. *Epidemiology and Control of Hypertension*. New York: Grune and Stratton; 1975:3–20.

siblings are close. Also of interest is that virtually no correlation exists between spouses. A strong correlation between spouses (who are generally not biologically related) would suggest a role for environmental factors. However, an alternate suggestion could be that people seek out individuals like themselves for marriage (termed "assortative mating"). Thus, individuals who are overweight, for example, may seek out other individuals who also overweight for marriage. In such a situation, we might arrive at a high spousal correlation for weight or body mass index, and this would happen even for conditions that are not environmentally determined.

A large twin study was reported by Lichtenstein and colleagues in 2000.[13] This study was conducted to estimate the relative contributions of environmental and genetic factors in the causation of cancer. Data from 44,788 twin pairs listed in the Swedish, Danish, and Finnish twin registries were used to assess cancer risks at 28 anatomic sites in twins. Twins of persons with stomach, colorectal, lung, breast, and prostate cancer had an increased risk of developing the same type of cancer. The findings of this and other cancer studies emphasize the need to consider the effects of both genetic and environmental factors (and their interactions) in addressing the etiology of different cancers.

ADOPTION STUDIES

We have said that one problem in interpreting the findings from twin studies is that even MZ twins who share the same genetic constitution also share much of their environment. In such studies, it is therefore difficult to tease out the relative contributions of genetic and environmental factors to the cause of disease. One common approach is to compare different groups of adopted children, their adoptive parents (or family members), and their biologic parents. For example, if we are interested in whether schizophrenia is primarily genetic or environmental in its origin, we can conduct a study using adopted children. There are three basic contrasts:

1. Offspring of normal biologic parents reared by schizophrenic adopting parents
2. Offspring of normal biologic parents reared by normal adopting parents
3. Offspring of schizophrenic biologic parents reared by normal adopting parents

We can examine offspring of normal biologic parents who are adopted and reared by schizophrenic parents. If the disease is purely genetic in origin, what would we expect the risk of schizophrenia to be in these adopted children? It should approximate what is seen in the rest of the population because the family environment would not have any effect in increasing risk. If the disease is largely environmental, we would expect that being reared in an environment with schizophrenic adoptive parents would increase the risk of schizophrenia in these adopted children. As a control group, we could also examine offspring of normal biologic parents reared by normal adoptive parents, and we would expect them to have the population rate of schizophrenia. Obviously for diseases with low prevalence, it will be difficult to find affected adopting parents, so the third option is most frequently used where the children of schizophrenic biologic parents who were adopted by otherwise normal parents are assessed for increased risk of disease.

When interpreting data from adoption studies, certain factors need to be kept in mind. The first is the age at which the adoption took place. For example, if the adoption occurred in late childhood, part of the child's environment may have been influenced by their biologic parents. Ideally, we would like to study children who are adopted at birth. Another complicating issue is that, after adoption, some children maintain relationships with their biologic parents, including visits and other exposures to the environment of the biologic parents, so that the separation between the environment of the biologic parents and that of the adoptive parents is not complete.

Many adoption studies have been conducted in Scandinavian countries, which have excellent disease registries, adoption registries, and record linkage systems. As an example, Table 16.4 shows data from a study of schizophrenia carried out by Kety and Ingraham in which they studied rates of schizophrenia in biologic and in adoptive relatives of adopted children.[14] Using data from a nationwide adoption registry and psychiatric hospitals, they identified 34 adoptees who later became schizophrenic, and also identified 34 adoptees without serious mental disease. They then examined the rates of schizophrenia in the biologic and in the adoptive relatives of the schizophrenic

adoptees and in control adoptees. The rate of schizophrenia in the biologic relatives of the schizophrenic adoptees was 5.0%, compared with 0.4% in the biologic relatives of adoptees without serious mental disease. The findings strongly suggest a genetic component for the etiology of schizophrenia.

Table 16.5 shows the correlation coefficients for parent-child aggregation of blood pressure, comparing biologic children with adopted children. Clearly, the correlations are much weaker (near 0) for correlations between parents and adopted children than correlations between parents and biologic children. The findings strongly suggest a genetic component for blood pressure, a quantitative trait.

Time Trends in Disease Incidence

If we observe time trends in disease risk, with incidence either increasing or decreasing over a relatively short period of time, and if we are convinced that the trend is real, the observation implicates environmental factors in the causation of the disease. Clearly, genetic characteristics of human populations generally do not change over relatively short periods. Thus, the change in mortality from coronary heart disease (CHD) in men from 1979 to 2004 seen in Fig. 16.4 may be primarily due to changes in exposure to environmental factors. (Mortality may have also decreased because of improvements in medical care of patients with CHD.)

Fig. 16.5 shows age-adjusted death rates for stomach cancer in men in several countries. The highest rate is seen in Japan, and the rates in the United States are quite low. Are these differences real? Could they be due to differences in quality of medical care or in access to medical care in different countries? Could they be due to international differences in how death certificates are completed? Results of other studies suggest that these differences are real and likely due to differences in the prevalence of an environmental factor known to be a probable necessary cause of stomach cancer, *Helicobacter pylori* infection. (Furthermore, as case fatality for stomach cancer is high, these between-country differences probably reflect differences in the incidence of this cancer.)

Fig. 16.6 shows comparable data for breast cancer in women. Here we see that one of the lowest rates in the world is in Japan. Are differences between countries

TABLE 16.4 Schizophrenia in Biologic and Adoptive Relatives of Adoptees Who Became Schizophrenic (National Study of Adoptees in Denmark)

	BIOLOGIC RELATIVES			ADOPTIVE RELATIVES		
		SCHIZOPHRENIC			SCHIZOPHRENIC	
	Total No.	No.	%	Total No.	No.	%
Adoptees who became schizophrenic (N = 34)	275	14	5.0	111	0	0
Control adoptees (no serious mental disease) (N = 34)	253	1	0.4	124	0	0

From Kety SS, Ingraham LJ. Genetic transmission and improved diagnosis of schizophrenia from pedigrees of adoptees. *J Psychiatr Res*. 1992;26:247–255.

TABLE 16.5 Correlation Coefficients for Parent-Child Aggregation of Blood Pressure

	BETWEEN PARENTS AND	
	Biologic Child	Adopted Child
Systolic	0.32 (P < .001)	0.09 (NS)
Diastolic	0.37 (P < .001)	0.10 (NS)

NS, Not significant.
Modified from Biron P, Mongeau JG, Bertrand D. Familial aggregation of blood pressure in 558 adopted children. *Can Med Assoc J*. 1976;115:773–774.

TABLE 16.6 Standardized Mortality Ratios for Cancer of the Stomach in Japanese Men, Issei, Nisei, and US White Men

Group	Standardized Mortality Ratio
Japanese men	100
Issei[a]	72
Nisei[a]	38
US white men	17

[a]Issei and Nisei are first- and second-generation Japanese migrants, respectively.
From Haenszel W, Kurihara M. Studies of Japanese migrants: I. Mortality from cancer and other disease among Japanese in the United States. *J Natl Cancer Inst*. 1968;40:43–68.

due to environmental or genetic factors? Again, environmental influences are probably more important in the etiology of breast cancer, even though some genes are known to cause this disease (e.g., *BRCA1* and *BRCA2*), but these recognized genes cannot explain a majority of the variation in risk.[15,16]

How can we tease apart the relative contributions of genetic and environmental factors to international differences in risk of disease? We can do so by studying migrants in a manner analogous to that just described for studying adoptees.

MIGRANT STUDIES

Let us assume that a Japanese individual living in Japan—a country with a high risk for stomach cancer—moves to the United States, a country with a low risk of stomach cancer. What would we expect to happen to this person's risk of stomach cancer? If the disease is primarily genetic in origin, we would expect the high risk of stomach cancer to be retained even when people move from a high-risk to a low-risk area. However, if the disease is primarily environmental in origin, we would expect that over time the risk for such a migrant group would shift toward the lower risk of the adoptive country.

Table 16.6 shows standardized mortality ratios (SMRs) for stomach cancer in Japanese men living in Japan, Japanese men who migrated to the United States ("Issei"), and the children of the Japanese migrants ("Nisei") born in the United States, compared with SMRs of US white males. We see the SMRs progressively shift toward the lower SMR of US white males. These data strongly suggest that a significant environmental component is involved. For example, as mentioned previously, it is well known that the prevalence of an important cause of stomach cancer, *Helicobacter pylori* infection, varies among countries.[17]

However, we should bear in mind that when people migrate to another country they and their families do not immediately shed the environment of their homeland. Many aspects of their original culture are retained,

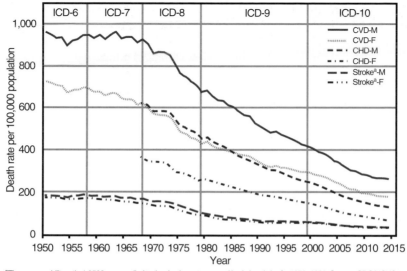

Fig. 16.4 Age-adjusted cardiovascular disease *(CVD)* mortality rates by sex, 1950–2014. *CVD,* Cardiovascular disease; *F,* female; *ICD,* International Classification of Diseases; *M,* male. (From Mensah GA, Wei GS, Sorlie PD, et al. Decline in cardiovascular mortality: possible causes and implications. *Circ Res.* 2017;120:366–380.)

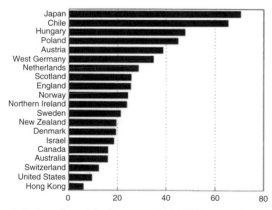

Fig. 16.5 Age-adjusted death rates per 100,000 for stomach cancer in 20 countries, men, 1976–77. (Data from Page HS, Asire AJ. *Cancer Rates and Risks.* 3rd ed. Washington, DC: US Government Printing Office; 1985, NIH Publication No. 85–691.)

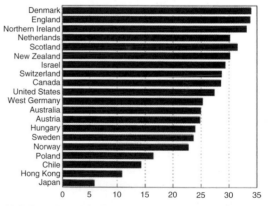

Fig. 16.6 Age-adjusted death rates per 100,000 for breast cancer in 20 countries, women, 1976–77. (Data from Page HS, Asire AJ. *Cancer Rates and Risks.* 3rd ed. Washington, DC: US Government Printing Office; 1985, NIH Publication No. 85–691.)

including certain dietary preferences. Thus, the microenvironment of the migrant, particularly environmental characteristics related to lifestyle, are generally a combination of their country of origin and those of the country of adoption. Another important consideration is the age at which the person migrated; in interpreting the findings from migrant studies, it is important to know how much of the person's life was spent in each country.

Let us turn to another example. The risk of multiple sclerosis has been shown to be related to latitude: the greater the distance from the equator, the greater the risk.[18] This observation is very intriguing and has stimulated much research. However, questions remain about the extent to which the relationship to latitude is a result of environmental factors, as well as about how we can determine which environmental factors might be involved.

Studies of people who have migrated from high-risk to low-risk areas are ideally suited to addressing some of these questions. One country that lent itself nicely to such a study is Israel, which, by latitude, is a low-risk country for multiple sclerosis. Israel had successive waves of immigration during the 20th century. Some of the migrants came from high-risk areas, such as the relatively north latitudes of the United States, Canada, and Northern Europe, whereas others came from low-risk latitudes closer to the equator, including areas of North Africa and the Arabian Peninsula.

Table 16.7 shows data for the incidence of multiple sclerosis in European and African and Asian migrants into Israel. This disease is not common; therefore the sample is small (only 67 cases among 668,880 migrants). Let us look at the rates for African and Asian migrants who moved from one low-risk area to another. Their risk remained low. Now examine the data for European migrants who migrated from a high-risk area (Europe) to a low-risk area (Israel). Europeans who migrated before the age of 15 years (top row) had a low rate, similar to that of African and Asian migrants. However, Europeans who migrated after the age of 15 years tended to retain the high rate of their country of origin. These findings suggested risk of multiple sclerosis is determined in childhood and the critical factor is whether childhood

years were spent in a high-risk or a low-risk area. A person who spent childhood years in a low-risk area retains a low risk; one who spent childhood years in a high-risk area retains a high risk, even after later migration to a low-risk area. This suggests some event in childhood may be of importance in causing multiple sclerosis.

What are the problems with migrant studies? First, migrants are not representative of the populations of their countries of origin. Therefore, we must ask what selection factors led certain people to migrate? For example, people who are seriously ill or disabled generally do not migrate. Other factors, including socioeconomic and cultural characteristics, are also related to which persons are likely to migrate and which persons are not. Consequently, given this problem of selection, we must ask whether we can legitimately compare the rates of stomach cancer among Issei and Nisei with the rates in native Japanese. Second, we need to ask what the age at migration was. How many years did the migrants spend in their country of origin and how many in their adopted country? Third, we should remember migrants do not completely shed the environment of their country of origin after they migrate. These and other factors need to be considered in interpreting the results of migrant studies. There is an obvious parallel with adoption studies, and as seen in Table 16.8, many of the issues that arise in interpreting the findings are similar for the two types of studies.

HOW GENETIC MARKERS ARE USED TO MAP GENES CONTROLLING RISK TO DISEASES, INCLUDING COMPLEX DISEASES

Genetic markers are variants in DNA sequence that can be typed directly. Markers are transmitted from

---

TABLE 16.7 Incidence of Multiple Sclerosis (MS) per 100,000 Among European, African, and Asian Immigrants to Israel by Age at Immigration

Age at Immigration	INCIDENCE OF MS IN MIGRANTS	
	European	African and Asian
<15 years	0.76	0.65
15–29 years	3.54	0.40
30–34 years	1.35	0.26

Modified from Alter M, Leibowitz U, Speer J. Risk of multiple sclerosis related to age at immigration to Israel. *Arch Neurol.* 1966;15:234–237.

TABLE 16.8 Issues in Interpreting the Results of Adoption and Migrant Studies

Adoption Studies	Migrant Studies
• Adoptees are highly selected.	• Migrants are highly selected.
• Age at adoption varies.	• Age at migration varies.
• Adoptees may retain various degrees of contact with their biologic parent(s).	• Migrants may retain many elements of their original environment, particularly those related to culture and lifestyle.

parent to offspring clearly following regular Mendelian patterns, and the chromosomal locations of genetic markers are generally known. If the marker is polymorphic in the population, then many people will carry one or another allele at the marker, and there will be reasonable numbers of heterozygotes and both homozygotes for biallelic markers. While blood groups (like the ABO blood type) qualify as a genetic marker, the most common form of genetic markers are single nucleotide polymorphisms (SNPs). Most SNPs do not have any direct physiologic effects, but a minority occur in coding or regulatory regions of a gene and may directly affect an individual's susceptibility to disease or response to medical treatments.

The ultimate purpose of mapping studies is to identify genes associated with susceptibility to a disease to enhance our understanding of disease pathogenesis and to facilitate development of appropriate preventive strategies. The search for disease susceptibility genes uses two main approaches:

1. Use of family studies to identify *linkage* or co-segregation between a certain marker and a possible disease gene.[19] The coinheritance of genetic markers and disease represents compelling evidence that such a gene does exist while localizing the potentially causal gene to a specific chromosomal region. However, if there are multiple genes that can cause the same disease, they would show evidence of *linkage heterogeneity*, where some families provide evidence of linkage to a given marker while others do not.

2. Search for an *association* between a marker allele and a disease using samples of unrelated people.

While even strong evidence of association remains somewhat less compelling evidence of direct causality, and such evidence is subject to possible confounding due to heterogeneity within the sample, the methods for testing the statistical association between disease and genetic markers build upon conventional epidemiologic study designs and are easy to implement.

Linkage Analysis in Family Studies

As mentioned earlier, when a person has a certain disease, it is valuable to examine his or her first-degree relatives for evidence of a greater-than-expected prevalence of disease. Excess risk in first-degree relatives suggests (though does not prove) the existence of some genetic component. It is also possible to examine high-risk families, such as the pedigree shown in Fig. 16.7, which shows a multiplex family with retinoblastoma across four successive generations. Such pedigrees not only give a visual picture of the familial nature of this disease, but can also be used to map the disease gene by testing for *co-segregation* with one genetic marker (or many markers, as in a genome-wide scan). Clearly this family is likely to reflect an autosomal dominant gene controlling risk. Note how this particular pedigree also demonstrates how even in high-risk families, the disease may skip generations and be transmitted by individuals (*male in the third generation who has a female offspring with disease*) who are not affected themselves (generally denoted as "incomplete penetrance" of the putative disease gene).

Assuming the disease gene has a rare, autosomal dominant mutation that causes retinoblastoma, linkage

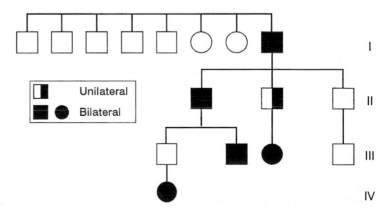

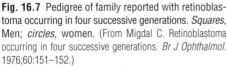

Fig. 16.7 Pedigree of family reported with retinoblastoma occurring in four successive generations. *Squares*, Men; *circles*, women. (From Migdal C. Retinoblastoma occurring in four successive generations. *Br J Ophthalmol.* 1976;60:151–152.)

can be tested between a genetic marker and the hypothetical disease gene. *Linkage analyses* seek to determine whether alleles from two loci (the hypothetical disease locus and some genetic marker) segregate together in a family and are passed as a unit from parent to child. Genes physically near each other on the same chromosome (i.e., the two linked genes) will tend to be transmitted together; that is, they will co-segregate. Genetic linkage can only be identified through family studies, and generally requires multi-generational families with many affected individuals (termed multiplex families). Some information about linkage can be obtained from nuclear families (two parents and several full siblings) if two or more of the offspring are affected. However, even when linkage is demonstrated in some families, it may not show any evidence of linkage in other families if two different genes control risk; that is, if there is linkage heterogeneity. Furthermore, the cases of disease in multiplex families needed for linkage analysis are not fully representative of all cases of disease. Linkage often sheds light on the biologic mechanisms underlying the transmission and pathogenesis of disease. For example, the causal gene for polycystic kidney disorder, an autosomal dominant disease, has been characterized. As seen in the family shown in Fig. 16.8, the 1-allele shows evidence of linkage with disease and is seen in the father and two

of his offspring, all of whom were affected. In the case of cystic fibrosis (Fig. 16.9), an autosomal recessive condition, the causal variant must be inherited from both the father and the mother. Thus, the disease is not seen in either parent, but only in the child who has both alleles.

ASSOCIATION STUDIES

Similar to the approach of testing for familial aggregation of disease, we can also test for an association between an SNP and a disease (or a continuous phenotype). This test of association is the same as that used in traditional epidemiology, but the genetic marker allele or genotype becomes the exposure of interest. We can test for association with a single gene, or a set of genes known to be potentially associated (candidate genes) or agnostically across the entire genome (genome-wide). The feasibility of studying the entire genome to identify genetic associations, in the form of genome-wide association studies (GWAS), has changed the overall approach for studying associations between genetic markers (most often SNPs) and disease. In the GWAS approach, using 1 to 5 million SNPs, we are looking for regions of the genome strongly associated with a disease (and therefore likely to harbor a causal gene), but the individual SNPs yielding evidence of association are generally not directly causal and most often they

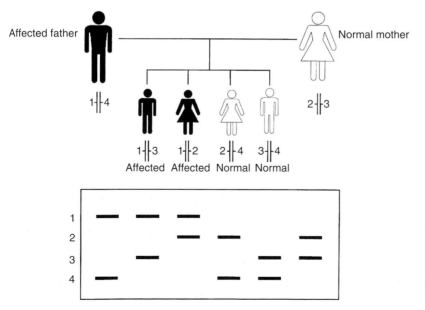

Fig. 16.8 DNA analysis of autosomal dominant disorders. Example: Polycystic kidney disorder. (From Taylor HA, Schroer RJ, Phelan MC, et al. *Counseling Aids for Geneticists.* 2nd ed. Greenwood, SC: Greenwood Genetic Center; 1989.)

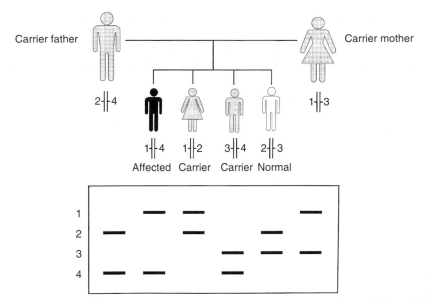

Fig. 16.9 DNA analysis of autosomal recessive disorders. Example: Cystic fibrosis. (From Taylor HA, Schroer RJ, Phelan MC, et al. *Counseling Aids for Geneticists.* 2nd ed. Greenwood, SC: Greenwood Genetic Center; 1989.)

are in noncoding regions of the genome. However, these significant SNPs may be correlated with some unobserved high-risk allele at an unknown causal gene, and can still be useful in mapping nearby genes that do control risk. GWAS have become possible in the last 10 years or so, largely due to technological advances in SNP genotyping; they have been widely used for a variety of common diseases where multiple genes and some environmental risk factors are known to play some role in causing disease.[20,21] The premise underlying GWAS is that common SNPs scattered throughout the genome can "tag" haplotypes with sufficient accuracy to reveal correlations between observed SNPs and unobserved causal genes when analyzed under the traditional case-control or cohort study design. The test statistic (usually a chi-squared test or a logistic regression model, topics not covered in this text) is simple, and significant genotype or allele frequency differences between groups of cases and controls should reveal meaningful differences reflecting either a direct or indirect association between a marker and some unknown causal gene. Because the number of SNPs used in GWAS is large (originally at least 100,000 SNPs but now typically 1 to 2.5 million SNPs per person in a study), the conventional critical value of the alpha error (P-value) of 5% for each SNP is no

longer appropriate because so many tests are being done in each study. To minimize the rate of false-positive results, a genome-wide significance level is set at $P = 5*10^{-7} - 5*10^{-8}$.

Many of the problems in methodology and interpretation of results addressed in earlier chapters apply to the associations between diseases and genetic markers. This includes biases (selection, information) and confounding. One important confounder for genetic association studies is ancestry. We know that, despite the genetic similarities between individuals (>99%), there are allele frequency differences between people originating from different parts of the world due to the natural variation among human sub-populations, or possibly selective or environmental pressures present through the history of different sub-populations. Thus, ancestry can be associated both with exposure (allele or genotype frequency) and with the disease outcome, and thus confound the study results. There are methods to address this important confounder, which may include simple stratification by self-reported ancestry or estimating the percentage of each person's ancestry based on genetic markers, including that in the statistical model. Selecting appropriate controls is always important. When presented with a list of associations with a disease and a genetic marker (blood group or SNP), we should ask how were the conclusions regarding such associations arrived at, and what comparison groups were used? Thus, the methodologic issues discussed in earlier chapters in the context of different types of epidemiologic study designs are highly relevant when investigating ways in which genetic factors relate to these diseases.

Despite their limitations, much has been accomplished through GWAS. Since the first GWAS-based discovery of the association of complement factor H (CFH) gene and age-related macular degeneration,[22] more than 2,000 robust associations between genes and complex diseases have been identified.[23] By combining multiple studies, it is now clear that multiple genes influence the risk of most complex diseases representing major public health burdens.[20] These replicated genetic risk factors should be useful in improving risk prediction (on a broad level), diagnostic classification, and eventually drug development (both for potential efficacy and to minimize adverse events). This progress has generated excitement about precision medicine where genetic information can guide clinical medicine (see below). Recently, Khoury and Evans[24] advocated for a similar emphasis on developing "precision prevention," characterized by strategies building up the role and importance of genetics in public health.

Interaction Between Genetic and Environmental Risk Factors

The question of genetic susceptibility to environmental factors and the possibility of interaction between them must also be addressed. In Chapter 14, we discussed the study by Grant and Dawson that describes an association of earlier age at onset of alcohol consumption to prevalence of lifetime alcohol abuse (Fig. 16.10). As seen in Fig. 16.11, when the subjects were divided into those with a positive family history of alcoholism and those with a negative family history, the overall relationship still held, although the prevalence was higher among those with a positive family history.[25] This observation suggests that, although the observed relationship between lifetime risk of alcohol abuse and age at initiating alcohol consumption may reflect environmental influences, the effect of family history suggests either an interaction with genetic factors or some influence of child rearing related to a family history of alcohol abuse.

One example of potential gene-environment interaction involves smoking and the factor V Leiden mutation. Smoking is a known risk factor for myocardial infarction (MI), and factor V Leiden is a common hereditary abnormality that affects blood

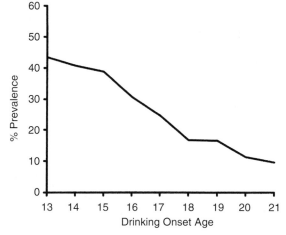

Fig. 16.10 Prevalence of lifetime alcohol dependence by age at drinking onset. (Modified from Grant BF, Dawson DA. Age at onset of alcohol use and its association with DSM-IV alcohol abuse and dependence: results from the National Longitudinal Alcohol Epidemiologic Survey. *J Substance Abuse.* 1997;9:103–110.)

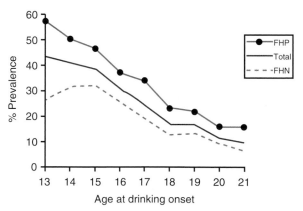

Fig. 16.11 Prevalence of lifetime alcohol dependence by age at drinking onset and family history of alcoholism. *FHN,* Family history negative; *FHP,* family history positive. (Modified from Grant BF. The impact of a family history of alcoholism on the relationship between age at onset of alcohol use and DSM-IV alcohol dependence: results from the National Longitudinal Alcohol Epidemiologic Survey. *Alcohol Health Res World.* 1998;22:144–147.)

clotting and increases the risk of venous thrombosis. Rosendaal and colleagues conducted a population-based case-control study of 472 young women including 84 who had an MI before the age of 45.[26] The factor V Leiden mutation was more prevalent in the MI case group, with a 2.4 increased odds ratio as compared to those without this mutation. However, when considering both smoking and carrier status, there is a suggestion of statistical interaction between smoking and the factor V Leiden as illustrated in Table 16.9. In particular, noncarrier women who smoked showed an odds ratio 9 times more likely to have a premature MI, but carrier women who smoked were 32 times more likely to have a premature MI compared to those women who did not smoke and were not carriers. Because the estimated combined effects of the genotype and smoking greatly exceeded what would be expected under either a multiplicative or an additive model, these findings suggest statistical interaction (or deviation from a simple combination of the marginal effects of genotype and environmental exposures). While this type of analysis is intriguing, it is often impossible to say definitively whether such statistical interaction represents true biologic interactions (e.g., synergistic or antagonistic relationships between the effects of genetic and environmental risk factors).[27] There is biologic plausibility, however, for each of these exposures, and their interaction is also biologically plausible. Detecting gene-environment interaction always requires larger sample sizes, and confirming its existence across populations may prove difficult because the allele frequencies and exposure rates can differ across populations, as discussed by Aschard.[28]

In 1995, Brennan and colleagues reported a study of cigarette smoking and squamous cell cancer of the head and neck.[29] They found that in patients with invasive cancer of the head and neck, smoking was associated with a marked increase in mutations in the p53 gene, which is normally a tumor suppressor. Such mutations are likely to contribute to both the inception and the growth of cancers. The investigators studied tumor samples from 127 patients with head and neck cancer and found p53 mutations in 42% (54 of 127) of patients. Patients who smoked at least one pack per day for at least 20 years were more than twice as likely to have mutations in p53 as patients who were nonsmokers. Patients who smoked and drank more than 1 oz of hard alcohol per day were 3.5 times more likely to have mutations in p53 than patients who neither smoked nor drank. As seen in Fig. 16.12, p53 mutations were found in 58% of patients who both smoked and drank; in 33% of patients who smoked but did not drink; and in 17% of patients who neither smoked nor drank. Furthermore, the type of mutation found in patients who neither smoked nor drank seemed likely to be endogenous rather than caused by environmental mutagens (i.e., exogenous). The findings suggest that cigarette smoking may tend to inactivate the p53 tumor suppressor gene and thus provide a molecular basis for the well-recognized relationship of cigarette smoking to head and neck cancer.

TABLE 16.9 Association of Smoking and Factor V Leiden on Risk of Myocardial Infarction in Young Women

Odds Ratio (95% CI)	FACTOR V GENOTYPE	
Current Smoker	Wildtype	Leiden
No	1.0 (ref)	1.1 (0.1, 8.5)
Yes	9.0 (5.1, 15.7)	32.0 (7.7, 133)

The risk of myocardial infarction is elevated in young women who smoke but is greatest in those with the factor V Leiden genotype. This statistical interaction between genotype and environment exceeds what would be expected by genetics or environment alone (OR = 32).

CI, Confidence Interval.

From Austin MA, Schwartz SM. Cardiovascular disease. In: Costa LG, Eaton DL, eds. *Gene-Environment Interactions: Fundamentals of Ecogenetics.* Hoboken, NJ: John Wiley & Sons; 2006. Modified from Rosendaal FR, Siscovick DS, Schwartz SM, et al. Factor V Leiden (resistance to activated protein C) increases the risk of myocardial infarction in young women. *Blood.* 1997; 89:2817–2821.

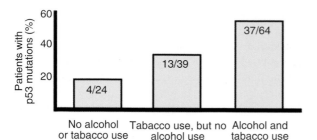

Fig. 16.12 Association of p53 gene mutations with cigarette smoking and alcohol consumption in 129 patients with squamous cell carcinoma of the head and neck. (From Brennan JA, Boyle JO, Koch WM, et al. Association between cigarette smoking and mutation of the p53 gene in squamous cell carcinoma of the head and neck. *N Engl J Med.* 1995;332:712–717.)

A further step in this approach is to identify a specific gene defect that is associated with a certain environmental exposure. An example is seen in findings linking a specific defect in the p53 gene to aflatoxin exposure in patients with hepatocellular carcinoma (HCC). In Chapter 14, the positive synergism of hepatitis B virus (HBV) and aflatoxin B₁ exposure in increasing the risk of HCC is discussed. To determine whether the frequency of a specific mutation in the p53 tumor suppressor gene (a "hot spot" mutation at codon 249) was related to the risk related to aflatoxin exposure, Bressac and coworkers screened HCC samples from 14 countries.[30] The mutation was found in 17% (12/72) of tumor samples from four countries in southern Africa and the southeast coast of Asia but in none of 95 samples from other geographic locations including North America, Europe, the Middle East, and Japan. The four countries in which the mutation was found, China, Vietnam, South Africa, and Mozambique, have the highest incidence of HCC in the world and share a similar warm and humid climate, which favors the growth of aflatoxin-producing molds. The rate of HBV carriage was high but did not vary significantly among the countries studied. However, the risk of aflatoxin exposure did vary among these countries and the presence of the mutation was found to correlate with the risk of exposure to aflatoxins.

Further support for these findings was provided by Aguilar and colleagues, who studied samples of normal liver from three geographic areas that varied in their prevalence of aflatoxin exposure: negligible levels (United States), low levels (Thailand), and high levels (Qidong, China).[31]

The frequency of the mutation paralleled the level of aflatoxin B₁ exposure, suggesting that aflatoxin has a causal and probably early role in the development of liver tumors.

Thus, studies combining epidemiologic and molecular methods may prove invaluable in confirming an etiologic role for certain environmental agents by demonstrating their specific gene effects. Moreover, such studies may also suggest biologic pathways and mechanisms that may be involved in the development of certain cancers and other diseases. However, combined epidemiologic and molecular studies may also help determine that a disease is not primarily caused by environmental factors. For example, Harris pointed out that the exact nature of the p53 mutation can be valuable in indicating that a certain cancer did not result from an environmental carcinogen but instead was caused by endogenous mutagenesis, such as was seen in the study just described, of patients with head and neck cancer who were nondrinkers and nonsmokers.[32] Germ line mutations in p53 can also indicate that a person has an increased susceptibility to cancer as originally proposed by Knudson in 1971.[33]

However, it must be remembered that statistical power to detect gene-environment effects will generally require much greater sample sizes compared to what is required to detect marginal effects of either the genetic or the environmental risk factor.[28] The rule of thumb is that a fourfold increase in sample size is needed to detect interactions, and sometimes even simple forms of interaction can be difficult to confirm in actual data sets. This is especially true when there is substantial error in measuring the environmental risk factor. Still, if evidence of gene-environment interaction can be obtained, it would open new opportunities for public health intervention, because modifying environmental risk factors is far easier than altering the genetic structure of a population.

Precision Medicine

Sequencing technology is now driving the current era of genetic epidemiology. Sequencing has the advantage of identifying **all** variants in a given region of the genome (i.e., rare and low frequency single nucleotide variants, as well as common tagging SNPs). This new phase has been driven by two forces: (1) the advancements in massive parallel or "next-generation sequencing" technology that is becoming affordable even for samples sizes seen in epidemiologic studies and (2) the impending completion of combined GWAS analyses for many (if not most) complex diseases across large studies, which has identified numerous genes as significantly influencing risk. We have not reached our goal of fully understanding complex diseases (and we might be far from it) if causal pathways involve mechanistic gene-gene and gene-environment interactions. We have gone from originally identifying the double helix in the middle of the 20th century to the ability to sequence the entire genome of many individuals in the first quarter of the 21st century.

Whole genome sequencing is particularly exciting because of its promise of deepening our understanding of genes and for its potential for facilitating the development of "personalized treatments" of individual patients. We previously discussed some limitations of randomized trials in developing new treatment modalities, particularly because the trials generally deal with groups rather than with individuals, and thus usually estimate average effects. Therefore, as pointed out earlier, the study results are often given for groups and leave the treating physician without information regarding how likely it is that a given individual whom he or she is treating will benefit from the new drug, or whether the patient will develop serious side effects from it. However, with the advent of the current new era in human genetics the hope has been that we will be able to develop therapies that are tailor-made for the individual patient on the basis of the characteristics of his or her genome. For example, the drug clopidogrel is used after the placement of a coronary stent following a heart attack. Clopidogrel depresses platelet activity, which reduces your risk of a heart attack. Loss of function of genetic variants in the CYP2C19 gene result in decreased metabolite production and is associated with the increased risk of a subsequent heart attack,[34,35] even when patients are treated with clopidogrel. However, adjustment of the dose of clopidogrel in patients who have these CYP2C19 alleles (found in nearly one-third of the general US population) or changing the medication to another drug decreases the risk of subsequent heart attacks similar to the level of patients without these alleles.[36–38] Thus, genetic information generated from populations can be used to treat the individual patient.

Prospects for the Future

Despite the excitement accompanying sequencing of the human genome and the results of genome-wide studies described earlier, for most complex diseases (in which both genetic and environmental factors have been implicated) the current data are still not yet sufficient to specifically delineate how genes control risk. Enhanced understanding of the molecular changes in cancer resulting from studies of genetic changes in cancer cells should improve our understanding of how individuals can vary in their susceptibility to cancers and facilitate the development of specific therapies for biologic pathways involved in different tumors. Such "targeted" or "individualized" therapies may help in understanding and treating subgroups of tissue-specific tumors. By targeting specific molecular pathways involved in different tumors, as well as the points at which tumor cells may be particularly vulnerable to certain therapies, individualized treatment should become more effective. Such treatment might also have fewer and less severe side effects than conventional therapies, which are not specific in their cytotoxic effects and affect both abnormal and normal cells.

Childs articulated a concept encompassing not only the different characteristics of histologically different tumors, but also the unique genetic and environmental characteristics of humans that may have led to a vulnerability to such tumors.[39] As a result, what might appear at first glance to be the same disease occurring in different individuals should perhaps be considered different diseases with the same phenotype because the disease in a person is a "package" of physical, laboratory, and other abnormalities, combined with a unique set of genetically and environmentally determined host factors influencing overall susceptibility. These susceptibilities may often include social and psychological factors in addition to recognized environmental factors. These factors may be operating at the level of the individual, the family, the community, or some other broad social grouping. Although this combination will differ from one individual to another, by current definitions and classifications of disease, many individuals may appear to have the same illness. Integration of knowledge of all these divergent areas may provide the foundation for earlier detection of high-risk individuals and could lead to more effective measures of prevention in coming years.

In 2000, Childs and Valle wrote:

The signs and symptoms of a patient today may well have been forged in the developmental and maturational matrix of the past. And in making that characterization, we discern the individuality and heterogeneity of that which we give the name of a disease. …

In medicine we have trouble accepting this kind of individuality. When we see a patient, we think first of the name of a disease and then of the variation expressed in the patient. This way of thinking is typological, and is to be distinguished from "population" thinking in which a population, say, of patients with the "same" disease, consists of variable individuals.[40]

Dalton and Friend published a schematic presentation of the cyclical nature of the process of incorporating new knowledge into therapies that are individualized for each patient (Fig. 16.13) and the process is described in the caption to this figure.[41] Although this approach

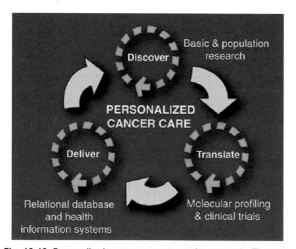

Fig. 16.13 Personalized cancer care as a continuous cycle. The cycle starts with the discovery of specific molecular alterations in tumors that are then linked to specific patient outcomes in clinical trials. The ability to capture molecular profiles and clinical information at the level of individual patients allows translation of the information into more personalized cancer care. Available relational databases and health information systems ensure more informed delivery of cancer therapies to future patients; it can also guide the discovery of new therapies. (From Dalton WS, Friend SH. Cancer biomarkers—an invitation to the table. *Science.* 2006;312:1165–1168.)

has great potential, its benefits have not yet been extensively realized in the treatment of most complex diseases. However, new technologies at the molecular and genetic levels are likely to have profound effects on health care and on the development of "*personalized medicine*," which will include new approaches to disease prevention and treatment of disease that will be made possible by technical advances and by the integration of new information derived from different biologic and sociologic disciplines.

Conclusion

This chapter has described some of the epidemiologic approaches used to assess the relative contributions of genetic and environmental factors in causing human disease. The link of epidemiology and genetics has become increasingly recognized, and a field called *genetic epidemiology* has emerged.[19] Excellent discussions have been published regarding the impact of the genomic era on epidemiologic research.[42,43]

Most epidemiologic studies are directed at identifying environmental factors in controlling the risk of disease, but when designing and conducting studies and interpreting their results, it is important to bear in mind that individuals in epidemiologic studies differ not only in environmental exposures but also in their genetic makeup, and this too influences risk. When appropriate, epidemiologic studies of risk factors, including case-control and other study designs, should be expanded to include gathering family histories and obtaining biologic samples whenever possible. Incorporating genetic advances and genetic markers into epidemiologic studies is proving increasingly valuable in identifying high-risk subgroups and tailoring therapies specific to the individual. They are likely to become increasingly important in improving disease prevention in the future.

REFERENCES

1. Massie J, Ioannou L, Delatycki M. Prenatal and preconception population carrier screening for cystic fibrosis in Australia: where are we up to? *Aust N Z J Obstet Gynaecol.* 2014;54(6):503–509.
2. Ashley-Koch A, Yang Q, Olney RS. Sickle hemoglobin (HbS) allele and sickle cell disease: a HuGE review. *Am J Epidemiol.* 2000;151(9):839–845.
3. Therrell BL Jr, Lloyd-Puryear MA, Eckman JR, et al. Newborn screening for sickle cell diseases in the United States: a review of data spanning 2 decades. *Semin Perinatol.* 2015;39(3):238–251.

4. Minkovitz CS, Grason H, Ruderman M, et al. Newborn screening programs and sickle cell disease: a public health services and systems approach. *Am J Prev Med*. 2016;51(1 suppl 1):S39–S47.

5. Mak CM, Lee HC, Chan AY, et al. Inborn errors of metabolism and expanded newborn screening: review and update. *Crit Rev Clin Lab Sci*. 2013;50(6):142–162.

6. Hogben L. *Nature and Nurture*. New York: WW Norton; 1939.

7. Jörgensen G, Lenz W, Pfeiffer RA, et al. Thalidomide-embryopathy in twins: a collaborative study. *Acta Genet Med Gemellol (Roma)*. 1970;19(1):205–210.

8. Grasby KL, Verweij KJH, Mosing MA, et al. Estimating heritability from twin studies. *Methods Mol Biol*. 2017;1666:171–194.

9. Kaij L. *Studies on the Etiology and Sequels of Abuse of Alcohol*. Lund: Hakan Ohlssons Boktryckeri; 1960.

10. Hrubec Z, Omenn GS. Evidence of genetic predisposition to alcoholic cirrhosis and psychosis: twin concordances for alcoholism and its biological end points by zygosity among male veterans. *Alcohol Clin Exp Res*. 1981;5:207–215.

11. Murray RM, Clifford C, Gurlin HM. Twin and alcoholism studies. In: Galanter M, ed. *Recent Developments in Alcoholism*. Vol. 1. New York: Plenum; 1983:25–47.

12. Pickens RW, Svikis DS, McGue M, et al. Heterogeneity in the inheritance of alcoholism: a study of male and female twins. *Arch Gen Psychiatry*. 1991;48:19–28.

13. Lichtenstein P, Holm NV, Verkasalo PK, et al. Environmental and heritable factors in the causation of cancer: analyses of cohorts of twins from Sweden, Denmark, and Finland. *N Engl J Med*. 2000;343:78–85.

14. Kety SS, Ingraham LJ. Genetic transmission and improved diagnosis of schizophrenia from pedigrees of adoptees. *J Psychiatr Res*. 1992;26:247–255.

15. King MC, Marks JH, Mandell JB, et al. Breast and ovarian cancer risks due to inherited mutations in BRCA1 and BRCA2. *Science*. 2003;302(5645):643–646.

16. Prevalence and penetrance of BRCA1 and BRCA2 mutations in a population-based series of breast cancer cases. Anglian Breast Cancer Study Group. *Br J Cancer*. 2000;83(10):1301–1308.

17. Malaty HM. Epidemiology of Helicobacter pylori infection. *Best Pract Res Clin Gastroenterol*. 2007;21(2):205–214.

18. Wood H. Multiple sclerosis: latitude and vitamin D influence disease course in multiple sclerosis. *Nat Rev Neurol*. 2017; 13(1):3.

19. Khoury MJ, Beaty TH, Cohen BH. *Fundamentals of Genetic Epidemiology*. New York: Oxford University Press; 1993.

20. Visscher PM, Wray NR, Zhang Q, et al. 10 years of GWAS discovery: biology, function, and translation. *Am J Hum Genet*. 2017;101(1):5–22.

21. Visscher PM, Brown MA, McCarthy MI, et al. Five years of GWAS discovery. *Am J Hum Genet*. 2012;90(1):7–24.

22. Klein RJ, Zeiss C, Chew EY, et al. Complement factor H polymorphism in age-related macular degeneration. *Science*. 2005;308(5720):385–389.

23. Manolio TA. Bringing genome-wide association findings into clinical use. *Nat Rev Genet*. 2013;14(8):549–558.

24. Khoury MJ, Evans JP. A public health perspective on a national precision medicine cohort: balancing long-term knowledge generation with early health benefit. *JAMA*. 2015;313(21):2117–2118.

25. Grant BF. The impact of a family history of alcoholism on the relationship between age at onset of alcohol use and DSM-IV alcohol dependence: results from the National Longitudinal Alcohol Epidemiologic Survey. *Alcohol Health Res World*. 1998;22:144–147.

26. Rosendaal FR, Siscovick DS, Schwartz SM, et al. Factor V Leiden (resistance to activated protein C) increases the risk of myocardial infarction in young women. *Blood*. 1997;89:2817–2821.

27. Austin MA, Schwartz SM. Cardiovascular disease. In: Costa LG, Eaton DL eds. *Gene-Environment Interactions: Fundamentals of Ecogenetics*. Hoboken, NJ: John Wiley and Sons; 2006:271–283.

28. Aschard H. A perspective on interaction effects in genetic association studies. *Genet Epidemiol*. 2016;40(8):678–688.

29. Brennan JA, Boyle JO, Koch WM, et al. Association between cigarette smoking and mutation of the p53 gene in squamous-cell carcinoma of the head and neck. *N Engl J Med*. 1995;332: 712–717.

30. Bressac B, Puisieux MS, Kew M, et al. p53 mutation in hepatocellular carcinoma after aflatoxin exposure. *Lancet*. 1991;338:1356–1359.

31. Aguilar F, Harris CC, Sun T, et al. Geographic variation of p53 mutational profile in nonmalignant human liver. *Science*. 1994;264:1317–1319.

32. Harris C. p53: at the crossroads of molecular carcinogenesis and risk assessment. *Science*. 1993;262:1980–1981.

33. Knudson AG Jr. Mutation and cancer: statistical study of retinoblastoma. *Proc Natl Acad Sci USA*. 1971;68:820–823.

34. Shuldiner AR, O'Connell JR, Bliden KP, et al. Association of cytochrome P450 2C19 genotype with the antiplatelet effect and clinical efficacy of clopidogrel therapy. *JAMA*. 2009;302(8):849–857.

35. Mega JL, Simon T, Collet JP, et al. Reduced-function CYP2C19 genotype and risk of adverse clinical outcomes among patients treated with clopidogrel predominantly for PCI: a meta-analysis. *JAMA*. 2010;304(16):1821–1830.

36. Cavallari LH, Lee CR, Beitelshees AL, et al. Multisite investigation of outcomes with implementation of CYP2C19 genotype-guided antiplatelet therapy after percutaneous coronary intervention. *JACC Cardiovasc Interv*. 2018;11(2):181–191.

37. Shuldiner AR, Palmer K, Pakyz RE, et al. Implementation of pharmacogenetics: the University of Maryland Personalized Anti-platelet Pharmacogenetics Program. *Am J Med Genet C Semin Med Genet*. 2014;166C(1):76–84.

38. Scott SA, Sangkuhl K, Stein CM, et al; Clinical Pharmacogenetics Implementation Consortium. Clinical Pharmacogenetics Implementation Consortium guidelines for CYP2C19 genotype and clopidogrel therapy: 2013 update. *Clin Pharmacol Ther*. 2013;94(3):317–323.

39. Childs B. *Genetic Medicine—A Logic of Disease*. Baltimore: Johns Hopkins University Press; 1999.

40. Childs B, Valle D. Genetics, biology and disease. *Annu Rev Genomics Hum Genet*. 2000;1:1–19.

41. Dalton WS, Friend SH. Cancer biomarkers—an invitation to the table. *Science*. 2006;312:1165–1168.

42. Millikan R. The changing face of epidemiology in the genomics era. *Epidemiology*. 2002;13:472–480.

43. Willett WC. Balancing life-style and genomics research for disease prevention. *Science*. 2002;296:695–698.

REVIEW QUESTIONS FOR CHAPTER 16

1 *If a greater proportion of monozygotic twin pairs are found to be concordant for a certain disease than are dizygotic twin pairs, the observation suggests that the disease is most likely caused by:*
a. Exclusively environmental factors
b. Exclusively genetic factors
c. Hereditary factors almost exclusively, with some nonhereditary factors possibly playing a role
d. Environmental and genetic factors almost equally
e. Gender differences in monozygotic twins

2 *When the incidence of a disease in adopted children is studied and compared with its incidence in biologic relatives and in adoptive relatives, all of the following are relevant concerns* except:
a. Age at onset
b. Amount of contact maintained by the adoptee with his or her biologic parents
c. Marital status of the biologic parents
d. Selection factors relating to who is adopted and who is not
e. *c* and *d*

Question 3 is based on the information given below:

In a familial study of schizophrenia, the following concordance rates were observed within various pairs of relatives:

Pair	Concordance Rate (%)
Husband–wife	5
Parent–child	40
Monozygotic twins	65
Dizygotic twins	42
Ordinary siblings	40

3 *A reasonable conclusion to be drawn from these data is:*
a. Genetic factors are unimportant in the etiology of schizophrenia
b. The data suggest a potentially important genetic component
c. The incidence of schizophrenia within relative pairs is highest in monozygotic twins
d. The prevalence of schizophrenia within relative pairs is highest in monozygotic twins
e. Twins are less likely to have schizophrenia than are ordinary siblings

Question 4 is based on the information given below:

In a study of Japanese migrants to the United States, the following standardized mortality ratios (SMRs) were found for disease X:

Group	Standardized Mortality Ratio
Native Japanese living in Japan	100
Japanese migrants	105
Children of Japanese ancestry	108
United States whites	591

4 *These findings suggest that:*

a. Environmental factors are the major determinants of these SMRs

b. Genetic factors are the major determinants of these SMRs

c. Environmental factors associated with the migrant culture are probably involved

d. Migrants are highly selected and are nonrepresentative of the population in their native country

e. International differences in coding death certificates for disease X are an important determinant of these SMRs

5 *If an association is found between the incidence of a disease and a certain genetically determined characteristic:*

a. The disease is clearly genetic in origin

b. Genetic factors are at least implicated in all cases of the disease

c. Genetic factors are implicated in at least some cases of the disease

d. A role for environmental factors is excluded

e. Expression of the disease is likely to be unavoidable

Glossary of Genetic Terms for Chapter 16

Term	Definition
Allele	An allele is one of two or more versions of a gene. An individual inherits two alleles for each gene, one from each parent. If the two alleles are the same, the individual is homozygous for that gene. If the alleles are different, the individual is heterozygous. Though the term allele was originally used to describe variation among genes, it now also refers to variation among noncoding DNA sequences.
Autism	Autism is a developmental brain disorder characterized by impaired social interactions, communication problems, and repetitive behaviors. Symptoms usually appear before the age of 3 years. The exact cause of autism is not known; however, it is likely influenced by genetics. Autism is one of a group of related developmental disorders called autism spectrum disorders (ASDs). Other ASDs include Asperger syndrome and Rett syndrome.
Autosomal Dominant	Autosomal dominance is a pattern of inheritance characteristic of some genetic diseases. "Autosomal" means that the gene in question is located on one of the numbered, or nonsex, chromosomes. "Dominant" means that a single copy of the disease-associated mutation is enough to cause the disease. This is in contrast to a recessive disorder, where two copies of the mutation are needed to cause the disease. Huntington disease is a common example of an autosomal dominant genetic disorder.
Candidate Gene	A candidate gene is a gene whose chromosomal location is associated with a particular disease or other phenotype. Because of its location, the gene is suspected of causing the disease or other phenotype.
Carrier	A carrier is an individual who carries and is capable of passing on a genetic mutation associated with a disease and may or may not display disease symptoms. Carriers are associated with diseases inherited as recessive traits. In order to have the disease, an individual must have inherited mutated alleles from both parents. An individual having one normal allele and one mutated allele does not have the disease. Two carriers may produce children with the disease.
Carrier Screening	Carrier screening is a type of genetic testing performed on people who display no symptoms for a genetic disorder but may be at risk for passing it on to their children. A carrier for a genetic disorder has inherited one normal and one abnormal allele for a gene associated with the disorder. A child must inherit two abnormal alleles in order for symptoms to appear. Prospective parents with a family history of a genetic disorder are candidates for carrier screening.
Chromosome	A chromosome is an organized package of DNA found in the nucleus of the cell. Different organisms have different numbers of chromosomes. Humans have 23 pairs of chromosomes—22 pairs of numbered chromosomes, called autosomes, and one pair of sex chromosomes, X and Y. Each parent contributes one chromosome to each pair so that offspring get half of their chromosomes from their mother and half from their father.
Complex Disease	A complex disease is caused by the interaction of multiple genes and environmental factors. Complex diseases are also called multifactorial. Examples of complex diseases include cancer and heart disease.
Deletion	Deletion is a type of mutation involving the loss of genetic material. It can be small, involving a single missing DNA base pair; or large, involving a piece of a chromosome.
DNA (Deoxyribonucleic Acid)	DNA is the chemical name for the molecule that carries genetic instructions in all living things. The DNA molecule consists of two strands that wind around one another to form a shape known as a double helix. Each strand has a backbone made of alternating sugar (deoxyribose) and phosphate groups. Attached to each sugar is one of four bases—adenine (A), cytosine (C), guanine (G), and thymine (T). The two strands are held together by bonds between the bases: adenine bonds with thymine, and cytosine bonds with guanine. The sequences of the bases along the backbones serve as instructions for assembling protein and RNA molecules.

Term	Definition
DNA Sequencing	DNA sequencing is a laboratory technique used to determine the exact sequence of bases (A, C, G, and T) in a DNA molecule. The DNA base sequence carries the information a cell needs to assemble protein and RNA molecules. DNA sequence information is important to scientists investigating the functions of genes. The technology of DNA sequencing was made faster and less expensive as a part of the Human Genome Project.
Dominant	Dominant refers to the relationship between two versions of a gene. Individuals receive two versions of each gene, known as alleles, from each parent. If the alleles of a gene are different, one allele will be expressed; it is the dominant gene. The effect of the other allele, called recessive, is masked.
Fraternal Twins	Fraternal twins are also dizygotic twins. They result from the fertilization of two separate eggs during the same pregnancy. Fraternal twins may be of the same or different sexes. They share half of their genes just like any other siblings. In contrast, twins that result from the fertilization of a single egg that then splits in two are called monozygotic, or identical, twins. Identical twins share all of their genes and are always the same sex.
Gene	The gene is the basic physical unit of inheritance. Genes are passed from parents to offspring and contain the information needed to specify traits. Genes are arranged, one after another, on structures called chromosomes. A chromosome contains a single, long DNA molecule, only a portion of which corresponds to a single gene. Humans have approximately 20,000 genes arranged on their chromosomes.
Gene Environment Interaction	Gene environment interaction is an influence on the expression of a trait that results from the interplay between genes and the environment. Some traits are strongly influenced by genes, while other traits are strongly influenced by the environment. However, most traits are influenced by one or more genes interacting in complex ways with the environment.
Gene Mapping	Gene mapping is the process of establishing the locations of genes on the chromosomes. Early gene maps used linkage analysis. The closer two genes are to each other on the chromosome, the more likely it is that they will be inherited together. By following inheritance patterns, the relative positions of genes can be determined. More recently, scientists have used recombinant DNA (rDNA) techniques to establish the actual physical locations of genes on the chromosomes.
Genetic Counseling	Genetic counseling is the professional interaction between a health care provider with specialized knowledge of genetics and an individual or family. The genetic counselor determines whether a condition in the family may be genetic and estimates the chances that another relative may be affected. Genetic counselors also offer and interpret genetic tests that may help to estimate the risk of disease. The genetic counselor conveys information in an effort to address concerns of the client and provides psychological counseling to help families adapt to their condition or risk.
Genetic Epidemiology	Genetic epidemiology is a relatively new medical discipline that seeks to understand how genetic factors interact with the environment in the context of disease in populations. Areas of study include the causes of inherited disease and its distribution and control.
Genetic Map	A genetic map is a type of chromosome map that shows the relative locations of genes and other important features. The map is based on the idea of linkage, which means that the closer two genes are to each other on the chromosome, the greater the probability that they will be inherited together. By following inheritance patterns, the relative locations of genes along the chromosome are established.
Genetic Marker	A genetic marker is a DNA sequence with a known physical location on a chromosome. Genetic markers can help link an inherited disease with the responsible gene. DNA segments close to each other on a chromosome tend to be inherited together. Genetic markers are used to track the inheritance of a nearby gene that has not yet been identified, but whose approximate location is known. The genetic marker itself may be a part of a gene or may have no known function.

Continued

Term	Definition
Genetic Screening	Genetic screening is the process of testing a population for a genetic disease in order to identify a subgroup of people who either have the disease or the potential to pass it on to their offspring.
Genome	The genome is the entire set of genetic instructions found in a cell. In humans, the genome consists of 23 pairs of chromosomes, found in the nucleus, as well as a small chromosome found in the cells' mitochondria. Each set of 23 chromosomes contains approximately 3.1 billion bases of DNA sequence.
Genome-Wide Association Studies (GWAS)	A genome-wide association study (GWAS) is an approach used in genetics research to associate specific genetic variations with particular diseases. The method involves scanning the genomes from many different people and looking for genetic markers that can be used to predict the presence of a disease. Once such genetic markers are identified, they can be used to understand how genes contribute to the disease and develop better prevention and treatment strategies.
Genomics	Genomics refers to the study of the entire genome of an organism whereas genetics refers to the study of a particular gene.
Genotype	A genotype is an individual's collection of genes. The term also can refer to the two alleles inherited for a particular gene. The genotype is expressed when the information encoded in the genes' DNA is used to make protein and RNA molecules. The expression of the genotype contributes to the individual's observable traits, called the phenotype.
Germ Line	A germ line is the sex cells (eggs and sperm) that are used by sexually reproducing organisms to pass on genes from generation to generation. Egg and sperm cells are called germ cells, in contrast to the other cells of the body that are called somatic cells.
Heterozygous	Heterozygous refers to having inherited different forms of a particular gene from each parent. A heterozygous genotype stands in contrast to a homozygous genotype, where an individual inherits identical forms of a particular gene from each parent.
Homozygous	Homozygous is a genetic condition where an individual inherits the same alleles for a particular gene from both parents.
Identical Twins	Identical twins are also known as monozygotic twins. They result from the fertilization of a single egg that splits in two. Identical twins share all of their genes and are always of the same sex. In contrast, fraternal, or dizygotic, twins result from the fertilization of two separate eggs during the same pregnancy. They share half of their genes, just like any other siblings. Fraternal twins can be of the same or different sexes.
Inherited	An inherited trait is one that is genetically determined. Inherited traits are passed from parent to offspring according to the rules of Mendelian genetics. Most traits are not strictly determined by genes, but rather are influenced by both genes and environment.
Linkage	Linkage is the close association of genes or other DNA sequences on the same chromosome. The closer two genes are to each other on the chromosome, the greater the probability that they will be inherited together.
Locus	A locus is the specific physical location of a gene or other DNA sequence on a chromosome, like a genetic street address. The plural of locus is "loci."
Mapping	Mapping is the process of making a representative diagram cataloging the genes and other features of a chromosome and showing their relative locations. Cytogenetic maps are made using photomicrographs of chromosomes stained to reveal structural variations. Genetic maps use the idea of linkage to estimate the relative locations of genes. Physical maps, made using recombinant DNA (rDNA) technology, show the actual physical locations of landmarks along a chromosome.
Mendel, Johann (Gregor)	Gregor Mendel was an Austrian monk who, in the 19th century, worked out the basic laws of inheritance, even before the term "gene" had been coined. In his monastery garden, Mendel performed thousands of crosses with garden peas. Mendel is considered the founder of the science of genetics.
Mendelian Inheritance	Mendelian inheritance refers to patterns of inheritance that are characteristic of organisms that reproduce sexually. The Austrian monk Gregor Mendel performed thousands of crosses with garden peas at his monastery during the middle of the 19th century. Mendel explained his results by describing two laws of inheritance that introduced the idea of dominant and recessive genes.

Term	Definition
Mutation	A mutation is a change in a DNA sequence. Mutations can result from DNA copying mistakes made during cell division, exposure to ionizing radiation, exposure to chemicals called mutagens, or infection by viruses. Germ line mutations occur in the eggs and sperm and can be passed on to offspring, while somatic mutations occur in body cells and are not passed on.
Newborn Screening	Newborn screening is testing performed on newborn babies to detect a wide variety of disorders. Typically, testing is performed on a blood sample obtained from a heel prick when the baby is 2 or 3 days old. In the United States, newborn screening is mandatory for several different genetic disorders, though the exact set of required tests differs from state to state.
Pedigree	A pedigree is a genetic representation of a family tree that diagrams the inheritance of a trait or disease though several generations. The pedigree shows the relationships between family members and indicates which individuals express or silently carry the trait in question.
Phenotype	A phenotype is an individual's observable traits, such as height, eye color, and blood type. The genetic contribution to the phenotype is called the genotype. Some traits are largely determined by the genotype, while other traits are largely determined by environmental factors.
Polygenic Trait	A polygenic trait is one whose phenotype is influenced by more than one gene. Traits that display a continuous distribution, such as height or skin color, are polygenic. The inheritance of polygenic traits does not show the phenotypic ratios characteristic of Mendelian inheritance, though each of the genes contributing to the trait is inherited as described by Gregor Mendel. Many polygenic traits are also influenced by the environment and are called multifactorial.
Polymorphism	Polymorphism involves one of two or more variants of a particular DNA sequence. The most common type of polymorphism involves variation at a single base pair. Polymorphisms can also be much larger in size and involve long stretches of DNA.
Sex Linked	Sex linked is a trait in which a gene is located on a sex chromosome. In humans, the term generally refers to traits that are influenced by genes on the X chromosome. This is because the X chromosome is large and contains many more genes than the smaller Y chromosome. In a sex-linked disease, it is usually males who are affected because they have a single copy of X chromosome that carries the mutation. In females, the effect of the mutation may be masked by the second healthy copy of the X chromosome.
Single Nucleotide Polymorphisms (SNPs)	SNPs are a type of polymorphism involving variation of a single base pair. Scientists are studying how SNPs in the human genome correlate with disease, drug response, and other phenotypes.
Trait	A trait is a specific characteristic of an organism. Traits can be determined by genes or the environment, or more commonly by interactions between them. The genetic contribution to a trait is called the genotype. The outward expression of the genotype is called the phenotype.
X-Linked	X-linked is a trait where a gene is located on the X chromosome. Humans and other mammals have two sex chromosomes, the X and the Y. In an X-linked or sex linked disease, it is usually males that are affected because they have a single copy of the X chromosome that carries the mutation. In females, the effect of the mutation may be masked by the second healthy copy of the X chromosome.

Data from National Human Genome Research Institute. Glossary of genetic terms. https://www.genome.gov/glossary/index.cfm. Accessed December 10, 2017.

APPLYING EPIDEMIOLOGY TO EVALUATION AND POLICY

In Section II, we reviewed the major types of study designs used in epidemiology and examined how the results of epidemiologic studies are used to demonstrate associations and derive causal inferences. Although the methodologic issues discussed are interesting and intriguing, much of the excitement in epidemiology stems from the fact that epidemiologic results should have direct application to problems involving human health. The challenges include deriving valid inferences from the data generated by epidemiologic studies, ensuring appropriate and clear communication of the findings and their interpretations to policy makers and the general public, and dealing with ethical problems that arise because of the close link of epidemiology to human health and to clinical and public health policy.

This section discusses the use of epidemiology in evaluating both health services (Chapter 17) and programs for screening and early detection of disease (Chapter 18). These two chapters also address some of the methodologic and conceptual challenges that commonly arise in both. We then turn to some other issues involved in the application of epidemiology to the development of policy (Chapter 19), including the relationship of epidemiology to prevention, risk assessment, epidemiology in the courts, and the sources and impact of uncertainty.

In the final chapter, we address some of the major ethical and professional considerations that arise both in conducting epidemiologic investigations and in utilizing the results of epidemiologic studies to improve the health of the community. Epidemiologic studies are a major approach for enhancing the effectiveness of both clinical care and public health interventions. Some of the major issues in this chapter include investigators' obligations to study subjects, protecting privacy and confidentiality, race and ethnicity in epidemiologic studies, conflict of interest, and interpreting the findings of epidemiologic studies as they are applied to the processes of developing and improving health policy in different communities (Chapter 20).

Chapter 17

Using Epidemiology to Evaluate Health Services

Learning Objectives

- To distinguish measures of process from measures of outcome, and to discuss some commonly used measures of outcome in health services research.
- To define efficacy, effectiveness, and efficiency in the context of health services.
- To compare and contrast epidemiologic studies of disease etiology with epidemiologic studies evaluating health services.
- To discuss outcomes research in the context of ecologic data, and to present some potential biases in epidemiologic studies that emerge when evaluating health services using group-level data.
- To describe some possible study designs that can be used to evaluate health services using individual-level data, including randomized and nonrandomized designs.

Perhaps the earliest example of an evaluation is the description of creation given in the book of Genesis 1:1–4, which is shown in the original Hebrew in Fig. 17.1. Translated, with the addition of a few subheadings, it reads as follows:

BASELINE DATA
In the beginning God created the heaven and the earth. And the earth was unformed and void and darkness was on the face of the deep.

IMPLEMENTATION OF THE PROGRAM
And God said, "Let there be light." And there was light.

EVALUATION OF THE PROGRAM
And God saw the light, that it was good.

FURTHER PROGRAM ACTIVITIES
And God divided the light from the darkness.

This excerpt includes all of the basic components of the process of evaluation: baseline data, implementation of the program, evaluation of the program, and implementation of new program activities on the basis of the results of the evaluation. However, two problems arise in this description. First, we are not given the precise criteria that were used to determine whether or how the program was "good"; we are told only that God saw that it was good (which, in hindsight, may be sufficient). Second, this evaluation exemplifies a frequently observed problem: the program director is assessing his own program. Both conscious and subconscious biases can arise in evaluation. Furthermore, even if the program director administers the program superbly, he or she may not necessarily have the specific skills that are needed to conduct a methodologically rigorous evaluation of the program.

Dr. Wade Hampton Frost, a leader in epidemiology in the early part of the 20th century, addressed the use of epidemiology in the evaluation of public health programs in a presentation to the American Public Health Association in 1925.[1] He wrote, in part, as follows:

The health officer occupies the position of an agent to whom the public entrusts certain of its resources in public money and cooperation, to be so invested that they may yield the best returns in health; and in discharging the responsibilities of this position he is expected to follow the same general principles of procedure as would be a fiscal agent under like circumstances. …

Since his capital comes entirely from the public, it is reasonable to expect that he will be prepared to explain to the public his reasons for making each investment, and to give them some estimate of the returns which he expects. Nor can he consider it unreasonable if the public

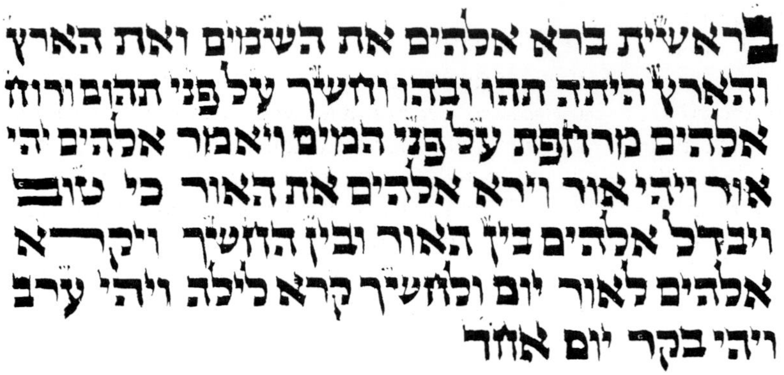

בְּרֵאשִׁית בָּרָא אֱלֹהִים אֵת הַשָּׁמַיִם וְאֵת הָאָרֶץ
וְהָאָרֶץ הָיְתָה תֹהוּ וָבֹהוּ וְחֹשֶׁךְ עַל פְּנֵי תְהוֹם וְרוּחַ
אֱלֹהִים מְרַחֶפֶת עַל פְּנֵי הַמָּיִם וַיֹּאמֶר אֱלֹהִים יְהִי
אוֹר וַיְהִי אוֹר וַיַּרְא אֱלֹהִים אֶת הָאוֹר כִּי טוֹב
וַיַּבְדֵּל אֱלֹהִים בֵּין הָאוֹר וּבֵין הַחֹשֶׁךְ וַיִּקְרָא
אֱלֹהִים לָאוֹר יוֹם וְלַחֹשֶׁךְ קָרָא לָיְלָה וַיְהִי עֶרֶב
וַיְהִי בֹקֶר יוֹם אֶחָד

Fig. 17.1 The earliest known evaluation (Genesis 1:1–4).

should wish to have an accounting from time to time, to know what returns are actually being received and how they check with the advance estimates which he has given them. Certainly any fiscal agent would expect to have his judgment thus checked and to gain or lose his clients' confidence in proportion as his estimates were verified or not.

However, as to such accounting, the health officer finds himself in a difficult and possibly embarrassing position, for while he may give a fairly exact statement of how much money and effort he has put into each of his several activities, he can rarely if ever give an equally exact or simple accounting of the returns from these investments considered separately and individually. This, to be sure, is not altogether his fault. It is due primarily to the character of the dividends from public health endeavor, and the manner in which they are distributed. They are not received in separate installments of a uniform currency, each docketed as to its source and recorded as received; but come irregularly from day to day, distributed to unidentified individuals throughout the community, who are not individually conscious of having received them. They are positive benefits in added life and improved health, but the only record ordinarily kept in morbidity and mortality statistics is the partial and negative record of death and of illness from certain clearly defined types of disease, chiefly the more acute communicable diseases, which constitute only a fraction of the total morbidity.[1]

Dr. Charles V. Chapin commented on Frost's presentation:

Dr. Frost's earnest demand that the procedures of preventive medicine be placed on a firm scientific basis is well timed. Indeed, it would have been opportune at any time during the past 40 years and, it is to be feared, will be equally needed for 40 years to come.[2]

Chapin clearly underestimated the number of years; the need remains as critical today, some 90+ years later, as it was in 1925.

Studies of Process and Outcome

Avedis Donabedian is widely regarded as the author of the seminal work on creating a framework of examining health services in relation to the quality of care. He identified three important factors simultaneously at play: (1) structure, (2) process, and (3) outcome. Structure relates to the physical locations where care is provided, the personnel, equipment, and financing. We will restrict our discussion here to the remaining two components, process and outcome.

STUDIES OF PROCESS

At the outset, we should distinguish between process and outcome studies. Process means that we decide what constitutes the components of good care, services, or preventive actions. Such a decision may first be made by an expert panel. We can then assess a clinic or health care provider, by reviewing relevant records or by direct observation, and determine to what extent the care provided meets established and accepted criteria. For example, in primary care we can determine what percentage of patients have had their blood pressure measured. The problem with such process measures is that they do not indicate whether the patient is better off; for example, monitoring blood pressure does not ensure that the patient's blood pressure is under control or that the patient will consistently take antihypertensive medications if they are prescribed. Second, because process assessments are often based on expert opinion, the criteria used in process evaluations may change over time as expert opinion changes. For example, in the 1940s, the accepted standard of care for premature infants required that such infants be placed in 100% oxygen. Incubators were monitored to be sure that such levels were maintained. However, when research demonstrated that high oxygen concentration played a major role in producing retrolental fibroplasia—a form of blindness in children who had been born prematurely—high concentrations of oxygen were subsequently deemed unacceptable.

STUDIES OF OUTCOME

Given the limitations of process studies, the remainder of this chapter focuses on outcome measures. *Outcome* denotes whether or not a patient (or a community at large) benefits from the medical care provided. Health outcomes are frequently considered the domain of epidemiology. Although such measures have traditionally been mortality and morbidity, interest in outcomes research in recent years has expanded the measures of interest to include patient satisfaction, quality of life, degree of dependence and disability, and similar measures.

Efficacy, Effectiveness, and Efficiency

Three terms that are often encountered in the literature dealing with evaluation of health services are *efficacy*, *effectiveness*, and *efficiency*. These terms are often used in association with the findings from randomized trials.

EFFICACY

Does the agent or intervention "work" under ideal "laboratory" conditions? We test a new drug in a group of patients who have agreed to be hospitalized and who are observed as they take their therapy. Or a vaccine is tested in a group of consenting subjects. Thus, efficacy is a measure in a situation in which all conditions are controlled to maximize the effect of the agent. Generally, "ideal" conditions are those that occur in testing a new agent of intervention using a randomized trial.

EFFECTIVENESS

If we administer the agent in a "real-life" situation, is it effective? For example, when a vaccine is tested in a community, many individuals may not come in to be vaccinated. Or, an oral medication may have such an undesirable taste that no one will take it (so that it will prove ineffective), despite the fact that under controlled conditions, when compliance was ensured, the drug was shown to be efficacious.

EFFICIENCY

If an agent is shown to be effective, what is the cost–benefit ratio? Is it possible to achieve our goals in a less expensive and better way? Cost includes not only money, but also discomfort, pain, absenteeism, disability, and social stigma.

If a health care measure has not been demonstrated to be effective, there is little point looking at efficiency, for if it is not effective, the least expensive alternative is not to use it at all. At times, of course, political and societal pressures may drive a program even if it is not effective (an often-cited example is DARE—Drug Abuse Resistance Education, which has never been shown to have an impact on adolescent and young adult drug use). However, this chapter will focus only on the science of evaluation and specifically on the issue of effectiveness in evaluating health services.

Measures of Outcome

If efficacy of a measure has been demonstrated—that is, if the methods of prevention and intervention that are of interest have been shown to work—we can then turn to evaluating effectiveness. What guidelines should we use in selecting an appropriate outcome measure to serve as an index of effectiveness? First, the measure must be clearly *quantifiable*; that is, we must be able to express its effect in quantitative terms. Second, the measure of outcome should be relatively *easy to define and diagnose*. If the measure is to be used in a population study, we would certainly not want to depend on an invasive procedure for assessing any benefits. Third, the measure selected should lend itself to *standardization* for study purposes. Fourth, the population served (and the comparison population) must be *at risk* for the same condition for which an intervention is being evaluated. For example, it would obviously make little sense to test the effectiveness of a sickle cell screening program in a white population in North America (as sickle cell disease primarily affects African Americans).

The type of health outcome end point that we select clearly should depend on the question that we are asking. Although this may seem self-evident, it is not always immediately apparent. Box 17.1 shows possible end points in evaluating the effectiveness of a vaccine program. Whatever outcome we select should be explicitly stated so that others reading the report of our findings will be able to make their own judgments regarding the appropriateness of the measure selected and the quality of the data. Whether the measure we have selected is indeed an appropriate one depends on clinical and public health aspects of the disease or health condition in question.

Box 17.2 shows possible choices of measures for assessing the effectiveness of a throat culture program in children. Measures of volume of services provided, numbers of cultures taken, and number of clinic visits have been traditionally used because they are relatively easy to count and are helpful in justifying requests for budgetary increases for the program in the following year. However, such measures are all process measures and tell us nothing about the effectiveness of an intervention. We therefore move to other possibilities listed in this box. Again, the most appropriate measures should depend on the question being asked. The question must be specific. It is not enough just to ask how good the program is.

Comparing Epidemiologic Studies of Disease Etiology and Epidemiologic Research Evaluating Effectiveness of Health Services

In classic epidemiologic studies of disease etiology, we examine the possible relationship between a putative cause (the independent variable or "exposure") and an adverse health effect or effects (the dependent variable or "outcome"). In doing so, we take into account other factors, including health care, that may modify the relationship or confound it (Fig. 17.2A). In health services research, we focus on the health service as the independent variable (the "exposure"), with a reduction in adverse health effects as the anticipated outcome (dependent variable) if the modality of care is effective. In this situation, environmental and other factors that may influence the relationship are also taken into account (see Fig. 17.2B). Thus, both etiologic epidemiologic research and health services research address the possible relationship between an independent variable and a dependent variable, and the influence of other factors on the relationship. Therefore, it is not surprising that many of the study designs discussed are common to both epidemiologic and health services research, as are the methodologic problems and potential biases that may characterize these types of studies.

BOX 17.1 SOME POSSIBLE END POINTS FOR MEASURING THE SUCCESS OF A VACCINE PROGRAM

1. Number (or proportion) of people immunized
2. Number (or proportion) of people at (high) risk who are immunized
3. Number (or proportion) of people immunized who show serologic response
4. Number (or proportion) of people immunized and later exposed in whom clinical disease does not develop
5. Number (or proportion) of people immunized and later exposed in whom clinical or subclinical disease does not develop

BOX 17.2 SOME POSSIBLE END POINTS FOR MEASURING SUCCESS OF A THROAT CULTURE PROGRAM

1. Number of cultures taken (symptomatic or asymptomatic)
2. Number (or proportion) of cultures positive for streptococcal infection
3. Number (or proportion) of persons with positive cultures for whom medical care is obtained
4. Number (or proportion) of persons with positive cultures for whom proper treatment is prescribed and taken
5. Number (or proportion) of positive cultures followed by a relapse
6. Number (or proportion) of positive cultures followed by rheumatic fever

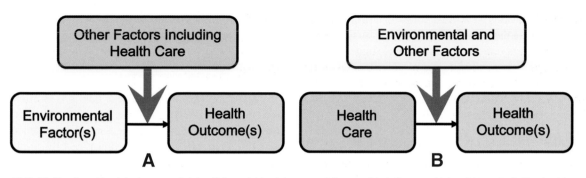

Fig. 17.2 (A) Classic epidemiologic research into etiology, taking into account the possible influence of other factors, including health care. (B) Classic health services research into effectiveness, taking into account the possible influence of environmental and other factors.

Evaluation Using Group Data

Regularly available data, such as mortality data and hospitalization data, are often used in evaluation studies. Such data can be obtained from different sources, and such sources may differ in important ways. For example, Fig. 17.3 shows the changes in the estimated proportion of the US population with influenza-like illness (ILI) over time—*trends*—using three different data sources: sentinel surveillance sites overseen by the Centers for Disease Control and Prevention (CDC), Google Flu Trends, and Flu Near You.[3]

Although the trends are fairly similar in this time period, we can see that Google Flu Trends estimated a higher proportion of the US population with ILI toward the end of 2012, nearly twice as high as the CDC estimates. This is potentially attributed to the varying methodology of data collection of each data source. The CDC generates its data from over 2,700 health care centers that capture over 30 million patient visits each year. Google Flu Trends uses data mining and modeling methodology generated from the flu-related search terms entered in Google's search engine. Flu Near You uses data entered by internet users volunteering information, not necessarily physicians, to report on a weekly basis whether they, or their family members, have ILI symptoms. It is possible that not all individuals who develop ILI symptoms will seek medical care, and hence are not captured by the CDC data, but they may perform a Google search for ways to alleviate ILI symptoms, for example. Since Flu Near You solely depends on voluntary self-report of ILI symptoms it might well underestimate prevalence. In

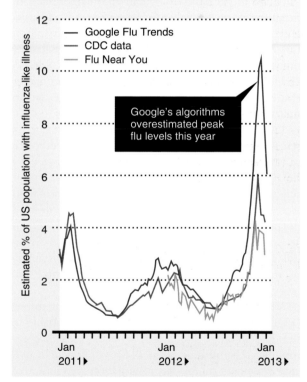

Fig. 17.3 Estimated proportion of US population with influenza-like illness January 2011–13. *CDC,* Centers for Disease Control and Prevention. (From Butler D. When Google got flu wrong. *Nature.* 2013;494:155–156.)

a recent flu season, New York State Governor Andrew M. Cuomo declared a Public Health Emergency in response to a severe flu season. It was suggested that this might have prompted numerous searches on Google by individuals who are not actually suffering from ILI symptoms, which in turn could have triggered the spike that we see in the figure.

OUTCOMES RESEARCH

The term *outcomes research* has been increasingly used to denote studies comparing the effects of two or more health care interventions or modalities—such as treatments, forms of health care organization, or type and extent of insurance coverage and provider reimbursement—on health or economic outcomes. The health end points may include morbidity and mortality as well as measures of quality of life, functional status, and patient perceptions of their health status, including symptom recognition and patient-reported satisfaction. Economic measures may reflect direct or indirect costs, and can include hospitalization rates, rehospitalization for the same condition within 30 days of discharge, outpatient and emergency room visits, lost days of work, child care, and days of restricted activity. Consequently, epidemiology is one of several disciplines needed in outcomes research.

Outcomes research often uses data from large data sets that were derived from large populations. Although in recent years some of the large data sets have been developed from cohorts that were originally set up for different research purposes, many of the data sets used were often originally initiated for administrative or fiscal purposes, rather than for any research goals. Often several large data sets, each having information on different variables, may be combined or linked (resulting in "meta-data") in order to have sufficient sample size to explore a question of interest.

With the advent of the electronic medical record (EMR), patient care data are increasingly available to the epidemiology and health services research communities. The purpose of the EMR is to provide health care providers all of the information pertaining to individual patients—findings from office visits, utilization of preventive services, prescribed medications, procedures, radiologic findings, laboratory test results—continuously over time (i.e., prospectively). However, the purpose of the EMR is not to serve as a research base but to direct patient care. Harnessing the EMR to evaluate health services research questions has great promise, but to date it has proven difficult to use and the methods to maximize its potential are still being developed and tested in the field.

The advantages of using large data sets (sometimes referred to as "big data") are that the data refer to real-world populations, and the issue of "representativeness" or "generalizability" is minimized. In addition, since the data sets exist at the time the research is initiated, analysis can generally be completed and results generated relatively rapidly. Moreover, given the large data sets used, sample size is not usually a problem except when smaller subgroups are examined. Given these considerations, the costs of using existing data sets are generally lower than the costs of primary data collection.

The disadvantages are that, since the data were often initially gathered for fiscal patient care and administrative purposes, they may not be well suited for research purposes and for answering the specific research question addressed in the study. Even when the data were originally gathered for research, our knowledge of the area may now be more complete and new research questions may have arisen that were not even conceived of when the original data collection was initiated. In general, data may be incomplete. Data on the independent and dependent variables may be very limited. Data may be missing on clinical details including disease severity and on the details of interventions, and diagnostic coding may be inconsistent across facilities and within facilities over time. Data relating to possible confounders may be inadequate or absent since the research now being conducted was often not even possible when the data were originally generated. Because certain variables that today are considered relevant and important were not included in the original data set, investigators may at times create surrogate variables for the missing variables, using certain variables that are included in the data set but that may not directly reflect the variable of interest. However, such surrogate variables vary in the extent to which they are an adequate measure of the missing variable of interest. For all these reasons, the validity of the conclusions reached may therefore be in doubt.

Another important problem that may arise with large data sets is that because the necessary variables may be absent in the available data set, the investigator may consciously or subconsciously change from the question he or she had originally wanted to address to a question that is of less interest, but for which the variables that are needed for conducting the study are present in the data set. Thus, rather than the investigator deciding what research question should be addressed, the data set itself may end up determining what questions are asked in the study.

Finally, using large data sets, investigators become progressively more removed from the individuals being studied. Over the years, direct interviews and reviews of patient records have tended to be replaced by large computerized databases. Using these sources of data, many personal characteristics of the subjects are never explored and their relevance to the questions being asked is virtually never assessed.

One area in which existing sources of data are often used in evaluation studies is prenatal care. The problems discussed earlier are exemplified in the use of birth certificates. These documents are often used because they are easily accessible and provide certain medical care data, such as the trimester in which prenatal care was begun. However, birth certificates for women with high-risk pregnancies have missing data more often than those for women with low-risk pregnancies. The quality of the data provided on birth certificates also may differ regionally and internationally, and may complicate any comparisons that are made.

An example of outcomes research using large data sets is a study by Ikuta et al. of Medicare beneficiaries in the United States.[4] Since Medicare health coverage is provided to virtually all elderly (ages 65 years and older) individuals in the United States, it is assumed that if a study population is limited to those who have Medicare coverage, financial obstacles to care and other variables such as age, gender, or racial/ethnic subpopulations are held constant among different groups. However, wide disparities still remain between blacks and whites in utilizing many Medicare services. The authors studied the national trends in the use of pulmonary artery catheterization (PAC) among Medicare beneficiaries during the period 1999–2013.[4] PAC is a procedure by which a tube is inserted in one of the large veins in the body, and then threaded through the heart to be ultimately placed in the pulmonary artery. This procedure used to be indicated as part of routine management

of heart failure and sepsis-related acute respiratory distress syndrome, among many others. However, given the rising evidence that PAC did not improve patient outcomes, the clinical practice guidelines of the American College of Cardiology and the Society of Critical Care Medicine now recommends *against* the routine use of PAC. The authors studied inpatient claims data from the Centers for Medicare and Medicaid Services from 1999 to 2013 and estimated the rate of use of a PAC per 1,000 admissions, 30-day mortality, and length of stay. They found a statistically significant 67.8% relative reduction in PAC use (6.28 per 1,000 admissions in 1999 to 2.02 per 1,000 admissions in 2013), in addition to year-to-year reductions in in-hospital mortality, 30-day mortality, and length of stay. However, the findings also showed that such rates varied substantially by gender (Fig. 17.4), race (Fig. 17.5), and age (Fig. 17.6). These results showed the added benefits in restricting the use of PAC in some patients. In the meantime, the authors admitted the limitations in the use of administrative data sets and the inability to generalize to younger and uninsured individuals.

POTENTIAL BIASES IN EVALUATING HEALTH SERVICES USING GROUP DATA

Studies evaluating health services using group data are susceptible to many of the biases that characterize etiologic studies, as discussed in Chapter 15. In addition,

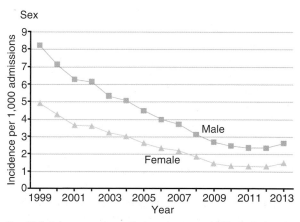

Fig. 17.4 Pulmonary artery catheter use rate per 1,000 admissions by gender between 1999 and 2013. (Modified from Ikuta K, Wang Y, Robinson A, et al. National trends in use and outcomes of pulmonary artery catheters among medicare beneficiaries, 1999–2013. *JAMA Cardiol.* 2017;2:908–913.)

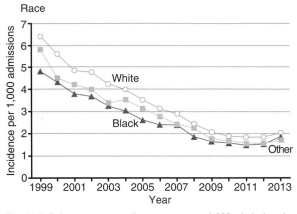

Fig. 17.5 Pulmonary artery catheter use rate per 1,000 admissions by race between 1999 and 2013. (Modified from Ikuta K, Wang Y, Robinson A, et al. National trends in use and outcomes of pulmonary artery catheters among medicare beneficiaries, 1999–2013. *JAMA Cardiol.* 2017;2:908–913.)

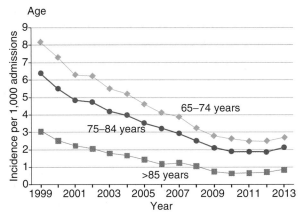

Fig. 17.6 Pulmonary artery catheter use rate per 1,000 admissions by age groups between 1999 and 2013. (Modified from Ikuta K, Wang Y, Robinson A, et al. National trends in use and outcomes of pulmonary artery catheters among medicare beneficiaries, 1999–2013. *JAMA Cardiol.* 2017;2:908–913.)

certain biases are particularly relevant for specific research areas and topics, and may be important depending on the specific epidemiologic design selected. For example, studies of the relationship of prenatal care to birth outcomes are prone to several important potential biases. In such studies, the question often addressed is whether prenatal care, as measured by the absolute number of prenatal visits, reduces the risk of prematurity and low birth weight. Several potential biases may be introduced into this type of analysis. For example, other things being equal, a woman who

delivers prematurely will have fewer prenatal visits (i.e., the pregnancy was shorter so that there was less time in which it was possible for her to "be at risk" for prenatal visits). The result would be an artefactual relationship between fewer prenatal visits and prematurity, only because the gestation was shorter. However, bias can also operate in the other direction. A woman who begins prenatal care in the last trimester of pregnancy will likely not have an early premature delivery, as she has already carried the pregnancy into the last trimester. This would lead to an observed association of fewer prenatal visits with a reduced likelihood of early premature delivery. In addition, women who have had medical complications or a poor pregnancy outcome in a prior pregnancy may be so anxious that they come for more prenatal visits (where problems with the fetus may be detected early), and they may also be at greater risk for a poor outcome. Thus, the potential biases can run in one or both directions. If such women are at a risk that is not amenable to prevention, an apparent association of more prenatal visits with an adverse outcome may be observed.

Finally, prenatal outcome studies based on prenatal care are often biased by self-selection; that is, the women who choose to begin prenatal care early in pregnancy are often better educated and from a higher socioeconomic status with more positive attitudes toward health care. Thus, a population of women, who to begin with are at lower risk for adverse birth outcomes, select themselves for earlier prenatal care. The result is a potential for an apparent association of early prenatal care with lower risk of adverse pregnancy outcome, even if the care itself is without any true health benefit.

TWO INDICES USED IN ECOLOGIC STUDIES OF HEALTH SERVICES

One index in evaluating health services that uses ecologic studies is avoidable mortality. *Avoidable mortality* analyses assume that the rate of "avoidable deaths" should vary inversely with the availability, accessibility, and quality of medical care in different geographic regions. The UK Office for National Statistics defines avoidable mortality as:

Avoidable deaths are all those defined as preventable, amenable, or both, where each death is counted only once. Where a cause of death falls within both the preventable and amenable definition, all deaths from that cause are counted in both categories when they are presented separately.[5]

Conditions include tuberculosis, hepatitis C, human immunodeficiency virus/acquired immunodeficiency syndrome (HIV/AIDS), selected malignant neoplasms, substance use disorders, cardiovascular and respiratory diseases, unintentional and intentional injuries, among others.

Ideally, avoidable mortality would serve as a measure of the accessibility, adequacy, and effectiveness of care in an area. Deaths from HIV/AIDS will be less frequent in communities with ample, friendly, and convenient HIV testing and counseling and high-quality AIDS service organizations, often found in urban areas. In rural areas, such services may be less accessible, and diagnoses may only be made when a patient presents with an AIDS-defining illness. Thus, patients are more likely to have a higher mortality rate in areas with poorer service coverage, which they would not have experienced had they lived in an urban environment. Changes over time could be plotted and comparisons made with other areas. Unfortunately, the necessary data for such an analysis are often lacking for many of the conditions suggested for avoidable mortality analyses. Moreover, data on confounders may not be available and the resulting inferences may therefore be open to question.

A second approach is to use *health indicators*. With this approach, certain sentinel conditions are assumed to reflect the general level of health care, and changes in the incidence of these conditions are plotted over time and compared with data for other populations. The changes and differences that are found are then related to changes in the health service sector and are used to derive inferences about causation. However, it is difficult to know which criteria need to be met in order for a given condition to be acceptable as a valid health indicator. A systematic process should be followed to allow the identification and implementation of a valid health indicator. Each indicator should have the following attributes: valid, reliable, relevant, realistic, measurable, well known, can be used in continuous assessment, and can effectively measure success and failure. The first phase of developing an indicator is usually through the identification of a proposed list of indicators by group of experts in the area, followed by shortlisting the list to the indicators that fulfill most

or all the attributes outlined above. The second phase includes pilot testing, which is primarily targeted to test the availability of the data and to estimate the time, effort, and finances to collect information of this indicator. The third phase of development is the full testing of the indicators on a larger scale and tuning the indicator based on feedback from health care personnel on the use of these indicators. The fourth and final phase is the full implementation of the mature indicators. At this stage, there should be a mandate for reporting the indicators and having systems in place for data collection, tabulation, analysis, and interpretation, coupled with a feedback mechanism to the intermediate and peripheral levels of the health care system.

The CDC maintains 26 Leading Health Indicators (LHIs) under 12 topics. The Healthy People 2020 LHIs are given in Box 17.3 and can be accessed on their website (healthypeople.gov). As mentioned earlier, avoidable deaths are all those defined as preventable, amenable, or both, where each death is counted only once. Where a cause of death falls within both the preventable and amenable definition, all deaths from that cause are counted in both categories when they are presented separately.

Evaluation Using Individual Data

Because of the limitations inherent in analyzing studies using grouped data (i.e., studies in which we do not have data on both health care [exposure] and particular health outcomes at the individual level), studies using individual data are generally preferable. If we wish to compare two populations, one receiving the care being evaluated (perhaps a new treatment) and one not receiving it (patients who are given "usual care"), we must ask the following two questions in order to be able to derive inferences about the effectiveness of care:

1. Are the characteristics of the two groups comparable—demographically, medically, and in terms of factors relating to prognosis?
2. Are the measurement methods comparable (e.g., diagnostic methods and the way disease is classified) in both groups?

Both issues have been discussed in earlier chapters because they also apply equally well to questions of etiology, prevention, and therapy, and they must therefore be considered in any type of study design.

BOX 17.3 THE HEALTHY PEOPLE 2020 LEADING HEALTH INDICATORS ARE COMPOSED OF 26 INDICATORS ORGANIZED UNDER 12 TOPICS

ACCESS TO HEALTH SERVICES
- Persons with medical insurance (AHS-1.1)
- Persons with a usual primary care provider (AHS-3)

CLINICAL PREVENTIVE SERVICES
- Adults receiving colorectal cancer screening based on the most recent guidelines (C-16)
- Adults with hypertension whose blood pressure is under control (HDS-12)
- Persons with diagnosed diabetes whose A1c value is greater than 9% (D-5.1)
- Children receiving the recommended doses of DTaP, polio, MMR, Hib, HepB, varicella, and PCV vaccines by age 19–35 months (IID-8)

ENVIRONMENTAL QUALITY
- Air Quality Index >100 (EH-1)
- Children exposed to secondhand smoke (TU-11.1)

INJURY AND VIOLENCE
- Injury deaths (IVP-1.1)
- Homicides (IVP-29)

MATERNAL, INFANT, AND CHILD HEALTH
- All infant deaths (MICH-1.3)
- Total preterm live births (MICH-9.1)

MENTAL HEALTH
- Suicide (MHMD-1)
- Adolescents with a major depressive episode in the past 12 months (MHMD-4.1)

NUTRITION, PHYSICAL ACTIVITY, AND OBESITY
- Adults meeting aerobic physical activity and muscle-strengthening objectives (PA-2.4)
- Obesity among adults (NWS-9)
- Obesity among children and adolescents (NWS-10.4)
- Mean daily intake of total vegetables (NWS-15.1)

ORAL HEALTH
- Children, adolescents, and adults who visited the dentist in the past year (OH-7)

REPRODUCTIVE AND SEXUAL HEALTH
- Sexually active females receiving reproductive health services (FP-7.1)
- Knowledge of serostatus among HIV-positive persons (HIV-13)

SOCIAL DETERMINANTS
- Students graduating from high school 4 years after starting ninth grade (AH-5.1)

SUBSTANCE ABUSE
- Adolescents using alcohol or illicit drugs in past 30 days (SA-13.1)
- Binge drinking in past month—adults (SA-14.3)

TOBACCO
- Adult cigarette smoking (TU-1.1)
- Adolescent cigarette smoking in past 30 days (TU-2.2)

An important issue in using epidemiology to study outcomes for the evaluation of health services is the need to address prognostic stratification. If a change in health outcome is observed after a certain type of care has been delivered, can we necessarily conclude that the change is due to the (new) health care provided, or could it be a result of differences in prognosis based on comorbidity—preexisting disease that may or may not be specifically related to the disease being studied, in severity, or in any other associated conditions that bear on prognosis? To address these issues, medical outcome studies must carry out a prognostic stratification by studying case mix and carefully characterizing the individuals studied on the basis of disease severity.

Let us now turn to some *study designs* used in the evaluation of health services.

RANDOMIZED DESIGNS

Randomization eliminates the problem of selection bias that results from either self-selection by the patient or selection of the patient by the health care provider. Usually, study participants are assigned to receive one type of care versus another rather than to receive care versus no care (Fig. 17.7). For many reasons, both ethical and practical, randomizing patients to receive no care usually is not considered.

Let us consider a study that used a randomized design to evaluate different approaches to health care for elderly patients who have had a stroke. Early, organized, hospital-based management has been strongly recommended for the care of patients with stroke. However, few data are available from well-conducted controlled studies to compare hospital care with specialized care at home (domiciliary care). An alternative

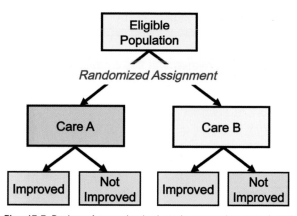

Fig. 17.7 Design of a randomized study comparing care A and care B.

to stroke units in the hospital is a specialized stroke team that can provide care anywhere in the hospital where stroke patients may be treated. It may not be possible for every hospital to offer care in a specialized unit to all patients who have a stroke because of space limitations and other administrative and financial issues, hence the formation of a "roaming" stroke team.

To identify the optimal organizational structure for the care of patients with stroke, Kalra and colleagues[7] conducted a randomized, controlled trial to compare the efficacy of three forms of care (Fig. 17.8). Patients were randomly assigned to one of the following groups: (1) care provided in a hospital stroke unit by a stroke physician and a multidisciplinary team; (2) care provided by a multidisciplinary stroke team with expertise in stroke management; or (3) care at home (domiciliary care) provided by a specialist team. The outcome was mortality or institutionalization, which was assessed at 3, 6, and 12 months after the onset of a stroke. Data were analyzed by intention-to-treat. At each of the three time points, patients treated in the hospital stroke unit were less likely to die or to be institutionalized than patients in the group treated by the stroke team or the group receiving domiciliary care. Cumulative survival in the three groups is shown in Fig. 17.9. The study supports the use of specialized stroke units for the care of patients with stroke.

As seen in Fig. 17.9, an interesting and somewhat surprising finding in this study is that survival was better in patients who were randomized to receive

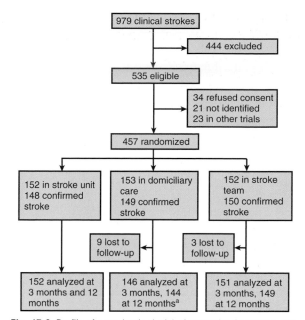

Fig. 17.8 Profile of a randomized trial of strategies for stroke care. [a]Fifty-one patients in this group were admitted to the hospital within 2 weeks of randomization, but are included in the intention-to-treat analysis. (Modified from Kalra L, Evans A, Perez I, et al. Alternative strategies for stroke care: a prospective randomized controlled trial. *Lancet.* 2000;356:894–899.)

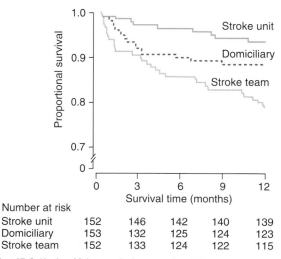

Fig. 17.9 Kaplan–Meier survival curves for different strategies of care after acute stroke. (From Kalra L, Evans A, Perez I, et al. Alternative strategies for stroke care: a prospective randomized controlled trial. *Lancet.* 2000;356:894–899.)

domiciliary care (care at home) than in those randomized to receive care in the hospital by a stroke team.

A possible explanation for this observation is that patients in the domiciliary care group whose condition deteriorated or who had developed new problems were withdrawn from domiciliary care and admitted to a stroke unit. These patients were still analyzed with the domiciliary care group because an intention-to-treat analysis was used that analyzes outcome according to the original randomization. These patients may have benefited from care in the stroke unit, and if so, their outcome would tend to improve the outcome results for the domiciliary care group because of the intention-to-treat analysis.

Drummond and colleagues[8] conducted a 10-year follow-up of a randomized, controlled trial of care in a stroke rehabilitation unit. They found that management in a stroke rehabilitation unit conferred survival benefits even 10 years after the stroke. The exact reasons are not clear, but the authors suggest that one explanation may be that long-term survival is related to early reduction in disability.

NONRANDOMIZED DESIGNS

Many health care interventions cannot be subjected to randomized trials for several reasons. First, such trials are often logistically complex and extremely expensive. Because so many different health care measures are in use at any one time, it may not be feasible to subject all of them to randomized evaluations. Second, ethical problems may be perceived to occur in health services evaluation studies. Specifically, randomization may be viewed as an unacceptable process by many patients and by their health care providers. Third, randomized trials often take a long time to complete; because health care programs and health problems change over time, when the results of the study are finally obtained and analyzed, they may no longer be entirely relevant. For these reasons, many health care researchers look for alternative approaches that may at least yield some information. One such approach discussed above—*outcomes research*—generally refers to the use of data from nonrandomized studies that often use large existing data sets (or so-called "big data").

Before–After Design (Historical Controls)

If randomization is not possible or will not be used for any reason, one possible study design to evaluate a program is to compare people who received care before a program was established (or before the health care measure became available) with those who received care from the program after it was established (or after the measure became available). What are the problems with the *before–after* design? First, the data obtained in each of the two periods are frequently not comparable in terms of either quality or completeness. When a new form of health service delivery is developed, evaluators of the program may want to include people who were treated in the past, before the program began, as a comparison group. The data on people treated after the new program begins may be collected using a well-designed research instrument, whereas data for past patients may include only that which may be available from health care records that had been designed and used only for clinical or administrative purposes. If we find a difference in outcome, we may not know if the observed difference is a result of the effect of the program or of differences in the quality of data from the two time periods.

Second, if we see a difference—for example, mortality is lower after a program was initiated than before the program was initiated—we do not know whether the difference is due to the program itself or to other factors that may have changed over time, such as housing, nutrition, other aspects of lifestyle, or the use of other health services.

Third, a problem of selection exists. Often, it is difficult to know whether the population studied after a program was established is actually similar to that seen before the program was established in terms of other factors that might affect outcome.

Does this mean that *before–after* studies have no value? No, it does not. But it does mean that such studies can only provide a suggestion—and are rarely conclusive—in demonstrating the effectiveness of a new health service.

A *before–after* design was used in a study to assess the impact of the Medicare prospective payment system (PPS) in the United States on quality of care.[9] The study was stimulated by concern that the PPS, with its closely regulated length of hospital stays and incentives for cost-cutting, might have adversely affected the quality of care. The *before–after* design was selected because the PPS was instituted nationwide, so a prospective cohort design could not be used. Data for almost 17,000 Medicare patients who were hospitalized in 1981–82 before the PPS was instituted were compared with data for patients hospitalized in 1985–86 after the PPS was in place. Quality of care was evaluated for five diseases: (1) congestive heart failure, (2) myocardial infarction, (3) pneumonia, (4) cerebrovascular accident, and (5) hip fractures. Outcome findings were adjusted for level of patient sickness on admission to the hospital. Although PPS was not found to be associated with an increase in either 30-day mortality or 6-month mortality, an increase was observed in instability at discharge (defined as the presence of conditions at discharge that clinicians agree should be corrected before discharge or monitored after discharge, and that may result in poor outcomes if not corrected).[10] The authors point out that other factors may also have changed during the time before and after institution of the PPS. Although the *before–after* design was probably the only design possible for the issue addressed in this study, the study is nevertheless susceptible to some of the problems of this type of design, which were discussed earlier.

When the change in the risk of the outcome is dramatic, the *before–after* design is akin to the so-called *natural experiment* (see Chapter 14, section titled "Approaches to Etiology in Human Populations"). It would, for example, be difficult to explain the marked decline in the rates of hospitalization for diabetes and meningitis by reasons other than the introduction of insulin and streptomycin, respectively.

Simultaneous Nonrandomized Design (Program–No Program)

One option to avoid the problems of changes that occur over calendar time is to conduct a simultaneous comparison of two populations that are not randomized, in which one population is served by the program and the other is not. This type of design is, in effect, a cohort study in which the type of health care being studied represents the "exposure." As in any cohort study, the problem arises as to how to select exposed and unexposed groups for study.

In recent years considerable interest has focused on whether higher hospital volume and higher surgeon volume relate to better patient outcomes and costs, and many studies have been carried out on these issues. An example of a simultaneous, nonrandomized study of hospital volume is one reported by Wallenstein and colleagues.[11] This study explored whether differences in patient outcomes in different hospitals related to the volume of hospital procedures performed. The authors studied hospitalizations of patients who underwent laparoscopic hysterectomy, the most common (600,000 surgeries annually) major gynecologic procedure in the United States. They examined the relationship of in-hospital complications (intraoperative, surgical site, and medical) as well as length of stay and cost during the index hospitalization to the volume of surgeries performed by physicians and overall in the hospital.[11] As seen in Table 17.1, a dose-response relationship was found: the highest in-hospital complications, length of stay, and costs occurred in hospitals that had the lowest volume of hysterectomies per year. The finding that hospitals that perform more hysterectomies have lower lengths of stay and costs has important potential policy implications and argues for the regionalization of gynecologic surgical services.

TABLE 17.1 Association Between Hospital Volume of Laparoscopic Hysterectomies Performed Per Year and Morbidity, Mortality, and Resource Utilization

	NUMBER OF PROCEDURES		
	<49.4/year	46.4–105/year	>105/year
Any complication (%)	5.8	5.0	4.7
Intraoperative complications (%)	2.4	2.2	2.1
Surgical site complications (%)	2.6	2.3	1.8
Medical complications (%)	1.4	1.1	1.2
Length of stay longer than 2 days (%)	10.0	7.8	5.3
Cost (dollars)	$6,527.00	$5,809.00	$5,561.00
Death (%)	0.02	0.01	0.01

Modified from Wallenstein ME, Ananth CV, Kim JH, et al. Effect of surgical volume on outcomes for laparoscopic hysterectomy for benign indications. *Obstet Gynecol.* 2012;119:709–716.

It is possible that the findings relating higher hospital volumes to better patient outcomes might be due to higher volumes of procedures performed by the surgeons at these hospitals rather than to the overall volumes of procedures performed at these hospitals. Birkmeyer and colleagues addressed this issue.[12] Using Medicare claims data for 1998 and 1999, they examined mortality among all 474,108 patients who underwent one of four cardiovascular procedures or four cancer resection procedures (Fig. 17.10). They found that for most procedures the mortality rate was higher in patients operated on by low-volume surgeons than in patients operated on by high-volume surgeons. This relationship held regardless of the surgical volume of the hospital in which the surgery was performed.

Comparison of Utilizers and Nonutilizers

One approach for a simultaneous, nonrandomized study is to compare a group of people who use a health service with a group of people who do not (Fig. 17.11).

The problem of self-selection inherent in this type of design has long been recognized. Haruyama and

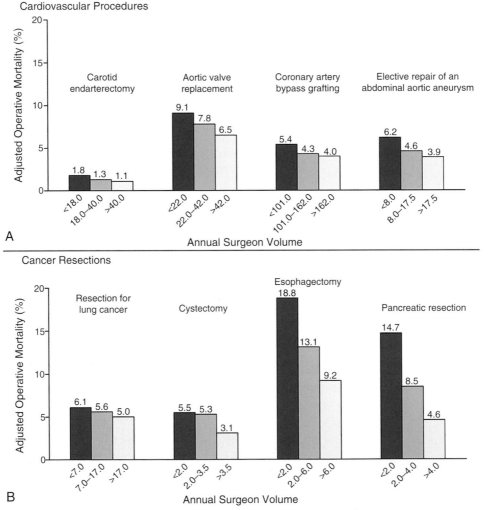

Fig. 17.10 Adjusted operative mortality among Medicare patients in 1998 and 1999 according to level of surgeon volume for four cardiovascular procedures (A) and four cancer resection procedures (B). Operative mortality was defined as the rate of death before hospital discharge or within 30 days after the index procedure. Surgeon volume was based on the total number of procedures performed. (From Birkmeyer JD, Stukel TA, Siewers AE, et al. Surgeon volume and operative mortality in the United States. *N Engl J Med.* 2003;349:2117–2127.)

colleagues studied the association between the personal utilization of general health checkups (GHCs) and medical expenditures (MEs) in a middle-aged Japanese population (Table 17.2).[13]

In this study, the authors recruited 33,417 residents of Soka City, Saitama Prefecture, Japan, and studied their GHC utilization from 2008 to 2010. The utilization of GHCs was divided into zero times (nonutilizers), one to three times (low-frequency utilizers), and four to six times (high-frequency utilizers). Compared with the nonutilizers, the high-frequency utilizers showed statistically significantly higher outpatient MEs. In addition, the low- and high-frequency utilizers showed statistically significantly lower inpatient MEs and total MEs than the nonutilizers. The authors concluded that outpatient MEs increased with the frequency of GHC attendance, and the early diagnosis facilitated by early outpatient consultation is more likely to lead to a slight increase in outpatient MEs but a decrease in inpatient MEs for serious diseases, resulting in a decrease in the total cost of health care.

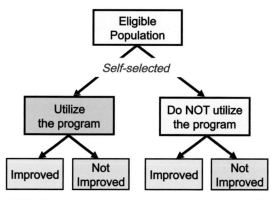

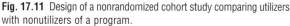

Fig. 17.11 Design of a nonrandomized cohort study comparing utilizers with nonutilizers of a program.

Another example of differences between characteristics of groups under comparison is given by a study conducted by Gierisch et al. on nonadherence to breast cancer screening with periodic mammographic examinations.[14] In this study, the nonadherent women were more likely than adherent women to be aged 40 to 49, and to have fair or poor self-rated health as well as difficulty in getting mammograms. As these variables are related to breast cancer (and all-cause mortality), they must be taken into consideration when using a nonrandomized design to examine the effectiveness of breast cancer screening.

Although we can try to address the selection problem by characterizing the prognostic profile of those who use care and those who do not, so long as the groups are not randomized, we are left with a gnawing uncertainty as to whether some factors were not identified in the study that might have differentiated utilizers and nonutilizers and, therefore, affected the health outcome.

Comparison of Eligible and Ineligible Populations

Because of the problem of possible selection biases in comparing groups of utilizers with nonutilizers, another approach compares persons who are eligible for the care being evaluated with a group of persons who are not eligible (Fig. 17.12).

The assumption being made here is that eligibility or noneligibility is not related to either prognosis or outcome; therefore no selection bias is being introduced that might affect the inferences from the study. For example, eligibility criteria may include the type of employer or the census tract of residence. However, even with this design, one must be on the alert for factors that may introduce selection bias. For example, clearly, census tract of residence may relate to socioeconomic status. The issue of finding an appropriate

TABLE 17.2 Odds Ratio (and 95% Confidence Intervals) of Any Medical Consultation (Defined as Seeing a Doctor in a Period of 1 Year) According to Subgroups of General Health Checkup Utilization in Middle-Aged Japanese Population, 2010			
	Nonutilizers	**Low-Frequency**	**High-Frequency**
Outpatient	1.00	2.90 (2.61–3.22)	4.37 (3.88–4.92)
Inpatient	1.00	0.79 (0.71–0.88)	0.75 (0.67–0.83)

Modified from Haruyama Y, Yamazaki T, Endo M, et al. Personal status of general health checkups and medical expenditure: a large-scale community-based retrospective cohort study. *J Epidemiol.* 2017;27(5):209–214.

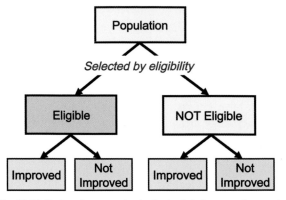

Fig. 17.12 Design of a nonrandomized cohort study comparing people eligible with people not eligible for a program.

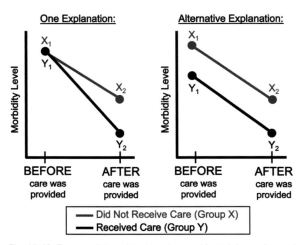

Fig. 17.13 Two possible explanations that would result in an observed difference in morbidity between Group X and Group Y after Group Y (shown in *black*) has received a health care service.

noneligible population for comparison may be critical. However, ineligible persons can be selected from similar neighborhoods that could compensate for the concern with ensuring comparability of socioeconomic status. In addition, as differences between eligible and ineligible individuals may also affect external validity, on occasion adjustment for the variables that differ between these individuals improves external validity.

Combination Designs

Fig. 17.13 shows a hypothetical result from a non-randomized study comparing the morbidity level in

a group that has *not* received a health service (Group X, shown in *red*) with the morbidity level in a group that *has* received the health service (Group Y, shown in *black*). Because the observed level of morbidity is lower for Group Y than for Group X, we might be tempted to conclude from these results that the health service reduces morbidity. However, as seen in Fig. 17.13 *(left of figure),* in order to reach this conclusion, we must assume that the original levels of morbidity in the two groups were comparable at a time before the care was provided to Group Y. If the morbidity levels for X_1 and Y_1 were similar, we could interpret the finding of a lower level of morbidity in Group Y (Y_2) than in Group X (X_2) at a time after which care has been administered as likely to have resulted from the care provided.

However, as seen in Fig. 17.13 *(right of figure),* it is possible that the groups might have been originally different and their prognoses may have differed at that time even before any care was provided. If such were the case, any differences in morbidity observed after care (i.e., Y_2 lower than X_2) might only reflect the original differences at the time before care was administered, and would not necessarily shed any light on the effectiveness of the care provided. Without data on morbidity levels in the two groups before the administration of care ("baseline"), the latter explanation of the observations cannot be ruled out.

In view of this problem, another approach to program evaluation is to use a *combination design,* which combines a *before–after* design with a *program–no program* design. This approach is demonstrated in the following example, in which outpatient care for sore throats in children was evaluated.

The study is designed to assess the effectiveness of outpatient care for sore throats in children by determining whether children who are eligible for care experience lower rates of complications of untreated "strep" throat, such as glomerulonephritis (inflammation of the kidney) or pediatric neuropsychiatric disorders associated with streptococcal infections (PANDAS), such as tics, than did children who are not eligible. The rationale was as follows: "Strep" throats are common in children. Untreated "strep" throats can lead to complications like kidney infection. If "strep" throats are properly treated, complications can be prevented. Therefore, if these programs are effective in treating "strep" throats, fewer

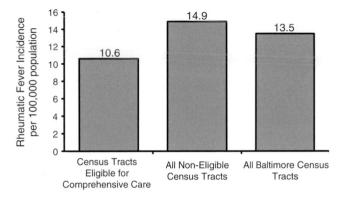

Fig. 17.14 Comprehensive care and rheumatic fever incidence per 100,000, 1968–70; Baltimore, black population, aged 5 to 14 years. (Modified from Gordis L. Effectiveness of comprehensive-care programs in preventing rheumatic fever. *N Engl J Med*. 1973;289:331–335.)

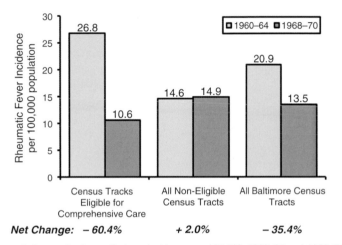

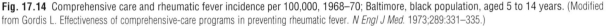

Fig. 17.15 Comprehensive care and changes in rheumatic fever incidence per 100,000, 1960–64 and 1968–70; Baltimore, black population, aged 5 to 14 years. (Modified from Gordis L. Effectiveness of comprehensive-care programs in preventing rheumatic fever. *N Engl J Med*. 1973;289:331–335.)

cases of complications should occur in children who receive the treatment.

It is possible to identify and compare subgroups of children and adolescents and to compare their rates of complications from untreated "strep." The groups could include residents of census tracts that meet eligibility criteria for comprehensive care and residents of census tracts that do not meet these eligibility criteria for comprehensive care. Both could then be compared to the city or town as a whole.

An historic example from Dr. Gordis's research[15] shows another complication of "strep" throat—rheumatic fever, which was much more common in the past century than today. Fig. 17.14 shows a *program–no*

program comparison of rheumatic fever rates in black children in Baltimore City. In children eligible for comprehensive care based on their census tracts, the rheumatic fever rate was 10.6 per 100,000, compared with 14.9 per 100,000 in those who were not eligible. Although the rate was lower in the eligible group in this simultaneous comparison, the difference was not dramatic.

The next analysis in this combination design examined changes in rheumatic fever rates over time in both eligible and noneligible populations.

As seen in Fig. 17.15, the rheumatic fever rate declined 60% in the eligible census tracts from 1960 to 1964 (before the programs were established) to

1968–70 (after the programs were operating). In the noneligible tracts, rheumatic fever incidence was essentially unchanged (+2%). Thus, both parts of the combination design are consistent with a decline related to the care available.

However, because many changes had occurred in Baltimore City during this time, it was not certain whether the care provided by the programs was indeed responsible for the decline in rheumatic fever. Another analysis was therefore carried out. In children, streptococcal throat infection can be either symptomatic or asymptomatic. Clearly, only a child with a symptomatic sore throat would have been brought to a clinic. If we hypothesize that the care in the clinic was responsible for the reduction in rheumatic fever incidence, we would expect the decline in incidence to be limited to children with symptomatic clinical sore throats who would have sought care, and not to have occurred in asymptomatic children who had no clinically apparent infections.

As seen in Fig. 17.16, the entire decline was limited to children with prior clinically overt infection; no change in rheumatic fever incidence occurred in those children with asymptomatic "strep" throat. These findings are therefore highly consistent with the suggestion that it was the medical care, or some factor closely associated with it, which was responsible for the decline in rheumatic fever incidence.

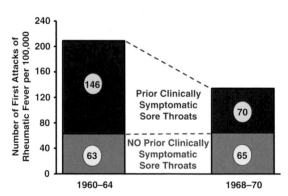

Fig. 17.16 Changes in the annual incidence of first attacks of rheumatic fever in relation to the presence or absence preceding clinically symptomatic sore throat. As seen in the figure, the entire decline in first attacks of rheumatic fever was due to a decline in first attacks of rheumatic fever that were preceded by clinically symptomatic sore throats. (Modified from Gordis L. Effectiveness of comprehensive-care programs in preventing rheumatic fever. *N Engl J Med.* 1973;289:331–335.)

Case-Control Studies

The use of the case-control design for evaluating health services, including vaccines and other forms of prevention and screening programs, has elicited increasing interest in the field of public health. Although the case-control design has been applied primarily to etiologic studies, when appropriate data are obtainable, this design can serve as a useful, but limited, surrogate for randomized trials. However, because this design requires definition and specification of cases, it is most applicable to studies of *prevention* of specific diseases. The "exposure" is then the specific preventive or other health measure that is being assessed. As in most health services research, stratification by disease severity and by other possible prognostic factors is essential for appropriate interpretation of the findings. The methodologic problems associated with such studies (which are discussed extensively in Chapter 7) also arise when the case-control design is used for evaluating effectiveness. In particular, these studies need to address the selection of controls and issues associated with confounders.

Conclusion

This chapter has reviewed the application of basic epidemiologic study designs to the evaluation of health services. Many of the issues that arise are similar to those that arise in etiologic studies, although at times they present a different twist. In etiologic studies, we are primarily interested in the possible association of a potential causal factor and a specific disease, and factors such as health services accessibility often represent possible confounders that must be taken into account. For example, in the Multi-Ethnic Study of Atherosclerosis, evaluation of determinants of atrial fibrillation must take into account the potential confounding effect of health insurance status (a marker of access to health care), as diagnosis of this condition is often made during a patient's encounter with a physician.[16]

In health care evaluation studies, we are primarily interested in possible associations of a health care or preventive activity and a particular disease outcome, and factors such as preexisting disease and other prognostic and risk factors become potential confounders that must be taken into consideration. Consequently, although many of the same design issues remain, the focus in evaluation research is often on different issues of measurement and assessment. The randomized trial remains the optimal method for demonstrating the effectiveness of a health intervention. However, ethical issues may remain in play, as it may be unethical to withhold a known or effective treatment in a randomized trial design. In initiating any evaluation study of health care, we should ask at the outset whether it is biologically and clinically plausible, given our current knowledge, to expect a specific benefit from the care being evaluated.

For practical reasons, nonrandomized observations are also necessary and must be capitalized in the attempt to expand our efforts at health services evaluation. Critics of randomized trials have pointed out that such studies have included—and can only include—a small fraction of all patients receiving care in the health care system so that generalizability of the results is a potential problem. Although this is true, generalizability is a problem with any study, no matter how large the study population. Nevertheless, even as we further refine the methodology of clinical trials, we also need improved methods to enhance the information that can be obtained from nonrandomized evaluations of health services.

The study of specific components of care, rather than a care program per se, is essential. In this way, if an effective element can be identified in a mix of many modalities, the others can be eliminated and the quality of care can be enhanced in a cost-effective fashion.

In Chapter 18, the discussion of evaluation is extended to a specific type of health services program: screening (early detection) for disease in human populations.

REFERENCES

1. Frost WH. Rendering account in public health. *Am J Public Health*. 1925;15:394–397.
2. Chapin CV. Comments on "Rendering An Account on Public Health," by Frost. *Am J Public Health*. 1925;15:397–398.
3. Butler D. When Google got flu wrong. *Nature*. 2013;494(7436): 155–156.
4. Ikuta K, Wang Y, Robinson A, et al. National trends in use and outcomes of pulmonary artery catheters among medicare beneficiaries, 1999-2013. *JAMA Cardiol*. 2017;2(8):908–913.
5. Office of National Statistics. *Review of Avoidable Mortality Definition*. Cardiff: Government of the United Kingdom; 2015.
6. Khoja T, Farag MK. *Synopsis of Indicators: Monitoring, Evaluation, and Supervision of Healthcare Quality*. Kingdome of Saudi Arabia: Ministry of Health; 1995.
7. Kalra L, Evans A, Perez I, et al. Alternative strategies for stroke care: a prospective randomized controlled trial. *Lancet*. 2000;356:894–899.
8. Drummond AE, Pearson B, Lincoln NB, et al. Ten year follow-up of a randomized controlled trial of care in a stroke rehabilitation unit. *BMJ*. 2005;331:491–492.
9. Kahn KL, Rubenstein LV, Draper D, et al. The effects of DRG-based prospective payment system on quality of care for hospitalized Medicare patients: an introduction to the series. *JAMA*. 1990;264:1953–1955.
10. Kosecoff J, Kahn KL, Rogerts WH, et al. Prospective payment system and impairment at discharge: the "quicker and sicker" story revisited. *JAMA*. 1990;264:1980–1983.
11. Wallenstein ME, Ananth CV, Kim JH, et al. Effect of surgical volume on outcomes for laparoscopic hysterectomy for benign indications. *Obstet Gynecol*. 2012;119:709–716.
12. Birkmeyer JD, Stukel TA, Siewers AE, et al. Surgeon volume and operative mortality in the United States. *N Engl J Med*. 2003;349:2117–2127.
13. Haruyama Y, Yamazaki T, Endo M, et al. Personal status of general health checkups and medical expenditure: a large-scale community-based retrospective cohort study. *J Epidemiol*. 2017;27(5):209–214.
14. Gierisch JM, Earp JA, Brewer NT, et al. Longitudinal predictors of nonadherence to maintenance of mammography. *Cancer Epidemiol Biomarkers Prev*. 2010;19(4):1103–1111.
15. Gordis L. Effectiveness of comprehensive-care programs in preventing rheumatic fever. *N Engl J Med*. 1973;289:331–335.
16. Lin GM, Colangelo LA, Lloyd-Jones DM, et al. Association of sleep apnea and snoring with incident atrial fibrillation in the Multi-Ethnic Study of Atherosclerosis. *Am J Epidemiol*. 2015;182: 49–57.

REVIEW QUESTIONS FOR CHAPTER 17

1 *All of the following are measures of process of health care in a clinic* except:

  a. Proportion of patients in whom blood pressure is measured

  b. Proportion of patients who have complications of a disease

  c. Proportion of patients advised to stop smoking

  d. Proportion of patients whose height and weight are measured

  e. Proportion of patients whose bill is reduced because of financial need

2 *The extent to which a specific health care treatment, service, procedure, program, or other intervention does what it is intended to do when used in a community-dwelling population is termed its:*

a. Efficacy

b. Effectiveness

c. Effect modification

d. Efficiency

e. None of the above

3 *The extent to which a specific health care treatment, service, procedure, program, or other intervention produces a beneficial result under ideal controlled conditions is its:*

a. Efficacy

b. Effectiveness

c. Effect modification

d. Efficiency

e. None of the above

4 *A major problem in using a historical control design for evaluating a health service using case-fatality (CF) as an outcome is that if the CF is lower after provision of the health service was started, then:*

a. The lower CF could be caused by changing prevalence of the disease

b. The lower CF may be a result of decreasing incidence

c. The lower CF may be an indirect effect of the new health service

d. The CF may have been affected by changes in factors that are not related to the new health service

e. None of the above

Question 5 is based on the information given below:

In-Hospital Case-Fatality (CF) for 100 Men Not Treated in a Coronary Care Unit (CCU) and for 100 Men Treated in a CCU, According to Three Clinical Grades of Severity of Myocardial Infarction (MI)						
	NON-CCU (NO. OF PATIENTS)			**CCU (NO. OF PATIENTS)**		
Clinical Grade	**Total**	**Died**	**CF (%)**	**Total**	**Died**	**CF (%)**
Mild	60	12	20	10	3	30
Severe	36	18	50	60	18	30
Shock	4	4	100	30	13	43

The results shown are based on a comparison of the last 100 patients treated before the CCU was installed and the first 100 patients treated within the CCU. All 200 patients were admitted during the same month.

You may assume that this is the *only* hospital in the town and that the natural history of MI was *unchanged* during this period.

5 *The authors concluded that the CCU was very beneficial for men with severe MI and for those in shock, because the in-hospital CFs for these categories were much lower in the CCU. This conclusion:*

a. Is correct

b. May be incorrect because CFs were used rather than mortality rates

c. May be incorrect because of a referral bias of patients to this hospital from hospitals in distant towns

d. May be incorrect because of differences in the assignment of the clinical severity grade before and after the opening of the CCU

e. May be incorrect because of failure to recognize a possible decrease in the annual incidence rate of MI in recent years

Chapter 18

Epidemiologic Approach to Evaluating Screening Programs

For all sad words of tongue or pen
The saddest are these:
"it might have been."[1]

—J.G. Whittier, 1856

If, of all words of tongue and pen,
The saddest are, "It might have been,"
More sad are these we daily see:
"It is, but hadn't ought to be."[2]

—Bret Harte, 1871

Learning Objectives

- To extend the discussion of the validity and reliability of screening tests introduced in Chapter 5.
- To revisit the natural history of disease and introduce the concepts of lead time and critical point.
- To describe the major sources of bias that must be taken into account in assessing study findings that compare screened and unscreened populations, including referral bias, length-biased sampling, lead time bias, 5-year survival, and overdiagnosis bias.
- To discuss various study designs for evaluating screening programs, including nonrandomized and randomized studies and the challenges of interpreting the results of these studies.
- To discuss problems in assessing the sensitivity and specificity of commercially developed screening tests.
- To introduce issues associated with cost-benefit analyses of screening.

In Chapter 1, we distinguished among primary, secondary, and tertiary prevention. In Section II, we discussed the design and interpretation of studies that aim to identify risk factors or etiologic factors for disease so that the occurrence of disease can be completely prevented—*primary prevention*. In this chapter, we address how epidemiology is used to evaluate the effectiveness of screening programs for the early detection of disease—*secondary prevention*. This subject is particularly important in both clinical practice and public health because there is increasing acceptance of a physician's obligation to include prevention along with diagnosis and treatment as major responsibilities in the clinical care of patients.

The validity and reliability of screening tests were discussed in Chapter 5. In this chapter, we will discuss some of the methodologic issues that must be considered in deriving inferences about the benefits that may come to those who undergo screening tests.

The question of whether patients benefit from the early detection of disease includes the following components:

1. Can the disease be detected early?
2. What are the sensitivity and the specificity of the test?
3. What is the predictive value of the test?
4. How serious is the problem of false-positive test results?
5. What is the cost of early detection in terms of funds, resources, and emotional impact?
6. Can the subject be harmed by having a screening test?
7. Do the individuals in whom disease is detected early benefit from the early detection, and is there an overall benefit to those who are screened?

In this chapter, we primarily address the last question. Several of the other issues in the preceding list are considered only in the context of this question.

The term *early detection of disease* means diagnosing a disease at an earlier stage than would usually occur in standard clinical practice. This usually denotes

353

detecting disease at a presymptomatic stage, at which point the patient has no clinical complaint (no symptoms or signs) and therefore no reason to seek medical care for the condition. The assumption in screening is that an appropriate intervention is available for the disease that is detected and that the medical intervention can be more effectively applied if the disease is detected at an earlier stage.

At first glance, the question of whether people benefit from early detection of disease may seem somewhat surprising. Intuitively, it would seem obvious that early detection is beneficial and that intervention at an earlier stage of the disease process is more effective and/or easier to implement than a later intervention. In effect, these assumptions represent a "surgical" view; for example, every malignant lesion is localized at some early stage, and at this stage it can be successfully excised before regional spread occurs or certainly before widespread metastases develop. However, the intuitive attractiveness of such a concept should not blind us to the fact that throughout the history of medicine, deeply felt convictions have often turned out to be erroneous when they were not supported by data obtained from appropriately designed and rigorously conducted studies. Consequently, regardless of the attractiveness of the idea of the beneficial aspects of early disease detection, both to clinicians involved in prevention and therapy and to those involved in community-based prevention programs, the evidence to support the validity of this concept must be rigorously examined.

As in evaluating any type of health service, screening can be evaluated using process or outcome measures. Box 18.1 provides a list of operational measures that includes process measures, as well as measurements of yield and information produced by the screening program.

We are particularly interested in the question of what benefit is gained by people who undergo screening in a screening program. However, just as is the case with evaluation of health services (discussed in Chapter 17), there is little advantage to improving the *process* of screening if persons who are screened derive no benefit. That is, if early detection does not lead to any improvement in survival, what is the gain to patients to be detected earlier? Perhaps just a longer remaining time to worry with poor quality of life! We will

BOX 18.1 ASSESSING THE EFFECTIVENESS OF SCREENING PROGRAMS USING OPERATIONAL MEASURES

1. Number of people screened
2. Proportion of target populations screened and number of times screened
3. Detected prevalence of preclinical disease
4. Total costs of the program
5. Costs per case found
6. Costs per previously unknown case found
7. Proportion of positive screenees brought to final diagnosis and treatment
8. Predictive value of a positive test in population screened

Modified from Hulka BS. Degrees of proof and practical application. Cancer. 1988;62:1776–1780. Copyright © 1988 American Cancer Society. Reprinted by permission of Wiley-Liss, Inc., a subsidiary of John Wiley & Sons, Inc.

BOX 18.2 ASSESSING THE EFFECTIVENESS OF SCREENING PROGRAMS USING OUTCOME MEASURES

1. Reduction of mortality in the population screened
2. Reduction of case-fatality in screened individuals
3. Increase in percent of cases detected at earlier stages
4. Reduction in complications
5. Prevention of or reduction in recurrences or metastases
6. Improvement of quality of life in screened individuals

therefore examine some of the problems associated with determining whether early detection of disease confers benefits to the individual who undergoes screening (in other words, whether the outcome is improved by screening).

What do we mean by *outcome?* To answer the question of whether patients benefit, we must precisely define what we mean by benefit, and what outcome or outcomes are considered to be evidence of patient benefit. Some of the possible outcome measures that might be used are shown in Box 18.2.

Natural History of Disease

To discuss the methodologic issues involved in evaluating the benefits of screening, let us examine in further detail the natural history of disease (first discussed in Chapter 6).

We will begin by placing screening in its appropriate place on the timeline of the natural history of disease and will do so in relation to the different approaches to prevention discussed in Chapter 1.

Fig. 18.1A is a schematic representation of the natural history of a disease in an individual. At some point, biologic onset of disease occurs. This may be a subcellular change, such as an alteration in DNA, which at this point is generally undetectable. At some later point the disease becomes symptomatic, or clinical signs develop (i.e., the disease now moves into a clinical phase). The clinical signs and symptoms (e.g., blood in the stool) prompt the patient to seek care, after which a diagnosis is made and appropriate therapy is instituted, the ultimate outcome of which may be cure, control of the disease, disability, or death.

As seen in Fig. 18.1B, the onset of symptoms marks an important point in the natural history of a disease. The period when disease is present can be divided into two phases. The period from biologic onset of the disease to the development of signs and symptoms is called the *preclinical phase* of the disease, which comes before the clinical phase of the disease.

The period from the time when signs and symptoms develop to an ultimate outcome such as possible cure, control of the disease, or death is referred to as the *clinical phase* of the disease. As seen in Fig. 18.1C and D, *primary prevention* (i.e., preventing the development of disease by preventing or reducing exposure to disease-causing agents) denotes an intervention before a disease has developed. (Prevention of risk factor exposure, such as immunization and prevention of smoking initiation, is also known as *primordial prevention*.) *Secondary prevention*, detecting disease at an earlier stage than usual, such as by screening, takes place during the *preclinical phase* of an illness (i.e., after the disease has developed but before clinical signs and symptoms have appeared). *Tertiary prevention* refers to

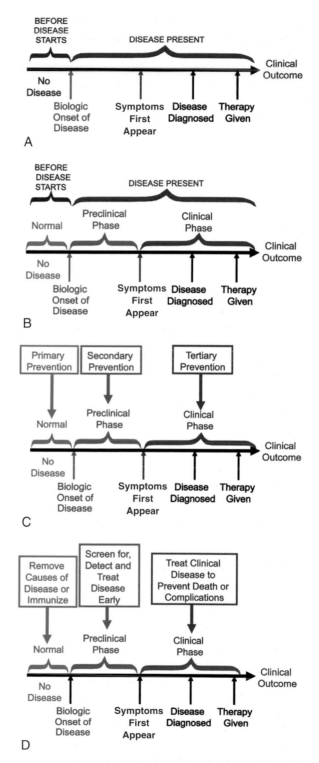

Fig. 18.1 (A) Natural history of a disease. (B) Natural history of a disease with preclinical and clinical phases. (C) Natural history of a disease with points for primary, secondary, and tertiary prevention. (D) Natural history of a disease with specific primary, secondary, and tertiary prevention measures.

treating clinically ill individuals to prevent complications of the illness (e.g., stroke rehabilitation), including death of the patient.

If we want to detect disease earlier than usual through programs of health education, we could encourage symptomatic persons to seek medical care sooner. However, a major challenge lies in identifying persons with disease who do not have any symptoms. Our focus in this chapter is on identifying disease in persons who have not yet developed symptoms and who are in the preclinical phase of illness.

Let us now take a closer look at the *preclinical phase* of the disease (Fig. 18.2). At some point during the preclinical phase, it becomes possible to detect the disease by using currently available tests (see Fig. 18.2A). The interval from this point to the development of signs and symptoms is the *detectable preclinical phase* of the disease (see Fig. 18.2B). When disease is detected by a screening test, the time of diagnosis is advanced to an earlier point in the natural history of the disease than would have happened if the screening was not done. The *lead time* is defined as the interval by which the time of diagnosis is advanced by screening for the early detection of disease compared with the usual time of diagnosis (see Fig. 18.2C). The concept of lead time is inherent in the idea of screening and then detecting a disease earlier than it would usually be found.

Another important concept in screening is if there is a *critical point* in the natural history of a disease (Fig. 18.3A).[3] This is a point in the natural history before which treatment is more effective and/or less difficult to administer. If a disease is potentially curable, cure may be possible before this point but not later on. For example, in a woman with breast cancer, one critical point would be that at which the disease spreads from the breast to the axillary lymph nodes. If the disease is detected and treated prior to spreading, the prognosis is much better than after spread to the nodes has taken place.

As shown in Fig. 18.3B, there may be multiple critical points in the natural history of a disease. For example, in the patient with breast cancer, a second critical point may be that at which disease spreads from the axillary nodes to other more distant parts of the body. Prognosis is still better when the disease is confined to the axillary lymph nodes than when systemic spread has occurred,

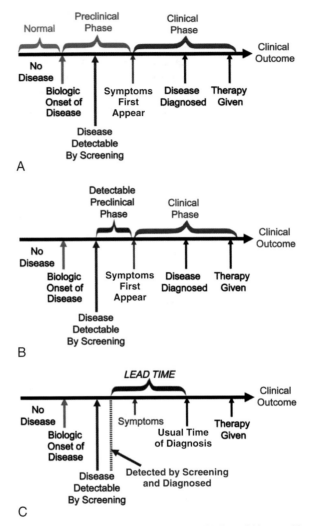

Fig. 18.2 Preclinical phase of the disease. (A) Natural history with point at which disease is detectable by screening. (B) Natural history with detectable preclinical phase. (C) Natural history with lead time.

but not as good as when the disease is confined to the breast. The concept of multiple critical points suggests that the earlier the diagnosis, the better the prognosis.

However, the critical point is somewhat theoretical because we usually cannot identify when the critical point is reached. However, it is a very important concept in screening. If we cannot envision one or more critical points in the natural history of a disease, there is clearly no rationale for screening and early detection. Early

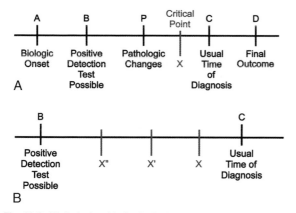

Fig. 18.3 (A) A single critical point in the natural history of a disease. (B) Multiple critical points in the natural history of a disease. (Modified from Hutchison GB. Evaluation of preventive services. *J Chronic Dis.* 1960;11:497–508.)

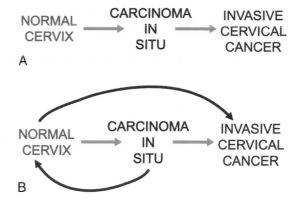

Fig. 18.4 (A) Natural history of cervical cancer: I. Progression from normal cervix to invasive cancer. (B) Natural history of cervical cancer: II. Extremely rapid progression and spontaneous regression.

detection presumes that a biologic point exists in the natural history of a disease before which treatment will benefit a person more than if he or she is treated after that point.

Pattern of Disease Progression

We might expect to see a potential benefit from screening and early detection if the following two assumptions hold:

1. All or most clinical cases of a disease first go through a detectable preclinical phase.
2. In the absence of intervention, all or most cases in a preclinical phase progress to a clinical phase.

Both assumptions are reasonably self-evident. For example, if none of the preclinical cases progress to clinical cases, there is no reason to perform screening tests. Alternatively, if none of the clinical cases passes through a preclinical phase, there is no reason to perform screening tests. Thus both assumptions are important in assessing any potential benefit from screening.

Let us look at the example of screening for cervical cancer. It has been some 80 years since the Papanicolaou (Pap) was developed to test for the presence of precancerous or cancerous cells of the cervix, the opening of the uterus. During this routine procedure, cervical cells are scraped from around the cervix and

then examined. The biology of cervical cancer has been well documented, going through a series of steps from dysplasia to carcinoma in situ, to invasive cervical cancer that often takes years to develop. Thus early detection often allows treatment to stop the progression of this cancer. More recently, with the documentation of the viral origins of cervical cancer (human papillomavirus [HPV] infection), cervical cancer screening is now done by HPV detection with less frequent Pap tests. Fig. 18.4A shows the progression from a normal cervix to cervical cancer. We might expect that detection and treatment of more cases at the in situ (noninvasive) stage would be reflected in a commensurate reduction in the number of cases that progress to invasive disease.

However, the two assumptions associated with early detection are open to question. In certain situations, and unlike what happens in cervical cancer, the preclinical phase may be so short that the disease is unlikely to be detected by any periodic screening program. In addition, there is increasing evidence that spontaneous regression may occur in some diseases; therefore not every preclinical case inexorably progresses to clinical disease. Importantly, this is the case with HPV detection in women—most of the HPV types detected in routine screening will generally revert (spontaneously disappear) in the following 6 months!

However, evaluating the benefits of cervical cancer screening is complicated by the problem that some cases progress through the in situ stage so rapidly and the preclinical stage is so brief, that for all practical purposes there is no preclinical stage during which disease can be detected by screening. In addition, nuclear DNA quantitation studies suggest that cervical intraepithelial abnormalities may exist either as a reversible state or as an irreversible precursor of invasive cancer. Data also suggest that some cases of cervical intraepithelial neoplasia detected by a Pap smear regress spontaneously, particularly in the earlier stages, but also in the later stage (carcinoma in situ). In one study, one-third of women with abnormal Pap smears who refused any intervention were later found to have normal Pap smears. In addition, data suggest that most, if not all, in situ cervical neoplasias are associated with different types of papillomaviruses. Only neoplasias associated with certain high-risk types of papillomavirus progress to invasive cancer, so we may be dealing with heterogeneity of both the causal agent and disease.

The simple model of progression from normal cervix to invasive cervical cancer seen in Fig. 18.4A would suggest that early detection followed by effective intervention would be reflected by a commensurate reduction in the number of invasive lesions that subsequently develop. A more accurate presentation of the natural history of cervical cancer may be that seen in Fig. 18.4B. The extent of both phenomena, spontaneous regression and extremely rapid progression, clearly influences the size of the decrease in invasive disease that might be expected to result from early detection and intervention and must therefore be taken into account in assessing the benefits of screening. Although these issues have been demonstrated for cervical cancer, they are clearly relevant to evaluating the benefits of screening for many diseases.

Methodologic Issues

To interpret the findings in a study designed to evaluate the benefits of screening, certain methodologic problems must be taken into account. Most studies of screening programs that have been reported are not randomized trials because of the difficulties of randomizing a population for screening. The question is, therefore, can we examine a group of people who have been screened and compare their mortality to a group of

people who have not been screened (i.e., use a cohort design to evaluate the effectiveness of screening)?

Let us assume that we can compare a population of people who have been screened for a disease with a population of people who have not been screened for the disease. Let us assume further that a viable and effective treatment is available and will be used effectively for those in whom disease is detected. If we find a lower mortality from the disease in those in whom disease was identified through screening than in those in whom disease was not detected in this manner, can we conclude that screening and early detection of disease have been beneficial? Let us turn to some of the methodologic issues involved.

SELECTION BIASES
Referral Bias (Volunteer Bias)

In coming to a conclusion about the benefits of screening, the first question we might ask is whether there was a selection bias in terms of who was screened and who was not. We would like to be able to assume that those who were screened had the same characteristics as those who were not screened (i.e., they were similar to one another in all ways except their screening history). However, there are many differences in the characteristics of those who participate in screening or take advantage of other health programs and those who do not. Many studies have shown volunteers to be healthier than the general population and to be more likely to comply (to be adherent) with medical recommendations. If, for example, persons whose disease had a better prognosis from the outset were either referred for screening or were self-selected, we might observe lower mortality in the screened group even if early detection played no role in improving prognosis. Of course, it is also possible that volunteers may include many people who are at high risk and who volunteer for screening because they have anxieties based on a positive family history or their own lifestyle characteristics. The problem is that we do not know in which direction the selection bias might operate and how it might affect the study results.

The problem of selection bias that most significantly affects our interpretation of the findings is best addressed by carrying out the comparison with a randomized experimental study in which care is taken that the two groups have comparable initial prognostic profiles (Fig. 18.5).

Length-Biased Sampling (Prognostic Selection)

The second type of problem that arises in interpreting the results of a comparison of a screened and an unscreened group is a possible selection bias; this does not relate to who comes for screening but rather to the type of disease that is detected by the screening. The question is: Does screening selectively identify cases of the disease which have a better prognosis? In other words, do the cases found through screening have a better natural history regardless of how early therapy is initiated? If the outcome of those in whom disease is detected by screening is found to be better than the outcome of those who were not screened, and in whom disease was identified during the usual course of clinical care, could the better outcome among those who are screened result from selective identification by screening of persons with a better prognosis? Could the better outcome be unrelated to the time of diagnostic and treatment interventions?

How could this come about? Recall the natural history of disease, with clinical and preclinical phases, as shown in Fig. 18.1B. We know that the clinical phase of illness differs in length for different people (i.e., there is a natural distribution of clinical illness parameters in every population). For example, some patients with colon cancer die soon after diagnosis, whereas others survive for many years. What appears to be the same disease may include individuals with different lengths of a clinical phase.

What about the preclinical phase in these individuals? Actually, each patient's disease has a single continuous natural history, which we divide into preclinical and clinical phases (Fig. 18.6) on the basis of the point in time at which signs and symptoms develop. In some, the natural history is brief, and in others the natural history is protracted. This suggests that if a person has a slowly progressive natural history with a long clinical phase, the preclinical phase will also be long. In contrast, if a person has a rapidly progressive disease process and a short natural history, the clinical phase is likely to be short, and it seems reasonable to conclude that the preclinical phase will also be short. There are in fact data to support the notion that a long clinical phase is associated with a long preclinical phase and a short clinical phase is associated with a short preclinical phase. Lung cancer serves as an example: it has a short clinical phase and most likely also a short preclinical phase, as suggested by the inconsistent results from clinical trials of smokers screened by computed tomography, with some trials showing an approximately 15% to 20% effectiveness and others showing no effectiveness whatsoever.[4]

Remember that our purpose in screening is to detect the disease during the preclinical phase because during the clinical phase the patient is already aware of the problem and even without screening will probably seek medical care for symptoms. If we mount a one-time screening program in a community, which group of patients are we likely to identify—those with a short preclinical phase or those with a long preclinical phase?

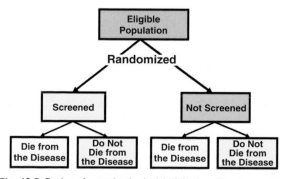

Fig. 18.5 Design of a randomized trial of the benefits of screening.

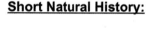
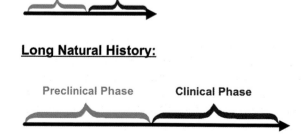

Fig. 18.6 Short and long natural histories of disease: relationship of length of clinical phase to length of preclinical phase.

To answer this question, let us consider a small population that is screened for a certain disease (Fig. 18.7). As shown in Fig. 18.7, each case has a preclinical and a clinical phase. The figure is drawn so that each preclinical phase is the same length as its associated clinical phase. Patients in the clinical phase will be identified in the usual course of medical care, so the purpose of the screening is to identify cases in the preclinical state (i.e., before any onset of signs or symptoms). Note that the lengths of the preclinical phases of cases represented here vary. The longer the preclinical phase, the more likely the screening program will detect the case while it is still preclinical. For example, if we screen once a year for a disease for which the preclinical phase is only 24 hours long, we will clearly miss virtually all of the cases during the preclinical phase. However, if the preclinical phase is 1 year long, many more cases will be identified during that time. Screening tends to selectively identify those cases that have longer preclinical phases of illness. Consequently, even if the subsequent therapy had no effect, screening would still selectively identify persons with a long preclinical phase, and they would consequently experience a longer clinical phase (i.e., those with a better prognosis). These people would have a better prognosis even if there were no screening program or even if there were no true benefits from screening.

This problem can be addressed in several ways. One approach is to use an experimental randomized design in which care is taken to keep the groups comparable in terms of the lengths of the detectable preclinical phase of illness. However, this may not be easy. In addition, survival would have to be examined for all members of each group (i.e., the screened and unscreened). In the screened group, survival would be calculated for those in whom disease is detected by screening and for those in whom disease is detected between screening examinations, the so-called *interval cases*. We will return to the importance of interval cases later in this chapter.

LEAD TIME BIAS

Another problem that arises in comparing survival in people who are screened with survival in those who are not screened is *lead time bias* (first illustrated in Fig. 18.2C)—how much earlier can the diagnosis be made if the disease is detected by screening compared with the usual timing of the diagnosis if screening were not carried out?

Consider four individuals with a certain disease shown by the four timelines in Fig. 18.8. The thicker part of each horizontal line denotes the apparent survival that is observed. The first timeline (A) shows the usual time of diagnosis and the usual time of death. The second timeline (B) shows an earlier time of diagnosis but the same time of death. Survival *seems* better because the interval from diagnosis to death is longer, but the patient is not any better off because death has not been delayed. The third timeline (C) shows earlier diagnosis

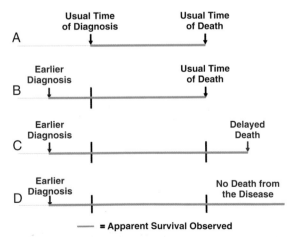

Fig. 18.8 (A) Outcome of diagnosis at the usual time, without screening. (B–D) Three possible outcomes of an earlier diagnosis as a result of a screening program.

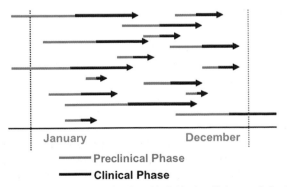

Preclinical Phase
Clinical Phase

Fig. 18.7 Hypothetical population of individuals with long and short natural histories.

and a delay in death from the disease—clearly a benefit to the patient (assuming that subsequent quality of life is good). Finally, the fourth timeline (D) shows earlier diagnosis, with subsequent prevention of death from the disease.

The benefits we seek in screening are delay or prevention of death. Although we have chosen to focus on mortality in this chapter, we could also have used morbidity parameters, recurrence, quality of life, or patient satisfaction as valid measures of outcome.

LEAD TIME AND 5-YEAR SURVIVAL

Five-year survival is a frequently used measure of therapeutic success, particularly in cancer therapy. Let us examine the possible effect of lead time on apparent 5-year survival.

Fig. 18.9A shows the natural history of disease in a hypothetical patient with colon cancer, which was diagnosed in the usual clinical context without any screening. Biologic onset of the disease was in 2008.

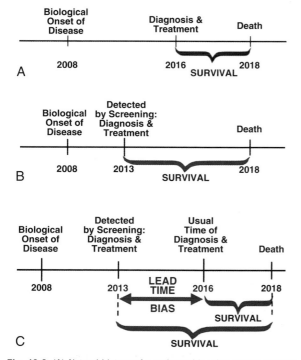

Fig. 18.9 (A) Natural history of a patient with colon cancer without screening. Disease diagnosed and treated in 2008. (B) Disease detected by screening 3 years earlier in 2013 (lead time). (C) Lead time bias resulting from screening 3 years earlier.

The patient became aware of symptoms in 2016 and had a diagnostic workup leading to a diagnosis of colon cancer. Surgery was performed in 2016, but the patient died of colon cancer in 2018. This patient has survived for 2 years (2016–18) and clearly is not a 5-year survivor. If we use 5-year survival as an index of treatment success, this patient is a treatment failure.

Consider what might happen to this patient if he resides in a community in which a screening program is initiated (see Fig. 18.9B). For this hypothetical example only, let us assume that there is actually no benefit from early detection (i.e., the natural history of colon cancer is unaffected by early intervention). In this case the patient is asymptomatic but undergoes a routine screening test in 2013, the result of which is positive. In 2013, surgery is performed, but the patient dies in 2018. The patient has survived 5 years and is now clearly a 5-year survivor. However, he is a 5-year survivor not because death has been delayed but because the diagnosis has been made earlier. When we compare this screening scenario with the scenario without screening (see Fig. 18.9A), it is apparent the patient has not derived any benefit from earlier detection in terms of having lived any longer. Indeed, the patient may have lost out in terms of quality of life because the earlier detection of disease by screening gave him an additional 3 years of postoperative and other medical care and may have deprived him of 3 years of normal life. This problem of an *illusion* of better survival only because of earlier detection is called the *lead time bias*, as shown in Fig. 18.9C.

Thus, even if there is no true benefit from early detection of a disease, there will *appear* to be a benefit associated with screening, even if death is not delayed, because of an earlier point of diagnosis from which survival is measured. This is not to say that early detection carries no benefit; rather, even without any benefit, the lead time associated with early detection suggests the appearance of a benefit in the form of enhanced survival. Lead time must therefore be taken into account in interpreting the results of nonrandomized evaluations.

Fig. 18.10 shows the effect of the bias resulting from lead time on quantitative estimates of survival. Fig. 18.10A shows a situation in which no screening activity is being carried out. Five years after diagnosis, survival is 30%. If we institute a screening program with a

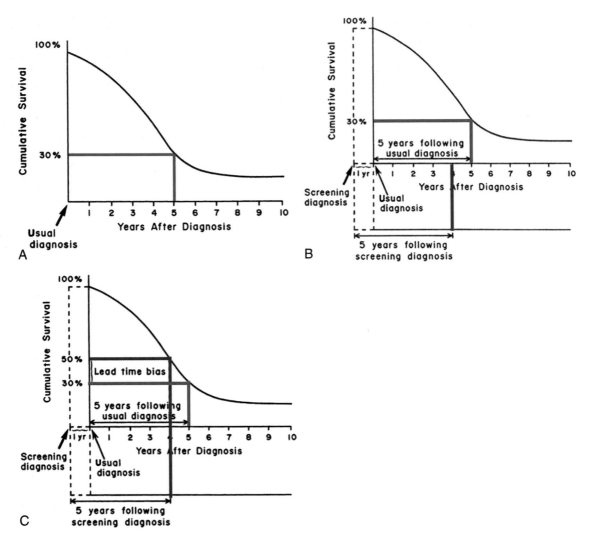

Fig. 18.10 (A) Lead time bias-I: 5-year survival when diagnosis is made without screening. (B) Lead time bias-II: Shift of 5-year period by screening and early detection (lead time). (C) Lead time bias-III: Bias in survival calculation resulting from early detection. (Modified from Frank JW. Occult-blood screening for colorectal carcinoma: the benefits. *Am J Prev Med.* 1985;1:3–9.)

1-year lead time, the entire frame is shifted to the left (see Fig. 18.10B). If we now calculate survival at 5 years from the new time of diagnosis (see Fig. 18.10C), survival appears to be 50% but only as a result of lead time bias. The problem is that the apparently better survival is not a result of screened people living longer, but it is rather a result of a diagnosis being made at an earlier point in the natural history of their disease. For many diseases, such as cancer, the patient cannot die before the onset of the clinical phase and thus the

time before early and usual diagnosis (i.e., the lead time) reflects what is also known as the "immortal time bias."

Consequently, in any comparison of screened and unscreened populations we must make an allowance for an estimated lead time in an attempt to identify any prolongation of survival above and beyond that resulting from the artifact of lead time. If early detection is truly associated with improved survival, survival in the screened group should be greater than survival in the control group *plus the lead time*. We therefore have to generate some estimate of the lead time for the disease being studied.[5]

Another strategy is to compare mortality from the disease in the entire screened group with that in the unscreened group, rather than just the cumulative survival or its reciprocal, the case fatality rate, in those in whom disease was detected by screening.

OVERDIAGNOSIS BIAS

Another potential bias is that of overdiagnosis. At times, people who initiate a screening program have almost limitless enthusiasm for the program. Even cytopathologists reading Pap smears for cervical cancer may become so enthusiastic that they may tend to overread the smears (in other words, to make false-positive readings). If they do overread, some normal women will be included in the group thought to have positive Pap smears. Consequently, the abnormal group will be diluted with women who are free of cancer. If normal individuals in the screened group are more likely to be erroneously diagnosed as positive than are normal individuals in the unscreened group (i.e., labeled as having cancer when in reality they do not), one could get a false impression of increased rates of detection and diagnosis of early-stage cancer as a result of the screening. In addition, because many of the persons with a diagnosis of cancer in the screened group would actually not have cancer and would therefore have a good survival, the results would represent an inflated estimate of survival after screening in persons thought to have cancer, resulting in a mistaken conclusion that screening had been shown to improve survival from cancer in this population.

The possible quantitative impact of overdiagnosis resulting from screening is demonstrated in a hypothetical example shown in Fig. 18.11. Fig. 18.11A shows Scenario 1, in which there is no screening. In this scenario, 1,000 patients with clinical lung cancer are followed for 10 years. At that point, 900 have died and 100 are alive. The 10-year survival for the 1,000 patients is therefore $\frac{100}{1,000}$, or 10%.

Fig. 18.11B shows Scenario 2, in which screening results in overdiagnosis. In this scenario, 4,000 people screen positive for lung cancer. Of these, 1,000 are the same patients with clinical lung cancer seen in Fig.

18.11A, and the other 3,000 are people who do not have lung cancer but are overdiagnosed by the screening test as being positive for lung cancer (false-positives).

After 10 years, these 3,000 people are still alive, as are the 100 people who had clinical lung cancer and survived as shown in Fig. 18.11A. The result is that of the 4,000 people who screened positive initially, 3,100 have survived for 10 years. As shown in the comparison of Scenario 1 and Scenario 2 in Fig. 18.11C, 10-year survival in Scenario 2 is now 78% compared with 10% in Scenario 1 in the original patient population of 1,000 who had clinical lung cancer. However, the apparently "better" survival seen in Scenario 2 is entirely due to the inclusion of 3,000 people who did not have lung cancer but were overdiagnosed by the screening method.

In effect, this is a misclassification bias, as discussed in Chapter 15. In this example, 3,000 people without lung cancer have been misclassified by the screening test as having lung cancer. Consequently, it is essential that in such studies of survival, the diagnostic process be rigorously standardized to minimize the potential problem of overdiagnosis.

Study Designs for Evaluating Screening: Nonrandomized and Randomized Studies

NONRANDOMIZED STUDIES

In discussing the methodologic issues involved in nonrandomized studies of screening, we have in essence been discussing nonrandomized observational studies of screened and unscreened persons—a cohort design (Fig. 18.12).

The case-control design has also been used as a method of assessing the effectiveness of screening (Fig. 18.13). In this design the "cases" are people with advanced disease—the type of disease we hope to prevent by screening. Several proposals have been made for appropriate controls for such a study. Clearly, they should be "noncases" (i.e., people without advanced disease). Although the "controls" used in early case-control studies for evaluating screening were people with disease at an early stage, many researchers believe that people selected from the population from which the cases were derived are *better* controls. We then determine the prevalence of a history of screening among both the cases and the controls, so that screening is

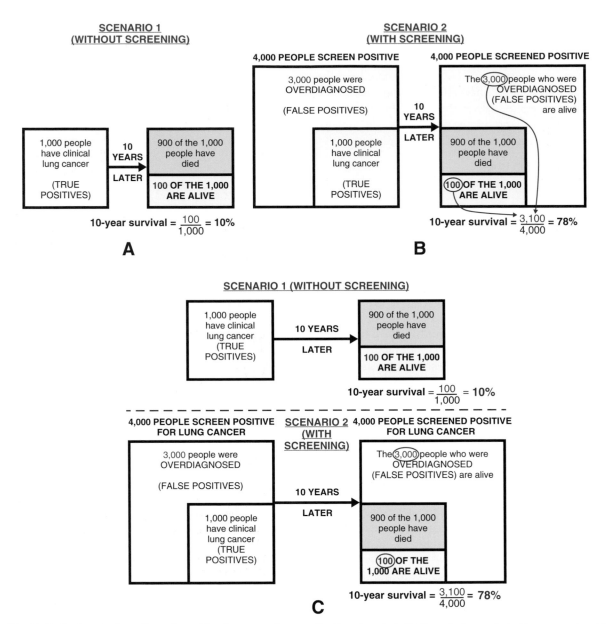

Fig. 18.11 The impact of overdiagnosis resulting from screening on estimation of survival. (A) Scenario 1—survival with no screening. (B) Scenario 2—when screening results in overdiagnosis: survival after 10 years. (C) Comparison of 10-year survival in Scenario 1 and Scenario 2. (Modified from Welch HG, Woloshin S, Schwartz LM. Overstating the evidence for lung cancer screening: the International Early Lung Cancer Action Program [I-ELCAP] study. *Arch Intern Med.* 2007;167:2289–2295.)

looked at as an "exposure." If screening is effective, we would expect to find a greater prevalence of screening history among the controls than among those with advanced disease, and an odds ratio can be calculated, which will be less than 1.0 if screening is effective.

RANDOMIZED STUDIES

In this type of study, a population is randomized, half to screening and half to no screening. Such a study is difficult to mount and carry out and may be fraught with ethical concerns. Perhaps the best known

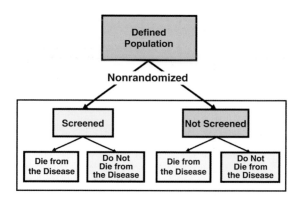

Fig. 18.12 Design of a nonrandomized cohort study of the benefits of screening.

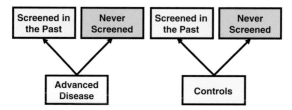

Fig. 18.13 Design of a case-control study of the benefits of screening.

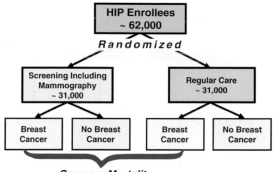

Fig. 18.14 Design of the Health Insurance Plan *(HIP)* randomized controlled trial begun in 1963 to study the efficacy of mammography screening. (Data from Shapiro S, Venet W, Strax P, et al., eds. *Periodic Screening for Breast Cancer: The Health Insurance Plan Project and Its Sequelae, 1963–1986*. Baltimore: Johns Hopkins University Press; 1988.)

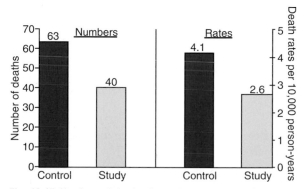

Fig. 18.15 Numbers of deaths due to breast cancer and mortality rates from breast cancer in control and study groups; 5 years of follow-up after entry into study. Data for study group include deaths among women screened and those who refused screening. (Data from Shapiro S, Venet W, Strax P, et al. Selection, follow-up, and analysis in the Health Insurance Plan Study: a randomized trial with breast cancer screening. *Natl Cancer Inst Monogr.* 1985;67:65–74.)

randomized trial of screening is the trial of screening for breast cancer using mammography that was carried out at the Health Insurance Plan (HIP) of New York.[6] Shapiro and colleagues conducted a randomized trial in women enrolled in the prepaid HIP program, an early health maintenance organization (HMO) in New York. This study has become a classic in the literature in reporting evaluation of screening benefits through a randomized trial design, and it serves as a model for future studies of this type.

The study was begun in 1963. It was designed to determine whether periodic screening using clinical breast examination by a physician and mammography reduced breast cancer mortality in women aged 40 to 64 years. Approximately 62,000 women were randomized into a study group and a control group of approximately 31,000 each (Fig. 18.14). The study group was offered screening examinations; 65% appeared for the first examination and were offered additional examinations at annual intervals. Most of these women had at least one of the three annual screening examinations that were offered. Screening consisted of physical breast examination, mammography,

and interview. Control women received the usual medical care in the prepaid medical program. Many reports have been published from this outstanding study, and we will examine only a few of the results here.

Fig. 18.15 shows the number of breast cancer deaths and the mortality rates in both the study group (women who were offered screening mammography) and the control group after 5 years of follow-up.

Note that the data for the study group include deaths among women screened and those who refused

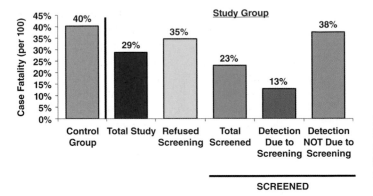

Fig. 18.16 Five-year case-fatality among patients with breast cancer. Case-fatality for those in whom detection was due to screening allow for a 1-year lead time. (Data from Shapiro S, Venet W, Strax P, et al. Ten- to 14-year effect of screening on breast cancer mortality. *J Natl Cancer Inst.* 1982;69:349–355.)

screening. Recall the presentation on the problem of unplanned crossover in randomized trials. In that context, it was pointed out that the standard procedure in data analysis was to analyze according to the original randomization—an approach known as "intention to treat." That is precisely what was done here. Once a woman was randomized to mammography, she was kept in that group for purposes of analysis even if she subsequently refused screening. Despite this, we see that breast cancer deaths are much higher in the control group than in the study group.

Fig. 18.16 shows 5-year case-fatality in the women who developed breast cancer in both groups. The case-fatality in the control group was 40%. In the *total study group* (women who were randomized to receive mammography, regardless of whether or not they were actually screened) the case-fatality was 29%. Shapiro and coworkers then divided this group into those who were screened and those who refused screening. In those who refused screening, the case-fatality was 35%. In those who were screened, the case-fatality was 23%.

Shapiro and colleagues then compared survival in women whose breast cancer was detected at the screening examination with that in women whose breast cancer was identified between screening examinations (i.e., no breast cancer was identified at screening, and before the next examination a year later, the women had symptoms that led to the diagnosis of breast cancer). If the cancer had been detected by mammography, the case-fatality was only 13%. However, if the breast cancer was an *interval case* (i.e., diagnosed between examinations), the case-fatality was 38%. What could explain this difference in case-fatality? The likely explanation

is that disease that was found between regular mammographic examinations was rapidly progressive. It was not detectable at the regular mammographic examination but was identified before the next regularly scheduled examination a year later because it was so aggressive. (Another possibility is that at least some apparent interval cases were in reality cases that had not been detected at the previous screening examination [i.e., they were false-negatives].)

These observations also support the notion discussed earlier in this chapter that a long clinical phase is likely to be associated with a long preclinical phase. Women in whom cancer findings were detected at screening had a long preclinical phase and a case-fatality of only 13%, indicating a long clinical phase as well. The women who had normal mammograms and whose disease became clinically apparent before the next examination had a short preclinical phase and, given the group's high case-fatality, also had a short clinical phase.

Fig. 18.17 shows deaths from causes *other than breast cancer* in both groups over 5 years. Mortality was much higher in those who did not come for screening than in those who did. Because the screening was only directed at breast cancer, why should those who came for screening and those who did not manifest different mortality rates for causes *other* than breast cancer? The answer is, clearly, volunteer bias—the well-documented observation that people who participate in health programs differ in many ways from those who do not: in their health status, attitudes, educational and socioeconomic levels, and other factors. This is another demonstration that for purposes of evaluating a health program, comparison of participants and nonparticipants is not a valid approach.

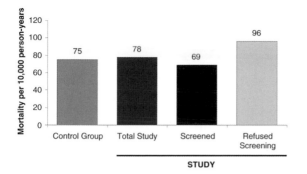

Fig. 18.17 Mortality from all causes *excluding breast cancer* per 10,000 person-years, Health Insurance Plan. (Data from Shapiro S, Venet W, Strax P, et al. Selection, follow-up, and analysis in the Health Insurance Plan Study: a randomized trial with breast cancer screening. *Natl Cancer Inst Monogr.* 1985;67:65–74.)

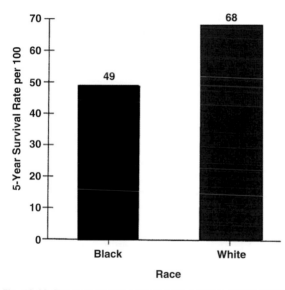

Fig. 18.18 Five-year relative survival rates, by race, among women with breast cancer diagnosed 1964–73 (Surveillance, Epidemiology, and End Results program). (Data from Shapiro S, Venet W, Strax P, et al. Prospects for eliminating racial differences in breast cancer survival rates. *Am J Public Health.* 1982;72:1142–1145.)

Before we leave our discussion of the HIP study, we might digress and mention an interesting application of these data carried out by Shapiro and coworkers.[7] Fig. 18.18 shows that, in the United States, 5-year relative survival from breast cancer is better in whites than in blacks.

The question has been raised whether this is due to a difference in the biology of the disease in blacks

and in whites or to a difference between blacks and whites in accessing health care, which may delay the diagnosis and treatment of the disease in black patients. Shapiro and colleagues recognized that the randomized trial of mammography offered an unusual opportunity to address this question. The findings are shown in Fig. 18.19. Let us first look only at the survival curves for the control group consisting of blacks and whites (see Fig. 18.19A). The data are consistent with those in Fig. 18.18: blacks and Hispanics had a worse prognosis than did whites. Now let us also look at the curves for whites and blacks in the study group of women who were screened and for whom there was therefore no difference in access to care or use of care, because screening was carried out on a predetermined schedule (see Fig. 18.19B). We see considerable overlap of the two curves: essentially no difference. This strongly suggests that the screening had eliminated the racial difference in survivorship and that the usually observed difference between the races in prognosis of breast cancer is in fact a result of poorer access to care or poorer use of care among blacks, with a consequent delay in diagnosis and treatment and hence survival.

FURTHER EXAMPLES OF STUDIES EVALUATING SCREENING

Mammography for Women 40 to 49 Years of Age

A major controversy in the 1990s centered on the question of whether mammography should be universally recommended for women in their 40s. The data from the Shapiro et al. study, as well as from other studies, established the benefit of regular mammography examinations for women 50 years and older. However, the data are less clear for women in their 40s. Many issues arise in interpreting the findings of randomized trials carried out in a number of different populations. Although a reduction of mortality has been estimated at 17% for women in their 40s who have annual mammograms, the data available are generally from studies that were not specifically designed to assess possible benefits in this age group. Moreover, many of the trials recruited women in their *late* 40s, suggesting the possibility that even if there are observed benefits, they could have resulted just as well from mammograms performed when they would have been aged 50 years or older.

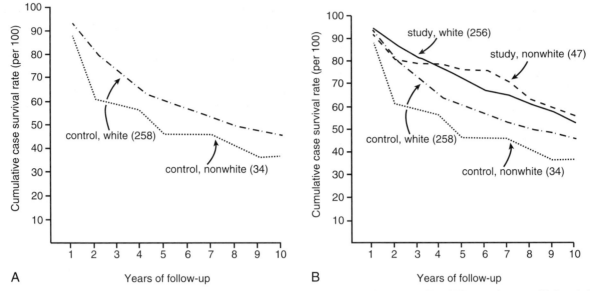

Fig. 18.19 (A) Cumulative case-survival rates, first 10 years after diagnosis by race, Health Insurance Plan (HIP) control groups. (B) Cumulative case-survival rates, first 10 years after diagnosis by race, HIP study and control groups. (From Shapiro S, Venet W, Strax P, et al. Prospects for eliminating racial differences in breast cancer survival rates. *Am J Public Health.* 1982;72:1142–1145.)

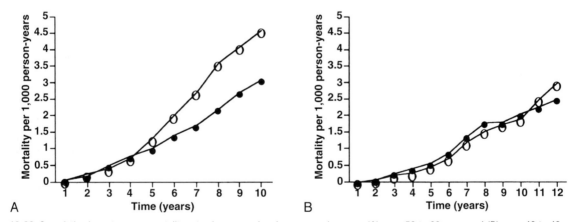

Fig. 18.20 Cumulative breast cancer mortality rates in screened and unscreened women (A) ages 50 to 69 years and (B) ages 40 to 49 years. ● = screened; ○ = unscreened. (From Kerlikowske K. Efficacy of screening mammography among women aged 40 to 49 years and 50 to 69 years: comparison of relative and absolute benefit. *Natl Cancer Inst Monogr.* 1997;22:79–86. [A] Modified from Tabar L, Fagerberg G, Duffy SW, et al. Update of the Swedish two-county program of mammographic screening for breast cancer. *Radiol Clin North Am.* 1992;30:187–210. [B] Modified from Nystrom L, Rutqvist LE, Wall S, et al. Breast cancer screening with mammography: overview of Swedish randomized trials. *Lancet.* 1993;341:973–978.)

A related issue is seen in Fig. 18.20. When mortality over time is compared in screened and unscreened women *50 years of age or older* (see Fig. 18.20A), the mortality curves diverge at approximately 4 years after enrollment, with the mammography group showing a lower mortality that persists over time. However, when screened and unscreened *women in their 40s* are compared (see Fig. 18.20B), the mortality curves do not suggest any differences in mortality for at least 11 to 12 years after enrollment. Further follow-up will be needed to determine if the divergence observed in the mortality curves would actually persist and represent a true benefit to women who have had mammograms in their 40s. However, interpreting these curves is complicated because women who have been followed for 10 or more years in these studies would have passed age 50. Consequently, even if mortality in screened women declines after 11 years, any such benefit observed could be due to mammograms that were performed *after* age 50 rather than to mammograms in their 40s. Further follow-up of women enrolled in many of these studies, and in newly initiated studies that are enrolling women in their early 40s, may help to clarify these issues.

In 1997 a consensus panel was created by the National Institutes of Health (lead by Professor Gordis) to review the scientific evidence for benefits of mammography in women ages 40 to 49. The panel concluded that the data available *did not* warrant a universal recommendation for mammography for all women in their 40s. The panel recommended that each woman should decide for herself (in consultation with her physician) whether to undergo mammography.[8] Her decision may be based not only on an objective analysis of the scientific evidence and consideration of her individual medical history, but also on how she perceives and weighs each potential risk and benefit, the values she places on each, and how she deals with uncertainty. Given both the importance and the complexity of the issues involved in assessing the evidence, a woman should have access to the best possible relevant information regarding both benefits and risks, presented in an understandable and usable form.

Most women will depend heavily on the knowledge and sophistication of their physicians rather than make the decision themselves on when to commence screening mammography. One important problem in this regard is that many physicians do not have sufficient knowledge of cancer screening statistics to provide the support needed by women and their families to carefully examine the results and conclusions, as well as the validity, of studies of mammography for women in their 40s. A study by Wegwarth and coauthors gave results of a national survey of primary care physicians in the United States and found that most primary care physicians mistakenly interpreted improved survival and increased detection with screening as evidence that screening saves lives. Few correctly recognized that reduced mortality in a randomized trial constitutes evidence of benefit of screening.[9]

The consensus panel added that for women in their 40s who choose to have mammography performed, the costs of the mammograms should be reimbursed by third-party payers or covered by HMOs so that financial impediments will not influence a woman's decision as to whether or not to have a mammogram. The recommendations of the panel were rejected by the National Cancer Institute, which had itself originally requested creation of the panel, and by other agencies. There were clear indications that strong political forces were operating at that time in favor of mammography for women in their 40s.

The controversy over mammography became an even broader one with the 2001 publication of a review by Olsen and Gøtzsche of the evidence supporting mammography *at any age*.[10] Among the issues raised by the investigators were concerns about possible inadequacy of some of the randomizations; possible unreliability of assessment of cause of death; their finding that in some trials exclusions of women from the studies were carried out after randomization had taken place and women with preexisting cancer were excluded only from the screened groups; and their assessment that the two best trials failed to find any benefit.

An accompanying *Lancet* editorial concluded by saying: "At present, there is no reliable evidence from large randomized trials to support screening mammography programmes."[11] A 2004 article countered the arguments raised by Olsen and Gøtzsche and concluded that the prior consensus on mammography was correct.[12]

However, the controversy continues unabated. In 2002 the US Preventive Services Task Force reviewed the evidence and recommended screening mammography every 1 to 2 years for women 40 years of age and older. Using an earlier version of the methodology than that described in Chapter 14, they classified the supporting evidence as "fair" on a scale of "good," "fair," or "poor."[13] In 2009 this task force again reviewed the question of mammography for women in their 40s and recommended that women aged 50 to 74 years should have screening mammography every 2 years, but they also concluded as follows: "For biennial screening mammography in women aged 40 to 49 years, there is moderate certainty that the net benefit is small." The task force gave its recommendation a "C" grade and pointed out that this grade is a recommendation against routine screening of women aged 40 to 49 years. They added, "The Task Force encourages individualized, informed decision making about when [at what age] to start mammography screening."[14] The "C" grade was confirmed in a more recent recommendation statement from the task force.[15]

In 2007 the American College of Physicians published new guidelines about mammography for women in their 40s, based on an extensive systematic review that addressed both benefits and potential harms.[16,17] The group concluded that the evidence of net benefit is *less clear* for women in their 40s than for women in their 50s and that mammography carries significant risks, saying: "We don't think the evidence supports a blanket recommendation." In 2011 the National Health Service in the United Kingdom issued its guidelines recommending that women aged 47 to 73 years undergo mammography every 3 years.[18]

In 2015 the American Cancer Society (ACS) updated its guidelines for breast cancer screening for women at "average risk."[19] The ACS recommended starting screening at age 45 years, with annual screening through age 54, after which biennial screening should be considered. As is clear, this is not an area where science, epidemiology, and public policy are totally aligned!

Thus the controversy between proponents and critics continues and is not likely to be settled to everyone's satisfaction by expert pronouncements. The problems in methodology and interpretation are complex and will probably not be resolved by further large trials. Such trials are difficult and expensive to initiate and conduct, and because of the time needed to complete them, these trials are also limited in that the findings often do not reflect the most recent improvements in mammographic technology. However, with so much of the data equivocal and a focus of controversy, progress will most likely come from new technologies for detecting breast cancer. Meanwhile, women are left with a decision-making challenge regarding their own choices concerning mammography, given the major uncertainties in the available evidence.

Screening for Cervical Cancer

Perhaps no screening test for cancer has historically been used more widely than the Pap smear. One would therefore assume that there has been overwhelming evidence of its effectiveness in reducing mortality from invasive cervical cancer. Unfortunately, there has never been a properly designed randomized, controlled trial of cervical cancer screening; there probably never will be, because cervical cancer screening has been accepted as effective for the early detection of cervical cancer both by health authorities and by women.

In the absence of randomized trials, several alternative approaches have been used. Perhaps the most frequent evaluation design has been to compare incidence and mortality rates in populations with different rates of screening. A second approach has been to examine changes over time in rates of diagnosis of carcinoma in situ. A third approach has been that of case-control studies in which women with invasive cervical cancer are compared with control women and the frequency of past Pap smears is examined in both groups. All of these studies are generally affected by the methodologic problems raised previously in this chapter. Given the recognition that HPV is in the causal chain to cervical cancer, prevention currently recommends HPV testing along with Pap testing. The ACS recommends starting screening at age 21 with annual Pap tests (either conventional cytology or liquid based), with HPV testing started at age 30 or the use of high-risk HPV screening alone.[20] However, even for high risk HPV types, infection may revert after HPV screening alone, resulting in a large number of false-positives. Accordingly, the US Preventive Services Task Force recommends screening in women aged 21 to 65 years with cytology (Pap test) every 3 years or, for women aged 30 to 65 years who want a less frequent screening, cytology combined with HPV every 5 years.[4]

Despite these reservations, the evidence indicates that many carcinomas in situ probably do progress to invasive cancer; consequently, early detection of cervical cancer in the in situ stage would result in a significant saving of life, even if it is lower than many optimistic estimates. Much of the uncertainty we face regarding screening for cervical cancer stems from the fact that no well-designed randomized trial was initially carried out before it became part of routine medical practice. This observation points out that in the United States, a set of standards must be met before new pharmacologic agents are licensed for human use, but another, less stringent, set of standards is used for new technology or new health programs. No drug would be licensed in the United States without evaluation through randomized, controlled trials, but unfortunately no such evaluation is required before screening or other types of programs and procedures are introduced. Of course, if universal prevention of HPV through vaccination of presexually active adolescents was applied, cervical cancer would end!

Screening for Neuroblastoma

Some of the issues just discussed are encountered in screening for neuroblastoma, which is a tumor that occurs in young children. The rationale for screening for neuroblastoma was outlined by Tuchman and colleagues[21]: (1) Outcome has improved little in the past several decades. (2) Prognosis is known to be better in children who manifest the disease before the age of 1 year. (3) At any age, children in advanced stages of disease have worse prognoses than those in early stages. (4) More than 90% of children presenting with clinical symptoms of neuroblastoma excrete higher than normal amounts of catecholamines in their urine. (5) These metabolites can easily be measured in urine samples obtained from diapers.

These facts constitute a strong rationale for neuroblastoma screening. Fig. 18.21 shows data from Japan, where a major effort at neuroblastoma screening was mounted. The percentages of children younger than 1 year in whom neuroblastoma was detected were compared before and after initiation of screening in Sapporo, a city in Hokkaido, and these data were compared with birth data from the rest of Hokkaido, where no screening program was mounted. After initiation of screening, a greater percentage of cases of neuroblastoma in children younger than 1 year was detected in Sapporo than in the rest of Hokkaido.

However, a number of serious problems arise in assessing the benefits of neuroblastoma screening. It is now clear that neuroblastoma is a biologically heterogeneous disease, and there is clearly a better prognosis from the start in some cases than in others. Many tumors have a good prognosis because they regress spontaneously, even without treatment. Furthermore, screening is most likely to detect slow-growing, less malignant tumors and is less likely to detect aggressive, fast-growing tumors.

Thus it is difficult to show that screening for neuroblastomas is, in fact, beneficial. In fact, two large studies of neuroblastoma screening appeared in 2002. Woods and colleagues[22] studied 476,654 children in Quebec, Canada. Screening was offered to all the children at ages 3 weeks and 6 months. Mortality from neuroblastoma up to 8 years of age among children screened in Quebec was no lower than among four unscreened cohorts (Table 18.1) and no lower than in the rest of Canada, excluding

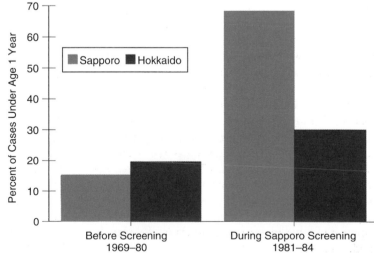

Fig. 18.21 Percentage of neuroblastoma cases younger than 1 year in Sapporo and Hokkaido, Japan, before and after screening. (Modified from Goodman SN. Neuroblastoma screening data: an epidemiologic analysis. *Am J Dis Child.* 1991;145:1415–1422; Based on data from Nishi M, Miyake H, Takeda T, et al. Effects of the mass screening of neuroblastoma in Sapporo City. *Cancer.* 1987;60:433–436. Copyright © 1987 American Cancer Society. Reprinted by permission of Wiley-Liss, Inc., a subsidiary of John Wiley & Sons, Inc.)

TABLE 18.1 Rate of Death From Neuroblastoma by 8 Years of Age in the Screened Quebec Cohort, as Compared With the Rates in Four Unscreened Cohorts

Control Cohort	No. of Deaths Expected in Quebec Based on the Control Cohort	Standardized Mortality Ratio for Quebec (95% CI)
Ontario	19.8	1.11 (0.64–1.92)
Minnesota	24.4	0.90 (0.48–1.70)
Florida	15.7	1.40 (0.81–2.41)
Greater Delaware Valley	22.8	0.96 (0.56–1.66)

There were 22 deaths due to neuroblastoma in the screened Quebec cohort.

CI, Confidence interval.

From Woods WG, Gao R, Shuster JJ, et al. Screening of infants and mortality due to neuroblastoma. *N Engl J Med.* 2002;346:1041–1046.

TABLE 18.2 Rate of Death From Neuroblastoma by 8 Years of Age in the Screened Quebec Cohort, as Compared With the Rates in Unscreened Canadian Cohorts

Control Cohort	No. of Deaths Expected in Quebec Based on the Control Cohort	Standardized Mortality Ratio for Quebec (95% CI)
Historical Cohorts		
Quebec	22.5	0.98 (0.54–1.77)
Canada	21.2	1.04 (0.64–1.69)
Concurrent Cohort		
Canada, excluding Quebec	15.8	1.39 (0.85–2.30)

There were 22 deaths from neuroblastoma in the screened cohort. All data were collected by Statistics Canada.

CI, Confidence interval.

From Woods WG, Gao R, Shuster JJ, et al. Screening of infants and mortality due to neuroblastoma. *N Engl J Med.* 2002;346:1041–1046.

Quebec, and in two historical cohorts (Table 18.2). Schilling and colleagues[23] studied 2,581,188 children in Germany who were offered screening at 1 year of age. They found that neuroblastoma screening did not reduce the incidence of disseminated disease and did not appear to reduce mortality from the disease, although mortality follow-up was not yet complete. Thus the data currently available do not support screening for neuroblastoma. The findings in these studies demonstrate the importance of understanding the biology and natural history of the disease and the need to obtain relevant and rigorous evidence regarding the potential benefits or lack of benefits when screening for any disease is being considered. The ability to detect a disease by screening cannot be equated with a demonstration of benefit to those screened.

Problems in Assessing the Sensitivity and Specificity of Screening Tests

New screening programs are often initiated after a screening test first becomes available. When such a test is developed, claims are often made—by manufacturers of test kits, investigators, or others—that the test has high sensitivity and a high specificity. However, as we shall see, from a practical standpoint, this may often be difficult to demonstrate.

Fig. 18.22A shows a 2 × 2 table, as we have seen in earlier chapters, tabulating reality (disease present or absent) against test results (positive or negative).

To calculate sensitivity and specificity, data are needed in all four cells. However, often only those with positive test results (*a* + *b*) (seen in the *upper row* of the figure) are sent for further testing. Data for those who test negative (*c* + *d*) are frequently not available, because these patients do not receive further testing. For example, as shown in Fig. 18.22B, the Western blot test serves as a gold standard for detecting human immunodeficiency virus (HIV) infection, and those with positive enzyme-linked immunosorbent assay (ELISA) results are sent for Western blot testing.

However, because those with negative ELISA results are generally not tested further, the data needed in the lower cells for calculating sensitivity and specificity of the ELISA are often not available from routine testing. To obtain such data, it is essential that some negative ELISA specimens also be sent for further testing, together with the ELISA-positive specimens.

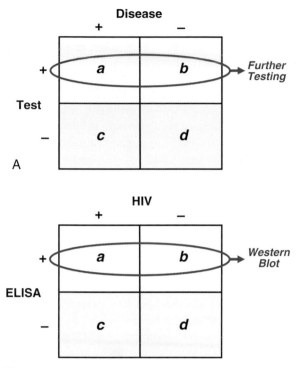

Fig. 18.22 (A) Problem of establishing sensitivity and specificity because of limited follow-up of those with negative test results. (B) Problem of establishing sensitivity and specificity because of limited follow-up of those with negative test results for human immunodeficiency virus (HIV) using the enzyme-linked immunosorbent assay (ELISA) test.

Interpreting Study Results That Show No Benefit of Screening

In this chapter, we have stressed the interpretation of results that show a difference between screened and unscreened groups. However, if we are unable to demonstrate a benefit from early detection of disease, any of the following interpretations may be possible:

1. The apparent lack of benefit may be inherent in the natural history of the disease (e.g., the disease has no detectable preclinical phase or an extremely short detectable preclinical phase).
2. The therapeutic intervention currently available may not be any more effective when it is provided earlier than when it is provided at the time of usual diagnosis.

3. The natural history and currently available therapies may have the potential for enhanced benefit, but inadequacies of the care provided to those who screen positive may account for the observed lack of benefit (i.e., there is efficacy but poor effectiveness).

Cost-Benefit Analysis of Screening

Some people respond to cost-benefit issues by concentrating only on cost, asking, if the test is inexpensive, why not perform it? However, although the test for blood in the stool, for example, in screening for colon cancer, costs only a few dollars for the filter paper kit and the necessary laboratory processing, to calculate the total cost of such a test we must include the cost of the colonoscopies that are done after the initial testing for those who are detected as "positive," as well as the cost of the complications that infrequently result from colonoscopy.

The balance of cost effectiveness includes not only financial costs but also nonfinancial costs to the patient, including anxiety, emotional distress, and inconvenience. Is the test itself invasive? Even if it is not, if the test result is positive, is invasive therapy warranted by the test result? What is the false-positive rate in such tests? In what proportion of persons will invasive tests be carried out or anxiety be generated despite the reality that the individuals do not have the disease in question? Thus the "cost" of a test is not only the cost of the test procedure but also the cost of the entire follow-up process that is set in motion by a positive result, even if it turns out to be a false-positive result. These considerations are reflected in the four major concerns voiced by the ACS in revising its guidelines for cancer screening (Box 18.3).[24]

Another view of cost-benefit was presented by Elmore and Choe.[25] In discussing screening mammography for women aged 40 to 49, they wrote:

Here's one way to explain the evidence (with the caveat that numbers are rounded and simplified): For every 10,000 women who receive regular screening mammography starting at age 40 years, 6 of them might benefit through a decreased risk for death due to breast cancer. Yet even this modest benefit requires multiple screening examinations and follow-up for all 10,000

BOX 18.3 CRITERIA USED BY THE AMERICAN CANCER SOCIETY FOR RECOMMENDATIONS ON CANCER-RELATED CHECKUPS

1. There must be good evidence that each test or procedure recommended is medically effective in reducing morbidity or mortality.
2. The medical benefits must outweigh the risks.
3. The cost of each test or procedure must be reasonable compared with its expected benefits.
4. The recommended actions must be practical and feasible.

women for more than a decade. Stated another way, 9,994 women receive no mortality benefit at all, because most women will not develop breast cancer and some women will have cancer detected when it is too late for a cure.[25]

Conclusion

This chapter has reviewed some of the major sources of bias that must be taken into account in assessing study findings that compare screened and unscreened populations. The biases of selection for screening and prognostic selection can be addressed, in large part, by using a randomized, controlled trial as the study design. Reasonable estimates of the lead time can be made if appropriate information is available. Few of the methods that are currently used to detect disease early have been subjected to evaluation by randomized trials, and most are probably not destined to be studied in this way. This is a result of several factors, including the difficulty and expense associated with conducting such studies and the ethical issues inherent in randomizing a population to receive or not receive modalities of care that are widely used and considered effective, even in the absence of strong supporting evidence. Consequently, we are obliged to maximize our use of evidence from nonrandomized approaches, and to do so, the potential biases and problems addressed in this chapter must be considered.

In approaching programs for early disease detection, we need to be able to identify groups who are at high risk. This would include not only those at risk for developing the disease in question but also those who are "at risk" for benefiting from the intervention. These are the groups for whom cost-benefit calculations will favor benefit. We must keep in mind that, even if a screening test, such as a Pap smear, is not in itself overly invasive, the intervention mandated by a positive screening test result may be highly invasive.

The overriding issue is how to make decisions when our data are inconclusive, inconsistent, or incomplete. We face this dilemma regularly, both in clinical practice and in the development of public health policy. These decisions must first consider the existing body of relevant scientific evidence. However, in the final analysis, the decision whether or not to screen a population for a disease is a *value judgment* that should take into account the incidence and severity of the disease, the feasibility of detecting the disease early, the likelihood of intervening effectively in those with positive screening results, and the overall cost-benefit calculation for an early detection program.

To improve our ability to make appropriate decisions, additional knowledge is needed regarding the natural history of disease and, specifically, regarding the definition of characteristics of individuals who are at risk for a poor outcome. Before new screening programs are introduced, we should argue strongly for well-conducted randomized, controlled trials, so that we will not be operating in an atmosphere of uncertainty at the time in the future when such trials have become virtually impossible to conduct. Nevertheless, given the fact that most medical and public health practices—including early detection of disease—have not been subjected to randomized trials and that decisions regarding early detection must be made on the basis of incomplete and equivocal data, it is essential that we as health professionals appreciate and understand the methodologic issues involved so that we can make the wisest use of the available knowledge on behalf of our patients. Even the best of intentions and passionate evangelism cannot substitute for rigorous evidence that supports or does not support the benefit of screening.

REFERENCES

1. Whittier JG, from Maud Muller: *The Panorama, and Other Poems.* Boston, Ticknor and Fields, 1856.
2. Harte B, from *"Mrs. Judge Jenkins: Sequel to Maud Muller" East and West Poems.* Boston, James R. Osgood and Company, 1871.
3. Hutchison GB. Evaluation of preventive services. *J Chronic Dis.* 1960;11:497–508.
4. Moyer VA, on behalf of the U.S. Preventive Services Task Force. Screening for lung cancer: U.S. Preventive Services Task

Force Recommendation Statement. *Ann Intern Med.* 2014;160: 330–338.

5. Szklo M, Nieto FJ. *Epidemiology: Beyond the Basics.* 3rd ed. Burlington, MA: Jones & Bartlett; 2014:141–145.

6. Shapiro S, Venet W, Strax P, et al, eds. *Periodic Screening for Breast Cancer: The Health Insurance Plan Project and Its Sequelae, 1963–1986.* Baltimore: Johns Hopkins University Press; 1988.

7. Shapiro S, Venet W, Strax P, et al. Prospects for eliminating racial differences in breast cancer survival rates. *Am J Public Health.* 1982;72:1142–1145.

8. *Breast Cancer Screening for Women Ages 40–49.* NIH Consensus Statement Online, 1997 January 21–23, cited 15:1–35, 2007.

9. Wegwarth O, Schwartz LM, Woloshin S, et al. Do physicians understand cancer screening statistics? A national survey of primary care physicians in the United States. *Ann Intern Med.* 2012;156:340–349.

10. Olsen O, Gøtzsche C. Cochrane review on screening for breast cancer with mammography. *Lancet.* 2001;358:1340–1342.

11. Horton R. Screening mammography: an overview revisited. *Lancet.* 2001;358:1284–1285.

12. Freedman DA, Petitti DB, Robins JM. On the efficacy of screening for breast cancer. *Int J Epidemiol.* 2004;33:43–55.

13. U.S. Preventive Services Task Force. Breast cancer screening: a summary of the evidence for the U.S. Preventive Services Task Force. *Ann Intern Med.* 2002;137:347–360.

14. U.S. Preventive Services Task Force. Breast cancer: screening; July 2010. http://www.uspreventiveservicestaskforce.org/uspstf09/breastcancer/brcanrs.htm. Accessed June 14, 2013.

15. Siu AL, on behalf of the U.S. Preventive Services Task Force. Screening for breast cancer: US Preventive Services Task Force recommendation statement. *Ann Intern Med.* 2016;164: 279–296.

16. Brewer NT, Salz T, Lillie SE. Systematic review: the long-term effects of false-positive mammograms. *Ann Intern Med.* 2007;146:502–510.

17. Qaseem A, Snow V, Sherif K, et al. Screening mammography for women 40 to 49 years of age: a clinical practice guideline from the American College of Physicians. *Ann Intern Med.* 2007;146:511–515.

18. Warner E. Breast-cancer screening. *N Engl J Med.* 2011;365: 1025–1032.

19. Oeffinger KC, Fontham ETH, Etzioni R, et al. Breast cancer screening for women at average risk. 2015 Guideline update from the American Cancer Society. *JAMA.* 2015;314(15):1599–1614.

20. American Cancer Society. *The American Cancer Society Guidelines for the Prevention and Early Detection of Cervical Cancer.* https://www.cancer.org/cancer/cervical-cancer/prevention-and-early-detection/cervical-cancer-screening-guidelines.html. Accessed February 20, 2018.

21. Tuchman M, Lemieux B, Woods WG. Screening for neuroblastoma in infants: investigate or implement? *Pediatrics.* 1990;86:791–793.

22. Woods WG, Gao R, Shuster JJ, et al. Screening of infants and mortality due to neuroblastoma. *N Engl J Med.* 2002;346:1041–1046.

23. Schilling FH, Spix C, Berthold F, et al. Neuroblastoma screening at one year of age. *N Engl J Med.* 2002;346:1047–1053.

24. Smith RA, Mettlin CJ, David KJ, et al. American Cancer Society guidelines for the early detection of cancer. *CA Cancer J Clin.* 2000;50:34–49.

25. Elmore JG, Choe JH. Breast cancer screening for women in their 40s: moving from controversy about data to helping individual women. *Ann Intern Med.* 2007;146:529–531.

REVIEW QUESTIONS FOR CHAPTER 18

Questions 1 through 4 are based on the following information:

A new screening program was instituted in a certain country. The program used a screening test that is effective in detecting cancer Z at an early stage. Assume that there is no effective treatment for this type of cancer and therefore that the program results in no change in the usual course of the disease. Assume also that the rates noted are calculated from all known cases of cancer Z and that there were no changes in the quality of death certification of this disease.

1 *What will happen to the apparent* incidence rate *of cancer Z in the country during the first year of this program?*
   a. Incidence rate will increase
   b. Incidence rate will decrease
   c. Incidence rate will remain constant

2 *What will happen to the apparent* prevalence rate *of cancer Z in the country during the first year of this program?*
   a. Prevalence rate will increase
   b. Prevalence rate will decrease
   c. Prevalence rate will remain constant

3 *What will happen to the apparent* case-fatality *for cancer Z in the country during the first year of this program?*
   a. Case-fatality will increase
   b. Case-fatality will decrease
   c. Case-fatality will remain constant

4 *What will happen to the apparent* mortality rate *from cancer Z in the country as a result of the program?*
   a. Mortality rate will increase
   b. Mortality rate will decrease
   c. Mortality rate will remain constant

5 *The best index (indices) for concluding that an early detection program for breast cancer truly improves the natural history of disease, 15 years after its initiation, would be:*

a. A smaller proportionate mortality for breast cancer 15 years after initiation of the early detection program compared to the proportionate mortality prior to its initiation

b. Improved long-term survival rates for breast cancer patients (adjusted for lead time)

c. A decrease in incidence of breast cancer

d. A decrease in the prevalence of breast cancer

e. None of the above

6 *In general, screening should be undertaken for diseases with the following feature(s):*

a. Diseases with a low prevalence in identifiable subgroups of the population

b. Diseases for which case-fatality is low

c. Diseases with a natural history that can be altered by medical intervention

d. Diseases that are readily diagnosed and for which treatment efficacy has been shown to be equivocal in evidence from a number of clinical trials

e. None of the above

Question 7 is based on the information given below:

The diagram below shows the natural history of disease X:

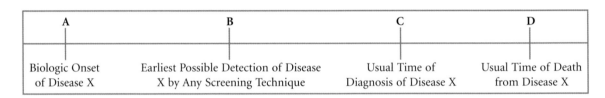

7 *Assume that early detection of disease X through screening improves prognosis. For a screening program to be most effective, at which point in the natural history in the diagram must the critical point be?*

a. Between A and B

b. Between B and C

c. Between C and D

d. Anywhere between A and C

e. Anywhere between A and D

8 *Which of the following is not a possible outcome measure that could be used as an indicator of the benefit of screening programs aimed at early detection of disease?*

a. Reduction of case-fatality in screened individuals

b. Reduction of mortality in the population screened

c. Reduction of incidence in the population screened

d. Reduction of complications

e. Improvement in the quality of life in screened individuals

Chapter 19

Epidemiology and Public Policy

All scientific work is incomplete—whether it be observational or experimental.

All scientific work is liable to be upset or modified by advancing knowledge.

That does not confer upon us a freedom to ignore the knowledge we already have, or to postpone the action that it appears to demand at a given time.[1]

—Sir Austin Bradford Hill, President's Address, Royal Society of Medicine, January 14, 1965

Experience is that marvelous thing that enables you to recognize a mistake when you make it again.[2]

—Franklin P. Jones, legendary American humorist (1908–1980)

Learning Objectives

- To review the role of epidemiology in disease prevention and to contrast two possible strategies for prevention: targeting groups at high risk for disease as compared with focusing on the general population.
- To define risk assessment and discuss the role of epidemiology in risk assessment, including measurement of possible exposures.
- To discuss how epidemiology can be used to shape public policy through the courts in the United States.
- To introduce the systematic review and meta-analysis as tools to summarize all the available epidemiologic evidence to influence public policy and to discuss how publication bias may affect the results of both systematic reviews and meta-analyses.
- To identify some possible sources of uncertainty in using the results of epidemiologic studies as a basis for making public policy.

A major role of epidemiology is to serve as a basis for developing policies that affect human health,

including primary and secondary prevention and control of disease. As seen in previous chapters, the findings from epidemiologic studies may be relevant to issues in both clinical practice and community health and to population approaches to disease prevention and health promotion. As discussed in Chapter 1, the practical applications of epidemiology are often viewed as being so integral to the discipline that they are incorporated into the very definition of epidemiology. Historically, epidemiologic investigations were initiated to address emerging challenges relating to human disease (most often communicable diseases) and the health of the public. Indeed, one of the major sources of excitement in epidemiology is the direct applicability of its findings to alleviate problems of human health. This chapter presents an overview of some issues and problems relating to epidemiology in its application in formulating and evaluating public policy.

Epidemiology and Prevention

The importance of epidemiology in prevention has been emphasized in several of the preceding chapters. Identifying populations at increased risk, ascertaining the cause(s) of their increased risk(s), and analyzing the costs and benefits of eliminating or reducing exposure to the causal factor or factors all require an understanding of basic epidemiologic concepts and of the possible interpretation of the findings of epidemiologic studies. In addition, assessing the strength of all available evidence and identifying any limits on the inferences derived or on the generalizability of the findings are critically important. Thus epidemiology is often considered to be the "basic science" of prevention.

How much epidemiologic data do we need to justify a prevention effort? Clearly there is no simple answer to this question. Some of the issues involved differ depending on whether primary or secondary prevention is being considered. If we are discussing primary prevention, the answer depends on the severity of the condition, the costs involved (in terms of dollars, human suffering, and loss of quality of life), the strength of the evidence implicating a certain causal factor or factors in the etiology of the disease in question, and the difficulty of reducing or eliminating exposure to that factor.

With secondary prevention, the issues are somewhat different. We must still consider the severity of the disease in question. In addition, however, we must ask whether we can detect the disease earlier than usual by screening and how invasive and expensive such detection would be. Additional considerations include whether a benefit accrues to a person who has the disease if treatment is initiated at an earlier-than-usual stage and whether there are harmful effects associated with screening. Epidemiology offers valuable approaches to resolve many of these issues.

In recent years considerable attention has been addressed to expanding what has been called the traditional risk-factor model of epidemiology, in which we explore the relationship of an independent factor (exposure) to a dependent factor (disease outcome) (Fig. 19.1). It has been suggested that this approach should be expanded in two ways: First, it should include measurement not only of the adverse outcome—the disease itself—but also of the economic, social, and psychological impacts resulting from the disease outcome on the individual, his or her family, and the wider community. Second, it is clear that exposure to a putative causal agent is generally *not* distributed uniformly in a population. The factors that determine whether a person becomes exposed must therefore be explored if prevention is to be successful in reducing the exposure (Fig. 19.2). The full model is even more complex, as seen in Fig. 19.3: The relationship is influenced by *determinants of susceptibility* of the individual to the exposure; these include genetic factors

together with environmental influences and social determinants. Although such an expanded approach is intuitively attractive and provides an excellent framework in which to analyze public health problems, we still have to demonstrate whether certain exposures or other independent variables are associated with increased risks of specific diseases.

In any case, deciding how much data and what types of data we need for prevention will be societally driven, reflecting society's values and priorities. Epidemiology, together with other disciplines, can provide

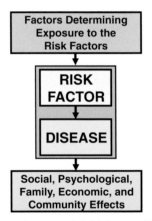

Fig. 19.2 Diagram of an expanded risk-factor epidemiology model to include determinants of exposure as well as social, psychological, family, economic, and community effects of the disease.

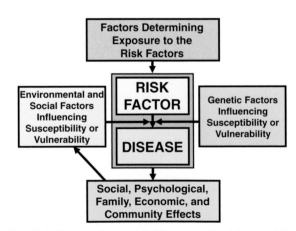

Fig. 19.3 Diagram of expanded risk-factor epidemiology model to include interrelationships of factors that determine susceptibility or vulnerability.

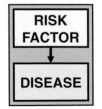

Fig. 19.1 Diagram of classic risk-factor epidemiology.

much of the necessary scientific data that are relevant to addressing questions of risks and prevention. However, the final decision on initiating or sustaining a prevention program will be largely determined by economic and political considerations as well as societal values. At the same time, it is hoped that such decisions will also be based on a firm foundation of scientific evidence provided by epidemiology and other relevant disciplines.

It is important to distinguish between *macroenvironmental* and *microenvironmental* exposures. Macroenvironmental exposures are exposures to things such as air pollution, which affect populations or entire communities. Microenvironmental exposures are environmental factors that affect a specific individual, such as diet (and the availability of healthy foods), smoking (by the individual or exposure to secondhand smoke), and alcohol consumption (personally and the availability of alcohol in the community). From the prevention standpoint, macroenvironmental factors are in many ways easier to control and modify, as this can be accomplished by legislation and regulation (e.g., setting environmental standards for pollutants). In contrast, modification of microenvironmental factors depends on modifying individual habits and lifestyle

and addressing the availability of healthy food, green space, and safe neighborhoods, which can often be a much greater challenge.

In dealing with microenvironmental factors, providing scientific evidence and risk estimates is frequently not enough to induce individuals to modify their lifestyles (e.g., stopping smoking). Individuals often differ in the extent to which they are willing to take risks in many aspects of their lives, including health. In addition, the behaviors of individuals may differ depending on whether they are confronted with the risk of an adverse outcome or the probability of a positive event (Fig. 19.4). In addition, individuals often place the blame elsewhere for health problems brought on by their own lifestyles. Thus risk communication, mentioned previously, must extend beyond communicating risk data to policy makers. It must also deal with communicating with the public in an understandable fashion in the context of people's perceptions of their risk, so that individuals will be motivated to accept responsibility and act on behalf of their own health to the greatest extent possible. Epidemiologists should therefore work with health educators to more appropriately educate the public about personal risk issues.

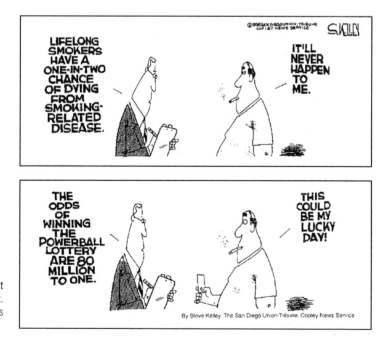

Fig. 19.4 Risk of what? How the end point may affect an individual's perception of risk and willingness to act. (Steve Kelley. © 1998 San Diego Union Tribune. Copley News Service.)

Population Approaches Versus High-Risk Approaches to Prevention

An important question in prevention is whether our approach should target groups that are known to be at high risk or whether it should extend primary prevention efforts to the general population as a whole. This issue was first brought up by Rose in 1985[3] and later amplified by Whelton in 1994[4] in a discussion of the prevention of hypertension as well as deaths from coronary heart disease (CHD).

Epidemiologic studies have demonstrated that the risk of death from CHD steadily increases with increases in both systolic and diastolic blood pressure; there is no known threshold. Fig. 19.5A and B shows the distribution of systolic blood pressures in the general population of men and women who are above 18 years of age in the United States (2001–2008), respectively.

Looking at the US general population above 50 years of age, Fig. 19.5C shows the risk of a composite end point of first occurrence of all-cause death, nonfatal myocardial infarction, or nonfatal stroke in relation to systolic blood pressure; the risk increases steadily with

higher levels of systolic blood pressure. Individuals below 60 years of age with systolic blood pressures of 160 mm Hg had more than 1.50 times the risk of the composite CHD end point than those whose systolic blood pressure was below 140 mm Hg.

Based on the Joint National Committee on the Prevention, Detection, Evaluation and Treatment of High Blood Pressure (JNC 7), values as low as those defining prehypertension (systolic and diastolic blood pressures ranging from 120 to 139 mm Hg and 80 to 99 mm Hg, respectively) may result in a 20% excess risk of strokes.[5]

It therefore seems reasonable to combine a high risk within a population approach: one set of preventive measures addressed to those at particularly high risk and another designed for the primary prevention of hypertension and addressed to the general population.

Such analyses can have significant implications for prevention programs. The types of preventive measures that might be used for high-risk individuals often differ from those that are applicable to the general population. Those who are at high risk and are aware that they are at high risk are more likely to tolerate more expensive,

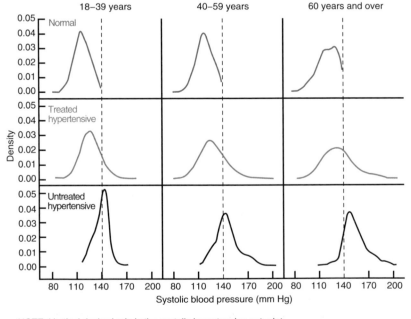

NOTE: Vertical dashed rule is the systolic hypertension cutpoint.

SOURCE: CDC/NCHS, National Health and Nutrition Examination Survey, 2001–08.

A

Fig. 19.5 (A) Mean systolic blood pressure for men aged 18 years and over, by age and hypertension status.

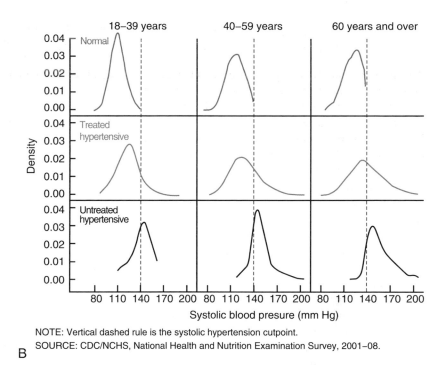

NOTE: Vertical dashed rule is the systolic hypertension cutpoint.
SOURCE: CDC/NCHS, National Health and Nutrition Examination Survey, 2001–08.

B

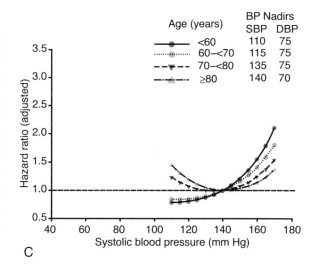

C

Fig. 19.5 cont'd (B) Mean systolic blood pressure for women aged 18 years and over, by age and hypertension status. (C) Adjusted hazard ratio of first occurrence of all-cause death, nonfatal myocardial infarction, or nonfatal stroke as a function of age (in 10-year increments), systolic blood pressure *(SBP)*. Reference systolic blood pressure for hazard ratio: 140 mm Hg, respectively. Blood pressures *(BP)* are the on-treatment average of all postbaseline recordings. The quadratic terms for systolic blood pressures were statistically significant in all age groups (all *P* < .001). The adjustment was based on sex, race, history of myocardial infarction, heart failure, peripheral vascular disease, diabetes, stroke/transient ischemic attack, renal insufficiency, and smoking. *DBP,* Diastolic blood pressure. (A and B, From Wright JD, Hughes JP, Ostchega Y, et al. Mean systolic and diastolic blood pressure in adults aged 18 and over in the United States, 2001–2008. *Natl Health Stat Report.* 2011;(35):1–22, 24. C, Modified from Denardo SJ, Gong Y, Nichols WW, et al. Blood pressure and outcomes in very old hypertensive coronary artery disease patients: an INVEST substudy. *Am J Med.* 2010;123(8):719–726.)

uncomfortable, and even more invasive procedures. However, in applying a preventive measure to a general population, the measure must have a low cost and be only minimally invasive; it needs to be associated with relatively little pain or discomfort if it is to be acceptable to the general population.

Fig. 19.6 shows the goal of a population-based strategy, which is a downward shifting of the entire curve of blood pressure distribution when a blood pressure–lowering intervention is applied to an entire community, such as reduction of the salt content of processed foods. Because the blood pressure of most

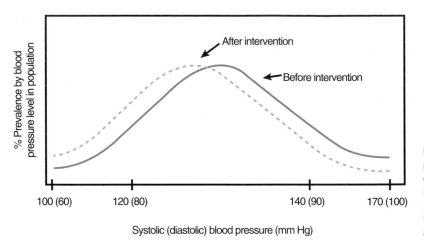

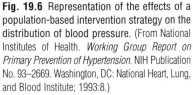

Fig. 19.6 Representation of the effects of a population-based intervention strategy on the distribution of blood pressure. (From National Institutes of Health. *Working Group Report on Primary Prevention of Hypertension.* NIH Publication No. 93–2669. Washington, DC: National Heart, Lung, and Blood Institute; 1993:8.)

members of the population is above the very lowest levels that are considered optimal, even a small downward shift (shift to the left) in the curve is likely to have major public health benefits, as Rose suggested some three decades ago.[3] In fact, such a shift would prevent more strokes in the population than would successful treatment limited to "high-risk" individuals. Furthermore, Rose[3] pointed out that the high-risk strategy is essential to protecting susceptible individuals. Ultimately, however, our hope is to understand the basic cause of the incidence of a disease—in this case, elevated blood pressure—and to develop and implement the necessary means for its (primary) prevention. Rose concluded as follows:

Realistically, many diseases will long continue to call for both approaches, and fortunately competition between them is usually unnecessary. Nevertheless, the priority of concern should always be the discovery and control of the causes of incidence.[3]

Epidemiology and Clinical Medicine: Hormone Replacement Therapy in Postmenopausal Women

Epidemiology can also be considered a basic science of clinical investigation. Data obtained from epidemiologic studies are essential in clinical decision making in many situations. An understanding of epidemiology is crucial to the process of designing meaningful studies of the natural history of disease, the quality of different diagnostic methods, and the effectiveness of clinical interventions. Epidemiology is highly relevant to addressing the many uncertainties and dilemmas in clinical policy, not all of which can easily be resolved.

A dramatic example is the use of hormone replacement therapy (HRT) by postmenopausal women. In 1966 Robert Wilson, a physician, published a book titled *Feminine Forever*, which advocated HRT for postmenopausal women. After the publication of this book, millions of postmenopausal women began taking estrogens in the hope of retaining their youth and attractiveness and avoiding the unpleasant, often encountered symptoms of menopause, such as hot flashes, night sweats, and vaginal dryness. The medical community largely accepted Wilson's recommendation for estrogen replacement, and even gynecology textbooks supported it. However, in the 1970s, an increased risk of uterine cancer was reported in women taking estrogen replacement. As a result, estrogen was subsequently combined with progestin, which counteracts the effect of estrogen on the uterine endometrial lining. This combination leads to monthly uterine bleeding that resembles a normal menstrual period.

A number of nonrandomized observational studies subsequently appeared and reported other health benefits, such as fewer heart attacks and strokes, less osteoporosis, and fewer hip fractures associated with HRT. Considering the entire body of evidence that had accumulated, support for the conclusion that estrogen protected women against heart disease appeared strong and generally consistent. Women were advised that when they reached 50 years of age, they should discuss with their physicians whether they should begin HRT to protect themselves against heart disease and other conditions associated with aging.

Recognizing that there was little supporting evidence from randomized trials using hard disease end points, such as risk of myocardial infarction, two randomized trials were initiated: the Heart and Estrogen/Progestin Replacement Study (HERS) and the Women's Health Initiative (WHI). The HERS study[6] included 2,763 women with known CHD. It found that, in contrast to accepted beliefs, combination HRT *increased* women's risk of myocardial infarction during the initial years after starting therapy. The study failed to find evidence that HRT offered protection during a follow-up period of almost 7 years (Fig. 19.7).

The WHI[7] was a randomized, placebo-controlled trial of 16,608 women designed in 1991 and 1992 to evaluate HRT for the primary prevention for heart disease and other conditions common in the elderly. The planned duration of the trial was 8.5 years. One component (study arm) of the trial was a randomized, placebo-controlled investigation of estrogen plus progestin in postmenopausal women who had an intact uterus. This component of the study was stopped 3 years early because, by that time, results had shown increased risks of heart attack, stroke, breast cancer,

and blood clots (Fig. 19.8). Although the study showed a reduced incidence of osteoporosis, bone fractures, and colorectal cancer, overall the dangers from HRT outweighed the benefits.

Only about 2.5% of the enrolled women had adverse events. On the basis of the study results, it has been estimated that, annually, for every 10,000 women taking

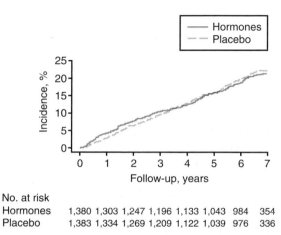

No. at risk								
Hormones	1,380	1,303	1,247	1,196	1,133	1,043	984	354
Placebo	1,383	1,334	1,269	1,209	1,122	1,039	976	336

Fig. 19.7 Kaplan-Meier estimates of the cumulative incidence of coronary heart disease events (death and nonfatal myocardial infarctions). (From Grady D, Herrington D, Bittner V, et al, for the HERS Research Group. Cardiovascular disease outcomes during 6.8 years of hormone therapy: heart and estrogen/progestin replacement study follow-up [HERS II]. *JAMA.* 2002;288:49–57.)

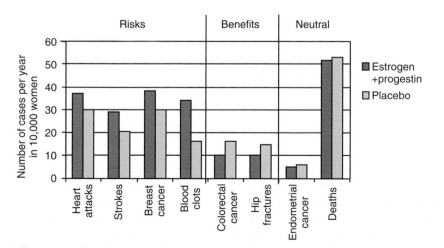

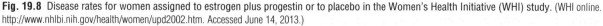

Fig. 19.8 Disease rates for women assigned to estrogen plus progestin or to placebo in the Women's Health Initiative (WHI) study. (WHI online. http://www.nhlbi.nih.gov/health/women/upd2002.htm. Accessed June 14, 2013.)

estrogen plus progestin, we would expect 7 more women to have a heart attack (37 women taking estrogen plus progestin would have a heart attack compared with 30 women taking placebo), 8 more women to have a stroke, 8 more women to have breast cancer, and 18 more women to have blood clots. At the same time, we would expect 6 fewer cases of colorectal cancer and 5 fewer hip fractures.

Many women who had been taking HRT were shocked by the results of the WHI. The findings strongly indicated that, in women taking estrogen plus progestin for protection against heart disease, the risks of cardiovascular end points were actually increased. These women were left uncertain as to whether to continue with HRT or whether to seek alternatives. Many also believed that they had been misled by the medical community because, for many years, they had been reassured about the effectiveness and safety of HRT by their physicians, *despite the absence of clear data* from placebo-controlled randomized trials. Complicating the decision-making process for women at the time of menopause is that the WHI did not address the question faced by many women who often take combination HRT for brief periods to prevent and relieve postmenopausal symptoms such as hot flashes.

A major methodologic question is why there was such a discrepancy between the results of the placebo-controlled randomized WHI study regarding risk of heart disease and the results of a large number of nonrandomized, observational studies that previously supported a protective benefit from combination HRT. This issue is of great importance because, in many areas of medicine and public health, we depend on the findings of nonrandomized, observational studies because the costs of randomized trials may be prohibitive, and randomized studies may not be feasible for other reasons.

Several explanations have been offered.[8–10] In the observational studies, the women who were prescribed HRT were often healthier women who had a better cardiovascular risk profile. Women who use HRT are often better educated, leaner, more physically active, less likely to be smokers, more health-conscious, and of higher socioeconomic status than women who do not. Often, women who were prescribed HRT were judged to be compliant, and compliers often have other healthier patterns of behavior. Thus, confounding by

lifestyle and other factors may have taken place in the observational studies. In addition, when adverse effects occurred early in the observational studies and led to the discontinuation of HRT, these events might not always have been identified in the periodic cross-sectional measurements used. An additional explanation related to cardiovascular risk is that the observational studies were conducted soon after menopause, when the beneficial effects of HRT—such as its favorable effects on lipids and endothelial function—are known to occur, whereas the WHI trial included much older women with extensive underlying atherosclerosis, among whom there is a predominance of the prothrombotic and inflammatory effects of HRT.[11]

Clearly in the future it will be essential to address these issues when nonrandomized observational studies are used as the basis for clinical guidelines development and dissemination and setting new public health policies.

Risk Assessment

A major use of epidemiology in relation to public policy is for risk assessment. Risk assessment has been defined as the characterization of the potential adverse health effects of human exposures to environmental hazards. Risk assessment is thus viewed as part of an overall process that flows from research to risk assessment and then to risk management, as shown in Fig. 19.9. Samet and colleagues[12] reviewed the relationship of epidemiology to risk assessment and described risk management as involving the evaluation of alternative regulatory actions and the selection of the strategy to be applied. Risk management is followed by risk communication, which is the communication of the findings of risk assessment to those who need to know the findings in order to participate in policy making and to take appropriate risk-management actions, including communications to the public at large.

The National Research Council (1983) listed four steps in the process of risk assessment[13]:

1. *Hazard identification:* Determination of whether a particular chemical is causally linked to particular health effects
2. *Dose-response assessment:* Determination of the relationship between the magnitude of exposure

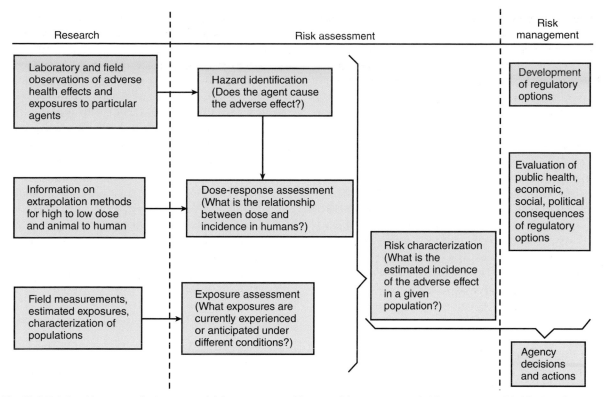

Fig. 19.9 Relationships among the four steps of risk assessment and between risk assessment and risk management. (Modified from Committee on the Institutional Means for Assessment of Risks to Public Health, Commission on Life Sciences, National Research Council. *Risk Assessment in the Federal Government: Managing the Process.* Washington, DC: National Academy Press; 1983:21.)

and the probability of occurrence of the health effects in question

3. *Exposure assessment:* Determination of the extent of human exposure before or after the application of regulatory controls

4. *Risk characterization:* Description of the nature—and often the magnitude—of human risk, including attendant uncertainty

Clearly epidemiologic data are essential in each of these steps, although epidemiology is not the only relevant scientific discipline in the process of risk assessment. In particular, toxicology plays a major role as well, and an important challenge remains to reconcile epidemiologic and toxicologic data when findings from the respective disciplines disagree.

A number of important methodologic problems affect the use of epidemiology in risk assessment. Because epidemiologic studies may address the relationship

BOX 19.1 SOURCES OF EXPOSURE DATA

1. Interviews
   a. Subject
   b. Surrogate
2. Employment or other records
3. Physician records
4. Hospital records
5. Disease registry records (e.g., cancer registries)
6. Death certificates

between an environmental exposure and the risk of a disease, rigorous assessment of each variable is critical. Perhaps the most significant problem is the assessment of exposures.

ASSESSMENT OF EXPOSURE

Data regarding exposure generally come from several types of sources (Box 19.1). Each type of source has advantages and disadvantages; the latter include lack of completeness and biases in reporting. Frequently investigators use several sources of information regarding exposure, but a problem often results when different sources yield conflicting information.

Another problem in exposure assessment is that macroenvironmental factors generally affect many individuals simultaneously, so that individual exposures may be difficult to measure. As a result, ecologic approaches are often chosen, in which aggregate rather than individual measurements are used (described in Chapter 7), and the aggregation is often carried out over large areas and populations. The characteristics of the community are therefore ascribed to the individuals residing in that community, but the validity of characterizing an individual exposure by this process is often open to question (recall the "ecological fallacy"). Furthermore, personal exposure histories can be quite difficult to obtain either retrospectively or prospectively and may be subject to considerable measurement error. In addition, the long latent or induction period between exposure and development of disease makes it necessary to ascertain long past exposures, which is particularly difficult. Sometimes it is possible to evaluate exposure of macroenvironmental factors at the individual level, as was done in an ancillary study within the Multi-Ethnic Study of Atherosclerosis (MESA Air). In this study, household levels of air pollution were estimated by considering distance from a major roadway[14] and by the use of a special device for the home monitoring of air pollution levels.[15]

A parallel set of problems is seen when we try to characterize the occupational exposures of an individual worker and to link an exposure at work to an adverse health outcome. First, because a worker is likely to be exposed to many different agents in an industrial setting, it is often difficult to isolate the independent risk that can be ascribed to a single specific exposure. Second, because there is often a long latent period between the exposure and the subsequent development of disease, studies of the exposure-disease relationship may be difficult; for example, unless a concurrent prospective study can be done (see Chapter 8), recall may be poor and records of exposure may have been lost. Third, increased disease risks may occur among those living near an industrial plant, so that it may be difficult to ascertain how much of a worker's risk results from living near the plant and how much is due to an occupational exposure in the work setting itself.

Perhaps the most fundamental problem in measuring exposures in epidemiologic studies is that sources and measures are often indirect. For example, considerable interest has arisen in recent years over the possible health effects of electromagnetic fields (EMFs). This interest followed the article of Wertheimer and Leeper in 1979,[16] which reported increased levels of leukemia in children living near high-voltage transmission lines. Subsequently, many methodologic questions were raised, and the question of whether such fields are associated with adverse health effects remains unresolved. For example, conclusions were discrepant in an update of two meta-analyses and a more recent meta-analysis done by the same first author![17,18]

In studying EMFs, several approaches are used for measuring exposure, including the wiring configuration in the home, spot or 24-hour measurements of the fields, or self-reports of electrical appliance use. However, the results of different studies regarding risk of disease differ depending on the type of exposure measurement used. In fact, actual magnetic field measurements, even 24-hour measurements, generate weaker associations with childhood leukemia than do those for wire configuration codes.[19] This observation raises a question about any possible causal link between exposure to magnetic fields and the occurrence of disease.

Even the best indirect measure of exposure often leaves critical questions unanswered. First, exposure is generally not dichotomous; data are therefore needed regarding the *dose* of exposure to explore a possible dose-response relationship. Second, it is important to know whether the exposure was continuous or periodic. For example, in the pathogenesis of cancer, a periodic exposure with alternating exposure and nonexposure periods may allow for DNA repair during the nonexposure periods. In the case of a continuous exposure, no such repair can take place. Finally, information about latency is critical: How long is the latent period and what is its range? This knowledge is essential to focus efforts on ascertaining exposure during a particular time period in which a causal exposure might well have occurred.

Because of these problems in measuring exposure using indirect approaches, much interest has focused on the use of biologic markers of exposures. (Use of such biomarkers has often been termed *molecular epidemiology*.)[20] The advantage of using biomarkers is that they overcome some problems of limited recall or lack of awareness of an exposure. In addition, biomarkers can overcome errors resulting from variation in individual absorption or metabolism by focusing on a later step in the causal chain.

Biomarkers can be markers of exposure, markers of biologic changes resulting from exposures, or markers of risk or susceptibility. Fig. 19.10 schematically represents the different types of exposures we may choose to measure.

We might also wish to measure ambient levels of possibly toxic substances in a general environment, the levels to which a specific individual is exposed, the amount of substance absorbed, or the amount of substance or metabolite of the absorbed substance that reaches the target tissue. Biomarkers bring us closer to being able to measure an exposure at a specific stage in the process by which an exposure is linked to human disease. For example, we can measure not only environmental levels of a substance but also DNA adducts that reflect the effect of the substance on biologic processes in the body after absorption.

Nevertheless, despite these advantages, biomarkers generally give us a dichotomous answer—a person was either exposed or not exposed. Biomarkers generally do not shed light on several important questions, such as the following:

- What was the total exposure dose?
- What was the duration of exposure?
- How long ago did the exposure occur?
- Was the exposure continuous or periodic?

An example of some of these shortcomings is salivary cotinine, which is a biomarker of nicotine absorption in smokers. As it is a marker only for recent smoking, it does not provide information on duration of exposure or whether the habit was continuous or periodic.

The answers to these questions are crucial in properly interpreting the potential biologic importance of a given exposure. For example, in assessing the biologic plausibility of a causal inference being made from observations of exposure and outcome, we need relevant data that will permit us to determine whether the interval observed between the exposure and the development of the disease is (biologically) consistent with what we know from other studies about the incubation period of the disease.

In addition to these concerns, a potential limitation of the use of exposure biomarkers is that, in a traditional case-control study, collection of a biologic sample and measurement of a biomarker are done only after the onset of the disease. Thus it is impossible to find out whether the exposure was present prior to the onset of the disease of interest. This shortcoming, however, is not present in case-control studies within a cohort in which biologic samples, such as serum or urine, are frozen and stored at baseline—that is, before incident cases develop during follow-up of the cohort.

It should be pointed out that use of biomarkers is not new in epidemiology. In Ecclesiastes it is written: "There is nothing new under the sun."[21] Even before the revolution in molecular biology, laboratory techniques were essential in many epidemiologic studies; these included bacterial isolates and cultures, phage typing of organisms, viral isolation, serologic studies, and assays of cholesterol lipoprotein fractions. With the tremendous advances made in molecular biology, a new variety of biomarkers has become available that is relevant to areas such as carcinogenesis. These biomarkers not only identify exposed individuals but also cast new light on the pathogenetic process of the disease in question.

Meta-Analysis

Several scientific questions arise when epidemiologic data are used for formulating public policy:

1. Can epidemiologic methods detect small increases in risk that are clinically meaningful?
2. How can we reconcile inconsistencies between animal and human data?
3. How can we use incomplete or equivocal epidemiologic data?

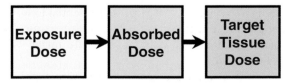

Fig. 19.10 What exposures are we trying to measure?

4. How can results be interpreted when the findings of epidemiologic studies disagree?

Many of the risks with which we are dealing may be quite small, but they may potentially be of great public health importance because of the large numbers of people exposed, with a resulting potential for adverse health effects in many people (recall the hypothesis proposed by Rose[3]). However, an observed small increase in relative risk above 1.0 may easily result from bias or from other methodologic limitations, and such results must therefore be interpreted with great caution unless the results have been replicated and other supporting evidence has been obtained.

Given that the results of different epidemiologic studies may not be consistent and that at times they may be in dramatic conflict, attempts have been made to systematize the process of reviewing the epidemiologic literature on a given topic. One process, the systematic review, uses standardized methodology to select and assess peer-reviewed articles to synthesize the literature regarding a specific health topic.[22] Systematic reviews may be accompanied by a process called meta-analysis, which has been defined as "the statistical analysis of a large collection of analysis results from individual studies for the purpose of integrating the findings."[23] Meta-analysis allows for aggregating the results of a set of studies included in a systematic review, with appropriate weighting of each study for the number of subjects sampled and for other characteristics. It can help to give an overall perspective on an issue when the results of studies disagree.

However, a number of problems and questions are associated with meta-analysis. First, should the analysis include all available studies or only published studies? Second, when the relative risks or odds ratios from various studies differ (i.e., the results are not homogeneous), meta-analysis results may mask important differences among individual studies. It is therefore essential that a systematic review resulting in a meta-analysis include only studies that meet well-established design and quality criteria. Third, the results of meta-analyses themselves may not always be reproducible by other analysts. Finally, a systematic review with or without meta-analysis is subject to the problem of publication bias (discussed later in this chapter). Fig. 19.11 shows a hypothetical "forest plot"

and the definition of its components. The forest plot is the type of presentation that is frequently used to show the results of individual studies as well as the results of the meta-analysis. Fig. 19.12 shows a forest plot on the relationship of socioeconomic status and depression. Note that of the 51 studies included in this meta-analysis, 5 suggest a negative association. Thus the results of this meta-analysis are not entirely homogeneous.

Meta-analysis was originally usually applied to randomized trials, but this technique is being used increasingly to aggregate nonrandomized, observational studies, including case-control and cohort studies. In these instances, the studies do not necessarily share a common research design. Hence the question arises as to how similar such studies need to be in order to legitimately be included in a meta-analysis. In addition, appropriate control of biases (such as selection bias and misclassification bias) is essential but often proves to be a formidable challenge in meta-analyses. In view of the considerations just discussed, meta-analysis remains a subject of considerable controversy.

A final problem with meta-analysis is that in the face of all the difficulties discussed, putting a quantitative imprint on the estimation of a single relative risk or odds ratio from all the studies may lead to a false sense of certainty regarding the magnitude of the risk. People often tend to have an inordinate belief in the validity of findings when a number is attached to them; as a result, many of the difficulties that arise in meta-analysis may at times be ignored.

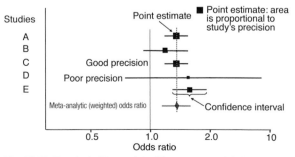

Fig. 19.11 Hypothetical forest plot, with components, labeled, showing the type of diagrammatic presentation frequently used to show results of individual studies *(A–E)* as well as the results of a meta-analysis.

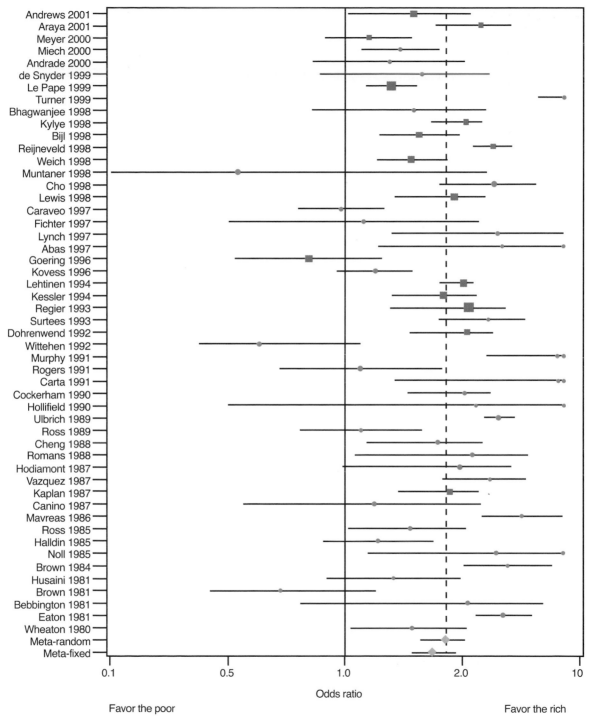

Fig. 19.12 Odds ratios for major depression in the lowest socioeconomic status group in 51 prevalence studies published after 1979. *Horizontal lines,* 95% confidence interval. Squares show original estimates; diamonds show meta-analyzed results. (From Lorant V, Deliège D, Eaton W, et al. Socioeconomic inequalities in depression: a meta-analysis. *Am J Epidemiol.* 2003;157(2):98–112.)

Publication Bias

Chapter 16 discussed the use of twin studies as a means of distinguishing the contributions of environmental and genetic factors to the root cause of disease. In that discussion it was mentioned that the degree of concordance and discordance in twins is an important observation for drawing conclusions about the role of genetic factors, but that estimates of concordance reported in the literature may be inflated by publication bias, which is the tendency for articles to be published that report concordance for rare diseases in twin pairs.

Publication bias is not limited to genetic studies of twins; it can occur in any area of epidemiology. It is a particularly important phenomenon in the publication of articles regarding environmental risks and on the results of clinical trials. Publication bias may occur because investigators do not submit the results of their studies when the findings do not support "positive" associations and increased risks (that is, "null findings"). In addition, journals may differentially select for publication studies that they believe to be of greatest reader interest, and they may not find studies that report no association to fall in this category. As a result, a literature review that is limited to published articles may preferentially identify studies that report increased risk. Clearly such a review is highly selective in nature and omits many studies that have obtained what have been called "negative" results (i.e., results showing no effect), which may not have reached publication.

Publication bias therefore has a clear effect on systematic review and meta-analysis. One approach to this problem is to try to identify unpublished studies and to include them in the analysis (pulling studies from the "gray" literature, often from conference presentations, often reporting null results, that do not lead to publication). However, the difficulty here is that, in general, unpublished studies are likely not to have passed journal peer review; therefore their suitability for inclusion in a meta-analysis may be questionable. Regardless of whether we are discussing a traditional type of literature review or a structured meta-analysis, the problem of potential publication bias must be considered.

It has been proposed that in order to prevent publication bias in systematic reviews (and thus, in meta-analyses), study registers, similar to the Cochrane collaboration, should be implemented. There are also strategies to evaluate publication bias in meta-analyses, including the Beggs funnel and tests of symmetry. These approaches are based on plotting the studies' values of the measure of association (e.g., relative risk or odds ratio) against their precision levels (measured by their standard errors, which are usually a function of their sample sizes). Using the relative risk as an example, as the standard errors increase, thus denoting decreasing precision, the relative risks become more variable, but it is expected that they follow a symmetric distribution around the between-study mean relative risk. If the distribution is asymmetric, publication bias is likely.

Epidemiology in the Courts

As mentioned earlier, litigation has become a major path for policy making in the United States. Epidemiology is assuming ever-increasing importance in the legal arena. Particularly in the area of toxic torts, it provides one of the major types of scientific evidence that is relevant to the questions involved. Issues such as effects of dioxin, silicone breast implants, tobacco smoking, and EMFs are but a few examples.

However, the use of data from epidemiologic studies is not without its problems. Epidemiology answers questions about *groups*, whereas the court often requires information about *individuals* (where it is necessary to causally link individual exposure and their disease status). Furthermore, considerable attention has been directed to the court's interpretation of evidence of causality. Whereas the legal criterion is often "more likely than not"—that is, that the substance or exposure in question is "more likely than not" to have caused a person's disease—epidemiology relies to a great extent on the US Surgeon General's guidelines for causal inferences.[24] It has been suggested that an attributable risk in the exposed greater than 50% might constitute evidence of "more likely than not."[25]

Until recently, evidence from epidemiology was only reluctantly accepted in the courts, but this has changed to a point where epidemiologic data are often cited as the only source of relevant evidence in toxic tort cases. For many years the guiding principle for using scientific evidence in the courts in the United States was the Frye test, which states that for a study to be admissible, "it must be sufficiently established to have gained general acceptance in the field in which it belongs."[26] Although terms such as "general acceptance" and "field in which it belongs" were left undefined, it did lead to an assessment of whether the scientific opinion expressed by an expert witness was generally accepted by other professionals in the discipline.

In 1993, in *Daubert v. Merrell Dow Pharmaceuticals,*[27] a case in which the plaintiff alleged that a limb deformity at birth was due to ingestion of the drug Bendectin during pregnancy, the US Supreme Court articulated a major change in the rules of evidence. The court ruled that "general acceptance" is not a necessary condition for the admissibility of scientific evidence in court. Rather, the trial judge is now considered a "gatekeeper" and is assigned the task of ensuring that an expert's testimony rests on a reliable foundation and is relevant to the "task at hand." Thus the judge "must make a preliminary assessment of whether the testimony's underlying reasoning or methodology is scientifically valid and can be properly applied to the facts at issue." Among the considerations cited by the court are whether the theory or technique in question can be and has been tested and whether the methodology has been subjected to peer review and publication.

Given their new responsibilities, judges presiding at trials in which epidemiology is a major source of evidence must have a basic knowledge of epidemiologic concepts—including, for example, study design, biases and confounding, and causal inference—if they are to be able to rule in a sound fashion on whether the approach used by the experts follows accepted "scientific method." Recognizing this need, the Federal Judicial Center has published the *Research Manual on Scientific Evidence* for judges, which includes a section on epidemiology.[28] Although it is premature to know the ultimate effect of the Daubert ruling, given the tremendous increase in the use of epidemiology in the courts, it will clearly require enhanced knowledge of epidemiology by many parties involved in legal proceedings that use evidence derived from epidemiologic studies.

Sources and Impact of Uncertainty

In 1983, the National Research Council in the United States wrote:

The dominant analytic difficulty [in conducting risk assessments for policy decision making] is pervasive uncertainty … data may be incomplete, and there is often great uncertainty in estimates of the types, probability, and magnitude of health effects associated with a chemical agent, of the economic effects of a proposed regulatory action, and of the extent of current and possible future human exposures.[29]

This insight remains as relevant today as when it was originally written. Uncertainty is a reality that we must accept and that must be addressed. Uncertainty is an integral part of science. What we believe to be "truth" today often turns out to be transient. Tomorrow a study may appear that contradicts or invalidates the best scientific information available to us today.

Uncertainty is relevant not only to risk assessments but also to issues of treatment, to issues of prevention such as screening, and to health economics issues. Clearly it is a relevant concern in the legal setting discussed earlier (Fig. 19.13).

Some of the possible sources of uncertainty are listed in Box 19.2. As seen there, the sources of uncertainty may be in the design of the study or in the conduct and implementation of the study, or they may result from the presentation and interpretation of the study findings. Many of these sources are addressed in earlier chapters.

One issue listed in Box 19.2 is whether, in a study of the effectiveness of a preventive measure, the results are described as a relative risk reduction or an absolute risk reduction. Often the *percent* reduction in mortality is selected because it gives a more optimistic view of

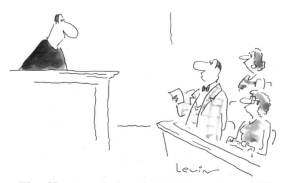

"Your Honor, we, the jury, find this one too close to call."

Fig. 19.13 One jury's approach to uncertainty. (Arnie Levin/The New Yorker Collection/The Cartoon Bank.)

BOX 19.2 EXAMPLES OF POSSIBLE SOURCES OF UNCERTAINTY IN EPIDEMIOLOGY

1. Uncertainty resulting from the design of the study
   a. The study may not have been designed to provide a relevant answer to the question of interest
   b. Biases that were not recognized or not adequately addressed
      (1) Selection bias
      (2) Information bias
   c. Measurement errors, which may lead to misclassification
   d. Inadequate sample size
   e. Inappropriate choice of analytic methods
   f. Failure to take into account potential confounders
   g. Use of surrogate measures that may not correctly measure the outcomes that are the major dependent variables of interest
   h. Problems of external validity (generalizability to the population of interest): the conclusions regarding potential interventions may not be generalizable to the target population
2. Uncertainty resulting from deficiencies in the conduct and implementation of the study
   a. Observations may be biased if observers were not blinded
   b. Poor quality of laboratory or survey methods
   c. Large proportion of nonparticipants and/or nonrespondents
   d. Failure to identify reasons for nonresponse and characteristics of nonrespondents
3. Uncertainty resulting from the presentation and interpretation of the study findings
   a. How were the results expressed?
   b. If the study assessed risk and possible etiology, were the factors involved described as risk factors or causal factors?
   c. If the study assessed the effectiveness of a proposed preventive measure, was the benefit of the measure expressed as relative risk reduction or absolute risk reduction? Why was it chosen to be expressed as it was, and how was the finding interpreted?

the effectiveness of a preventive measure. If, however, absolute risk reduction is used, such as the *number* of individuals per 1,000 whose lives would be saved, the result appears less impressive (recall the disease risks associated with HRT presented earlier in this chapter). If the rate of adverse events, such as mortality from the disease that is observed without screening, is low, a percent reduction will always seem more impressive than an absolute risk reduction because the *number* of events that could potentially be prevented is small even if the *percent* reduction is higher. If, for example, the mortality in those screened is 2 per 100,000 and in those not screened is 1 per 100,000, the reduction resulting from screening is 50%, but the absolute difference is merely 1 per 100,000.

A more relevant measure of the effectiveness (and efficiency) of a preventive or curative measure is the number needed to undergo the intervention to prevent one case or one death from the disease. This measure is based on the absolute difference. For example, if the difference between a new preventive strategy and the current (standard of care) strategy is 20%, the number needed to have the intervention in order to prevent the occurrence of one incident case is $([100 \times 1] \div 20) = 5$. However, if the difference is only 2%, this number becomes $([100 \times 1] \div 5) = 20$. Note that the effectiveness is the same if the mortality rates are, for example, 60% and 40% or 6% and 4% in two studies evaluating different novel interventions to prevent the same disease: $([60\% - 40\%] \div 60\%) = 33.3\%$ in the first study, and $([6\% - 4\%] \div 6\%) = 33.3\%$ in the second study. It is, however, clear that the first study deals with a more important public health problem for which prevention would be more efficient, as one case can be prevented by subjecting fewer individuals to the new approach.

Another issue that contributes to uncertainty in policy making that is not generally related to specific epidemiologic studies is how we deal with *anecdotal evidence,* such as that provided by a person who states that she was screened for breast cancer 10 years earlier, received early treatment, and is alive and apparently well 10 years after the screening. There is often a tendency to accept such evidence as supporting the effectiveness of the screening in reducing mortality from the disease. However, anecdotal evidence has two major problems. First, it does not take into account slow-growing tumors that might have been detected by screening but might not have affected survival even if the patient had not been screened. Second, it does not take into account very fast-growing tumors that screening would have missed, so that the person would not have received early treatment. That is, for those giving anecdotal evidence of survival after screening, there is no comparison group of individuals who were screened but did *not* survive. As an unknown sage has said, "The plural of *anecdote* is not 'data.' " Nevertheless, despite these major limitations, anecdotal evidence given by patients who have survived serious illnesses may have a strong emotional impact, which may significantly influence policy makers.

Ultimately the impact of scientific uncertainty on the formulation of public policy will depend on how the major stakeholders consider uncertainty. Among the different groups of stakeholders are scientists (including epidemiologists), policy makers, politicians, and the public (or the target populations). Each of these groups may have a different level of sophistication, a different level and type of self-interest, and may view data differently and be influenced to varying degrees by colleagues, friends, and various constituencies in society. Moreover, individuals have different personalities with different levels of risk tolerance and different ways of dealing with uncertainty. An important mediator is the set of values that every individual has relating to issues such as the value of a human life and the principles that should guide the allocation of limited resources in a society. The result is a complex interaction of uncertainty, resulting from characteristics of a study, interacting with a network of relationships relating to the elements just described. A schematic of some of the interrelationships influencing the effect of uncertainty on public policy is shown in Fig. 19.14. These factors are clearly major concerns in formulating appropriate public health and clinical policy. It is important that they be taken into account if a plan of action is to be successfully developed and implemented to address health issues in the population.

Policy Issues Regarding Risk: What Should the Objectives Be?

Public policy is generally recognized to be largely developed through the processes of legislation and regulation. As discussed earlier, in the United States, litigation has also become an important instrument for developing and implementing public policy. Ideally,

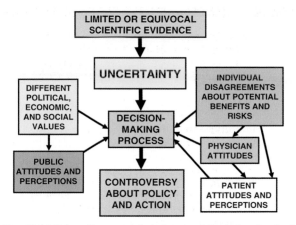

Fig. 19.14 Schematic presentation of some of the factors involved in the impact of uncertainty on the decision-making process for health policy.

each of these processes should reflect societal values and aspirations.

Certain major societal issues must be considered in making decisions about risk. Among the questions that must be confronted are the following:

1. What percentage of the population should be protected by the policy?
2. What level of risk is society willing to tolerate?
3. What level of control of risk is society willing to pay for?
4. Who should make decisions about risk?

At first glance, it might seem appealing to protect the entire population from any amount of risk, but realistically this is difficult if not impossible to accomplish. Regardless of what we learn from risk data about populations, there are clearly rare individuals who are extraordinarily sensitive to minute concentrations of certain chemicals. If the permissible amount of a chemical is to be set at a level that protects *every* worker, it is possible that entire manufacturing processes might have to be halted. Similarly, if we demand zero risk for workers or for others who may be exposed, the economic base of many communities might be destroyed. Policy making therefore requires a balance between what *can* be done and what *should* be done. The degree of priority attached to elimination of all risk and the decision as to what percentage of risk should be eliminated clearly are not scientific decisions but rather depend on societal values. It is hoped that such societal decisions will capitalize on available epidemiologic and other scientific knowledge in the context of political, economic, ethical, and social considerations.

Conclusion

The objectives of epidemiology are to enhance our understanding of the biology, pathogenesis, and other determinants of disease to improve human health and to prevent and better treat disease. A thorough understanding of the methodologic issues that arise is needed to better interpret epidemiologic results properly as a basis for formulating both clinical and public health policy. The appropriate and judicious use of the results of epidemiologic studies is fundamental to an assessment of risk to human health and to the control of these risks. Such use is therefore important to both primary and secondary prevention. Policy makers are often obliged to develop policy in the presence of incomplete or equivocal scientific data. In clinical medicine, in both the diagnostic and therapeutic processes, decisions are often made with incomplete or equivocal data; this has perhaps been more of an overt impediment in public health and community medicine. No simple set of rules can eliminate this difficulty. As H. L. Mencken wrote: "There is always an easy solution to every human problem—neat, plausible, and wrong."[30] A major challenge remains to develop the best process for formulating rational policies under such circumstances—a process that is relevant for both clinical medicine and public health.

REFERENCES

1. Hill AB. The environment and disease: association or causation? *Proc R Soc Med*. 1965;58:295–300.
2. Jones FB. *Saturday Evening Post*, November 29; 1953.
3. Rose G. Sick individuals and sick populations. *Int J Epidemiol*. 1985;14:22–38.
4. Whelton PK. Epidemiology of hypertension. *Lancet*. 1994;344:101–106.
5. Chobanian A, et al. The seventh report of the Joint National Committee on prevention, detection, evaluation and treatment of high blood pressure: the JNC 7 report. *JAMA*. 2003;289:2560–2572.
6. Grady D, Herrington D, Bittner V, et al, for the HERS Research Group. Cardiovascular disease outcomes during 68 years of hormone therapy: heart and estrogen/progestin replacement study follow-up (HERS II). *JAMA*. 2002;288:49–57.
7. The Women's Health Initiative. Risks and benefits of estrogen plus progestin in healthy postmenopausal women: principal results The Women's Health Initiative randomized controlled trial. *JAMA*. 2002;288:321–333.
8. Grodstein F, Clarkson TB, Manson JE. Understanding the divergent data on postmenopausal hormone therapy. *N Engl J Med*. 2003;348:645–650.
9. Michels KB. Hormone replacement therapy in epidemiologic studies and randomized clinical trials—are we checkmate? *Epidemiology*. 2003;14:3–5.
10. Whittemore AS, McGuire V. Observational studies and randomized trials of hormone replacement therapy: what can we learn from them? *Epidemiology*. 2003;14:8–10.
11. Manson JE, Bassuk SS, Harman SM, et al. Postmenopausal hormone therapy: new questions and the case for new clinical trials. *Menopause*. 2006;13:139–147.
12. Samet JM, Schnatter R, Gibb H. Epidemiology and risk assessment. *Am J Epidemiol*. 1998;148:929–936.
13. National Research Council Committee on the Institutional Means for Assessment of Risks to Public Health. *Risk Assessment in the Federal Government: Managing the Process*. Washington, DC: National Academy Press; 1983:21.
14. Auchincloss AH, Diez Roux AV, Dvonch JT, et al. Associations between recent exposure to ambient fine particular matter and blood pressure in the Multi-Ethnic Study of Atherosclerosis (MESA). *Environ Health Perspect*. 2008;116:486–491.
15. Cohen MA, Adar SD, Allen RW, et al. Approach to estimating participant pollutant exposures in the Multi-Ethnic Study of Atherosclerosis and Air Pollution (MESA Air). *Environ Sci Technol*. 2009;43(13):4687–4693.
16. Wertheimer N, Leeper E. Electrical wiring configurations and childhood cancer. *Am J Epidemiol*. 1979;109:273–284.
17. Kheifets L, Monroe J, Vergara X, et al. Occupational electromagnetic fields and leukemia and brain cancer: an update of two meta-analyses. *J Occup Environ Med*. 2008;50:677–688.
18. Kheifets L, Ahlbom A, Crespi CM, et al. Pooled analysis of recente studies on magnetic fields and childhood leukaemia. *Br J Cancer*. 2010;103:1128–1135.
19. Calvente I, Fernandez MF, Villalba J, et al. Exposure to electromagnetic fields (non-ionizing radiation) and its relationship with childhood leukemia: a systematic review. *Sci Total Environ*. 2010;408(16):3062–3069.
20. Bonassi S, Taioli E, Vermeulen R. Omics in population studies: a molecular epidemiology perspective. *Environ Mol Mutagen*. 2013;54(7):455–460.
21. *Ecclesiastes 1:9*.
22. Porta M. *A Dictionary of Epidemiology*. 5th ed. New York: Oxford University Press; 2008.
23. Glass GV. Primary, secondary and meta-analysis of research. *Educ Res*. 1976;5:3–8.
24. U.S. Department of Health, Education and Welfare. *Smoking and Health: Report of the Advisory Committee to the Surgeon General* Washington, DC, Public Health Service; 1964.
25. Black B, Lilienfeld DE. Epidemiology proof in toxic tort litigation. *Fordham Law Rev*. 1984;52:732–785.
26. *Frye v. United States, 293 F 1013 (D.C. Cir 1923)*.
27. *Daubert v. Merrell Dow Pharmaceuticals, Inc, 113 S Ct 2786*; 1993.
28. Green M, Freedman M, Gordis L. Reference guide on epidemiology. In: *Reference Manual on Scientific Evidence*. 3rd ed. Washington, DC: The National Academies Press; 2011:549.
29. National Research Council Committee on the Institutional Means for Assessment of Risks to Public Health. *Risk Assessment in the Federal Government: Managing the Process*. Washington, DC: National Academy Press; 1983:11.
30. Mencken HL. The divine afflatus. *New York Evening Mail*. November 16, 1917. (Essay reprinted in Mencken HL: *Prejudices*, series 2 New York, Alfred A Knopf; 1920.)

Chapter 20

Ethical and Professional Issues in Epidemiology

No man is an Island, entire of itself;
every man is a piece of the Continent, a part of the
main …
any man's death diminishes me, because I am
involved in Mankind;
And therefore never send to know for whom the bell
tolls;
It tolls for thee.

—John Donne, English clergyman and poet (1572–1631),
Meditation XVII

Learning Objectives

- To discuss the ethical obligations that investigators have to people who volunteer to participate in epidemiologic studies.
- To consider how the privacy and confidentiality of health records is protected in epidemiologic studies and how access to epidemiologic data is governed.
- To describe the scientific and ethical implications of classifying race and ethnicity in epidemiologic studies.
- To introduce issues associated with conflict of interest.
- To review how the findings of epidemiologic studies are interpreted and communicated to the public.

In the lines cited at the beginning of this chapter, John Donne emphasizes the interconnectedness of all people. Epidemiology also teaches us major lessons about connections and relationships. The previous chapters have demonstrated that disease does not arise in a vacuum. Many contagious diseases clearly depend on human (and frequently animal) contacts for transmission and for the propagation of epidemics. Moreover, in recent years, more and more diseases that for a long period were thought not to

have an infectious etiology are being identified as being of infectious origin to varying degrees. For example, the microorganism *Helicobacter pylori* has been implicated in the etiology of peptic ulcer and gastric cancer (see Chapter 14). Many cases of cancer of the cervix are linked to human papillomavirus (HPV), especially types 16 and 18; the foundation thus exists for promoting prevention programs through immunization against HPV among youth for lifelong prevention.

A major focus of epidemiology is on the impact of the environment on the risk of human disease. This reflects a combination of factors: First, we are at risk from effects of nature, including flooding and other natural disasters such as the tsunami that affected Japan in 2011, causing massive damage at the Fukushima Daiichi Nuclear Power Plant; Hurricane Maria in 2017, which devastated Puerto Rico and the US Virgin Islands; and the earthquake in Mexico City, which killed some 2000 inhabitants in 2017. Second, we are also vulnerable to the environmental and ecologic damage resulting from certain human attitudes, lifestyles, and behaviors. The negative effects that human activities have on our planet are often not adequately considered, and some influential decision makers are in abject denial of their existence. These activities and effects include air pollution, depletion of the ozone layer, global warming, climate change, the pollution of natural water supplies, deforestation, and overdevelopment, among many others. The negative effects of many of these types of problems are only now beginning to be fully understood and appreciated, with the legacy of environmental damage being left to future generations. As these problems are studied, increased understanding is also needed of individual variations in genetically determined human vulnerability to environmental agents.

Another aspect of interdependence that is relevant to epidemiologists is their need to develop collaborative relationships with other epidemiologists as well as with professionals in other fields. We have learned that many epidemiologic investigations require multidisciplinary approaches; that is, professionally, epidemiologists cannot be most productive and effective as "islands." Thus the lesson of "connectedness" expressed in John Donne's lines seems integral both to the dynamics of the diseases and conditions investigated by epidemiologists and to the everyday practice of epidemiology. It also applies to the participation of epidemiologists in formulating and implementing health-related policy, as demonstrated by the story of Semmelweis presented in Chapter 1.

Today, we live in a depersonalized era in which individuals often consider their own advancement to be life's major goal. A sense of community and concern for others is often lost. John Donne's worldview, stressing people's interdependence, at times seems alien to some current views of the world, one of which is humorously seen in Fig. 20.1. One of the best articulations of the need to simultaneously balance the competing interests and needs of the individual and the community was given by Hillel, a Talmudic sage who lived some 2,000 years ago. He said: "If I am not for myself [If I don't take care of myself], who will be for me? But if I am only for myself [in other words, if I take care only of myself], what am I worth? And if not now, when?"

Another factor that has an impact on epidemiology and epidemiologists is the rapid pace of societal change and technologic progress. A story is told of Adam and Eve in the Garden of Eden. After being expelled from

Eden, Adam turned to Eve and said, "Eve, my dear, we are living in a time of change."[1] In the 21st century, we too are living in a time of dramatic change. The rapidly evolving social and scientific context in which epidemiologic research is being conducted has led to new challenges for those working in epidemiology, for those who use the results of epidemiologic studies, and for the general public. In addition, major technologic advances, including tremendous increases in computing capacity and dramatic advances in laboratory technology (for example, recall Chapter 16 on the significant advances in genetics in the past several years), have made it possible to rapidly analyze large numbers of biologic samples and maintain enormous data sets. These advances have made possible many population-based studies that would not have been conceivable even a decade or two ago. The electronic medical record (EMR) is replacing paper charts in hospitals and includes outpatient and inpatient visits, results of laboratory tests, electrocardiography (ECG) readings, and computed tomography/magnetic resonance imaging (CT/MRI) scans. How to use these data (which have not been collected for research purposes) for epidemiologic studies is a major challenge to "big data" analysis. At the same time, these technologic advances have introduced new and different issues related to privacy, confidentiality, and the individual.

In light of the preceding discussion, this chapter briefly reviews some ethical and professional issues that are critical for epidemiologic research and for applying the results of this research to the improvement of human health. The issues to be discussed include several that relate to the actual conduct of epidemiologic studies and others that relate to broader societal issues and go beyond actual epidemiologic research itself.

Ethical Issues in Epidemiology

Clearly, in any scientific pursuit, fraud, deceit, or misrepresentation elicits universal disapproval and condemnation from members of the discipline, other professionals, and the lay public. Such issues are not presented in this chapter. Today some of the most difficult ethical dilemmas in epidemiology are likely to be more subtle, involving judgments, philosophies, attitudes, and opinions for which consensus may be more difficult to obtain.

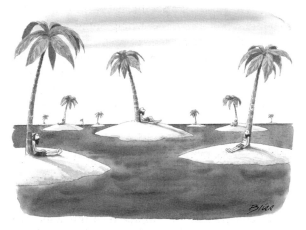

Fig. 20.1 "No man is an island"—a different view. (Harry Bliss/The New Yorker Collection/The Cartoon Bank.)

Does epidemiology differ from other scientific and medical disciplines with regard to ethical issues? Although epidemiology shares many characteristics with other scientific disciplines, it differs in some important ways. It is a discipline that largely grew out of medicine and public health, and even in its earliest years, its findings had immediate policy implications for clinical care or public health action. John Snow's studies of cholera in London (see Chapter 1) and his removal of the handle from the Broad Street pump, which his studies had implicated in the cholera outbreak (whether the pump handle was actually removed before or after the peak of the outbreak), reflected the clear policy implications of his findings.

The ultimate objective of epidemiology is to improve human health; epidemiology is a basic science of disease prevention. Hence the relationship of epidemiology to the development of public policy is integral to the discipline. As a result, the ethical and professional issues go beyond those that might apply to a scientific discipline, such as biophysics or physiology, and must be viewed in a broader context. First, epidemiologic findings have direct and often immediate societal relevance. Second, epidemiologic studies are generally funded from public resources and often have major implications for the allocation of limited societal resources. Third, epidemiologic research often involves human subjects in some way, and subjects who participate in epidemiologic studies generally derive no personal benefit from participating in these studies or from the study results.

Investigators' Obligations to Study Subjects

What are the investigators' obligations to the subjects in the nonrandomized observational studies with which most epidemiologists generally deal? First, to the greatest extent possible, a truly informed consent consistent with the principle of individual autonomy should be obtained from every subject. But can a truly informed consent be obtained from a subject in an epidemiologic study? If we believe that a full disclosure to the subjects of the study's objectives and hypotheses will introduce a response bias or other type of bias, clearly the consent cannot be a fully "informed" one. Another issue in consent relates to privacy and confidentiality. For many years, in good conscience, epidemiologists assured subjects that their data would be kept confidential, and that this commitment was unqualified. However, research data have become subject to court subpoena in recent years, with only a few exceptions. Therefore the assurance of confidentiality given in informed consent statements must now include qualifications to allow for breaches in confidentiality that could be legally mandated and that would therefore be beyond the control of the investigator. New privacy regulations went into effect in the United States in 2003, which significantly affect the rights of patients regarding health information (Fig. 20.2). We all too often hear about data breaches and the release of confidential information that can be used to harm research participants or cause damage to their reputations and bank accounts or that involve other types of fraud. We return to the subject of privacy and confidentiality later in this chapter.

Another issue pertains to balancing the rights of the individual and the welfare of society. In a very early study of men at high risk for infection with the human immunodeficiency virus (HIV), the participants were given an assurance of confidentiality. In the baseline interview that was subsequently administered, subjects were asked whether they had donated blood during the previous 2 years. Several subjects who were found to be HIV-positive reported having given blood within the 2 years prior to the HIV testing. The concern that emerged was that the donated blood might have been used in a transfusion. Although the blood may have been discarded by the blood bank, there was no way to check on this without breaching confidentiality and violating the original commitment to the subjects. Perhaps the investigators should have anticipated such a problem at the time the interview was developed, before obtaining the subjects' informed consent. But even with foresight, these types of problems arise. In this case, how do we balance the original commitment to the subjects with a need to determine whether anyone had received blood from these donors, so that further transmission of HIV might be prevented?

A third obligation to the subjects relates to communicating the results of the study to them at the study's completion. Our approach to this issue may differ depending on whether the subject has been found to have developed a health problem linked to an

OMB # 0920-0950

NATIONAL HEALTH AND NUTRITION EXAMINATION SURVEY

CONSENT/ASSENT AND PARENTAL PERMISSION FOR EXAMINATION AT THE MOBILE EXAMINATION CENTER

Print name of participant _____ _____ _____

                                    First   Middle   Last

PARENT OR GUARDIAN OF SURVEY PARTICIPANT WHO IS UNDER 18 YEARS OLD:

For the Parent or Guardian of the Survey Participant who is a minor (unless the participant is an emancipated minor)

I have read the Examination Brochure and the Health Measurements List, which explain the nature and purpose of the survey. I freely choose to let my child take part in the survey.

_____ _____
Signature of parent/guardian   Date

FOR PARENT OR GUARDIAN OF SURVEY PARTICIPANT 12-17 YEARS:

☐ I agree to have my child's interview about his/her current health status, diet, and health behaviors recorded for quality control.

☐ I do not agree to have my child's interview about his/her current health status, diet, and health behaviors recorded for quality control.

SURVEY PARTICIPANT WHO IS 12 YEARS OLD OR OLDER:

I have read the Examination Brochure and the Health Measurements List, which explain the nature and purpose of the survey. I freely choose to take part in the survey.

_____ _____
Signature of participant   Date

If you are 18 and older and do not want a written report of your exam results, check here ☐

_____

I observed the interviewer read this form to the person named above and he/she agreed to participate by signing or marking this form.

_____ _____
Witness (if required)   Date

Name of staff member present when this form was signed: _____

> **Assurance of Confidentiality**: We take your privacy very seriously. All information that relates to or describes identifiable characteristics of individuals, a practice, or an establishment will be used only for statistical purposes. NCHS staff, contractors, and agents will not disclose or release responses in identifiable form without the consent of the individual or establishment in accordance with section 308(d) of the Public Health Service Act (42 U.S.C. 242m(d)) and the Confidential Information Protection and Statistical Efficiency Act of 2002 (CIPSEA, Title 5 of Public Law 107-347). In accordance with CIPSEA, every NCHS employee, contractor, and agent has taken an oath and is subject to a jail term of up to five years, a fine of up to $250,000, or both if he or she willfully discloses ANY identifiable information about you. In addition, NCHS complies with the Federal Cybersecurity Act of 2015 (6 U.S.C. §§ 151 & 151 note). This law requires the federal government to protect federal computer networks by using computer security programs to identify cybersecurity risks like hacking, internet attacks, and other security weaknesses. If information sent through government networks triggers a cyber threat indicator, the information may be intercepted and reviewed for cyber threats by computer network experts working for, or on behalf of, the government.
> **02/2017**

— — — — — —
                                                SP ID

Fig. 20.2 Sample consent form. (National Health and Nutrition Examination Survey [NHANES] Consent/Assent and Parental Permission for Examination at the Mobile Examination Center. Retrieved from Centers for Disease Control and Prevention https://wwwn.cdc.gov/nchs/data/nhanes/2017-2018/documents/2017_adult_consent_form.pdf. Accessed November 2, 2018.)

exposure being studied or whether the subject has only been found to be at increased risk for future development of disease as a result of exposure. In either case, clearly and concisely communicating the results regarding risk to the subjects can be viewed as one possible expression of the *ethical principle of beneficence*—the obligation of the investigator to help the subjects further their important legitimate interests, such as disease prevention and control, for themselves and for their families and friends. However, according to this principle, we must not only provide the benefits such as prevention of disease but also balance the benefits and costs or harm (*principle of utility*).

If, for example, a subject has been exposed to a factor that is shown in a study to be a strong marker of the subclinical phase of a malignant neoplasm, should the subject be given this information? On the one hand, given that no effective treatment for that neoplasm is available and that there is no strong evidence that early detection of the disease is beneficial, might we be increasing a person's anxieties by transmitting this information without providing any benefit to that person?

On the other hand, we could argue that a participant in any study is entitled to receive the findings of the study even if the findings have no direct bearing on the person's health or even if they may lead to heightened anxiety. Why should we as investigators make this decision for participants? Indeed, many epidemiologists now offer all participating subjects the option of requesting a report of the study findings when the study has been completed.

Protecting Privacy and Confidentiality

Concerns about privacy and confidentiality in our society have increased with the increasing erosion of individual privacy through computerized records. Protection of privacy and confidentiality within the framework of medical investigation, including epidemiologic research, has become an important issue. The origins of such concerns are quite old. Hippocrates wrote in the now commonly used Oath of Physicians:

that whatsoever I shall see or hear ... of the lives of men and women ... which is not fitting to be spoken ... I will keep inviolably secret.

As Hippocrates qualified "whatsoever I shall see or hear" with the phrase "which is not fitting to be spoken," he apparently considered certain types of information to be of a nature that *is* "fitting to be spoken." Presumably, under certain circumstances, Hippocrates would have advocated the carefully monitored sharing of personal information in the interest of societal benefit. For example, if a case of smallpox was diagnosed in an American city, Hippocrates would probably support reporting this case to health authorities. Thus, individual autonomy regarding privacy and confidentiality is an important principle, but it is not unlimited.

In regard to privacy and confidentiality in epidemiologic studies, attention has focused on the use of medical records (both paper charts, in the past, and the EMR more commonly today). Let us ask why medical records are needed in epidemiologic studies. These records are needed for two main purposes: (1) to generate aggregate data or validate information obtained by other means without having to contact patients and/or (2) to identify individual patients for subsequent follow up using means such as interviews or laboratory tests.

Because epidemiology's objectives of improving human health are clearly laudable, one might be tempted at first glance to dismiss any concerns about misuse of medical record data and about intrusions into individual privacy by epidemiologists. However, the words of Supreme Court Justice Louis D. Brandeis ring as true today as when they were first written in 1928:

Experience should teach us to be most on guard to protect liberty when the Government's purposes are beneficent. Men born to freedom are naturally alert to repel invasion of their liberty by evil-minded rulers. The greatest dangers to liberty lurk in insidious encroachment by men of zeal, well-meaning but without understanding.[2]

The *ethical principle of autonomy* argues strongly for a meaningful informed consent in many areas related to research, including privacy and confidentiality. Concerns about protection of confidentiality in the research arena are valid. Over the years, these concerns have led to two major legislative proposals that look reasonable at first but in actuality would seriously damage epidemiologic research and impede progress in both public health and clinical practice. The two proposals are as follows:

1. Patient consent should be required before investigators are allowed access to medical records.
2. Data from medical records should be made available to investigators without any information that would identify an individual.

Both proposals are consistent with the ethical principle of *nonmaleficence*—doing no harm—to the subjects participating in a research study. However, if society has a vested interest in the findings from epidemiologic and other biomedical studies, it is necessary to strike a balance between the interests of the individual and those of the community at large.

Let us consider each of these two proposals separately. Why would the first proposal, which requires patient consent before investigators are allowed access to medical records, make many studies impossible?

*   As a first step in a study, records must often be reviewed to identify which patients meet the study criteria for recruitment (for example, which patients have the disease in question and are therefore eligible for inclusion in a case-control study).
*   Many epidemiologic studies are conceived only many years after a patient has been hospitalized (e.g., a new test may have become available that was not in use when the patient became ill), so informed consent could not have been obtained from the patient at that time. By the time the study is later developed, which could be years or decades later, many patients may have died or may no longer be traceable.
*   Certain patients refuse to be interviewed in epidemiologic studies, but the nonparticipants can be characterized using data in their medical records, so that any biases resulting from their nonparticipation can be assessed. If records were not available because of patient refusals, a potential selection bias would then be introduced, and its magnitude and direction could not be assessed.

Turning to the second proposal, why is information from medical records that identifies individual patients essential for most epidemiologic studies?

*   Reviewing medical records is often the first step in identifying a large enough group of persons with a disease who could then be followed up.

*   Identifying information is essential for linking the records of specific individuals from different sources (such as hospital records, physicians' records, employment records, and death certificates, as in studies of occupational cancer).

As seen in Fig. 20.3, linkage of records is critical for generating unbiased and complete information about each subject, not only in occupational studies (as shown here) but also in many types of epidemiologic investigations. An example is a nonconcurrent cohort study (see Chapter 8) to evaluate the relationship of estrogen receptor status in breast cancer to mortality by using data from medical records and conducting linkage with the National Death Index.

Thus we see that the use of medical records is frequently essential for epidemiologic studies. Indeed, many significant advances in protecting human health that resulted from epidemiologic research could not have been made if access to medical records had been restricted.[3] At the same time, however, we must be concerned about protecting individual privacy and confidentiality. For many years, epidemiologic studies have used the following procedures designed to protect the confidentiality of subjects:

*   Informed consent is required from study participants for all phases of research except review of medical records. The informed consent language must be consistent with the educational level of the participants (generally set at an eighth-grade comprehension level).
*   All data obtained are stored under lock and key.

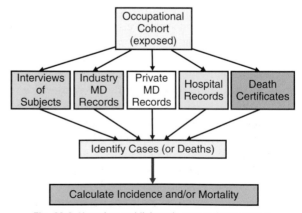

Fig. 20.3 Use of record linkage in occupational studies.

- Only study numbers are used on data forms; no personal identifiers are available on data forms or in computer files. Analysts are provided only with deidentified data for analysis. The key for linking study numbers with individual names is kept separately under lock and key by the principal investigator or his or her proxy (study coordinator).
- Individual identifying information is destroyed at the end of the study unless there is a specific justification for retaining this information. Such retention must be approved by the institutional review board (IRB) or committee on human research.
- All results are published only in aggregate or group form so that individuals are never identified.
- Unless it is essential for the study, individual identifying information is not entered in computer files, and individual identifiers (such as small-area geographic locations) are not included in routine tabulations generated from computerized data.
- The importance of maintaining privacy and confidentiality is regularly emphasized to the research staff.

When people consent to participate in epidemiologic studies, they have voluntarily agreed to some invasion of their privacy for the common good of society, hoping for advances in health promotion and disease prevention as a result of the studies they are making possible. Therefore investigators have an ethical obligation to protect the privacy and confidentiality of the subjects in these studies to the greatest extent possible. The policies described earlier that are currently in force have been highly successful in achieving this goal.

Recognizing the importance of the use of medical records in epidemiologic research and the effectiveness of current measures to protect privacy and confidentiality, the Privacy Protection Study Commission recommended that patient consent not be required for the use of medical records in epidemiologic research.[4] However, on April 14, 2003, the picture changed dramatically in the United States when new federal privacy regulations went into effect pursuant to the Health Insurance Portability and Accountability Act of 1996 (HIPAA).[5] The act was introduced in response to increasing public concern about lack of individual control over medical information and the general erosion of individual privacy in the United States. Electronic transfer of medical information and fears about potential misuse of genetic information made available by new laboratory methods also led to the development of these new regulations.

The HIPAA regulations provide the first systematic nationwide privacy protection for health information in the United States. The regulations give patients more control over their health information and set boundaries for the use and release of health records. With some exceptions, signed authorization is now required from each individual for the release of his or her protected health information. Protected health information can be disclosed to public health authorities without individual authorization for public health purposes, including (but not limited to) public health surveillance, investigations, and interventions. Protected health information can also be released for health research without individual authorization under certain conditions, including the following: (1) if an IRB has provided a waiver, (2) for activities preparatory to initiation of research, and (3) for research on a decedent's information.[6] The regulations are extremely complex. It will take time before the full impact of the new regulations on clinical and public health investigations and activities and on epidemiologic research can be assessed. Extensive discussions of the regulations have been published.[7–9]

Access to Data

When a study has been completed, who "owns" the data? Who should have access to the data—either "raw" or partially "cooked"—and under what conditions? We live in an era in which we can be confident that virtually any research data generated that deal with a controversial issue will be reanalyzed by real or alleged experts who support different positions. Some of the relevant questions regarding sharing of data include the following:

- At what point has a study truly been completed?
- Should the policy on sharing research data be dependent on who has paid for the study?
- Should the policy depend on who is requesting the data and on that person's possible motivations in making the request?
- Under what conditions should identifiers of individual participants be included with the data?

Generally data sharing requires removing all individual identifiers from the data.

- How can the investigator's interests be protected?
- Can all of the data be accessed or are only summary data made available?
- How extensive should data sharing be—should it be limited to requested variables or must the entire data set be shared?
- Can anyone request the data, or are the data restricted?
- Who will pay for the expenses involved in sharing data?

The challenge is to strike an appropriate balance between the interests of the investigator on the one hand and those of society on the other, for they do not inevitably coincide.

Race and Ethnicity in Epidemiologic Studies

An important issue that has received increasing attention in recent years is the use of race and ethnicity designations in epidemiologic studies. These variables are used both to describe populations and to test hypotheses in which race may serve as an independent variable, as in the many epidemiologic studies on racial disparities in health status. A PubMed review of the search terms *race, ethnicity, health* in October 2017 generated 17,603 publications and *race ethnicity disparities* yielded 12,001 records. Clearly race and ethnicity are the focus of many medical and epidemiologic investigations. However, there is concern about the use of these terms in epidemiologic research.

In an important paper published in 2008, Jay Kaufman and Richard Cooper discuss the concept of race as used in epidemiology and propose a set of cautions in its use. Race and ethnicity cannot be treated as dichotomous variables, as "human variation is continuous, not discrete," and ultimately, "existing racial classification schemes are the result of historical and political processes and that there is nothing natural, objective, or scientific about them."[10]

As a descriptor, race is often used to characterize the individuals who are studied in clinical trials or to describe inclusions and exclusions of populations in different types of epidemiologic studies. Race and ethnicity used as this type of variable can be helpful for this purpose and may be important for assessing the potential generalizability of the findings beyond the population studied.

When variables that designate race or ethnicity are included in studies designed to test hypotheses, the focus is often on possible associations of race with certain health outcomes. However, as Bhopal and Donaldson[11] have pointed out, biologically, race is ill defined, poorly understood, and may be of questionable validity. DNA research indicates that genetic diversity is a continuum with no clear breaks that can delineate racial groups.[12] Race has been described as "an arbitrary system of visual classification" that does not demarcate distinct subgroups of the human population.[13] Beginning with the 2000 US census, new guidelines permit respondents to identify themselves with more than one racial group. In the future, this policy may complicate the use of census data on race in epidemiologic studies.

An alternate approach is to use ethnicity rather than race. However, classifying people by ethnicity is also not simple or straightforward. Ethnicity is a complex variable that implies shared origins or social backgrounds; shared culture and traditions that are distinctive, maintained between generations, leading to a sense of identity and group; or shared language or religious tradition.[14] What have been the results of using racial designations in epidemiologic research? Many believe that, given the ambiguities involved in defining race, research using disease rates according to race has not significantly advanced our fundamental understanding of the causes and pathogenesis of human disease.[15] However, some have argued that even if such designations have not enhanced our understanding of the biologic mechanisms of disease, the use of racial variables in research has helped to identify subgroups—particularly minority and immigrant groups—to whom additional health care resources need to be directed. For example, race-specific mortality data in the United States have shown that[16]:

- A black infant is more than twice as likely as a white infant to die in the first year of life.
- Black people are more likely to have end-stage renal disease but less likely to receive kidney transplants than white people.
- Blacks are more likely to develop hypertension.
- Death rates for most causes of death are much higher for black people than for white people.

In studies of the health needs and health care priorities of various populations, the race of a population group may be described, an explicit comparison may be made with other racial and ethnic groups, or a comparison may be implied but not explicitly stated. Death rates by race are frequently used for setting national and state health objectives. The Centers for Disease Control and Prevention state that, "death rates by race and Hispanic origin are important for monitoring the health status of these population groups and for informing policies and programs directed to reducing disparities."[16]

One problem in using racial variables is that in so doing, even well-meaning investigators may inadvertently stigmatize certain population subgroups. As a result, certain racial designations may, in effect, become surrogates for undesirable lifestyle characteristics such as criminal behavior and drug abuse. As Bhopal has pointed out, "by emphasizing the negative aspects of the health of ethnic minority groups, research may have damaged their social standing and deflected attention from their health priorities."[15]

What conclusions can we draw? No variable, including race, should be included uncritically as a matter of routine in any epidemiologic study. Perhaps the best approach in planning any epidemiologic study in which race will be addressed is to ask a number of questions, including the following:

- Why is race being studied?
- On what basis will study participants be classified by race?
- How valid will the designations of race be, and how will they contribute to increasing our biologic knowledge of the disease in question or to enhancing preventive activities in certain disadvantaged groups?
- If race is being used as a surrogate for certain lifestyle factors, such as diet, could information on diet or other lifestyle factors be obtained directly, without using race as a surrogate?
- At the same time, we should also ask whether any damage may be done by using racial designations in a given study and whether such designations may unintentionally serve as virtual surrogates for undesirable lifestyles or characteristics.
- Is the construct validity of certain variables the same across races or ethnicities? For example,

education is often used as a proxy for socioeconomic status (SES). Does education express SES to the same extent in blacks and whites in the United States?

In any study, racial variables that are used should have a definite purpose that can be precisely articulated and should meet the same standards of reliability and validity that we would expect of any other variables we measure in our study. The potential benefit of using such variables in a study should clearly exceed any potential harm that may result. Race may be an appropriate and potentially valuable variable to address in epidemiologic studies provided the above issues have been adequately considered and addressed.

Jean-Claude Moubarac conducted a comprehensive review of the use of race and ethnicity in reports on health disparities in epidemiology and public health.[17] He presented a review of 280 articles published between 2009 and 2011 and identified four major remaining issues. First, researchers generally failed to differentiate race from ethnicity. Second, authors frequently ascribed ethnicity from racial categories. Third, common measurement procedures underlying each concept were rarely specified clearly. And fourth, there was a general failure to ascribe limits to the race and ethnicity taxonomies commonly used. Thus, it is clear that far greater precision is needed if race and ethnicity are to be appropriately investigated in epidemiology in the future.

Conflict of Interest

Both actual and perceived biases may result from conflict of interest. Such conflict can arise at each stage of a study, from an initial decision as to whether a specific study should be undertaken in the first place through analysis and interpretation of the data and dissemination of the results. Epidemiologic investigation in the United States today is performed by epidemiologists who work in academia, industry, and government. These three environments differ in several ways. Funding for epidemiologic research in government and industry is generally internal, whereas academic epidemiologists must seek external financial support from government, industry, or foundations. As a result, research performed by academic epidemiologists is generally subjected to more rigorous peer review as part of the grant application process. Even more important, however, is that the employer of the academic epidemiologist generally has no vested interest in what the results of the study turn out to be. This contrasts with other settings in which the employer may be significantly affected—politically, economically, or legally—by the nature of the research findings. Consequently, overt or subtle pressure by an employer not to initiate a study or to prolong the process leading to reporting of the results (or their suppression) can introduce a serious bias into reviews of the literature concerning issues such as occupational hazards. Moreover, these biases may be impossible to assess.

The potential bias resulting from such studies that have not been conducted and that might well have revealed associations of specific exposures with adverse outcomes has not been named. In this context, some may be reminded of a dialogue in Sir Arthur Conan Doyle's Sherlock Holmes story *Silver Blaze* in which Holmes investigates the disappearance of a racehorse with that name and the murder of its trainer. As Holmes is about to leave the village during the investigation, the local inspector turns to him and asks:

"Is there any point to which you wish to draw my attention?"

"To the curious incident of the dog in the night time." [replies Holmes]

"The dog did nothing in the night time."

"That was the curious incident," remarked Sherlock Holmes.[18]

(Holmes later described how he successfully identified the villain. He explained that when the intruder entered the stable "the dog did nothing in the night time" and did not even bark much, indicating that "obviously, the midnight visitor was someone whom the dog knew well.")

With this conversation in mind, the potential bias introduced by studies that are not done might be called *Silver Blaze bias*. Holmes understood why the dog failed to act and was able to apply this knowledge to solve the problem at hand. Similarly, there may be much to learn when a manufacturer fails to conduct what seems to be a clearly needed study of possible adverse effects of a product. But when such an association has been suggested, it is often difficult to determine whether certain epidemiologic studies were not initiated because

of vested interests and concerns about the potential results of the study. In the absence of evidence documenting an explicit decision not to conduct a certain study, this type of bias is often difficult or impossible to quantify or even detect.

Although academic settings are not immune to their own problems and pressures, problems relating to epidemiologic research that arise in an academic setting are less likely to be linked to the potential impact of the study's specific findings. Nevertheless, the possibility of conflict of interest relating to any epidemiologic study must be considered, regardless of the specific setting in which the research was conducted. Indeed, such conflict may be related more to sources of funding than to the research setting itself. However, the possibility must be recognized that, infrequently, institutional as well as individual conflicts of interest may influence the publication and dissemination of results. Efforts should be expended to ensure that, to avoid publication bias, the results of the study—whatever they may turn out to be—are published in a peer-reviewed journal in a timely fashion. Requirements for registering clinical trials are a major step in that direction (see discussion in Chapter 11). Sponsorship of the study should be clearly acknowledged in the article that reports the results of the study, as should any financial or other interests of the investigators or their families that may be affected by the study results.

Interpreting Findings

Many critical issues regarding how epidemiologic studies are conducted arise in connection with the appropriateness of the study design and with the interpretation and reporting of findings. Epidemiologists are often accused of endlessly reporting new risks, many of which are not large and are not confirmed in subsequent studies. The public finds many reported but often unconfirmed risks in the media, which leads them to become skeptical of newly reported risks because they are unable to sort out true and important risks from unconfirmed or trivial ones (Fig. 20.4); they frequently then become unwilling to take responsibility for their own health care if the facts are in doubt.[19] The question again arises: How do we assess the importance of a single study that shows an increased risk? How many confirmatory studies are needed?

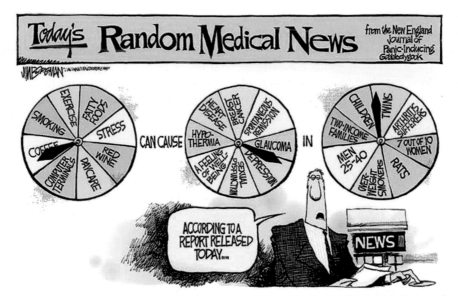

Fig. 20.4 One view of the seemingly endless stream of reported risks confronting the public. (JIM BORGMAN © Cincinnati Enquirer. Reprinted with permission of ANDREWS MCMEEL SYNDICATION. All rights reserved.)

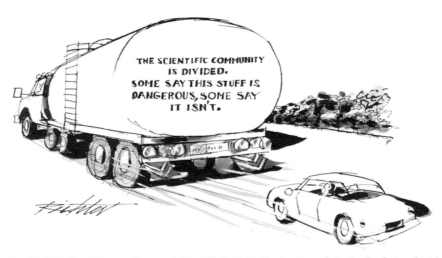

Fig. 20.5 Dealing with scientific uncertainty. (Mischa Richter/The New Yorker Collection/The Cartoon Bank.)

An additional problem is that in earlier years, initial solitary epidemiologic findings or scientific controversies were generally addressed and often resolved within the scientific community before findings were disseminated to the public. Today, both initial unconfirmed reports and scientific controversies are often aired in the press or in the popular media (and increasingly in social media) even before the studies have appeared in peer-reviewed journals (Fig. 20.5). The dilemma is that although enhanced public education and increased public awareness of scientific issues are laudable, anxiety levels are often unjustifiably raised by single studies that are widely reported and often later refuted. The problem is exacerbated by a reported bias in newspapers against reporting the results of studies that show no effect.[20]

Significant uncertainty is associated with the findings regarding certain questions, such as whether mammography is beneficial for women in their 40s and whether prostate-specific antigen testing is beneficial to men with localized prostate cancer. Dealing with uncertainty is difficult—and often painful—for people who are struggling to make a personal decision about whether to follow suggested interventions. Epidemiologists should help the public to understand uncertainty and to cope with the challenge of making decisions in the face of equivocal and incomplete information.

An additional question is: At what point does a reported trivial increase in a risk ratio, even if it is statistically significant, become a biologically significant risk that merits public concern? This question relates to the overall issue of public perceptions of risk. These perceptions are reflected in Tables 20.1 and 20.2. For many of the risks listed, the degree of public concern and the change in behavior do not seem commensurate with the magnitude of the risk.

If the absolute risk is low, even if the relative risk in exposed individuals is significantly increased, the actual risk to exposed individuals will still be very low. It is interesting that the public often prefers to address "hot" issues (such as a reported risk from alar in apples), for which the evidence may be tenuous, while ignoring well-established risk factors such as smoking, alcohol consumption, and sun exposure, for which lifestyle changes that are dependent on individual initiative are clearly warranted by the available evidence.

Epidemiologists have a major function in communicating health risks and interpreting epidemiologic data for nonepidemiologists; if epidemiologists do not participate in this activity, it will be left to others with far less training and expertise. This is an essential part of the policy-making process. Studies of human populations often yield different findings, and epidemiologists often hesitate to draw conclusions on the basis of existing data. In academic settings, epidemiologists can criticize the design of studies and their findings, and the typical refrain is to recommend additional research to resolve an issue. However, policy makers working at the front lines do not have this luxury of delay—they

TABLE 20.1 Involuntary Risks

Involuntary Risk	Risk of Death per Person per Year
Struck by automobile (United States)	1 in 20,000
Struck by automobile (United Kingdom)	1 in 16,600
Floods (United States)	1 in 455,000
Earthquake (California)	1 in 588,000
Tornadoes (Midwest)	1 in 455,000
Lightning (United Kingdom)	1 in 10 million
Falling aircraft (United States)	1 in 10 million
Falling aircraft (United Kingdom)	1 in 50 million
Release from an atomic power station	
At site boundary (United States)	1 in 10 million
At 1 km (United Kingdom)	1 in 10 million
Flooding of a dike (The Netherlands)	1 in 10 million
Bites of venomous creatures (United Kingdom)	1 in 5 million
Leukemia	1 in 12,500
Influenza	1 in 5,000
Meteorite	1 in 100 billion

From Dinman BD. The reality and acceptance of risk. *JAMA*. 1980;244:1226. Copyright 1980, American Medical Association.

TABLE 20.2 Voluntary Risks

Voluntary Risk	Risk of Death per Person per Year
Smoking: 20 cigarettes/day	1 in 200
Drinking: 1 bottle of wine/day	1 in 13,300
Soccer, football	1 in 25,500
Automobile racing	1 in 1,000
Automobile driving (United Kingdom)	1 in 5,900
Motorcycling	1 in 50
Rock climbing	1 in 7,150
Taking oral contraceptive pills	1 in 5,000
Power boating	1 in 5,900
Canoeing	1 in 100,000
Horse racing	1 in 740
Amateur boxing	1 in 2 million
Professional boxing	1 in 14,300
Skiing	1 in 430,000
Pregnancy (United Kingdom)	1 in 4,350
Abortion: Legal <12 weeks	1 in 50,000
Abortion: Legal >14 weeks	1 in 5,900

From Dinman BD. The reality and acceptance of risk. *JAMA*. 1980;244:1226. Copyright 1980, American Medical Association.

must make immediate decisions (to regulate or not to regulate). Even a decision not to regulate at this time represents a policy decision. Such decisions should ideally capitalize on existing epidemiologic findings. However, policy makers cannot act in a rational fashion by waiting for findings from future studies to direct their actions regarding current pressing health issues. Epidemiologists must therefore draw the best conclusions possible on the basis of currently available data, fully realizing that a better study, or even a perfect study, may appear tomorrow and may contradict today's conclusions.

Epidemiologists have several roles in the process of policy making, including generating and interpreting the data, presenting specific policy options that are consistent with the data, projecting the impact of each option, developing specific policy proposals, and evaluating the effects of policies after they have been implemented. Should an epidemiologist be both a researcher and an advocate for a specific policy? Does advocacy for a position imply a loss of objectivity and of scientific credibility? These are difficult questions, but many clear issues, such as the health hazards resulting from cigarette smoking, urgently need the participation of epidemiologists in the struggle to eliminate this source of the danger to the public's health. The question then is not only whether it is ethical for an epidemiologist to be an advocate but whether it is ethical for an epidemiologist *not* to be an advocate when the evidence of risk is so convincing. Thus the epidemiologist must serve as an educator as well as a researcher. The epidemiologist's educational efforts are directed at many target populations, including other scientists, other health professionals, legislators, policy makers, lawyers, judges, and the public. Each group must be dealt with differently, depending on its specific needs and on the objectives toward which the educational effort is directed. Epidemiologists must learn to work with the media, including radio, television, magazines, and newspapers, and, increasingly, with social media, in order to further their educational efforts. Epidemiologists should also familiarize themselves with what is known about how risks are perceived by patients, health care providers, and the general public so that they can help these groups deal with the findings of epidemiologic studies and with their implications for preventive measures including lifestyle changes.[21]

Conclusion

The ethical and professional issues facing epidemiology primarily relate to epidemiologists' obligations to participants in their epidemiologic studies as well as the overall challenge of a discipline that lies at the interface of science and public policy. The issues are complex, often subtle, and without simple direct answers. Given the pivotal position of epidemiology in the development of both clinical and public health policy and its implications for environmental regulation, individual lifestyle changes, and rapid changes in clinical practice, the findings from epidemiologic studies attract widespread attention and high public visibility. As new questions are addressed by epidemiology in the future, the ethical and professional dilemmas facing the discipline will also continue to evolve. It is critical that dialogue continues between epidemiologists and those who use the results of epidemiologic studies, including physicians and policy makers, as well as the public who will be affected by new health and prevention policies.

REFERENCES

1. Cited in Strong WS. Copyright in a time of change. *J Electronic Pub.* 1999;4(3):http://quod.lib.umich.edu/j/jep/3336451.0004.302/--copyright-in-a-time-of-change?rgn=main;view=fulltext. Accessed August 20, 2013.
2. Brandeis L. *Dissenting opinion in Olmstead v. United States, 277 U.S. 438* (1928).
3. Gordis L, Gold E. Privacy, confidentiality, and the use of medical records in research. *Science.* 1980;207:153–156.
4. *The Report of the Privacy Protection Study Commission: Personal Privacy in an Information Society.* Washington, DC, US Government Printing Office, 1977.
5. *Health Insurance Portability and Accountability Act of 1996.* Pub. L. No. 104–191, 110 Stat. 1936 (1996).
6. Centers for Disease Control and Prevention. HIPAA Privacy Rule and public health: guidance from CDC and the U.S. Department of Health and Human Services. *MMWR.* 2003;52(suppl): 1–20.
7. Gostin LO. National health information privacy: regulations under the Health Insurance Portability and Accountability Act. *JAMA.* 2001;285:3015–3021.
8. Gostin LO, Hodge JG Jr. Personal privacy and common goods: a framework. *Minn Law Rev.* 2002;86:1439–1480.
9. Kulynych J, Korn D. The new federal medical-privacy rule. *N Engl J Med.* 2002;347:1133–1134.
10. Kaufman JS, Cooper RS. Race in epidemiology: new tools, old problems. *Ann Epidemiol.* 2008;18(2):119–123.
11. Bhopal R, Donaldson L. White, European, Western, Caucasian, or what? Inappropriate labeling in research on race, ethnicity and health. *Am J Public Health.* 1998;88:1303–1307.
12. Marshall E. DNA studies challenge the meaning of race. *Science.* 1998;282:654–655.

13. Fullilove MT. Abandoning "race" as a variable in public health research—an idea whose time has come. *Am J Public Health.* 1998;88:1297–1298.

14. Senior PA, Bhopal R. Ethnicity as a variable in epidemiological research. *BMJ.* 1994;309:327–330.

15. Bhopal R. Is research into ethnicity and health, racist, unsound or important science? *BMJ.* 1997;314:1751–1756.

16. Rosenberg HM, Maurer KD, Sorlie PD, et al. Quality of death rates by race and Hispanic origin: a summary of current research, 1999. National Center for Health Statistics. *Vital Health Stat.* 1999;2(128):1–13.

17. Moubarac JC. Persisting problems related to race and ethnicity in public health and epidemiology research. *Rev Saude Publica.* 2013;47(1):104–115.

18. Doyle AC. Silver Blaze. In: *The Complete Sherlock Holmes.* New York: Doubleday; 1930.

19. Taubes G. Epidemiology faces its limits. *Science.* 1995;269:164–169.

20. Koren G, Klein N. Bias against negative studies in newspaper reports of medical research. *JAMA.* 1991;13:1824–1826.

21. Klein MP, Stefanek ME. Cancer risk elicitation and communication: lessons from the psychology of risk perception. *CA Cancer J Clin.* 2007;57:147–167.

Answers to Review Questions

Note to reader: To find complete rationales for all answer options, please go to http://www.studentconsult.com and activate/access your full online version of the book and ancillary content.

Chapter 1

No Review Questions.

Chapter 2

1. b
2. a
3. b
4. d
5. c
6. c

Chapter 3

1. e
2. 10%
3. c
4. c
5. d
6. b
7. c
8. c
9. d
10. d

Chapter 4

1. 5/1,000
2. 30%
3. e
4. b
5. b
6. a
7. 2.5 or 250
8. d
9. c

10. d
11. 9.6/1,000
12. e
13. d
14. a
15. b

Chapter 5

1. 72.0%
2. 84.0%
3. 69.2%
4. d
5. d
6. b
7. 3.3%
8. b
9. 70.0%
10. 57.1%
11. 0.4
12. b

Chapter 6

The answers to questions 6 through 8 are based on calculating and completing the table provided (as shown later in this section).

1. 54.8%
2. c
3. c
4. b
5. c
6. 0.982 or 98.2%
7. 0.006 or 0.6%

8. c
9. a
10. b

Chapter 7

1. c
2. a
3. c
4. b
5. c
6. d
7. e
8. d
9. c
10. c
11. c

Chapter 8

1. d
2. a
3. c
4. a
5. c
6. d
7. b

Chapter 9

No Review Questions.

Chapters 10 and 11

1. e
2. e
3. c

4. b
5. b
6. a
7. c
8. 57
9. 9a. b
   9b. c
   9c. e
   9d. d
   9e. a
10. 0.67
11. 43

Chapter 12

1. 15.3
2. d
3. e
4. e
5. 4.5
6. 6.3
7. 1:7 (0.143)
8. e
9. e
10. 1.94
11. 1.50
12. The odds of prostate cancer are 50% higher among never aspirin users compared to ever aspirin users.
13. b

Chapter 13

1. b
2. 27.5/1,000
3. 84.6%
4. 3.6/1,000
5. 78.3%

Chapter 14

1. c
2. a
3. e
4. b
5. d

Chapter 15

1. e
2. c
3. c
4. 12
5. 18.7
6. 9
7. 6.2
8. d
9. b

Chapter 16

1. c
2. c
3. b
4. b
5. c

Chapter 17

1. b
2. b
3. a
4. d
5. d

Chapter 18

1. a
2. a
3. b
4. c
5. b
6. c
7. b
8. c

Chapters 19 and 20

No Review Questions.

For questions 6 through 8 in Chapter 6:

Survival of Patients With AIDS Following Diagnosis							
(1) Interval Since Beginning Treatment (Months)	**(2)** Alive at Beginning of Interval	**(3)** Died During Interval	**(4)** Withdrew During Interval	**(5)** Effective Number Exposed to Risk of Dying During Interval: Col (2) − $\frac{1}{2}$ [Col (4)]	**(6)** Proportion Who Died During Interval: $\frac{\text{Col (3)}}{\text{Col (5)}}$	**(7)** Proportion Who Did Not Die During Interval: 1 − Col (6)	**(8)** Cumulative Proportion Who Survived From Enrollment to End of Interval: Cumulative Survival
x	l_x	d_x	w_x	l'_x	q_x	p_x	P_x
1–12	248	96	27	234.5	0.4094	0.5906	0.5906
13–24	125	55	13	118.5	0.4641	0.5359	0.3165
25–36	57	55	2	56.0	0.9821	0.0179	0.0057

Index

Page numbers followed by "*f*" indicate figures, "*t*" indicate tables, and "*b*" indicate boxes.

Cigarette smoking, 16
  cohort study of, 178, 179*t*
  coronary heart disease and, 158, 158*t*,
    243, 243*t*, 262, 263*t*, 264, 265*t*
  esophageal cancer and, 298*f*, 299
  lung cancer and, 158–159, 159*t*,
    162–163, 265*t*, 277, 279*f*, 297*f*,
    297*t*, 302*t*–303*t*
  maternal, 272*f*–273*f*
  squamous cell cancer and, 321, 322*f*
Circumcision, 166, 166*t*
Classification system, 57*f*
Clinical disease, 21–23
Clinical practice, 7, 7*f*–8*f*
Coffee drinking, pancreatic cancer and,
  163, 163*t*–164*t*, 164*f*–165*f*, 271, 272*f*,
  295*f*
Cohort effect, 85–86, 85*t*–86*t*
Cohort studies, 178–192, 179*f*
  bias in, 185–186
  breast cancer and progesterone
    deficiency, 182–183, 183*f*
  case-control studies *versus*, 158–159,
    187–190, 187*f*, 193–194, 194*f*, 196*f*
  childhood health and disease, 183–185,
    184*f*
  Collaborative Perinatal Study, 184
  concurrent, 180
  definition of, 174*t*, 270–271
  design of, 178–179, 179*f*, 179*t*, 186*f*,
    241*f*
  examples of, 181–183, 182*t*
  follow-up period for, 181
  Framingham Study, 181–182, 244
  historical, 181
  information biases in, 186
  nested case-control studies, 187–189,
    188*f*–189*f*
  nonrandomized, 347*f*–348*f*, 365*f*
  odds ratio in, 243*t*, 246–248, 247*f*
  problems associated with, 181, 181*f*
  prospective, 174*t*, 181, 181*f*, 195*t*
  randomized trials *versus*, 186
  relative risk calculations, 243–245, 243*t*
  retrospective, 158–159, 174*t*, 181, 181*f*,
    195*t*
  selection biases in, 185
  of smoking and coronary heart disease,
    178, 179*t*
  study populations, 179–180, 179*f*–180*f*
  types of, 180–181, 180*f*
  unmatched, 250–251, 250*f*, 251*t*
Collaborative Perinatal Study, 184
Colon cancer, 50*f*, 361, 361*f*
Combination designs, for health services
  evaluations, 348–350, 348*f*

Common-vehicle exposure, 26
Community health, 3–5
Comparative effectiveness research, 226
Complex diseases, 308–313, 328*t*–331*t*
Concordance rate, in twins, 310, 310*f*–312*f*
Concordant pairs, 251
Concurrent cohort study, 180
Confidentiality, 399–401, 400*f*
Conflict of interest, 403–404
Confounding, 271–272, 294–299,
  295*f*–296*f*, 295*t*–296*t*, 296*b*
Continuous contamination, 26
Continuous variables tests, 97–99, 98*f*
Controls
  best friend, 162
  definition of, 157–174
  historical, 200
  hospitalized persons as, 162–163, 162*f*,
    169
  multiple, 169–171
  neighborhood, 161
  nonhospitalized persons as, 161–162
  problems in, 163–165
  selection of, 160–165
  simultaneous nonrandomized, 200–201
  sources of, 161–165
Coronary Drug Project, 213, 213*t*–214*t*
Coronary heart disease, 229
  cholesterol levels and, 244*t*, 272, 272*f*
  cross-sectional study of, 154
  cumulative incidence of, 383*f*
  hypertension and, 380, 380*f*–381*f*
  myocardial infarction, 245*f*
  smoking and
    case-control study of, 158, 158*t*
    cohort study of, 178, 179*t*, 243, 243*t*,
     263*t*, 264, 265*t*
Cost effectiveness, 373
Cost-benefit analysis, of screening tests,
  373–374
Courts, 390–391
Cowpox, 13–14
Crenezumab, 18–19
Criteria, 286
Critical point, 356, 357*f*
Crossover studies, 208–211, 210*f*
  planned, 208, 209*f*
  unplanned, 208–211, 210*f*
Cross-products ratio, 248
Cross-sectional studies, 154–157, 155*f*,
  174*t*
Cross-sectional view, 85–86
Cross-tabulation, 36–38, 38*t*
Crude mortality, 80–82
Cutoff level, 97, 99
Cystic fibrosis, 319*f*

D

DALY. *See* Disability-adjusted life year
Data
  access to, 401–402
  group, 337–341, 337*f*
    biases in, 339–340
    disadvantages of, 338
    outcomes research, 338–339
    prenatal care use of, 339
  individual, 341–350
Daubert v. Merrell Dow Pharmaceuticals, 391
Death(s)
  changes in definition of, 77–78
  coding of, 76–77
  leading causes of, 67*f*, 265*f*
  underlying cause of, 76
Death certificate, 76, 78*b*, 79*f*–80*f*
Death rates, 17*f*. *See also* Mortality rate(s)
Defined population, 223
Deletion, 328*t*–331*t*
Dementia, proportion of prevalence of,
  55–56, 57*f*
Denominators, problems with, 56–58
Determinants of susceptibility, 378
Developing countries
  disease occurrence in, 3–5
  surveillance in, 42–43
Diabetes mellitus
  mortality rates for, 80*f*
  screening tests for, 99, 100*f*
Diagnosis
  methods of, 124
  population-based approach to, 6–7
  tissue confirmation for, 124
Diagnostic tests, validity and reliability of,
  94–122
Diarrheal disease, 34–35
Dichotomous screening tests, 95–97, 97*t*,
  101*f*
Differential misclassification, 292
Differential recall, 167
Direct age adjustment, 82–84, 82*t*
Direct causation, 274, 274*f*
Direct transmission, 20, 21*b*
Disability-adjusted life year (DALY), 87, 88*t*
Discordance rate, in twins, 310
Discordant pairs, 251
Disease
  biologic onset of, 123
  clinical, 21–23, 355–356
  detectable preclinical phase of, 356
  distribution of, 35
  early detection of, 353–354, 374
  exposure and, association between, 178,
    179*f*, 241–242, 270*f*, 299
  factors that cause, 20, 21*t*